2·9

PLEASE ENTER ON LOAN SLIP:

AUTHOR: Rees, T.J.

TITLE: Cosmetic facial surgery

ACCESSION NO: SA(M) 714

Thomas D. Rees, M.D., F.A.C.S.

CLINICAL ASSOCIATE PROFESSOR OF SURGERY (PLASTIC SURGERY), INSTITUTE OF RECONSTRUCTIVE PLASTIC SURGERY, NEW YORK UNIVERSITY MEDICAL SCHOOL; ATTENDING SURGEON, UNIVERSITY HOSPITAL, MANHATTAN EYE, EAR AND THROAT HOSPITAL, AND DOCTORS HOSPITAL; VISITING SURGEON, BELLEVUE HOSPITAL, NEW YORK; CONSULTANT, U.S. NAVAL HOSPITAL, ST. ALBANS, NEW YORK.

Donald Wood-Smith, M.D., F.R.C.S.E.

ASSISTANT PROFESSOR OF SURGERY (PLASTIC SURGERY), INSTITUTE OF RECONSTRUCTIVE PLASTIC SURGERY, NEW YORK UNIVERSITY MEDICAL SCHOOL; ATTENDING SURGEON, MANHATTAN EYE, EAR AND THROAT HOSPITAL, MANHATTAN VETERANS ADMINISTRATION HOSPITAL, AND NEW YORK UNIVERSITY HOSPITAL; VISITING SURGEON, BELLEVUE HOSPITAL; CONSULTING SURGEON, DEPARTMENT. OF OPHTHALMOLOGY, NEW YORK EYE AND EAR INFIRMARY, NEW YORK, NEW YORK.

COSMETIC FACIAL SURGERY

Illustrations by Daisy Stilwell

Photography by Don Allen

W. B. SAUNDERS COMPANY

PHILADELPHIA · LONDON · TORONTO

W. B. Saunders Company: West Washington Square
Philadelphia, Pa. 19105

1 St. Anne's Road
Eastbourne, East Sussex BN21 3UN, England

833 Oxford Street
Toronto, M8Z 5T9, Canada

Cosmetic Facial Surgery   ISBN 0-7216-7518-2

Print No.:   9   8   7   6   5   4   3

This book is sincerely dedicated to the young plastic surgeon who, finding himself faced with an increasing demand for cosmetic plastic surgery, wishes to perfect his knowledge and techniques in this fascinating specialty.

CONTRIBUTORS

RICHARD J. COBURN, D.M.D., M.D.
Clinical Assistant in Surgery, Harvard Medical School;
Clinical Associate in Surgery, Mount Sinai School of
Medicine, New York

SIDNEY HOROWITZ, D.D.S.
Professor of Dentistry and Director of the Division of
Orofacial Development, School of Dental and Oral
Surgery, Columbia University, New York

SEAMUS LYNCH, M.D.
Director, Department of Anesthesiology, Manhattan
Eye, Ear and Throat Hospital; Attending Anesthesi-
ologist, New York Hospital

FRANCES C. MACGREGOR, M.A.
Clinical Associate Professor of Surgery (Sociology),
Institute of Reconstructive Plastic Surgery, New York
University Medical Center, New York

NORMAN ORENTREICH, M.D., F.A.C.P.
Clinical Associate Professor of Dermatology, New
York University School of Medicine; Associate
Attending in Department of Dermatology, University
Hospital, New York University Medical Center

CHARLES P. VALLIS, M.D., F.A.C.S.
Instructor in Plastic Surgery, Tufts University School
of Medicine, Boston

FOREWORD

It has been a source of deep satisfaction for me to watch the progressive development and increasing surgical skills of each member of the relatively large staff of the multi-hospital complex whose headquarters are the Institute of Reconstructive Plastic Surgery. It is, therefore, with great pride that I write to introduce this text written by two associates, Dr. Thomas D. Rees and Dr. Donald Wood-Smith. With their collaborators they have assembled in one volume the most useful techniques of cosmetic surgery, which are elegantly and explicitly illustrated by Daisy Stilwell, our medical artist. In so doing, they have made an important contribution to plastic surgery by making available to every practicing plastic surgeon the methodology of diagnosis and treatment in this aspect of plastic surgery which requires painstaking attention to detail. Furthermore, historical reviews in capsule form help readers avoid the errors of the past while enabling them to capitalize on the best ideas of their predecessors.

As Frances C. Macgregor has so well stated in her chapter on sociopsychological considerations, the high premium on physical attributes, on youth and the social pressures to conform, characteristic of our culture, have led to the recognition of this type of surgery by the medical profession as well as by our society in general. It was not always so.

I congratulate the authors on their important contribution and the W. B. Saunders Company for the quality of the publication.

JOHN MARQUIS CONVERSE, M.D.

PREFACE

Cosmetic facial surgery, a subspecialty of plastic surgery, is firmly established, is growing at an ever-increasing rate and is now accepted by both the public and the medical profession. Social pressures encourage people to improve their appearance, as long as the methods used are within reasonable bounds. Those who still look upon cosmetic surgery with suspicion or disfavor are old-fashioned or uninformed.

In New York, as in some other large cities, the nature of the patient population is such that a plastic surgeon's practice turns toward cosmetic surgery. But regardless of where he practices, every plastic surgeon does his share of cosmetic operations. Perusal of existing books on the subject will demonstrate a paucity of meaningful current material, and much of what is available contains drawings and descriptions of operative techniques that appear to be the fanciful results of fertile imaginations. These techniques, often passed from surgeon to surgeon, seem never to be discarded, but rather elaborated upon as the years go by. Many published cosmetic surgical techniques are not only ineffective, but liable to produce unfortunate results if practiced by the unwary or inexperienced.

There is nothing mysterious about the techniques of cosmetic facial surgery, which in principle is straightforward general surgery. However, success depends on exhaustive attention to detail, excellence in surgical performance, and a highly developed sense of perfection. Careful preoperative selection of patients, based on sound judgment of what can and cannot be achieved by the proposed surgical technique, plays an equally vital role. Meticulous preoperative preparation and postoperative care are also important. Perhaps in no other branch of surgery are these picayune details so vital, for the result of cosmetic facial surgery is measured by the patient's as well as the surgeon's satisfaction.

The germination of this book was hastened by the observation that many young plastic surgeons, fresh from excellent training programs in reconstructive surgery, are insecure in the field of cosmetic surgery, which may assume major importance early in their practices. Medical conferences and symposia on the subject of esthetic surgery are always well attended; the discussion periods are brisk and lively. The increasing public demand for cosmetic facial operations has also added impetus to the need for training. This is particularly true in smaller cities, where the demand for cosmetic surgery is increasing rapidly.

The purpose, therefore, has been to produce a practical work for the learning surgeon. To be effective, such a book must be mainly the result of personal experience, rather than being drawn from publications of others, but at the same time it must rely on the pioneering work of many surgeons. Only those techniques that we consider to be useful, and to offer the best chance of success, have been emphasized (with the exception of some historical comments which are presented as such). Where a choice of techniques exists, only those that have proved effective in our hands have been included, although we have added some that have strong appeal and have been reported by sources considered to be reliable, but which we have not had the opportunity to use.

The material for this book has been collected during the senior author's 16 years of practice. Collation began in 1965 and the actual writing in 1968. As the material began to take shape it became apparent that help was required by colleagues to round out the book, particularly in special areas where personal experience was wanting. We are deeply indebted to the contributions made by our co-authors. Only through their willingness to share their knowledge and experience was it possible to enlarge the scope of this book to include much meaningful material that would otherwise have been excluded.

With few exceptions, the patient photographs were drawn from the senior author's practice. This was not intended as a forum for presenting good results, as moderate, limited and even poor results have also been included in order to make specific points. The procedures outlined in this book, taking into consideration the built-in limitations of human protoplasm and surgical method, have produced consistently acceptable results.

Finally, it is only fair to say that any book of this type is the summation of the acquired experience of many. It is impossible not to omit by oversight or necessity the work of others. To our friends in plastic surgery all over the world, we can only say that we and our co-authors hope you will not take offense at such omissions and will forgive us if we did not include something dear to your heart. Certainly no personal slight was intended.

THOMAS D. REES, M.D.

DONALD WOOD-SMITH, M.D.

ACKNOWLEDGMENTS

It is our collective hope that this book on cosmetic plastic surgery will provide a working reference for the young surgeon who is curious about this relatively new art. The operations described herein are rarely original. Any operative procedure, as performed by a particular surgeon, must be viewed as a composite concept of the work of others. For this we make no excuse, but thank our many teachers and our contemporary of world renown, Dr. John Marquis Converse. The senior author is also particularly indebted to the late great teachers of plastic surgery Sir Archibald McIndoe of England and Dr. Herbert Conway of New York. Because of our close association with them, these men have shared their own techniques with us. We are also indebted to the many others who have shared tidbits of valuable information.

This book must be considered a tribute to the excellence of medical illustration and photography at its best. Mr. Don Allen of New York, who is by far the finest medical photographer in our opinion, took most of the photographs. His work is consistent and true. Realistic photographs such as those printed here are of inestimable value to the surgeon. They demonstrate details of contour which vanish completely from the face of the supine or anesthetized patient. Medical photographs are usually abhorrent to the patient, who expects a flattering portrait but instead sees every defect clearly. We have stopped showing the pre- and postoperative photographs to patients unless there is a divergence of opinion as to what has been accomplished by surgery; even then such differences may not be resolved, because "no one looks that bad."

A very few photographs, however, were taken by us admitted amateurs, producing 35 mm. slides that were later converted to black-and-white prints. The results are obvious in reproduction and in contrast to the excellent work of Mr. Allen, who must shudder to see them side by side with his work.

The illustrations prepared by Miss Daisy Stilwell fulfill the requirements of medical illustration at its best. They are widely heralded for their clarity and simplicity. Her ability to execute a line drawing, with just the right note of emphasis by way of slight shading, pertinent arrows or subtle emphasis, is well known from many previous publications on plastic surgery in which she has had a part.

We wish to thank the *National Geographic Society* and the *American Museum of Natural History* for opening their files so that we could peruse and borrow photographs to illustrate the changing concepts of beauty. It can readily be seen in this first chapter that beauty is indeed "in the eye of the beholder," or at least that beauty is measured by different standards in different cultures. One need only acknowledge the ever-changing styles of dress and hair to accept the fact that man is a vain animal. Even those youngsters who seek to escape the styles they associate with their elders have developed their own ideals, which readily indicate their desire to be physically acceptable within the framework of their own time and group. The "mod" culture has thus produced its own concepts of vanity.

Grateful mention must also be made here of our long-suffering secretaries and assistants who over the years continue to deserve strong praise and gratitude. Typing manuscripts, collecting photographs, checking releases, as well as the myriad other duties heaped upon them having to do with this book (which they came to refer to as "*the* book") were often extra burdens on top of the day-to-day load of assisting a busy practice. It must have been especially distressing to arrive at the office on Monday morning, fresh from the week-end, to find Dictabelts, tapes, or corrected manuscript drafts piled high. Nevertheless, they must have enjoyed it, judging from their eager performance. Of these steadfast girls we owe much to Miss Julie Trowbridge, Mrs. Anne Petz, Miss Pauline Porowski, Miss Linda Wilrick and to Miss Mary Dean, Miss Carole Cannataro and Miss Sandra Sledz, of the senior author's staff, who helped so much. We are also indebted to Mrs. Kim Richman for her valuable editorial assistance.

Finally, much credit must also be given to Nan Rees and Miss Monika Krebs for their ceaseless toil and many hours of time taken from more enjoyable pastimes on weekends.

From previous experience we can say that working with publishers can be an unnerving and sometimes exasperating experience. To our delight the opposite was true throughout the production of this book. The spirit of cooperation, patience and devotion to the task shown by Albert E. Meier and John L. Dusseau of the W. B. Saunders Company was altogether a rewarding personal experience. Almost every change request was cheerfully agreed to. We are deeply indebted to them for their cooperation and for their helpful advice. What could have become an unpleasant chore became a joy.

CONTENTS

Chapter 1

CONCEPTS OF BEAUTY

Thomas D. Rees, M.D.

An old adage says that "beauty is in the eyes of the beholder." The evidence is clear that man's concept of beauty has changed many times through the ages, and it is likely that changes will continue for the rest of man's tenure on earth. The art of body adornment with paints or scarification dates from ancient times, probably from when primitive man first discovered the unusual effects that results from smearing his body with mud or painting it with pigments. He may have discovered this by looking at his image in the original looking glass, a pond of water.

Adornment of the self through the use of cosmetics, clothes, hairstyles or jewelry is widely accepted today, but the ancient tribal customs of scarification and tattooing are generally unacceptable in modern culture. Scarification in our society is generally considered to be a form of self-mutilation, usually indicating psychopathology. Tattooing is still a widespread form of decoration, but is considered to be in social bad taste in most so-called civilized countries. Just where the boundaries lie between self-mutilation and self-decoration is unclear. It is not difficult therefore to understand why self-mutilation is a common symptom of the neurotic or confused mind, for this type of activity may be nothing more than an attempt by the individual to call attention to himself.

Thus primitive man incises, paints, and decorates himself as an acceptable social form of ego manifestation, while modern "civilized" man is permitted only lesser degrees of self-adornment and resorts to more severe forms of self-beautification (or self-mutilation) when

he becomes frustrated, hostile or aggressive and can perceive no other way of expressing inner feelings (Rees and Daniller, 1969).

Behavior similar to self-mutilation has been noted in other primates such as the chimpanzee following the production of stress or a frustrating situation (Phillips and Muzaffer, 1961). Children and babies not uncommonly register frustration brought on by delay in feeding or when harshly reprimanded by severely scratching or even mutilating their faces.

Phillips and Muzaffer define self-mutilation as a socially unacceptable alteration of physical form, but the term "socially unacceptable" clearly can mean different things in different cultures and to different people. Schedter (1962) reminded us that Greek mythology refers to a band of fierce women, called Amazones. who amputated their right breasts lest they interfere with drawing the bow. Atresia of the breast brought on by compression from tight chest binding was in vogue in ancient Hellenistic circles to improve elan and poise. It came in vogue again in Chaucer's day, and again in the 1920's. The small firm breast as opposed to the voluptuous breast popularized by certain movie stars has become fashionable again in the early 1970's and it is conceivable that breast binding could once again be introduced; however, there is little possibility that it would be so ubiquitously accepted. Tight corsets were the vogue in the late nineteenth century to produce the "wasp waist." The result of this bit of physical restraint was a high incidence of pulmonary pathology.

There is considerable evidence to suggest

1

that in pre-Columbian culture persons with such deformities as harelip, dwarfism and spinal deformities (hunchback, etc.) were revered and even accorded special privileges. There is evidence that spinal deformities were induced to enhance a fashionable concept of physical beauty, according to Waisman (1967). Various deforming incisions were made in virtually every part of the body to enhance a popular concept of beauty in pre-Columbian times as well as in Africa, Asia and the South Pacific, where such practices persist to this day.

Perforations of the nose, ears, cheeks and lips through which various articles of adornment such as shells, wooden plugs and stakes, precious and semi-precious stones, and more recently metals of different types could be worn, is also an ancient and widespread custom. Even in higher cultures such as those of India and China, nose and ear perforation for the wearing of jewelry was a highly acceptable form of self-adornment.

The use of makeup was probably one of the first forms of self-decoration. The use of cosmetics, particularly on the face, was highly developed and entirely socially acceptable among the upper classes in ancient Crete. It should therefore surprise no one that body painting has recently enjoyed a brief vogue.

Lest we forget our heritage and tend to look with disdain on our more "primitive" brothers, several examples of interesting forms of self-adornment (or is it self-mutilation?) have been selected as represented in different cultures. The authors wish to express their deep gratitude to the publishers and staff of the National Geographic Magazine and the American Museum of Natural History for their help and cooperation in making these reproductions available.

After viewing some of the methods of obtaining beauty on the following pages it should seem apparent that modern cosmetic facial surgery is by all standards a mild form of torture to obtain the sought after ends. This is not meant to infer, however that there is any direct relationship between cosmetic surgery and what follows.

Vanity, it would seem, is shared by all members of the human race despite cultures imposed by genetics, religion, geography, or historical custom.

REFERENCES

Phillips, R. H., and Muzaffer, A.: Recurrent self-mutilation. Psychiatric Quart., 35:3, 1961.

Rees, T. D., and Daniller, A.: Self-mutilation: Some problems in reconstruction. Plast. Reconstr. Surg., 43:300, 1969.

Schedter, D. C.: Breast mutilation in the Amazones. Surgery, 51:554–560, 1962.

Waisman, A. I.: Ancient surgery of the Americas. Internat. Surg., 47:129, 1967.

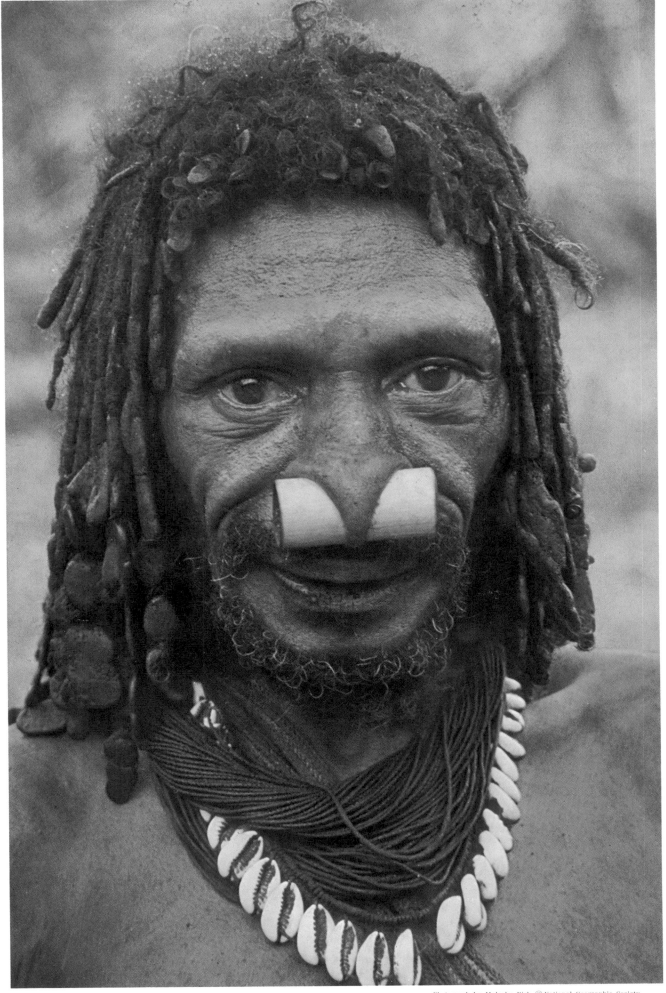

Nose, lip, or ear perforations, through which jewelry or ornamentation can be worn, are popular in many parts of the world, including New Guinea and much of Africa. The practice is almost ubiquitous among "stone age" New Guineans such as this man.

3

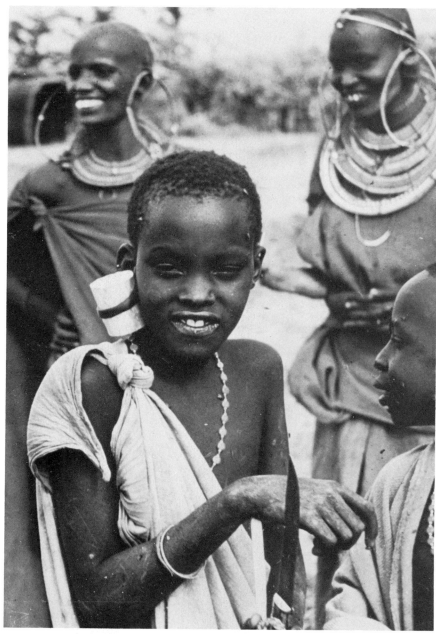

In many African tribes, the ears are perforated in childhood and gradually stretched to form great loops. These are considered decorative in themselves, but they also support various objects. Wooden plugs of graduated sizes are used to stretch the loops, as seen in this Masai boy.

Massive earrings of solid gold are seen in the ear loops of a Fulani maid, a resident of Mali in the sub-Sahara. Her permanent "lipstick" is an effect of tattooing. The mountain maid of Mandara wears in her ear a spent cartridge case left behind by the German rulers of the Cameroons before World War I.

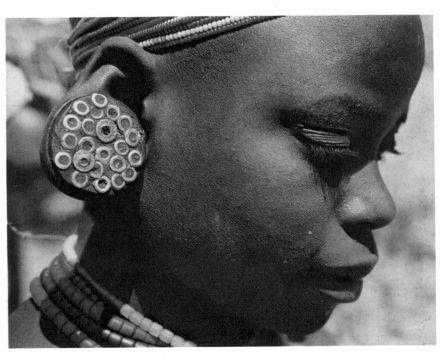

5

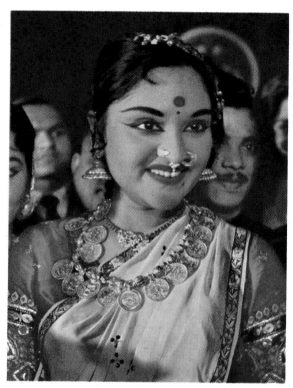

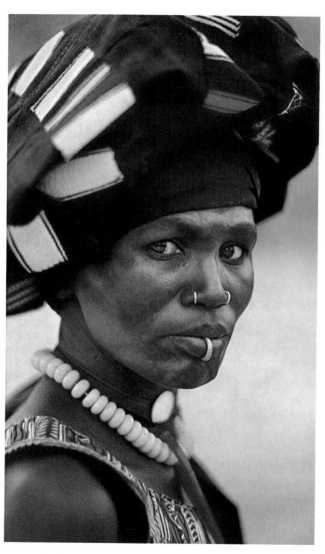

An Indian dancing girl wears precious stones in perforations of the alae of the nose as well as the columella. Tribesmen of the Bergen Country of Mali often adorn themselves with metal ornaments through perforations of the nose and lips.

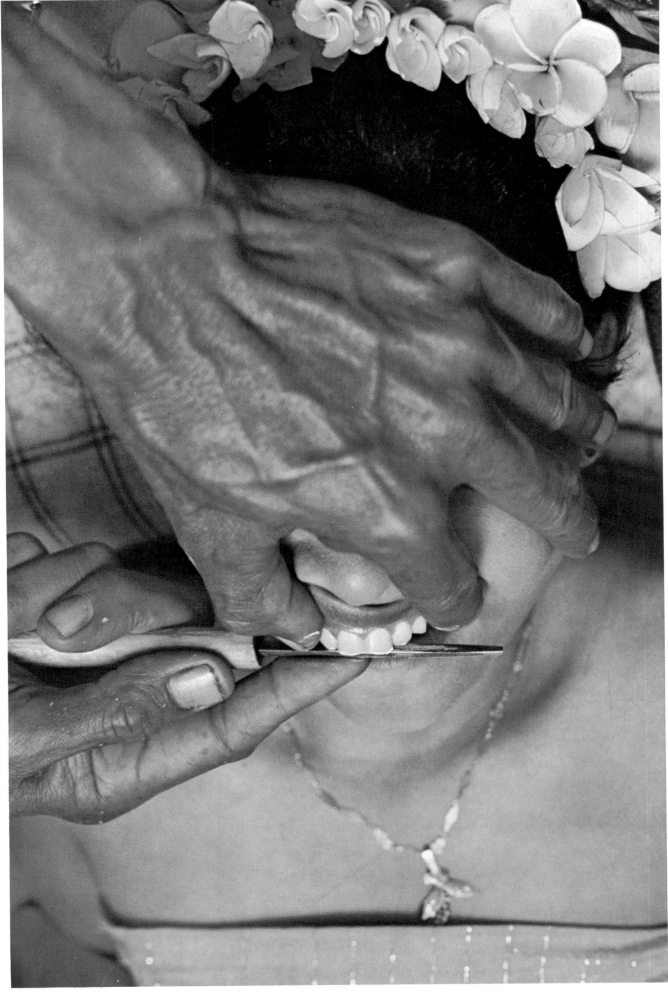

If modern surgery to improve one's appearance seems like an ordeal, consider the filing of teeth as it is practiced in Micronesia, Indonesia, and elsewhere. The young man in this picture lives in Bali.

7

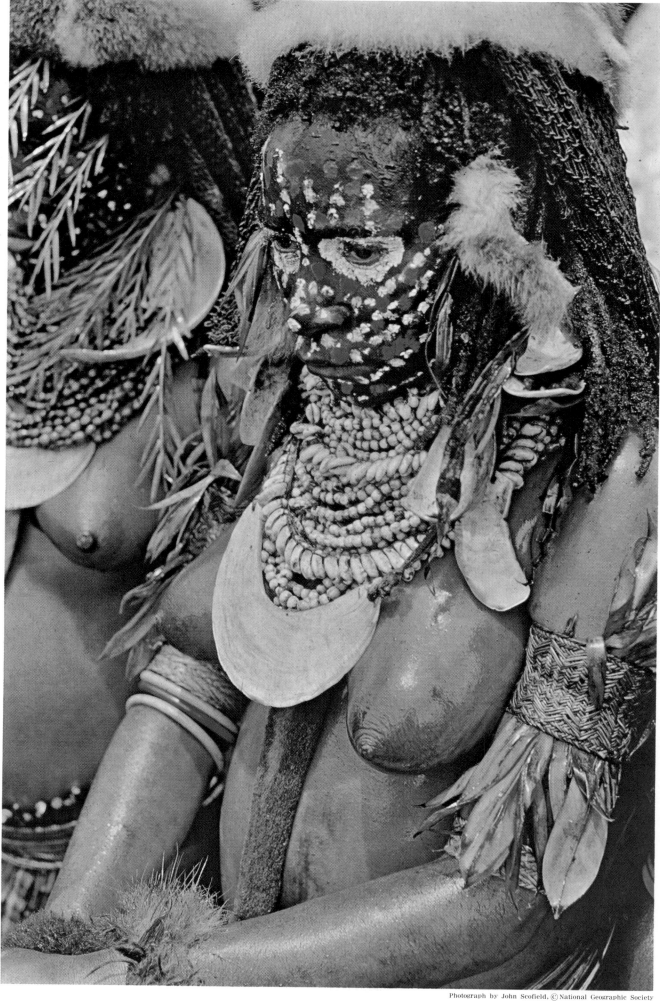

A lady of New Guinea in full ornamental regalia. Clearly most of these decorations have been fashioned from the local environment, with liberal use of shells, leaves, palm fronds, mud, and natural pigments. The arm bands probably came from traders.

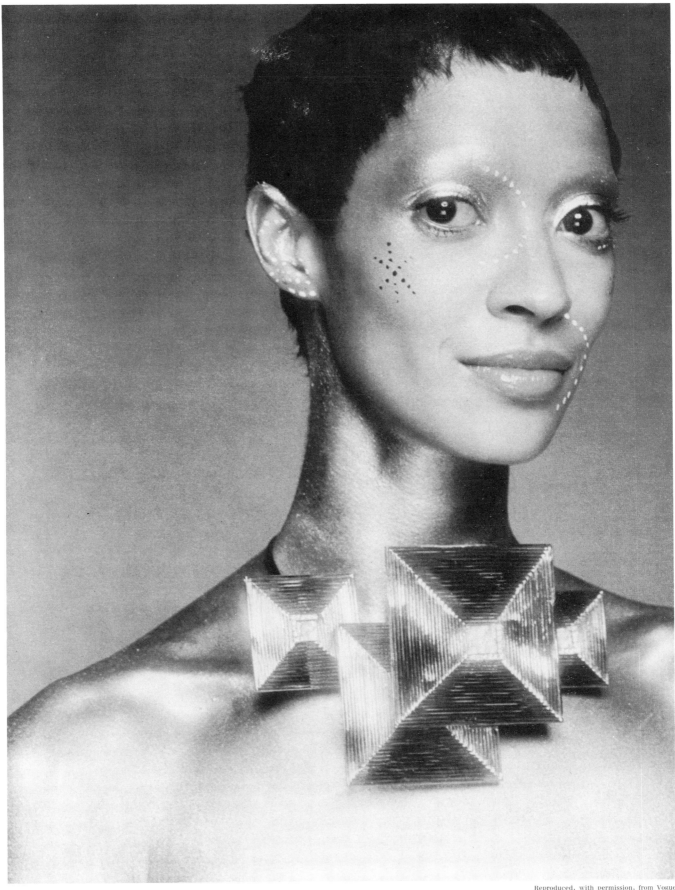

A modern civilized woman adorned with body paint, exotic make-up that is not entirely out of the realm of fashion possibilities these days.

This Kenyan has availed himself of ancient as well as modern techniques for self-adornment. The wearing of plugs or other objects in perforated and stretched ear lobes is a very old custom in Africa, as is painting of the face. Coral and glass beads worn on strings around the neck or head are of relatively recent origin, introduced by Arab and Indian traders. The sunglasses and a neck band made from a chrome-plated headlight rim are the most recent additions to the ensemble.

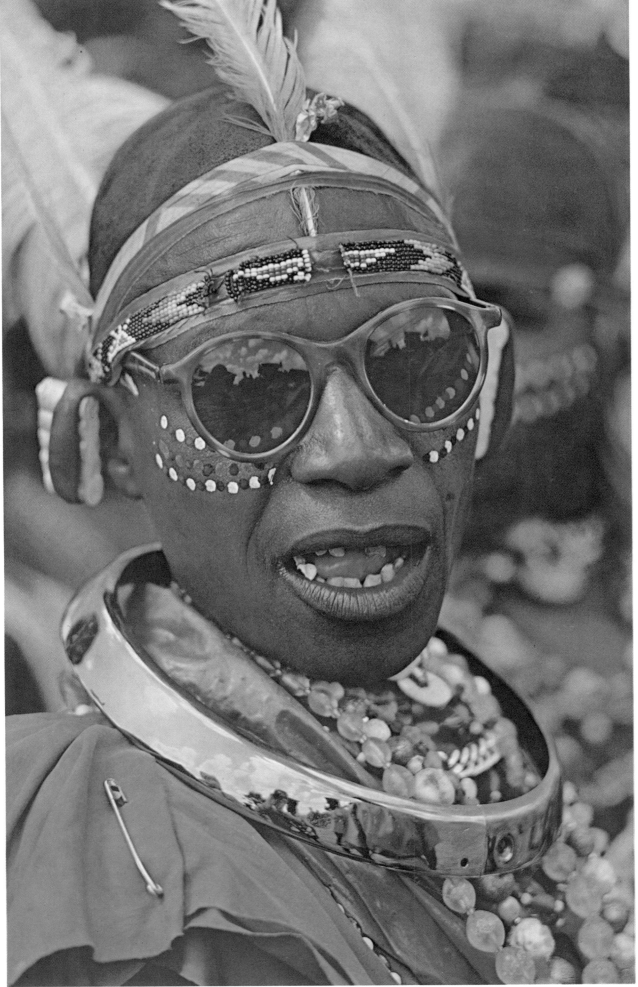

Photograph by Bruce Dale. © National Geographic Society

(See opposite page for legend.)

11

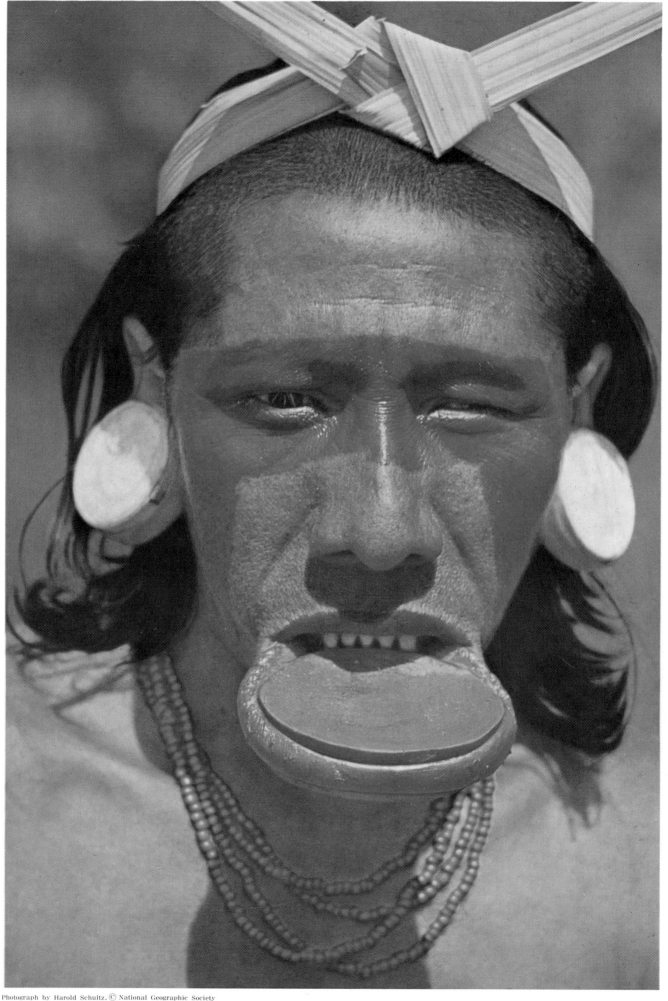

12

(See opposite page for legend.)

An African lady photographed during a transcontinental safari in 1938. Her lower lip measured 25 inches in circumference, and in this photograph it encircles a can that once contained 400 feet of motion picture film. The writer who visited her reported that her skin was so elastic that when pulled it snapped back "like a rubber band." This form of "mutilation" was probably begun centuries ago; tradition tells us that its original purpose was to make Ubangi women unattractive to slave traders. In the years since then the fashion has caught on, and these women are now considered appealing. Note the scarification marks on the forehead, and the scalloped ears.

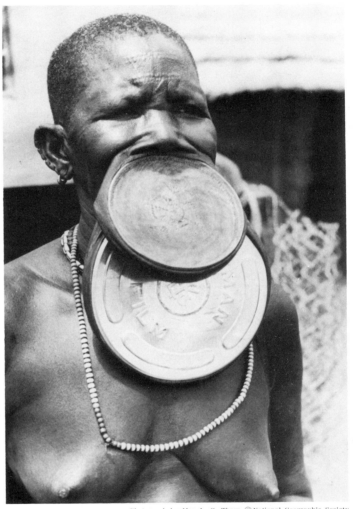

Photograph by Mrs. L. C. Thaw. © National Geographic Society

Stretching the lip is popular in both hemispheres, as the photos on these two pages suggest. The Brazilian gentleman on page 12, who belongs to the Suyá tribe, wears his lip disk in style, complete with red dye painting of the lip and face, earplugs of twisted palm leaves, a palm frond headband, and file-pointed teeth. He is a member of a vanishing tribe.

13

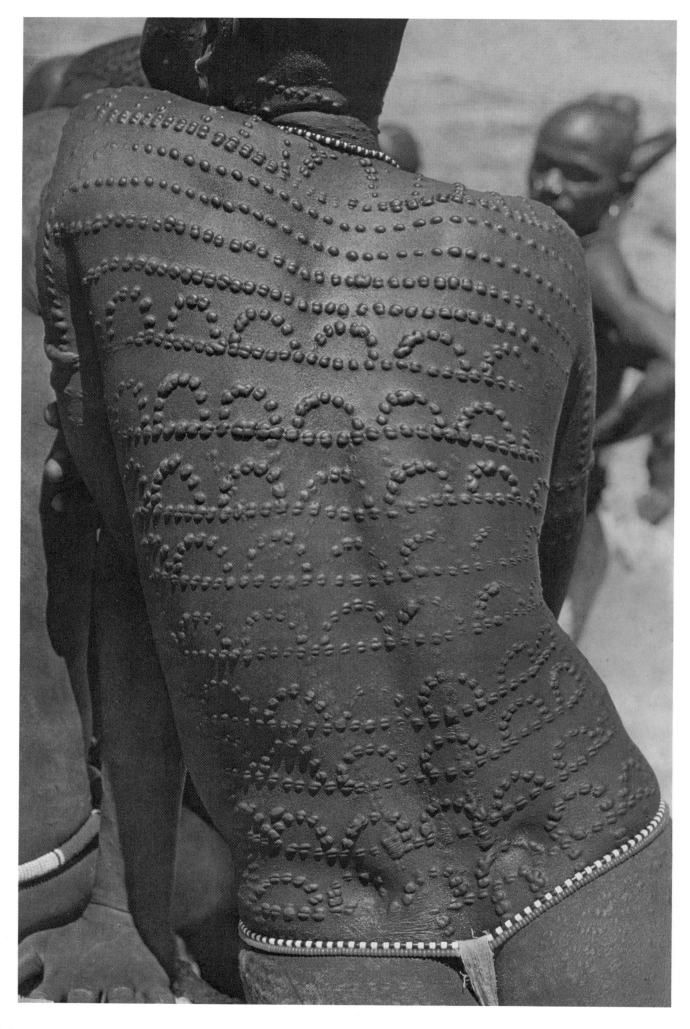

14

The people of the Masakin Qisar, a Nuba tribe, live in a remote part of the Sudan. Clothing is sparse or absent in the blistering sun of the region. For centuries these people have scarified the skin of their women as a method of beautification in the absence of the finery of clothes. Such scars, also found elsewhere in the world, often have significance. The three freshly cut rows of incisions across the left shoulder of the young girl pictured on this page are a particularly favored design because, lying over the heart, they are believed to make one's love life more favorable.

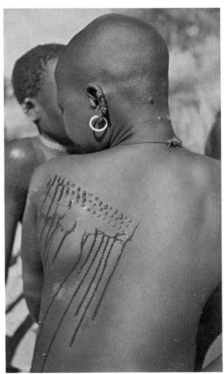

Both photographs by Oscar Luz. © National Geographic Society

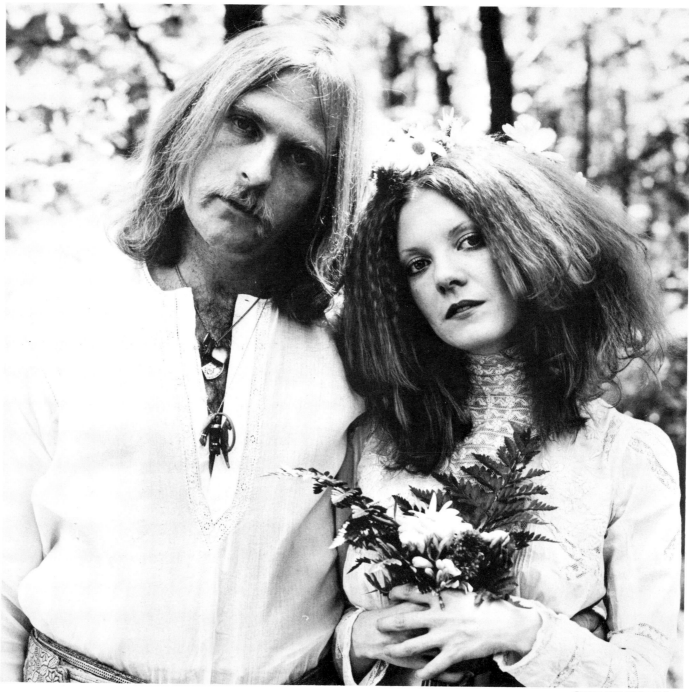

The "Look," 1973.

16

Chapter 2

SELECTION OF PATIENTS

Thomas D. Rees, M.D.

The chapter which follows this, by Frances Macgregor, is reproduced in its entirety from the Surgical Clinics of North America, April, 1971. Mrs. Macgregor has been actively engaged in the social and psychological study of plastic surgery patients for many years. She has profound understanding of the subject founded on long experience and piercing observation. Her interest inevitably focused on the selection of cosmetic patients for surgery. I urge the interested reader to review previous publications of Mrs. Macgregor's. These are listed in her bibliography along with additional key publications by other investigators on this very important subject.

The aim of cosmetic surgery is, after all, to make the patient happy. Generally if the patient is happy, so is the surgeon. When a happy result is not achieved, frustration and misunderstanding ensue and can lead to unpleasantness and, sometimes, to litigation. Communication is the key to all human intercourse. The total experience of a cosmetic surgical operation from consultation until the final follow-up visit depends for success upon a series of communications. It is distressing how rarely true communication occurs.

Plastic surgeons have long sought a simple "A, B, C" guide that could characterize preoperatively the personality of a patient and therefore predict behavior patterns. Hopefully a battery of behavioral examinations could define a "personality profile" that would indicate those individuals apt to be pleased by physical improvement through surgery and those who would not; or stated in another way, such a profile might indicate those with a realistic self-image. Such a quick and easy test has not been developed, probably because of the complicated natures of humans. It is this very diversity that makes the study of personality so fascinating yet so elusive.

There is no substitute for thorough personal interviewing and consultation prior to surgery. A primary aim of consultation is to establish meaningful communication between patient and surgeon at a personal level as well as to diagnose and plan treatment.

Communication actually begins long before the patient and surgeon confront each other across the consulting room desk. It begins with the first telephone call from the patient to the surgeon's aide, secretary or receptionist.

The first alarm that a patient may prove troublesome is often signaled during this first telephone contact. The patient who is "pushy," obnoxious or rude to the receptionist on the telephone is frequently egocentric, over-demanding, uncooperative and difficult to communicate with. Those patients who apply extraordinary pressure to obtain an early appointment and who are unwilling to accept an appointment at the normal allotted time almost certainly will expect "superservice" all along the way. Such patients are not only overdemanding about their appointments, but may well prove overdemanding about the results they expect from surgery. Concerted attempts to interfere with the normal office operation structure should always be viewed with caution and suspicion.

No surgeon likes to keep patients waiting; however, precise schedules in active day-to-day practice can rarely be adhered to. The patient who shows extreme irritation at these minor vexations should be viewed by the surgeon and his staff as one who is more apt to be unduly irritated and troublesome if some problems develop during or after the course of surgery. Everyone has the right to be impatient with delay; however, excessive signs of impatience evidenced by the patient on the first visit may herald a difficult relationship and result in an unhappy patient.

Rudeness is inexcusable. Patients who are rude to the office staff will most assuredly be rude to the hospital staff. They can make life unbearable for nurses, aides, surgeon and assistants.

It is a good practice to leave a new patient alone in the consulting room for a few moments before the actual consultation. Much can be learned from his or her behavior during this short period. Those who "help themselves" from the surgeon's bookshelves, desk drawers or personal effects are literally putting up a red flag, heralding difficulties to come. Such incursions should be duly noted by the surgeon and, if the bounds of propriety are significantly overstepped, other parameters of the patient's behavior should be investigated.

Appearance can sometimes provide definite symptoms of a disturbed or disoriented patient. Psychiatrists have long recognized that sloppiness of appearance can be a sign of disorganization or incipient psychosis. On the other hand, the "untidy" patient can show a reversal of this attitude following a successful cosmetic operation. Increased attention to personal appearance often is a pleasing dividend to a successful physical improvement.

The patient who is immaculately attired and coiffured can also be cause for concern, as these characteristics may indicate an overly perfectionistic individual who may be a "poor risk" for cosmetic surgery because the surgical result can rarely live up to the expectations of perfection. Such patients should be thoroughly

apprised of the limitations of the proposed procedures. It is sometimes wise to dictate a frank and thorough description of the possible shortcomings and complications of the operative procedure in the patient's presence.

I have found it useful throughout the past several years to address a personal letter to patients seeking cosmetic surgery which outlines in some detail what may and may not be expected from the operation. This is given to the patient for study prior to consultation. This form of communication has also proved helpful in answering many of the routine questions posed by most patients. It therefore not only serves to inform the patient, but discusses in a general way that complications can and do occur and that the results of surgery are considerably less than perfect. A copy of the letter is included in this chapter (pp. 20–22).

Those patients who are overly solicitous of the surgeon's attention or those who demonstrate overt tendencies toward seductiveness are usually disturbed and insecure individuals for whom striking a "sexy" attitude is a cover-up for deep-seated insecurities and neurotic tendencies. The surgeon is well advised to beware of such individuals and to insist on a preliminary psychiatric interview before making a surgical decision. In this context it may be said that while the surgeon often sees patients who show many symptoms indicating deep-seated neurosis or instability, it is not so easy or practical to obtain psychiatric evaluation. Those clinics which have full-time psychiatric help are fortunate indeed; however, the average practicing surgeon does not have this type of specialized help at his beck and call. He must often make many judgments on his own. Such judgments are often predicated on a sixth sense borne of long experience, but they can also be erroneous. The safest rule to apply is, when in doubt, do not operate. Psychiatrists are in short supply everywhere, and those with specialized knowledge applicable to plastic surgery are rare indeed. This is perhaps one of the most poorly understood areas in the field of cosmetic surgery and one which deserves much attention. Current studies are limited to a very few medical centers where psychiatrists interested in this subject are available.

We sincerely hope that current investigations will outline definitive studies for the future in this sensitive field to help to simplify the process of patient selection.

Many patients harbor personality disorders that can be improved by cosmetic surgery. Nevertheless, the risks are significant, and the gamble should be undertaken only when an educated calculation indicates that the odds are favorable for a happy outcome.

The surgeon should be leery of the patient who does most of the talking and very little listening. This type of individual is usually self-centered and unable to accept advice and instructions regarding the proposed operation, the results that can be expected and the possible complications. This problem of communication between surgeon and patient will continue into the hospital and throughout the postoperative period.

Patients who are hospitalized often feel neglected in the absence of constant attention. It is therefore important that the surgeon try to make clear to the patient what can be expected in the hospital. It is also important to make sure that all arrangements for office visits and follow-up care are clarified to avoid misunderstanding.

Those patients who complain of a very minor superficial defect are particularly difficult to please. Such patients frequently have an unreal image of themselves. Any attempts at surgical correction of minor defects are almost certainly destined to failure. Fredricks (1970) discussed several other points that should put surgeons on guard: the patient who speaks in a flat, monotone, and the overly hostile patients, particularly those who are excessively critical of previous surgeons who have "done them wrong." He also wisely warned the surgeon to guard against having his own ego massaged. It is sometimes difficult not to go against one's best judgment when the patient insists that the surgeon can accomplish a task that appears almost impossible, and that no one else could accomplish such a "miracle" of surgery.

Many circumstances can lead to cancellation of a surgical date; however, repeated cancellations indicate that the patient is not emotionally prepared, and further investigation is required before proceeding.

This discussion of the delicate interrelationship between patient and surgeon could easily fill an entire volume. Suffice it to say that the subject is of paramount importance in the field of cosmetic surgery but is poorly understood. Investigation in depth of this fascinating area has only just begun. It is hoped that much fruitful work will be forthcoming that will provide more definable guidelines to help in the selection of patients for whom the outcome of surgery will be more successful and to define those patients who need psychological guidance or psychiatric treatment.

Psychological Considerations

Generally speaking, patients, especially women, who are in the age group to be candidates for rhytidectomy (that is, 40 and over) are in a period of life when the disappointments tend to outweigh the pleasant surprises. For most the anticipation of new explorations and the joy of discovery are fading, and for some, already gone. Children, around whom their entire life may have revolved, have left home. The middle years have arrived, and with them the inevitable physical decline into old age and death. The sense of death as an inevitable fact becomes real to most people about this time. Before, it had been something that affected only others, the old or the infirm. In addition to this growing, distressing realization, especially in this second half of the 20th century, is the ever-growing emphasis on youth — its power and its desirability. Although their physical health is better protected so that most people actually "feel young" throughout middle age, they realize that youth has gone, never to be regained. Nevertheless, the pressure everywhere is to remain, and above all to *look*, young. It is not hard to understand, therefore, why facial rehabilitative surgery is undergoing an incredible boom.

Perhaps the hardest lesson for the young surgeon to learn, but one of the most important, is how to recognize which of this burgeoning number of patients seeking cosmetic surgery will become postoperative problems. He must learn to detect which patients will be unsatisfied or unhappy with the results, for these patients can and will make life miserable for everyone — for themselves, their families, the surgeon and the surgeon's staff. Experience is the greatest teacher in learning how to weed out the poor candidate for cosmetic surgery, but intuition plays an important role. The latter, unfortunately, cannot be taught, and some surgeons continue to have great difficulty developing the highly tuned psychic receiving apparatus that makes it possible to pick up early danger signals.

Ideally all cosmetic patients should have the benefit of a preliminary psychiatric evaluation. However, this is realistically, and logistically, impossible. There simply are not enough psychiatrists, psychologists or related specialists available to carry out such extensive interviewing, and those who are in practice are far overburdened as it is. It thus remains necessary in most instances for the surgeon to make his own evaluation. Those patients about whom he has doubts should either be rejected or, if pos-

19

To   : My Patients
From : Thomas D. Rees, M.D.
Re   : Some Facts for Patients About Cosmetic Facial
       and Eyelid Surgery

You will do yourself a service if you read what follows carefully, for here you will find answers to many of the questions that are most often asked about plastic surgery of the face, neck and eyelids. Most of these questions are universally asked by patients interested in this type of surgical correction.

The purpose of cosmetic surgery is to make you look as good as it is possible for you to look. It cannot do more than that. If you are expecting a transforming miracle from surgery, you will unquestionably be disappointed. Plastic surgery is a combination of art and science. Surgery is altogether not an exact science, and because some of the factors involved in producing the final result (such as the healing process), are not entirely within the control of either the surgeon or patient, it is impossible to warranty or guarantee results. Surgical results from facial and eyelid plastic surgery, however, are more predictable in some patients than in others. This is determined by a number of factors such as the physical condition of the face, the thickness and condition of the skin, the presence or absence of facial fat, the relative "age" of the skin, the numbers and types of wrinkles present, the underlying bone structure, heredity and hormonal influences, and others.

It is not possible, by surgical operation, to make someone who is over 40 years old look as if he or she is 20 years old or younger! While this may seem obvious, I mention it because some patients through misconceptions or misinformation believe the clock can be turned back in this miraculous fashion. It cannot.

Surgery intended to improve sagging skin or wrinkles necessarily leaves scars. Despite what you may have heard, all surgical scars are permanent and cannot be erased. The job of the plastic surgeon is to place scars in natural lines of the face and eyelids, where they are least noticeable and are more easily camouflaged by make-up or hair styles. While such scars are permanent, they are rarely noticeable or cause any trouble.

Preconsultation Letter for Patients

- 2 -

Now for some specific questions:

1. How long will the surgical results last?

Plastic surgery of the face, neck and eyelids retards the aging process and actually slows it up. It "slows down the clock, but does not stop it." It is not a question of a sudden "falling down." How soon you will want, or require, another operation is highly individualized. I can only speak in averages. In general, the operation of facial and neck lift, which is for the improvement of the jowls along the jaw line and the loose skin of the neck, may need to be redone in about five to eight years. Some very few patients are encountered who, for one reason or another, age more rapidly so that another operation may be desired in a shorter period of time than five years. Of course there are some who never require it again. The operation to improve or correct "bags" of the eyelids usually lasts longer. In most instances, the pouches beneath the lower lids do not recur. As one grows older the skin becomes looser and redundant and a trim of loose skin may be necessary at a later time. In those patients in whom there is exceedingly marked aging and excessive skin of the neck, face and jaw, sometimes (but extremely rarely) it is necessary to perform a second operation within a year to achieve the maximum improvement possible. If this seems to be the situation in your case, I will so inform you in advance.

2. Is facial surgery considered to be a major operation?

This type of surgery very rarely produces serious complications. It is, however, a surgical procedure and, as such, can be subject to unpredictables. Fortunately these are usually minor and amenable to treatment. These will be discussed with you in detail if you so desire.

3. Why are preoperative photographs important?

Just as the chest surgeon cannot operate in an intelligent way without x-rays of the chest, the plastic surgeon cannot operate on the face or eyelids without medical photographs.

- 3 -

These photographs are not meant to flatter you. You probably will find it a harsh photograph unsuitable for framing. The photos will show your face in every detail. This aids greatly in the surgical performance of technical variations in the surgery.

4. **What type of anesthesia is used during the operation?**

Either local or general anesthesia can be used, according to preference. I prefer to use a combination of light general anesthesia and local anesthesia, which I find is more comfortable for the patient. This technique permits a light anesthesia. A high level of oxygen is maintained throughout the surgery, which promotes safety. Local anesthesia is preferred by some patients and is completely adequate for this purpose. General anesthesia requires the services of an expert anesthesiologist, who charges separately. His fee is explained in the preoperative instructions. Whether you have a local or general anesthesia, there will be no pain during the operation.

5. **How long is the operation?**

The actual surgical time will vary, depending on the amount of surgery necessary for each patient. A face lift usually requires about two hours and eyelid surgery one hour.

6. **How long is the hospital stay?**

The usual hospital stay is three days. Admission is usually one day prior to the operation at about 2 p.m. and discharge time is about 10 a.m. the second or third day after surgery. Admission to the hospital may seem unnecessarily early, but is necessary in order to perform the required laboratory work and examinations by the resident surgeon and anesthesiologist.

Although the room accommodations are booked well in advance of admission, it may not always be possible to have the accommodation you desire on admission to the hospital. Every attempt will be made on my part to handle this problem to your advantage.

- 4 -

7. **Are bandages applied?**

Bandages are applied to the head and neck after a face lift. These are removed 48 hours after surgery. Bandages may or may not be applied to the eyelids for a few hours. Following removal of the bandages, ice compresses are applied to the eyes for several hours. Although this will not prevent all bruising and swelling it will help to minimize it. After you leave the hospital these ice compresses may be continued at home from time to time if you find them comforting. Bandages are applied for several reasons, one being to keep the operated area as immobile as possible; therefore, it is also important that telephone calls and visitors should be kept to a minimum for the first 48 hours after the operation. Postoperative pain is rare, and whatever discomfort there may be is usually mild and short-lived and is easily handled with routine medication.

8. **When are the stitches removed?**

Most eyelid stitches will be removed on the second day after operation. The remainder are removed on the third or fourth day. Some stitches in front of the ears are removed on the sixth or seventh day after a face lift. In most instances, all remaining stitches are removed by the tenth day. Removing stitches is quick and uncomplicated. But you must remain in the New York area for a minimum of 10 days following facial surgery and one week following eyelid surgery so that the removal may be done.

9. **When can make-up be applied?**

Eye make-up may usually be applied three days following the removal of the last sutures. This includes mascara, eye shadow and artificial eyelashes. Facial make-up can usually be applied about the tenth day. At this time, you may have to use some type of covering cream if there are still bruises below the eyes. It is important to remove all make-up very thoroughly, using an upward motion, at the end of the day. Oiled eye pads are recommended for the removal of eye make-up. My office staff will provide detailed instructions on use of make-up during the postoperative period.

- 5 -

10. **When may I get my hair done?**

On the fourth day following surgery you may comb your hair
out by using a solution of warm water and a large-tooth
comb. Your first shampoo will not be possible until the
eighth day following surgery. You may do this yourself or
go to a hairdresser who is acquainted with the special procedure of the first hairset after plastic surgery. My
office can recommend someone suitable. Rollers may be used,
but loosely. A hair dryer may also be used but must be kept
at the "comfort zone" (never hot), since at this time you
may not have full sensation in the areas operated upon.
Tinting and coloring usually may be done about three weeks
following the operation.

11. **Is hair shaved in preparation for the operation?**

The hair is not shaved. At the time of surgery a small margin of hair behind the ears is trimmed where the incision
will be. A similar area is trimmed inside the hairline
above the ears. Neither area is visible once the hair is
combed over the incision.

12. **Who takes care of me after surgery?**

Except over the weekends, you will be visited every day in
the hospital by me. If for unforeseen reasons I am unable
to visit you, you will be seen by one of my staff. There is
an expert team of associates and assistants always in atten-
dance, and they are continuously in touch with me. It is
also not possible for me to visit you the night of admission
to the hospital. Therefore, it is important that any unresolved questions be discussed prior to admission, if necessary, by a further visit to the office.

13. **Who actually performs the operation?**

I perform all surgery on my patients. I do have assistants
who play an active role in your operation by assisting me
just as the anesthetist and the nurse do. However, the actual
operative procedure is performed by me.

- 6 -

14. **What happens in the postoperative period?**

You must remember that before you see the improvement you are
expecting you will go through a standard postoperative period
in which you will look quite battered and bruised, followed
by another temporary period of time when you may look "strange"
to yourself. This varies considerably with each individual.
When both facial and eyelid surgery are performed together
you should set aside three weeks for recovery. At the end of
this time most patients are able to appear in public, although
the scars may need camouflaging with make-up. In some patients this time may be shortened by a few days and in others a
slightly longer period is required. I think you should also
bear in mind that in some patients undergoing facial and eyelid surgery there is a temporary period of slight emotional
depression immediately following the surgery, during the period of time when you look your worst. This is quite normal
and should not alarm you. It is not easy to look bruised and
swollen, particularly when natural expectations are toward
improvement of your appearance. Fortunately this period
usually passes rather quickly.

15. **Are private nurses available?**

Although not a necessity, some patients feel happier knowing
that someone will be with them following surgery. Some hospitals require the patient to book private nurses at the
time of admission. At other hospitals we are able to arrange
for nurses in advance. In spite of booking well in advance
of surgery, because of the critical shortage of such help
there is no guarantee that nurses will be available.

If you have any other questions be sure to get them answered
in advance by me or my office staff. Many members of my
office staff have been with me for years and are thoroughly
informed, trained and able to answer questions that may occur
to you. Well meaning friends are not a good source of information. Find out everything you want to know. A well informed
patient is a happy one.

Thomas D. Rees, M.D., F.A.C.S.

sible, referred for psychiatric appraisal before agreement to operate is reached.

Questionable candidates do not always present a cut and dried, black and white case. It is the group of patients in this "gray" area that causes most concern to the surgeon, and it is precisely in this group of patients that intuitiveness, experience and a certain degree of luck are needed to achieve a happy result for all.

Much has been written on the subject, but in our opinion only the surface has been scratched in our understanding of the psychological nuances involved in evaluating the prospective cosmetic patient. Probably there will never be a clear-cut evaluation technique that is thorough enough to prevent postoperative problems from arising, for cosmetic surgery deals with the very core of human behavior and that most delicate of all human perceptions, the self-image. Despite all that has been published about the self-image, our understanding of it is exceedingly superficial. It is often astonishing to the young surgeon to find out just how people really do visualize themselves, and how far removed this self-visualization can be from the interviewer's or surgeon's evaluation. There is no doubt that we all somewhat distort our self-image, so this should be expected to some degree in any patient. The line of demarcation between the normal range of distortion and the bizarre, however, is an important one in plastic surgery, because any cosmetic operation results in a certain change in self-image. When such a change is to the good as far as the patient is concerned, all is well. When the change is viewed as a negative one by the patient, despite the fact that the surgeon and even other observers may feel differently, the result can be disastrous for both patient and surgeon. Sometimes the result can even be a tragedy.

How can the surgeon who is not a trained psychiatrist, and who does not have the services of a trained psychiatrist or psychologist instantly available, effectively evaluate the emotional status of the patient requesting a change of physical appearance? The problem arises almost every day for most plastic surgeons and consumes a considerable portion of their time and interest. It also has, of course, a direct economic bearing on the surgeon's life, as there is no doubt that most law suits in the field of esthetic surgery arise from a misunderstanding between patient and surgeon on this all-important question of the patient's self-image. Most money settlements to patients who have had cosmetic surgery are not on the basis of out-and-out malpractice, but more on what is termed "breach of contract." The doctor did not produce the result that the patient expected or liked. Clearly the surgeon and the patient were miles apart in understanding and interpretation of what was to have been done. Such suits and settlements have driven the insurance premium rates for malpractice sky high, and in some cases insurance policies covering plastic surgery have been cancelled altogether. With the threat of litigation constantly hanging over the surgeon's head, it behooves him to develop his techniques of patient evaluation to the highest degree possible.

In the authors' view the ability to evaluate cosmetic patients on the basis of the flimsy and superficial knowledge gathered during one or two rather short interviews unfortunately falls more into the category of intuitiveness than behavioral science. Perhaps this is why some surgeons are constantly facing problems in their selection of patients while others seem to have little difficulty. The ability to penetrate the superficial mask of human behavior and to sense deep-seated disturbance is a gift that many doctors do not have. Such doctors might be better off in another field of medicine than in plastic surgery where this ability is vital in day-to-day practice. Some surgeons who have little native ability in this area are able to learn and to train their intuitive abilities so that they make fewer and fewer mistakes. Eventually, with experience, some of these surgeons become quite skilled in this regard.

A great deal of intensive research is needed in the area of psychosocial evaluation of the plastic surgery patient. As more and more patients seek cosmetic reconstruction, the demand for this knowledge increases. At present very few centers have even a semblance of such research programs. Among those that do are The Johns Hopkins University and the Institute of Reconstructive Plastic Surgery at New York University. Some of the problems retarding research in this area are the limited manpower available and the chronic lack of funds. It is surprising that more psychiatrists and psychologists have not realized the opportunities for study in patients seeking cosmetic surgery. Such patients are often quite eager and cooperative about psychiatric probing. Frequently they are aware that there is a relationship between their self-image and their desire to change their appearance, and they are often willing to explore that relationship.

Assuming a lack of scientific criteria and a dearth of psychiatric aid, what are some of the more superficial indications that can guide the young surgeon in his patient selection? Some of these have been described by various authors (Macgregor, 1950, 1953, Knorr et al., 1968). The young surgeon is advised to review these papers quite carefully. Certain well recognized syndromes, such as that of the "insatiable cosmetic patient," exist. These patients are not hard to recognize. As mentioned previously, it is the patient with more subtle problems who causes difficulty.

The first interview with the patient is the best time to detect potential problems. This interview is highly important and should be carried out under certain rather rigid circumstances and in a controlled environment. This is of great importance, since it is the initial consultation that sets the tone of the relationship between surgeon and patient. The first consultation should be conducted in a private consultation room without the presence of nurses, assistants or others. The consulting room should be comfortably decorated and esthetically pleasing so that the patient can feel relaxed.

It is preferable that the first interview be conducted without interruptions. A cut-off switch should be placed on the telephone. The secretary should hold all calls, if possible, enabling the surgeon to devote his entire attention to the patient. Some surgeons prefer seeing new patients at specific consultation times which do not conflict with follow-up practice or day-to-day office routine. While this may not be necessary, every effort should be made to provide peace and tranquility in this first interview, which rarely needs to exceed 20 or 30 minutes. Interviews lasting longer than 30 minutes or those in which the patient demands more time should arouse some suspicion in the surgeon that all is not quite right. If more time is required, the surgeon should arrange a second interview or consultation, particularly for those patients about whom he is unsure. Often a second interview can be arranged after photographs have been taken, or after other indicated studies, such as x-rays, urine tests and blood work, consultation with other specialists, and so forth, have been finished. This hiatus between consultations can be of great value for both surgeon and patient. The passing time allows seeds of suggestions and questions planted at the first interview to germinate and sometimes brings forth valuable information at the second interview.

Several situations tend to contraindicate, temporarily at least, face lifting procedures in men or women. These include patients in the throes of a severe emotional crisis, such as a marital problem or divorce, or grief following death of a loved one, and persons of late middle age who have just experienced a sudden change in job situation. If the emotional status of these patients becomes stabilized, however, they may benefit greatly, psychologically as well as physically, from the operation.

There are certain other signs which will indicate a disturbed or unsatisfactory cosmetic patient. These are admittedly generalities and may be subject to severe criticism by psychiatric colleagues. Nevertheless, many have stood the test of time and experience. The following are presented here only as the opinion (or bias) of the author.

Perhaps the most commonly observed psychological contraindication to surgery is in the patient who brings to the surgeon photographs of celebrities he or she would like to resemble. Most people who admire the appearance of others in this way are attractive in their own right, but have the unrealistic attitude that choosing a face is like choosing a hair style.

The patient who is disheveled and unkempt, or who appears in inappropriate or sloppy dress with uncombed hair or signs of poor personal hygiene, should be viewed with slight suspicion. Although many patients assume a drastically different view of themselves following successful cosmetic surgery and take an increased interest in clothes, make-up and hair styling, it does not necessarily follow that a sloppy and disorganized-appearing individual will benefit from such surgery. There is no guarantee that she will take a fresh interest in grooming when little such interest appeared preoperatively. Furthermore, total disinterest in self-grooming or appearance may be symptomatic of serious underlying mental disorder. Borderline psychotics frequently are disorganized in this way. The dishevelment of the withdrawn psychotic is even more apparent. However, it must be noted that everyone who is poorly groomed is not psychotic or even potentially so.

The surgeon's personal biases in reference to what is a neat appearance must also be reckoned with. The hippies and, in fact, much of the younger generation who dress casually in a studied sloppiness do not consider themselves disheveled in any way. Their self-images are well developed. It is only that the society to which they are conforming is not the one to which the surgeon belongs. It is not known at this point where cosmetic surgery will fit in this new society. Rhinoplasty, for one, may well be on the decline in this group of individuals, since their desire for the "natural look" includes their easy acceptance of even a huge hooked

24

nose. Since the greater part of this group has not yet approached the middle years when other generations have sought face lifts, it is yet to be seen if they will continue to desire the "natural look" during the transition from youth to middle age.

The patient who seeks consultation at the insistence of a friend or relative and does not seem convincingly self-motivated is a questionable candidate. Every effort should be made to establish that the patient herself truly wants the operation. The surgeon should be wary of those patients who present with statements such as, "I don't really want to be here or have this operation, but my boyfriend thinks I should." If the patient even implies that the surgery is being done solely to please someone else, the surgeon is well advised to refuse to operate.

The patient who tends to ask repeated questions, but apparently does not listen to the surgeon's answers, is also a potential problem. Often such patients ask a question, and then follow with another before the surgeon has even finished answering the first. Problems will undoubtedly arise with such patients in the area of advised consent. They are best avoided.

Perhaps one of the most telling examples of the patient who should be turned down can be detected within the first seconds of the interview. It is the patient who, almost immediately on sitting down, begins to deprecate another surgeon, or surgeons, or doctors in general. Many such patients have severe conflicts with authority, and physicians represent the ultimate authority in their minds. They are almost never satisfied with surgery, either primary or secondary. It is often very tempting for the young surgeon to accept such a patient, particularly when a facial deformity seems obviously amenable to surgical correction. The temptation increases when such patients often warmly infer that all other doctors are incapable except the surgeon with whom they are consulting. This is both flattering and ego-building to the unwary. Such patients, however, are destructive and usually quite neurotic. Even if the surgery is successful, the relationship will be an unpleasant and exasperating one.

The perfectionist presents a separate problem which is difficult to resolve. Perfectionistic patients are often recognized by their immaculate dress, their highly detailed and probing questions, their desire to know every detail, and above all their very detailed description of exactly what they would like to have done, sometimes complete with drawings, tracings and photographs. These patients are very apt to be disappointed in the minor details of the surgical correction, but often in the end are pleased with the overall result. Superperfectionists cannot be pleased. The expectations of such patients cannot be fulfilled, and they should be informed of this quite directly and turned away. Perfectionists of lesser degree require more time and attention by the surgeon, including more than one interview to emphasize and to explain everything in great detail, especially the inadequacies, drawbacks, defects and shortcomings of the operative procedure and the results.

If the surgeon decides to operate on a perfectionistic patient he must do so accepting a certain risk that the patient may not be happy, or may arrive at some measure of happiness or acceptance only after many weeks and a good deal of "niggling" annoyance and irritation to the surgeon and his staff. On the other side of the ledger, however, is the astonishing fact that in some rare instances perfectionists become the most devoted patients a surgeon can have. Suffice it to say that, prior to surgery, the relationship between such a patient and the surgeon must be firmly established and every detail explored to the utmost.

Another patient to avoid in most instances is the one who is rude, arrogant, difficult, insulting or otherwise very unpleasant to the secretary or receptionist. Often such patients are the epitome of politeness and attention to the surgeon. When a secretary informs the surgeon of such rude behavior, he should be on guard and should make a very careful evaluation of the situation before accepting the patient.

The patient who seems to ignore preoperative instructions as to medication, photographs, and other details may also prove to be a problem. Some such patients are simply a bit absentminded, but others may have quite severe neuroses. Losing instructions, or making repeated phone calls to the office staff to inquire about the same points, is a fairly reliable tip-off to the surgeon that he had better make sure that he has investigated all aspects of his relationship with the patient before surgery is undertaken. It is such patients who are required by many surgeons to sign an advised consent form, although the legality of such forms is open to considerable question. Usually this type of patient is also the one who forgets her purse or umbrella in the office or misses her appointment one or more times. Sometimes they do not even show up at the hospital at the appointed time, offering some lame excuse. Such patients may not be real trouble, but they can generate more than their share of minor irritation, including their failure to pay their fee either before or after surgery.

There are many other patient types that could be discussed. However, the interested reader is now invited to delve more deeply into the literature on the subject. The foregoing, rather superficial, discussion is meant more as an aid to the surgeon beginning in the field of cosmetic surgery than to the "old hands," although it is clear that these lessons have to be learned several times by most before they really sink in.

REFERENCES

Knorr, N. J., Hoopes, J. E., and Edgerton, M. T.: Psychiatric-surgical approach to adolescent disturbance in self image. Plast. Reconstr. Surg. *41*:248–253, 1968.

Macgregor, F. C., Abel, T. M., Bryt, A., Lauer, E., and Weissmann, S.: Facial Deformities and Plastic Surgery: A Psychosocial Study. Springfield, Ill., Charles C Thomas, 1953.

Macgregor, F. C., and Schaffner, B.: Screening patients for nasal plastic operations: Some sociologic and psychiatric considerations. Psychosomat. Med. *12*:277–291, 1950.

Chapter 3

SOCIAL AND PSYCHOLOGICAL CONSIDERATIONS

Frances C. Macgregor, M.A.

The legitimization of cosmetic surgery by our society in general and the medical profession in particular is relatively recent. Originally sought and performed furtively, plastic surgery for cosmetic purposes is as acceptable today as orthodontics, wigs, hair coloring or any other form of personal enhancement. No longer is it regarded as a luxury reserved for "vain" wealthy women or aging actors, but rather as a social or economic necessity, or both. The medical profession's acceptance of cosmetic surgery as a therapeutic procedure is reflected in the growing number of plastic surgery clinics and the health care plans which now make it possible for almost anyone to obtain partial or complete correction of his defect. With the advent of Medicaid, for example, even a person on relief can obtain a face lift without charge.

The changing attitudes toward cosmetic surgery and the increasing demands for it have resulted from several factors. Dominant among these are the high premium on physical attributes and the cultural pressure to conform. As the role of visual impression grows in importance, appearance becomes of major concern. "Exposure" is now a formula for getting ahead, and the face is one's passport. Since what we see often takes precedence over what we hear, even a politician's fate may hinge upon the art of the make-up man.

Another factor is the current devaluation of the middle and older age groups in what has become a youth culture. With respect to employment, this trend, coupled with the traditional view that as a man ages he becomes incompetent, has created problems of such proportion that signs of aging such as wrinkles, baggy eyes, jowls or a double chin are impediments that prevent many persons from getting or holding jobs, regardless of their capability.

Further impetus to the demand for cosmetic surgery has been given by scientific research findings on the social and psychological consequences of facial disfigurement: namely, that existing stereotypes—mostly negative or stigmatic—about the personality or character of a person with a receding chin, hook nose, malformed ears or facial scars can adversely affect his mental health and chances for success in life.

While in many ways beneficial to patient and surgeon alike, legitimization of cosmetic surgery has nonetheless accelerated its hazards and complications. The public today is sophisticated about medical care and in evaluating its competence. When dissatisfied, patients are outspoken about their rights and do not hesitate to seek legal aid. The plastic surgeon, therefore, is more vulnerable than ever. His difficulties are not necessarily related to surgical skill, but lie in the area of human relations and communication. He must deal with a heterogeneous patient population, representing a wide range of sociocultural differences, and the matter of correct evaluation and selection of candidates is beset with pitfalls both for him and for his patients.

Unfortunately there exists no "personality profile" or statistical chart, as some plastic surgeons have been heard to long for, by which —computerlike—one could learn in seconds whether a patient will be a psychological risk. The surgeon would like to be able to determine the patient's real motivation for surgery, whether he will cooperate or pose a management problem, what his subjective expectations are, whether he will be punitive or litigious if things go wrong, and so on. At best, a personality profile is a concept that rests on normative assumptions. While statistical frequency may be interpreted as statistically "normal," it does not follow that the patient with personality characteristics that correspond to a statistical norm is "normal" in a mental health sense. Even if one had a chart covering all types of personalities with mathematical weighting of characteristics which, when submitted to statistical analysis, would indicate or contraindicate surgery, other variables (social class and ethnic background, for example) would still make such an instrument one of dubious value.

Because of the nature and complexity of human relationships, the possibility of mistakes cannot be eliminated; the more aware the surgeon is of factors that affect his decisions or color his judgments, however, the greater the potential reduction in unhappy surprises or outcomes for himself and the patient.

What Can Go Wrong and Why

Since lack of relevant information is one of the major causes not only of errors in evaluation but also of misunderstandings in the management of soundly selected patients, the importance of knowing the individual cannot be over-emphasized. To know him well enough even to decide judiciously whether or not to operate often requires more interviewing time than many surgeons feel is either possible or essential. Though some surgeons supplement their direct contact with the patient by chart reading and consultations with colleagues, these patients, too, may receive insufficient attention because of daily pressures and priorities. Neglect is not implied, but unawareness of certain pertinent facts is often apparent.

For instance, it is generally assumed that when a cosmetic defect about which a patient complains is evident and operable, it is both unnecessary and unprofitable to investigate or discuss with him his problems, motives and expectations. This assumption is erroneous. In contrast to the conspicuously disfigured patient, whose needs are obvious, the one who presents a "minor" defect requires particular attention. The former's complaints are situationally real, whereas with the latter, one cannot be sure. He poses special problems.

SPECIAL PROBLEMS OF COSMETIC SURGERY PATIENTS

As evidenced by research findings, patients with slight defects tend to assess these defects as being more conspicuous than they are. Such patients are also apt to be the most demanding (Macgregor, 1967). Additionally, the smaller the defect that troubles the patient, the more likely he is to focus on minute details and post-operatively to magnify any residual imperfections.

Cursory consultations with such patients seldom expose their underlying motives. Given reasons such as wanting to look better or wanting to get or hold a job or a spouse are so highly sanctioned today as to obviate questioning. In many instances the stated reasons may be the real ones. But in as many others they may be oversimplifications or a less significant element in motivation for the request. For example, one investigation of rhinoplasty patients showed that—while not verbalized to the surgeons—a dominant factor in the requests of approximately half of the 89 persons interviewed was the desire to reduce or eradicate ethnic visibility (Macgregor, 1967).

It is not uncommon for the presenting complaints of patients with mild or moderate deformities to be symptomatic of emotional disturbance unrelated to the deformity (Macgregor and Schaffner, 1950). In a psychiatric analysis of women seeking rhinoplasty, Meyer and his associates (1960) concluded that preconscious and unconscious factors play an important part in patient motivation, and interpretations of these center around the following: conflicts in sexual identification, ambivalence in patients' identifications with parents, the symbolic (sexual) meaning of the nose and the wish for surgery, concepts of body image, and the incidence of psychopathology among patients.

Some unstable individuals select one body part, which they claim to be ugly or deformed, as an unconscious method of avoiding their

28

own personality shortcomings. They are convinced that this single flaw causes all their problems and that plastic surgery will magically transform their lives. In a study of 50 rhinoplasty patients, Linn and Goldman (1949) found a high incidence of neurosis, while Jacobson et al. (1960) found that the male patient seeking surgery for mild congenital deformity is apt to have serious emotional illness. As for mammoplasty, according to Knorr, Hoopes and Edgerton (1968), many adolescent and adult females who request breast augmentation exhibit hysterical character traits and are prone to depression.

Besides the person who presents a single complaint, it is not unusual to meet in one's practice a patient obsessed with real or imagined defects who shifts attention from one body part to another, and moves from one surgeon to another seeking relief which often ends in disaster. The following case is illustrative and also underscores the importance of careful interviewing prior to acceptance of any patient.

Miss G., age 30, was convinced that her slightly large nose was the source of all her troubles. The surgeon accepted her request for rhinoplasty without attempting to review her history or to learn what she expected of surgery. Though he considered his results good, she did not and demanded a second operation and then a third. When he refused her a fourth procedure she sought other surgeons. Two told her that further surgery was not advisable. Another, recognizing her disturbed state, suggested psychotherapy, but Miss G. argued that her first doctor hadn't thought she was "crazy," since he had agreed with her and operated three times. When seen at still another surgeon's office she believed her nose to be actually disfigured and was highly agitated. To the social scientist who interviewed Miss G. it was apparent that she needed immediate psychiatric care. She resisted this idea but a few days later was committed to an institution because she had become violent and threatened suicide.

Had Miss G.'s first surgeon taken time to talk with her, he would have found strong evidence that her complaints were symptomatic of emotional illness, and that psychiatry—not surgery—was indicated. In adolescence she had been obsessed with what she considered her "ugly" complexion (acne). Spending hours in front of the mirror, she aggravated the condition with heavy makeup. Because of this preoccupation and her refusal to go out socially, she was a problem to her family. When the acne finally subsided she became absorbed with the size of her breasts. Though they were not abnormally large, she underwent reduction mammoplasty. She next focused upon her nose, blaming it for her unhappiness and difficulties with others. By accepting her for rhinoplasty the surgeon unwittingly validated her complaint, with results that eventuated in her complete breakdown.

CRITERIA FOR REJECTING CANDIDATES

Most plastic surgeons have rules of thumb for deciding that a person is a risky candidate psychologically. Strict adherence to these rules, however, can preclude objective judgment, thereby depriving some people of the attention they deserve.

HISTORY OF PSYCHIATRIC TREATMENT. Because symptom removal has long been regarded with suspicion by psychiatry, a common caveat is a history of psychiatric treatment. As already indicated, there is good reason to examine each potential patient's emotional status. But not all forms of neurosis result from basic personality disturbances. Some may be realistic responses to external situations. Yet for most surgeons the fact that a person has a record of emotional instability makes him immediately suspect, even when his complaint is valid. There is doubt whether surgery will satisfy him, whether he will become a management problem or—worse still—whether surgery will precipitate a psychological breakdown. His chances of being accepted are even less if he has the reputation of being hostile or a "personality problem."

J. B., age 22, was such a person. When first seen by plastic surgeons in a Veterans Administration Hospital, where he had been admitted for a complaint diagnosed as "psychosomatic," he was arrogant and defensive, and had untenable relationships with both personnel and patients. The surgeons described him as a "pain in the neck."

To a psychiatrist J. B. had disclosed his feelings about his face and how it interfered with his relationships. He had what has been called the "FLK syndrome" (funny-looking kid). His large ears stood out from the sides of his rather small head. His upper jaw protruded, making the teeth so prominent that he could not bring his lips together. In contrast, the lower jaw receded.

An otoplasty was permitted, but two surgeons discouraged additional surgery and orthodontic treatment, lest these trigger a psychotic episode. In any event, they regarded J. B. as "too difficult" and predicted that he would be "a lot of trouble." "I wouldn't touch him," said one. "He's a kook," said another. The psychiatrist didn't consider J. B.'s appearance significant in the etiology of his personality disorder and was skeptical about the psychological effectiveness of surgery. One resident surgeon, however, was inclined to operate. Because of conflicting opinions, the patient was referred to the social scientist member of the rehabilitation team.

A review of J. B.'s life history showed that his emotional problems had stemmed in large measure from ridicule and social rejection. At school his peculiar face on his small, thin body provoked the

29

nicknames of "Long-legged Spider," "Elephant Ears," and "Buck Teeth"—epithets that he ruefully admitted were "appropriate, but this makes an impression. I always looked odd, and therefore I was considered odd."

Frequent family moves and new schools compounded his difficulties. Though bright, J. B. dropped out before finishing the eighth grade. "You can't go to school if you're not accepted by the kids, and you can't learn something if everyone around you is making faces at you and you have arguments every morning. Kids are naturally going to pick on you. If you don't look right, you're singled out as the bad guy."

When he become interested in girls, his frustration continued. "I used to go up to a girl at a dance, but I was always rejected. When I was young, everyone else went out with girls—I didn't."

Convinced that he would have to go through life looking "odd," his efforts to cope with a hostile environment took the following forms: He developed "a very short, sharp tongue." He rationalized leaving school on the grounds that he was "creative" and so musically gifted that he didn't need formal training; that since he was "talented" his looks were not "the most important." To cover his real feelings of inferiority and insecurity, he became arrogant and "put on an air of superiority and super-security." His isolation from others, he convinced himself, was self-imposed, since he had "superior intelligence and most other people were boring and unintelligent." Though his evaluation of his appearance was realistic, the defenses and strategems he used to cope with his situation only led to further social rejection, withdrawal and severe maladjustment.

J. B.'s growing intolerance of others multiplied his problems when he was drafted into the army. Hating it, he manifested symptoms such as shortness of breath and inability to perform routine physical activities. After hospitalization for bronchitis and pneumonia, he refused to return to duty. Placed in a mental hospital, he was eventually given a psychiatric discharge.

His behavior at the hospital where he had undergone otoplasty tended to substantiate the surgeons' impressions of J. B.'s instability. His neurosis, however, was situational, and his days were fraught with unmitigated humiliation. Surgery could not be expected to heal his psychic wounds, but correction of his appearance would remove a stigmatic barrier to his relations with others and help him to gain some self-esteem. For these reasons the social scientist endorsed surgery.

Postoperatively there was a striking change in J. B.'s face. Striking also was his dress: "mod" clothes, square gold-rimmed glasses, and ornate rings. He was delighted with the surgical results. He had begun to date and for the first time spoke hopefully of marriage. While his improved appearance gave him an almost immediate sense of well-being and more confidence when meeting people, he had sufficient insight to realize that he lacked the skills of normal social interaction.

J. B. got a job as assistant nurse in a department of physical medicine. He found the patients interesting and enjoyed his work. Within a few months his former hostility and arrogance had almost vanished.

POSSIBILITY OF LITIGATION. Another criterion for rejecting candidates is the possibility of punitive action by those who may find fault with their postoperative results, even though these may be satisfactory from the surgeon's point of view. In a specialty that has one of the highest records for malpractice suits, and consequently exceedingly high rates for insurance coverage, surgeons are perforce wary of accepting any patient who they suspect may retaliate if his or her expectations are not fulfilled. Patients who have had cosmetic surgery elsewhere but wish additional operations tend to be viewed with caution. Blame, derogatory remarks about the original doctor, and vindictive attitudes are seen as warnings signs, while any hint of legal action is so threatening that most surgeons close the door on further consideration of the patient's needs. This fear, realistic and justifiable as it may be in some cases, is so generalized that some patients who merit help are denied it. Caught in the rigid system of medical values and the stigma attached to those who seek any form of retribution, such persons are left to work out their problems alone. Even experienced specialists may make injudicious decisions when biases have priority and positions are taken without an effort to ascertain facts.

A case in point is that of S. F., in whose infancy a skin infection on her nose had left conspicuous pitting, about which she became exceedingly self-conscious. At age 24 she consulted a plastic surgeon who performed dermabrasion and rhinoplasty, which unfortunately resulted in further scarring and also notched alae. Four years later she requested evaluation at a plastic surgery clinic and was accepted for another dermabrasion. Dubious about this procedure because of its previous failure to eradicate the pitting, she asked instead for a skin overgraft. Although advised of the risk involved (possible scarring and a differentiation in skin color), she chose to take the chance, preferring this possible outcome to the pitting. Moreover, she volunteered to sign any document exonerating the surgeons should the operation fail.

While awaiting arrangement of her surgical appointment, S. F. mentioned to another patient that she had sued her first surgeon. The recipient of this information, an "old patient," told the head nurse. The surgeons' immediate reaction was to cancel the operation.

The story about the law suit was correct, but S. F. had not instigated it. While she had been disappointed with the surgical results, so had the surgeon. Two days before operating he had broken his

30

leg. According to S. F. he was in great pain and therefore hadn't done "as good a job as he might have. I felt sorry for him and I didn't blame him for what happened. He even offered to perform another operation." At the time S. F. was a secretary in a law firm. It was her employers who instituted procedures on her behalf, on the grounds that the surgery had been "botched up." She described the trial as "a terrible ordeal. I would never want to go through anything like it again." She still felt sorry for the surgeon and held no grudge. Her employers, however, had persisted and won the suit.

When the details of this case were reported to the surgeons who had refused to operate, S. F. was brought to the clinic conference for re-evaluation. While several members of the group favored surgery, others more skeptical and worried about legal action vetoed the idea. The patient, whose hopes had been raised, left the clinic in tears.

SURGEONS' MOTIVATIONS

Though the plastic surgeon may sometimes be overly cautious in selection, he may also err on the side of suggesting surgery. For instance, his high sensitivity to the slightest deviation or asymmetry and his zeal to make "beautiful people" may tempt him to propose esthetic improvements. Referred as the "Pygmalion complex," this enthusiasm to make alterations is a potential pitfall and can obscure the difference between "desire to cure and the need to cure" (Meyer, 1964). Surgeons' suggestions may also be motivated by professional self-interest such as eagerness to obtain operating experience or to recruit patients—phenomena not uncommon in resident training programs of teaching hospitals or in building up a practice.

While in some instances correction can safely be initiated and should be, the surgeon needs to be conscious of his motivations. To suggest that an individual's appearance can be improved is to point up a deficiency, a responsibility that must be carefully weighed. Should the person be nonreceptive, he will only be disconcerted. On the other hand, he may be more than ready to comply; but if he is dissatisfied with the outcome, the doctor may have to bear the full onus.

Such a consequence was aborted in the case of R. L., age 39, who said she had come to the clinic because the previous week, while she was being treated in the ENT clinic for a sinus infection, a plastic surgery resident observed that rhinoplasty would make her look better. She asserted she had never thought of having an operation, but "since the doctor thought it would be a good idea" she was "willing" to have it.

Interviewing disclosed that R. L. actually had long desired to have her nose altered but had refrained for fear the results would fall short of her standards of perfection. In the event of an imperfect result, she would have only herself to blame, a situation that she seemed psychologically unable to handle. Discussion of her work experience and social relationships revealed a vindictive need to hold others responsible whenever she failed. Fortuitously, in this instance, the resident's casual suggestion of a rhinoplasty had provided a solution to her dilemma. Should the operation fail to fulfill her hopes, he could be a convenient scapegoat. Considering the psychological hazard involved, it was decided not to operate.

CONFLICTING CONCEPTS OF "SUCCESS"

Another source of problems in cosmetic surgery is the dichotomy between the surgeon's concept of a satisfactory result and the patient's expectations. Since the surgeon's training is necessarily concerned with reconstruction or correction that approximates in form and contour the anatomic "ideal," he assumes that the patient has the same objective. That there are cultural variations in concepts of the "ideal" may be forgotten. Confident in his judgment of what can and should be done, the surgeon is dismayed and puzzled when a patient views technically successful results as disappointing.

Arbitrary ascription of physicians' standards in the controversial area of cosmetic surgery, where patients' responses are so often the criteria for "success," is to invite complications, as shown in the following case:

Tired of being called "Ski Snoot" and teased about her "Bob Hope" nose, 29 year old N. H. requested correction of its retroussé tip. The surgeon achieved what he considered an excellent result, but N. H. first wept hysterically, then became depressed. Though the modified tip pleased her, she had not expected the elimination of a slight dorsal concavity. To her this was a calamity because she was Irish and extremely proud of her heritage. Equating Irishness with a turned-up nose, she had tacitly valued the dorsal curvature. The surgeon's perception and creation of the "best" esthetic effect—in this instance a straight dorsum—destroyed what the patient prized—her Irish identity.

Preoperative consensus could forestall such deleterious outcomes. Of central importance to satisfactory results as well as to doctor-patient relationships is a clear understanding of the patient's perception of his defect, what it means to him, and what he expects surgery to achieve esthetically and subjectively. The surgeon should insist on as much specificity as possible from patients about what they want or don't want done and why, and in turn explain as definitively as he can what alterations he has in mind.

RELIANCE ON OTHER PROFESSIONALS

Because of the exigencies of treatment, it is important for plastic surgeons to have other professionals on whom they can rely in making judgments in the patients' best interests. Most medical centers have psychiatrists, clinical psychologists, and psychiatric social workers available for referral and consultation, and it has become customary to turn to these specialists when questions arise regarding psychological diagnosis and management. They are also the ones most often included as participants in rehabilitation and research programs. Their use of such methods as interviews, psychological tests and projective techniques often provides useful adjunctive information and insights in the team approach to comprehensive care.

In depending on these disciplines for psychosocial evaluations solutions to behavioral problems, the plastic surgeon should also be cognizant of certain limitations. The traditional training of psychiatrists, psychologists and social workers is rooted in Freudian theory and individual psychology, and as such has focused on personality development, the unconscious and the intrapsychic processes of persons who manifest some form of psychopathology or behavior considered abnormal. This orientation, aimed at understanding the individual, is concerned primarily with such idiosyncratic features as his emotional life, personality structure, primary sexual identification and the like. Interpretations of behavior considered deviant (which implies the existence of norms) tend to be couched in negative terms: repression, guilt, hostility, fixation, neurosis, and so on. Such interpretations fail to consider the person in the context of his social, cultural and religious background, the influence of the social world in which he lives, and the impact of these factors on his attitudes and behavior.

Today the narrowness and shortcomings of the individual psychological approach to behavior are recognized, and there is increasing attention to broader perspectives that include those of sociology and anthropology. According to the noted psychiatrist Jurgen Reusch (1966), emphasis must "shift away from man as an isolated entity and towards consideration of man in his environment." His social needs must be considered, and his interdependence

with his environment—including interaction with his surroundings. In similar vein, Murphy (1968) states: "The conception of personality as a self-contained . . . whole . . . goes badly with the world of reality."

For the person with cosmetic defects, his "world of reality" has unique import and must be taken into account. A facial flaw in particular can have profound consequences for his personal adjustment and social interaction. Frequently his problems are sociogenic rather than psychogenic. Referral to the psychiatrically oriented consultant, therefore, for diagnosis and solution of patients' problems is not always the answer. The following are two cases in point:

C. A., a young mother of three children, had incurred a slight facial scar in a car accident. In view of her low socioeconomic level and her established role as a housewife, her intense anxiety about her appearance seemed to the surgeons disproportionate and symptomatic of emotional disturbance. It was suggested that she needed a psychiatrist more than she did cosmetic surgery. C. A. happened to be Puerto Rican, and interviewing by a social science researcher revealed that indeed she had reason to be disturbed. In her sociocultural milieu, a scar on a woman's face is a sign that one has been branded for unfaithfulness. She was distressed more for her husband, whom she loved, than she was about herself, since his acquaintances were assuming he had slashed her cheek because she had committed adultery. The stigma which Puerto Ricans attach to such scars was the sole reason both for her visit to the clinic and for what the surgeons had perceived as an "over-reaction." Fortunately in this instance a serious diagnostic mistake was averted.

Sarah was a 14 year old girl whose lack of psychological readiness for surgery was the subject of a clinic conference. The surgeon suggested that the excessive anxiety of the mother was a factor in the child's resistance to a minor operation. The psychiatrist who had been called in to see Sarah declared that in his opinion the mother was not so much anxious as outright hostile toward her daughter. What kind of mother was it, he asked, who would slap her child's face on learning that the child's menses had begun? This fact he had learned from Sarah herself while questioning her about the menarche. For him this was substantial and sufficient evidence of the mother's hostility, even cruelty. What he had failed to take into consideration, or to explore, was the possibility that there might be some other explanation for the mother's behavior.

Both Sarah and her mother were Orthodox Jews from Eastern Europe, among whom it is the custom for the mother to slap her daughter's face at the time of the menarche "to bring the roses to the cheeks," or to bring good luck. By assessing behavior in terms of his own cultural standards of what is normal or abnormal, the psychiatrist was led to a false interpretation. The mother's behavior in this situation was not aberrant. Because it was a custom of their culture, it had no deeper psychological implication for the child than the ritualistic and facetious spanking an American child is given on his birthday (Macgregor, 1960).

In using the services of other professionals, plastic surgeons should have a knowledge of and weigh the special orientations and biases of such professionals. Indiscriminate and unquestioning reliance on any single discipline for interpretations of behavior can result in judgmental errors. On the other hand, appreciation of the training, value orientation, role and function of each specialist enables the surgeon to make optimal use of all whom he may have occasion to consult.

Summary

While social acceptance of cosmetic surgery and growing demands for it have proved eminently beneficial for patient and surgeon alike, they have also highlighted potential psychological pitfalls. Selection of a candidate requires assessment of his physical defect in the context of his emotional state, sociocultural background, motives and expectations. Persons with apparently "minor" deformities may pose special problems and should be carefully screened. Vital too is the surgeon's awareness of his own personal biases, and his examination of his criteria and motivations for accepting or rejecting patients. Though mutual satisfaction cannot be guaranteed, preoperative consensus based on understanding what the patient perceives and wants, and what the surgeon can recommend as technically feasible, helps to minimize possibly conflicting concepts of "success."

Knowledge of the orientations and limitations of other professionals can enable the plastic surgeon to use their services judiciously in making psychosocial evaluations and managing behavioral problems. Traditional reliance on disciplines that stress Freudian theory and individual psychology needs to be augmented by broader perspectives, including those of sociology and anthropology.

REFERENCES

Jacobson, W. E., Edgerton, M. T., Meyer, E., Canter, A., and Slaughter, R.: Psychiatric evaluation of male patients seeking cosmetic surgery. Plast. Reconstr. Surg. 26:356–372, 1960.

Knorr, N. J., Hoopes, J. E., and Edgerton, M. T.: Psychiatric-surgical approach to adolescent disturbance in self image. Plast. Reconstr. Surg. 41:248–253, 1968.

Linn, L., and Goldman, I. B.: Psychiatric observations concerning rhinoplasty. Psychosomat. Med. 11:307–314, 1949.

Macgregor, F. C.: Social and cultural components in the motivations of persons seeking plastic surgery of the nose. J. Health Soc. Behav. 8:125–135, 1967.

Macgregor, F. C.: Social Science in Nursing: Applications for the Improvement of Patient Care. New York, Russell Sage Foundation, 1960.

Macgregor, F. C., Abel, T. M., Bryt, A., Lauer, E., and Weissmann, S.: Facial Deformities and Plastic Surgery: A Psychosocial Study. Springfield, Ill., Charles C Thomas, 1953.

Macgregor, F. C., and Schaffner, B.: Screening patients for nasal plastic operations: Some sociologic and psychiatric considerations. Psychosomat. Med. 12:277–291, 1950.

Meyer, E.: Psychiatric aspects of plastic surgery. In Converse, J. M. (ed.): Reconstructive Plastic Surgery. Philadelphia, W. B. Saunders Company, 1964, Vol. 1, pp. 365–383.

Meyer, E., Jacobson, W. E., Edgerton, M. T., and Canter, A.: Motivational patterns in patients seeking elective plastic surgery. I. Women who seek rhinoplasty. Psychosomat. Med. 22:193–201, 1960.

Murphy, G.: cited in Norbeck, E., Price-Williams, D., and McCord, W. M. (eds.): The Study of Personality: An Interdisciplinary Appraisal. New York, Holt, Rinehart and Winston, 1968.

Ruesch, J.: The future of psychologically oriented psychiatry. In Masserman, J. H. (ed.): Sexuality of Women. New York, Grune & Stratton, 1966, pp. 144–163.

Chapter 4

HYPNOSIS, ANALGESIA, AMNESIA, ANESTHESIA

SEAMUS LYNCH, M.D.

Be gentle with me, . . .
Treat me tenderly,
I need the gentle touch,

. . . .

They've been so many who didn't understand

. . . .

but give it gently.
   Please.

             ROD MCKUEN, TWO
             Listen to the Warm

      Gentleness is an art when inducing and sustaining a pain-free unconscious state. The administration of an anesthetic is the application of a measured physiologic insult to a patient, administered, however, under precise pharmacologic control. Unnecessary fluctuations of blood pressure and pulse, irregularity of respiratory depth and rate, bucking and coughing (on the endotracheal tube), increased bleeding in the wound, straining and movement during application of the surgical dressing, bulky and obtrusive endotracheal equipment are all signs of the crude, casual and careless approach to anesthesia so frequently encountered in the operating room. Problems that are considered of little consequence in general surgery are of major importance to the patient undergoing cosmetic surgery, probably because postoperative pain is minimal, particularly in an operation such as facial or eyelid plasty. The loss of a capped incisor or a broken bridge, the ecchymoses produced by an intravenous needle poorly placed in the dorsum of the hand or hours of retching and vomiting can only tarnish the image of both the surgeon and the anesthesiologist. Such problems can be virtually eliminated by a gentle, knowledgeable and sympathetic approach to anesthesia, particularly by the application of the concept of the esthetic anesthetic.

Preoperative Evaluation

      It is essential that the anesthesiologist visit and examine the patient undergoing cosmetic plastic surgery on the day before the operation. The purpose of this visit is to gain the confidence of the patient and to relieve any fears and anxieties. The choice of premedication and the anesthetic agents is made at this time. Halothane certainly will not be administered to the patient with a history of jaundice, just as methoxyflurane (Penthrane) would not be considered for the patient with a history of chronic kidney disease. Because of the increased risk involved, elective surgery should not be attempted following a myocardial infarction unless a minimum of six months has passed since the cardiac injury. The patient who is accustomed to a daily alcohol intake, who uses tranquilizers, or who routinely takes sedatives for insomnia will require heavier premedication and, most likely, higher concentrations of anesthetic agents to produce a satisfactory anesthetic state. A detailed oral examination is mandatory because of the many delicate dental restorations so commonly observed today. Most potential errors in the management of anesthesia can be avoided by careful preoperative evaluation and planning.

Premedication

The patient who has been properly premedicated arrives in the operating room in a drowsy, amnesic and cooperative state, with no circulatory or respiratory depression. This optimum condition usually is achieved by a combination of drugs; because of its pharmacologic activity, each drug plays an important role in the final result. Drugs used for premedication include barbiturates, belladonna alkaloids, tranquilizers and narcotics.

BARBITURATES. A short-acting barbiturate such as secobarbital (Seconal) or Pentobarbital (Nembutal), 50 to 100 mg., is an ideal hypnotic agent. It is given orally 90 minutes prior to the induction of anesthesia.

NARCOTICS. Morphine sulfate, 8 to 10 mg., and meperidine (Demerol), 50 to 100 mg., are the commonly used narcotics. They enhance the sedative effect of the barbiturate and, because of their analgesic action, reduce the amount of anesthetic agent necessary during the operative procedure.

BELLADONNA ALKALOIDS. Atropine sulfate and scopolamine hydrobromide, 0.4 to 0.6 mg., are important in proper preoperative medication. Their primary value is in drying secretions in the airway. They also diminish the reflex activity of the pharynx, the larynx and the heart. Because it is an excellent drying agent and has an important specific amnesic effect on the patient, scopolamine is preferred. Atropine sulfate, however, effects greater control on the reflex activity of the myocardium. The narcotic and belladonna drugs are miscible and are administered by subcutaneous injection one hour prior to surgery.

TRANQUILIZERS. The addition of a phenothiazine such as prochlorperazine (Compazine), 10 to 20 mg., or perphenazine (Trilafon), 5 to 10 mg., enhances the hypnotic effects of the barbiturates and the narcotics without producing significant hypotension. As shown by Bellville, Bross and Howland (1960), their particular value is in their potent antiemetic properties, since reduction in postoperative nausea and vomiting is best for both patient and surgeon. The patient has a smooth and pleasant emergence from the anesthetic, and the surgeon need not contend with vomitus-soaked dressings.

Valium. Valium is a benzodiazepine derivative. It is an excellent tranquilizer in a 10- to 20-mg. dose injected intramuscularly. It is also a useful adjunct for the relief of skeletal muscle spasm. The patient under Valium is relaxed and calm and has a significant degree of amnesia. Its main drawback is that there is a small incidence of phlebitis.

Innovar. Innovar is the combination, in a 50:1 ratio, of a tranquilizer and a short-acting narcotic analgesic. Droperidol (Inapsine) is the tranquilizer and neuroleptic agent and sublimaze (Fentanyl) the narcotic. Each cubic centimeter contains Fentanyl 0.05 mg. and Inapsine 2.5 mg. Innovar can be used intramuscularly as premedication or intravenously during surgery to produce the state of neuroleptanalgesia (Fox and Fox, 1966). The neuroleptic state is characterized by (1) mental withdrawal; (2) hypomotility, a disinclination to move; (3) homeostatic stabilization by blockade of the adrenergic receptors; and (4) potent antiemesis.

PENTAZOCINE (TALWIN). Talwin is a potent analgesic. Talwin, 30 mg., is usually equivalent in effect to morphine, 10 mg., or meperidine, 75 to 100 mg. Analgesia occurs within 15 to 20 minutes after intramuscular injection and should last three hours. The usual narcotic antagonists, such as nalorphine, are not effective to reverse the respiratory depression caused by Talwin. Although it is not under narcotic control, dependency can occur.

PROPRANOLOL (INDERAL). Propranolol is a β-adrenergic blocking agent which is used in the treatment of various supraventricular cardiac arrhythmias such as atrial fibrillation, flutter and paroxysmal tachycardia, since it prolongs the A-V nodal refractory period. Inderal is of interest to the anesthesiologist because of its use for the aftercare of the patient who has had a myocardial infarction and for those patients with angina pectoris, since propranolol blocks the catecholamine ability to increase myocardial work and oxygen consumption. Propranolol causes a depression of A-V conduction and direct myocardial depression, so caution is warranted when anesthetizing patients who are being treated with this drug. Propranolol is dispensed as 10- to 40-mg. tablets. The daily maintenance dose is 20 to 80 mg. It is available also in ampule form for intravenous use, 1 mg. per cc. The dose here is 0.5 cc. to a maximum of 4 cc.

Principles of Safe Local Analgesia

The safe administration of local analgesia depends upon the following factors: (1) reasonable premedication; (2) the application or injection of the proper dose and concentration of the selected agent; (3) avoidance of intravenous injections of solutions; (4) use of vasoconstrictor drugs; and (5) being prepared at all times to treat adverse reactions.

REASONABLE PREMEDICATION

The desire to have the patient unaware of the discomfort of the surgical procedure during local anesthesia leads the surgeon to attempt to produce the state of general anesthesia by ordering heavy premedication. The induction of varying degrees of stupor and coma is unwise and unsafe and is best left in the hands of the anesthesiologist, who has the knowledge to sustain and, indeed, to resuscitate a patient so deeply anesthetized. Premedication is designed merely to produce a state of calm relaxation while unusual or uncomfortable situations occur. The patient should sustain all vital functions, including responsiveness.

Snoring is a sign of respiratory obstruction and, therefore, of hypoxia and hypocarbia. It is much safer to undermedicate than to risk the complications of iatrogenic coma. A barbiturate, Seconal or Nembutal, 100 mg., given orally 90 minutes before surgery, and Demerol, 50 to 100 mg., with Valium, 10 mg., or Compazine, 10 mg., intramuscularly, one hour preoperatively, should be more than adequate for most patients. If on arrival in the operating room the patient should still be apprehensive, it is quite easy to control the nervousness by starting an intravenous infusion and adding small amounts of narcotic or tranquilizer as required. Intermittent intravenous injections of 10 to 25 mg. of meperidine and 5 to 10 mg. of Valium should control any restless patient. The surgeon must remember that it is almost impossible to predetermine the exact amount of premedication that will produce the desired effect on each patient. Continuous titration of small doses intravenously will invariably produce the required precise degree of control.

DOSE CONCENTRATION

Exceeding the toxic dose of an agent is a common error. All anesthetic agents have well established maximum dose levels, as indicated in Table. 1

INADVERTENT INTRAVENOUS INJECTION

When a drug is injected intravenously, a high blood level results and may lead to cardiovascular and respiratory collapse. It behooves the surgeon, when injecting local anesthetic solutions, to aspirate—that is, to pull back on

TABLE 1

Drug	Maximum dose	Topical	Infiltration
Procaine (Novocaine)	1 gm.	Has no topical action	200 cc. of 0.5% = 1 gm. 100 cc. of 1% = 1 gm. 50 cc. of 2% = 1 gm.
Lidocaine (Xylocaine)	0.5 gm.	10 cc. of 2% = 200 mg. 5 cc. of 4% = 200 mg.	100 cc. of 0.5% = 0.5 gm. 50 cc. of 1% = 0.5 gm. 25 cc. of 2% = 0.5 gm.
Hexylcaine (Cyclaine)	0.5 gm.	10 cc. of 5% = 0.5 gm.	100 cc. of 0.5% = 0.5 gm. 50 cc. of 1% = 0.5 gm. 25 cc. of 2% = 0.5 gm.
Cocaine	20 mg.	4 cc. of 5% = 20 mg. 2 cc. of 10% = 20 mg.	Not used as it is too toxic
Tetracaine (Pontocaine)	200 mg.	4 cc. of 2% = 80 mg. 8 cc. of 1% = 80 mg.	80 cc. of 0.25% = 200 mg.

TABLE 2

ANESTHETIC VOLUME	EPINEPHRINE (1:1000 SOLUTION)	DILUTION	RECOMMENDED FOR:
100 cc.	2 cc.	1:50,000	Rhinoplasty
100 cc.	1 cc.	1:100,000	Blepharoplasty
100 cc.	0.5 cc.	1:200,000	Facial plasty (large volumes of solution are required)

the plunger—before injecting the local anesthetic, unless the needle is moving; and secondly, when injecting in a known vascular area, to reduce both the volume and the concentration of the drug.

USE OF VASOCONSTRICTOR AGENTS

These agents, by causing local vasoconstriction (chemical tourniquet effect), reduce the rate of absorption of the local anesthetic agent and so reduce the incidence of adverse reactions. They also prolong the duration of the anesthetic. The dangers of these agents, particularly epinephrine (which is the best), is in the use of unnecessarily high concentrations. Solutions of 1:100,000 will produce the maximum degree of vasoconstriction. Stronger solutions will not increase the vasoconstrictor effect and will only invite the complications of adrenaline intoxication, which are nervousness, cold sweats, hypertension and tachycardia, and severe arrhythmias. Errors in the preparation of local analgesic agents containing epinephrine should be avoided. Table 2 outlines the proper concentrations.

ADVERSE REACTIONS

Toxic effects of local agents are usually due to high blood levels of the anesthetic agents. There are many classifications available (Bonica, 1953; Moore, 1957). It is important that the surgeon recognize the seriousness of the situation at the earliest possible moment. If a patient who has been loquacious or restless suddenly settles down and becomes quiet, the surgeon should immediately examine the patient and check his respiration, pulse and blood pressure, since tachycardia, tachypnea and hypotension are the adverse signs most frequently encountered. A patient under local anesthesia should never be left unattended; means of

monitoring the patient's vital signs must be available. Such essential monitoring can be done by trained technicians or by electronic devices, many of which are available on the market.

The treatment of adverse reactions is symptomatic. Reactions to toxicity exhibit themselves by symptoms referable to the central nervous system, the respiratory system and the cardiovascular system. Actually these symptoms of toxicity are exhibited by muscular twitching, tremors and convulsions, hypopnea or apnea, and severe hypotension, and are the result of the depressing effects that local anesthetic agents have on the medulla and the myocardium, and to their dilatation effects on the vasculature. Treatment is urgent but symptomatic. Oxygen should be given immediately. Should convulsions occur, a small dose of an intravenous barbiturate (Sodium Nembutal, 1 or 2 cc.) is administered. If apnea occurs, artificial respiration by positive pressure on the rebreathing bag and endotracheal intubation are necessary. Circulatory depression, as indicated by hypotension and a weak pulse, requires an intravenous or intramuscular injection of a vasopressor such as ephedrine hydrochloride, 50 mg. Cardiac arrest should be treated by current methods.

Anesthetic Agents

THIOPENTAL SODIUM

Thiopental sodium (Pentothal) is a very versatile agent for use in plastic surgery, with few contraindications to its use. Contrary to popular belief, it is not a true anesthetic. Although it belongs to the barbiturate family of drugs, thiopental sodium has no analgesic effect within its clinical range. When combined with a low-potency, nonflammable agent such as nitrous oxide, it can produce excellent anesthesia for a wide range of plastic cosmetic surgical procedures. Such a combination allows the free use of electrocoagulation. Neither Pentothal nor nitrous oxide sensitizes the heart to the arrhythmic effects of epinephrine; indeed, Pentothal affords protection against such effects. It is apparent that this combination of agents allows the surgeon wide latitude in surgical technique and provides the patient with a safe and smooth anesthetic.

CYCLOPROPANE

Cyclopropane is of little value in plastic cosmetic surgery. It is highly flammable, and the use of epinephrine is contraindicated during its administration because of the frequent occurrence of severe ventricular arrhythmias. McLoughlin (1954) demonstrated that cyclopropane increases the the amount of bleeding in the wound. Its use should be reserved for the patient in shock from hemorrhage; then, cyclopropane is the agent of choice.

HALOTHANE

Halothane is the most valuable anesthetic agent available today. It is nonflammable, allowing free use of electrocoagulation. It obtunds the pharyngeal, laryngeal and tracheal reflexes in light planes of anesthesia, so that coughing and straining are rarely encountered. Currently there is a difference of opinion as to whether epinephrine can be used safely during the administration of halothane (Katz et al., 1962). We employ halothane freely for the maintenance of anesthesia, without restricting the concomitant use of epinephrine. However, the concentration of epinephrine should not exceed 1:100,000. Significant cardiac irregularities have not occurred in our series. The ability of halothane to produce hypotension is a significant asset to the working conditions of the plastic cosmetic surgeon.

SODIUM METHOHEXITAL

Sodium methohexital (Brevital) is a rapid, ultra short-acting barbiturate. It differs chemically from the established barbiturate anesthetics in that it contains no sulfur. It is used in a 1 per cent solution. The usual induction dose of 5 to 12 cc. (50 to 100 mg.) produces anesthesia for five to seven minutes.

METHOXYFLURANE

Methoxyflurane (Penthrane) is a halogenated ethyl methyl ether which is nonflammable and nonexplosive. It is a valuable agent but its odor is usually considered unpleasant by the operating room personnel. Induction is much slower than with halothane. Because of the occasional occurrence of high-output kidney failure (Crandell et al., 1966), it should not be used for operations on the elderly or when prolonged surgery is anticipated.

SUCCINYLCHOLINE CHLORIDE

Succinylcholine chloride is a short-acting muscle relaxant whose primary value is to relax the patient's jaw, pharynx and larynx to facilitate atraumatic intubation of the trachea. Since its action is not selective for those muscles, the patient is totally paralyzed for the duration of its effect. Prior to intubation, and immediately following, therefore, the anesthesiologist must breathe artificially for the patient until spontaneous respirations return, usually after a period of five to ten minutes.

KETAMINE HYDROCHLORIDE

Ketamine hydrochloride is an intravenous or intramuscular anesthetic which produces a profound dissociated sleep. Muscle tone of the tongue and pharyngeal muscles remains as in the awake state, and the respiration is not depressed, so that the endotracheal tube and controlled respiration are rarely needed. It would seem to be the ideal anesthetic for cosmetic surgery. Unfortunately blood pressure and pulse rates are elevated with ketamine and there is increased bleeding in the wound. Its main drawback is its high incidence of delirium, nightmares, delusions and schizoid reactions during the awakening period. It seems to distort the perception of time. Such bad trips may last only a few seconds, but to the patient it seems to go on for hours. This "nightmare" anesthetic has no place in cosmetic surgery.

Attention to Detail
AIRWAY MANAGEMENT

By its very nature, any surgical procedure on the head or neck usually demands the use of an endotracheal tube. It provides a free and unobstructed airway, even in the presence of blood in the pharynx, and enables the anesthesiologist to be at a considerable distance from the surgical site. If resuscitation should be necessary during the course of surgery, it can be instituted immediately, thereby avoiding dangerous delays while efforts at intubation are attempted under conditions other than ideal. In expert hands, complications from the use of an endotracheal tube are rare and of minor significance. The simple technique of oral intubation is performed quickly and atraumatically while the patient is totally relaxed by succinylcholine. It is important to use an adequate dose of this drug (60 to 100 mg.). A smaller dose will not produce complete relaxation, and pressure from the laryngoscope blade can damage the incisors or produce tears of the soft tissue in the hypopharynx. Its duration of action is directly related to the dose level, and recovery from a small dose is quite rapid. Such quick return of muscle activity following intubation does not allow sufficient time for the topical anesthetic agent to attain its peak effect and results in coughing and straining with the endotracheal tube in place. At the end of the operation, the tube must not be removed from the trachea while the patient is in a light plane of anesthesia, as this causes coughing and bucking. It is much better practice to maintain the level of anesthesia that was obtained during the operative procedure until the dressing has been applied and the surgeon is ready to leave the operating room. At this time the tube is removed rapidly during the expiratory phase of the respiratory cycle. This technique will almost always avoid coughing and bucking on the tube.

REDUCTION IN BULK OF EQUIPMENT

The presence of large, bulky equipment which encroaches on the operative field is a most annoying problem to the cosmetic plastic surgeon. To keep bulk at a minimum, we prefer the use of a soft rubber Magill endotracheal tube with a curved metal adapter at its proximal end. The tube is cut to exact length so that following insertion only this metal piece, resting on the patient's lower lip, is visible. The metal piece, in turn, is attached to a small cylindrical malleable connecting piece, and then to hoses leading to the machine. These hoses are extra long, allowing the anesthesiologist to sit below the level of the knee, in the case of oral intubation. Thus, there is no equipment in the way,

and the whole field is open to the surgeon. A minimal number of short adhesive strips may be used to secure the tube. If distortion of the face is a problem, adhesive strips are not used, since distortion is virtually eliminated when the tube lies freely. If the operation requires the tube to be moved from side to side, as in the case of full-face dermabrasion, it can easily be moved by the surgeon.

CARBON DIOXIDE RETENTION

Depressed respiration produces an elevated blood carbon dioxide level. Because of its vasodilating effect, this in turn increases the amount of oozing in the surgical field. The cosmetic plastic surgeon wants a bloodless field, if possible, as bleeding under a flap or graft prolongs the patient's convalescence. It is therefore most important that the patient's ventilation be augmented at all times by the technique of assisted or controlled respiration.

AIRWAY OBSTRUCTION

The fact that the patient has been intubated successfully does not guarantee that the airway will remain patent for the duration of the anesthesia. Under certain conditions the tube may become kinked by hyperextension or hyperflexion of the neck, or the lumen may be partially or completely occluded by a blood clot or inspissated mucus within or by the pressure of retractors or pharyngeal packs from without. When total obstruction occurs, it is readily diagnosed because breathing ceases; obstruction is easily and quickly remedied.

Unfortunately when the obstruction is not complete and a partial airway remains, only the alert anesthesiologist will be aware of the situation and take the steps necessary to relieve the obstruction. Partial obstruction can be recognized by the "rocking-boat" action of the patient's abdomen and chest, similar to that of asthmatic breathing. When such partial obstruction is uncorrected, the patient must exert considerable effort to overcome the resistance to breathing, and this results in annoying oozing of blood in the surgical field. This increased bleeding results from the elevation of the venous and the arterial blood pressures and the increase of carbon dioxide in the blood. If the surgeon notices any sudden change in the amount of bleeding in the wound, he must immediately ask the anesthesiologist to inspect the airway. Also, any change in the breathing pattern of the patient warrants an immediate check of the system. A kinked tube or a malfunctioning valve may be the cause of the obstruction.

COUGHING

Coughing and straining with the endotracheal tube in place produce an elevation in the blood pressure and a rise in the peripheral venous pressure which undoubtedly increase the amount of bleeding. They can even cause a recurrence of bleeding in areas under hemostatic control. It is essential that the anesthesiologist institute adequate topical anesthesia. On the other hand, the surgeon should be aware that an otherwise smooth anesthesia can be marred by abrupt motions of the head and neck. These actions move the tube in the trachea and invariably lead to coughing and straining by the patient. The surgeon must warn the anesthesiologist of his intentions so that the anesthesiologist can either deepen the level of anesthesia or administer small amounts of short-acting muscle relaxant, after which the move can be made with no fear of causing annoying disturbances.

PREMATURE RECOVERY

In cosmetic surgery, premature recovery of the patient is undesirable. The patient must not be allowed to awaken until the procedure is completely finished and the dressings have been applied. The anesthesiologist must realize that the application of the dressing is of great importance to the success of the surgical procedure. It is impossible to apply a dressing properly if the patient is coughing, vomiting or resisting vigorously. It must be remembered that this straining may cause bleeding under a skin graft or flap. To maintain a quiescent patient until the end of the procedure, either an adequate depth of anesthesia must be maintained to the completion of the dressing or a small amount of succinylcholine must be administered.

RECOVERY PERIOD

In the recovery room the patient is closely watched by the anesthesia and the recovery room staffs for signs of airway impairment, particularly if pressure dressings on the face and neck compromise the airway. If there are signs of delirious emergence from the anes-

thesia, it may be controlled by the intravenous injection of a mixture containing Demerol, 10 mg., and Trilafon, 1 mg., in each cubic centimeter. One cubic centimeter of solution is given every five minutes until the desired effect is realized. If the restlessness is obviously not due to pain, Valium in 5- to 10-mg. doses intramuscularly is also an excellent agent to tranquilize the patient. This allows a quiet, relaxed awakening which is greatly appreciated by the surgeon, the patient and the nursing staff.

Often the surgeon has the idea that tight dressings will stop the bleeding. Heavy packs and tight dressings may cause soft tissue obstruction of the pharynx and so actually interfere with the patient's breathing. Once the endotracheal tube is removed, the anesthesiologist should be prepared to cut away the dressings if there should be any indication of impaired breathing.

Induced Hypotension

The desire of the plastic surgeon for a bloodless field in which to operate is as old as the specialty itself. Throughout the years great effort has been expended in order to produce a dry, bloodless field in the anesthetized patient. The most dramatic approach is the application of induced hypotension to general anesthesia as fostered by Enderby (1958) in England.

Hypotension is induced by drugs that cause generalized peripheral vasodilation. Combined with posture, such as the head-up position for operations on the head and neck, hypotension allows pooling of blood in the dependent areas away from the surgical site. The venous return to the heart is reduced and the cardiac output falls, vastly reducing the amount of bleeding in the surgical wound. Such vasodilation is produced by drugs that block the automatic ganglia. Those commonly used are hexamethonium (Vegolysen), pentolinium tartrate (Ansolysen), trimethaphan camphorsulfonate (Arfonad), and homatropinium (Trophenium).

An important part of the technique advocated by Enderby is controlled respiration. Positive pressure applied to the airway by intermittent manual pressure on the rebreathing bag can, by raising the intrapleural pressure, further reduce the venous return to the right heart. This has a very marked hypotensive effect when used in combination with the ganglion-blocking agents.

HALOTHANE AND HYPOTENSION

Halothane produces hypotension by causing generalized peripheral vasodilation and by reducing the cardiac output. This action of halothane is probably due to a diminished sympatho-adrenal response as the norepinephrine effect on the myocardium is reduced (Severinghaus and Cullen, 1958; Enderby, 1960; Black and McArdle, 1962). We have applied this property of halothane clinically in a series of 750 patients undergoing plastic surgery when induced hypotension was deemed desirable.

The patient is premedicated in the usual manner and induced with thiopental. Following intubation, the patient is placed in a 20- to 30-degree head-up tilt, and administration of halothane in oxygen in a semiclosed system is begun. A sufficiently high concentration is administered to reduce the blood pressure to the desired level. This concentration may vary from 1 to 3 per cent, depending upon the individual response of the patient. At this time the surgeon infiltrates the surgical field with a mixture containing procaine, 0.5 per cent, and epinephrine 1:200,000. The purpose of this infiltration is twofold: (1) In light planes of general anesthesia, surgical stimuli tend to elevate the blood pressure. Procaine, by blocking these stimuli, allows a significantly lower concentration of halothane to be used in attaining the desired level of hypotension. (2) The epinephrine by its local vasoconstrictor effects eliminates the need for profound hypotension, that is, below 60 mm. Hg. It must be stressed that higher concentrations of epinephrine are unnecessary and dangerous. There were no serious arrhythmias from the described mixture in our series. However, in four patients in whom 1:35,000 epinephrine was inadvertently used, hypertension, tachycardia, multiple ventricular extrasystoles and ventricular tachycardia were noted.

Following surgical incision, an evaluation of the bleeding in the wound is made and the blood pressure is lowered by increasing the inhaled concentration of halothane to achieve the minimal reduction compatible with the control of bleeding. Systolic levels of 60 to 70 mm. Hg are easily maintained and give a satisfactory bloodless field in the majority of cases. It has been noted, however, that in corrective nasal plastic operations and in scalp and forehead flap procedures a more profound hypotension is necessary to control bleeding. In such cases the systolic blood pressure is reduced below 60 mm. Hg.

In 15 per cent of our patients, halothane used alone does not lower the blood pressure sufficiently. Rather than incorporate the use of controlled respiration, a small amount of Arfonad (50 to 100 mg.) is administered by infusion. This rapidly produces the required blood pressure level. Because halothane potentiates the action of the ganglion-blocking agents, very small amounts of Arfonad are needed in its presence (Enderby, 1960).

When the surgical procedure is completed, the level of anesthesia and hypotension is maintained until after the dressings have been applied. The patient is transported to the recovery room and retained there in the same degree of head-up tilt as in the operating room. Oxygen is administered by oral or nasal catheter until the patient has reacted fully. The blood level of halothane is reduced rapidly as soon as the administration of this agent is stopped, and the blood pressure gradually returns to normal within one hour. It has not been found necessary to restore the blood pressure by the use of vasopressors.

This technique has been administered to patients varying in age from 16 to 83 years. There has been no complication associated with hypotension, and there were no deaths.

On the other hand, it is such an exacting and demanding technique with so little margin for error that it cannot be recommended for general use. In expert hands this technique can be applied safely with no significant increase of risk to the patient (Enderby, 1961; Linacre, 1961).

Special Techniques

RHINOPLASTY

Injections in and around the nose are the major fear of the patient undergoing rhinoplasty. This discomfort can be eliminated by a very simple technique which satisfies both the patient and the surgeon in that it produces the conditions that each desires. Such a patient welcomes the opportunity to be unconscious during that short critical period during which the surgeon establishes the local anesthesia of the nose, as there is complete avoidance of the fears and apprehensions of discomfort that the patient associates with these injections.

Methohexitone (Brevital), the ultra short-acting oxybarbiturate, is ideally suited to induce such a short period of sleep. The surgeon packs the nasal passages and inserts the pledgets of

41

topical anesthetic and vasoconstrictor and then retires to scrub. During this interval, the anesthesiologist injects a solution of 1 per cent Brevital in 1-cc. increments, to a total of 4 to 6 cc., the end point being reached when the patient can no longer communicate with the anesthesiologist. The patient sleeps while the surgeon establishes the local anesthetic. During this period, there may be some motions or phonations on the part of the patient, but there is never any recollection of the injection. Once the local anesthetic is established, no additional Brevital is given. Within three to five minutes the patient can respond to questions, and the procedure continues in the usual manner.

CHEMABRASION

Full-face chemabrasion is not tolerated well by the patient unless he is placed under very heavy narcosis, with an ensuing prolonged arousal time. Pentothal sodium seems to be ideally suited for this short operation. The patient is premedicated in the usual manner. On his arrival in the operating room, a dilute solution of thiopental, 0.4 per cent, is administered by continuous intravenous infusion. As soon as the eyelid reflex is obtunded, chemabrasion is begun. Very fine control of the depth of anesthesia is maintained, so that the patient is awake following the application of the adhesive strips. A recovery room stay is rarely necessary.

NEUROLEPTANALGESIA

Neuroleptanalgesia is a euphemistic term that describes the condition of induced narcosis which produces profound analgesia and psychomotor sedation, while allegedly leaving the cortical and cardiovascular functions intact. The principal application of neuroleptanalgesia in cosmetic surgery is as a supplement to local anesthesia. Although the combination of any narcotic and tranquilizer may produce the condition of neuroleptanalgesia, the drug Innovar has become almost synonymous with this state of induced psychic indifference. It is of interest that when Innovar is properly administered, the patient can cooperate and respond to questions, yet when not stimulated by conversation, the neuroleptic state of calm detachment returns. Operations such as blepharoplasty, facial plasty, and revision of scars lend themselves to this technique, since regional anesthesia is so readily established by the surgeon.

The patient is premedicated in the usual manner. On his arrival in the operating room an intravenous infusion is started and Innovar is injected in increments of 1 cc. through the infusion tubing until the patient is in the neuroleptic state. At this time should there be any signs of respiratory obstruction, a soft nasal airway is inserted and the head adjusted for optimum breathing. At this time, also, the surgeon administers the local anesthetic and operates. If the patient shows signs of awareness or movement, additional 1-cc. increments of Innovar are given. For example, in blepharoplasty, the tugging during extirpation of the herniated fat usually elicits a pain response. At this phase of the procedure the anesthesiologist should anticipate this pain response and should administer an additional 1 cc. of Innovar. It must be stressed that Innovar is composed of a potent narcotic and a tranquilizer and should be used only when the patient's vital signs are constantly monitored by an anesthesiologist who is prepared, at a moment's notice, to institute endotracheal intubation, controlled respiration and cardiovascular resuscitation.

Innovar can be used also for the establishment of the total anesthetic state should endotracheal intubation be required for the safe conduct of the operation. Here, the induction is by thiopental and succinylcholine, as previously described. The anesthesia is maintained with nitrous oxide by inhalation and with intermittent injections of Innovar in increments of 0.5 to 1.0 cc. This technique is of special value in the patient for whom halothane may be contraindicated, for example, a patient with a history of previous liver disease (Bunker et al., 1969). However, unlike anesthesia with halothane, it behooves the surgeon, if there be any need to move the patient's head, to alert the anesthesiologist to this fact, so that a deeper plane of anesthesia can be established before this movement is made. If this is not done, bucking will surely occur, resulting in increased bleeding in the wound. It should be stressed that with halothane the surgeon is virtually guaranteed that the patient will not cough or buck. Such a guarantee cannot be made with Innovar. This unnecessary complication is much more likely to occur when Innovar is the nucleus of the anesthetic technique. A very satisfactory alternative to Innovar is the supplementation of local analgesia with a combination of diazepam (Valium) and meperidine (Demerol). Valium, 10 mg., is injected intravenously as soon as the intravenous infusion is established. Demerol is then given to the patient in a solution containing 10 mg. per cc. The solution is injected intermittently in 1-cc. increments until the appropriate neuroleptic state is achieved.

POSTOPERATIVE HEMATOMA

It is unfortunate that, despite great care on the part of the surgeon to achieve hemostasis during the facial plastic operation, a small proportion of these patients must return to the operating room in the immediate postoperative period because of hematoma. This frequently requires removing most of the sutures to find the source of bleeding. It is not only difficult but indeed hazardous to attempt local anesthesia for this purpose. A more prudent course is to induce general anesthesia, thereby establishing a clear airway, eliminating the risk of toxic reaction to the local anesthetic agent because of the vascularity of the area and, lastly, allowing the surgeon to effect hemostasis in an orderly manner.

Epilogue

The physician who undertakes the administration of potent drugs in order to render a patient semiconscious or unconscious assumes a great responsibility which cannot be undertaken in a capricious manner. Such degrees of insensibility can be produced only by prescribing potent sedatives, hypnotics, tranquilizers and narcotics. The pharmacologic effects of these drugs on the patient can never be predicted accurately. It would seem prudent that the surgeon relieve himself of this unnecessary responsibility in order that he may direct his attention entirely to his surgical endeavors.

If you need a friend
I'm sailing right behind.
Like a bridge over troubled waters
I will ease your mind;
Like a bridge over troubled waters
I will ease your mind.

PAUL SIMON

REFERENCES

Bellville, J. W., Bross, D. D. J., and Howland, W. S.: Postoperative nausea and vomiting. Clin. Pharmacol. Ther. *1*:590, 1960.

Black, G. W., and McArdle, W.: Effects of halothane on the peripheral circulation in man. Brit. J. Anaesth. *34*: 2, 1962.

Bonica, J. J.: The Management of Pain. Philadelphia, Lea & Febiger, 1953.

Bunker, J. P., Forrest, W. H., Jr., Mosteller, F., and Vandam, L. D. (eds.): National Halothane Study: The study of the possible association between halothane anesthesia and postoperative hepatic necrosis. Bethesda, Md., National Institutes of Health and of General Medical Sciences, 1969.

Crandell, W. B., Pappas, S. G., and Macdonald, A.: Nephrotoxicity associated with methoxyflurane anesthesia. Anesthesiology *27*:591, 1966.

Enderby, G. E. H.: The advantages of controlled hypotension in surgery. Brit. Bull. *14*:1, 1958.

Enderby, G. E. H.: Halothane and hypotension. Anaesthesia *15*:25, 1960.

Enderby, G. E. H.: A report on the mortality and morbidity following 9,107 hypotensive anesthetics. Brit. J. Anaesth. *33*:109, 1961.

Fox, J. W. C., and Fox, E.: Neuroleptanalgesia: A review. N. Carolina Med. J. *27*:471, 1966.

Katz, R. M., Matteo, R. S., and Papper, E. M.: Injection of epinephrine during general anesthesia with halogenated hydrocarbons and by cyclopropane in man. Anesthesiology *23*:597, 1962.

Linacre, J. L.: Induced hypotension in gynecological surgery. Brit. J. Anaesth. *33*:45, 1961.

McLoughlin, G.: Bleeding from cut skin and subcutaneous tissue surfaces during cyclopropane anesthesia. Brit. J. Anaesth. *26*:84, 1954.

Moore, D. C.: Regional Block. Springfield, Ill., Charles C Thomas, 1957.

Severinghaus, J. W., and Cullen, S. C.: Depression of myocardium and body O_2 consumption with Fluothane in man. Anesthesiology *19*:165, 1958.

43

Chapter 5

BLEPHAROPLASTY

Thomas D. Rees, M.D.

"Doing the eyelids is like slip-covering a chair;
it makes the rest of the room look tired." — A patient

History

The beginnings of eyelid surgery go back to the 10th Century in Arabia. Even at that early date the surgeon Avicenne (980–1036) — and somewhat later, Ibn Roshd (1126–1198) — noted the effect of excess skin folds of the upper eyelids in impairing vision and thus, according to Sichel (1844), devised ways to excise them. Reports of such skin folds did not appear in the European literature until 1792 when Beer described them in his textbook published in Vienna. The first illustration of this eyelid deformity was not published until 25 years later, in a subsequent edition of Beer's text.

In 1818 Von Graefe first used the word "blepharoplasty" to describe reconstructive techniques used to repair deformities caused by excision of eyelid carcinoma. Apparently, however, he did not envision the potential of the procedure to similarly correct eyelid defects caused by heredity or the ravages of age.

During the early 1800's European surgeons began to develop many new and imaginative techniques of cosmetic and reconstructive surgery. The pages of the *Journal Universel et Hebdomadaire de Médecine et de Chirurgie Pratique et des Institutions Médicales* of the 1830's are filled with colorful descriptions of procedures devised by Serre, Morax, Roux, Goyrand and others for the repair of eyelids and adjoining facial structures. Although many of their methods have since proved to be more fancy than fact, this was, nonetheless, the dawn of the coming era of eyelid surgery.

Reports of excess skin folds of the eyelid were also published by Mackenzie (1830), Alibert (1832), Graft (1836), and Dupuytren (1839), who noted poetically as well as accurately: "on rencontre cette singulière maladie chez des jeunes filles d'une constitution lymphatique, ayant la peau blanche, les cheveux blonds et les formes empâtées." (One finds this curious disease in young girls of a lymphatic constitution, with a white skin, blond hair and thick features.) Apart from Graf and Dupuytren, these authors confined their interest to the upper eyelids only. All advised excision of the excess skin alone.

Sichel (1844) provided one of the first accurate descriptions of herniated orbital fat. He stated (in translation): "The lid is smooth and swollen, and presents a tumor that may be elastic on palpation. Most commonly, this tumor is circumscribed between the adherent part of the lid and its transverse fold. Often it hangs in front of the inferior aspect of the lid as a bulge or a little transverse bag. Its weight, more considerable than the one of a simple skin fold, makes movements of the lid more difficult. . . . It is a rare condition. . . . It is most often found in children."

In 1899 a description of a case of "fat hernia" of the upper lid was published by Schmidt-Rimpler, but this diagnosis was discounted in 1930 by Elschnig, who remarked that it was, in all probability, merely a lipoma.

In 1880 Hotz defined the difference between ptosis atonica and the excess skin folds caused by old age. He pointed out that in ptosis

44

atonica, the skin does not remain attached on top of the tarsus as it does in elderly people. Fuchs (1899) attributed this to the fact that the bands of fascia connecting the skin with the tendons of the levator and with the upper margin of the orbit were not sufficiently rigid. Thus, in ptosis atonica, the skin could not be properly drawn up when the lid was raised, but hung down in the form of a flabby pouch.

Three years earlier Fuchs had reported a case of recurrent swelling of the eyelids of four years' duration in a girl of 20. This had produced wrinkles and vasodilatation of the superficial veins of the skin with marked redness and atrophy, prolapse of the orbital fat, and ptosis of the skin above the tarsus and in front of the eye. He called this condition "blepharochalasis."

A certain amount of confusion still exists regarding the term "blepharochalasis." In recent years it has been increasingly used as a diagnostic term to describe almost any degree of excess skin or fat of the eyelids, when, classically, the diagnosis should be reserved for those patients—usually young and female—with advanced skin folds of the eyelids with the atrophic changes described previously, associated with recurrent bouts of swelling or edema. Panneton (1936 a and b) further limited the term to apply only to the most advanced stages of "baggy eyelids" of familial origin.

The familial nature of the disorder was emphasized by Panneton (1936 a and b) when he reported 51 cases in a family of 79 members. Based on this family study, he advanced the hypothesis that baggy eyelids were the first stage of an inherited deformity, the second stage of which corresponded to a mild ptosis atonica, and the third stage to blepharochalasis.

True blepharochalasis is apparently a rare entity, for in a review of the world literature, Panneton (1936 a) mentioned only 93 reported cases, and indicated that only 63 of these truly met his criteria for the disease. Not aware of the earlier reports of Graf (1836), Kreiker (1929), Elschnig (1930) and Stein (1930), Panneton described what he believed to be the first case of blepharochalasis of the lower eyelids published in the literature.

All the authors thus far mentioned advocated removal of excess skin and protruding fat only when it was markedly obvious. Cosmetic surgery of baggy eyelids did not develop until later.

The earliest attempts to correct "l'oeil poché" were designed to remove excess skin only. Contributions were made by Miller (1908, 1924), Kolle (1911), Bourguet (1921, 1929), Noël (1926), Hunt (1926), Bettman (1928), Joseph (1928), Kahn (1934), Barsky (1938), Arruga (1952), and others.

Some of the prescribed incisions were more conjecture than reality. Miller, for example, imagined 13 different incisions to correct 13 possible deformities. Some of these operative procedures were apparently maintained in secrecy by their originators. Passot (1919) complained of such secrecy, particularly among German surgeons, protesting that ". . .ceux-ci, gardant secrètes leurs méthodes, ont, par ce silence, laissé peser sur leur procédé une vague suspicion. . . ." (By keeping their methods secret, they allow a certain suspicion to exist about their procedures.) However, he did pay special tribute to the open publications of Kolle (1911), which he considered scholarly.

One of the procedures widely employed in Europe throughout this period was popularly known as the "temporal lift," a technique which has recently again gained popularity in the lay press as the "mini-lift." As early as 1921 this type of surgery was condemned by Bourguet. The efficacy of the technique, which provides for the excision of temporal and preauricular skin to correct small wrinkles of the skin lateral to the eyelids—so-called "crow's-feet"—is still disputed by most surgeons.

Bourguet (1929) was apparently the first to advocate fat removal in eyelid surgery, doing so in the same paper in which he identified the two different fat compartments of the upper eyelids. He was followed by Claoué (1931), Passot (1931) and Fomon (1939), who proposed a transconjunctival approach. Closure of the defect in the orbital septum with fascia lata strips was advised by Sakler (1937).

From the 1940's on, most publications, including textbooks by May (1947), Padgett and Stephenson (1948) and Spaeth (1948), described fat excision as an integral part of the operative procedure. But it was not until 1951 that a full description of the fat compartments of the eyelids was provided by Castanares. Later in 1951 the term "supraorbital adipocele" was proposed by Holden, and in 1952 Fox suggested "dermachalasis" as a descriptive addition to the diagnostic terminology.

Despite the various terms proposed over the years to describe the condition of baggy eyelids, i.e., ptosis atonica, ptosis lipomatosis, blepharochalasis, dermachalasis, herniated orbital fat, and so forth, there is still no general agreement as to what the various degrees of this condition should be properly called. From the

45

foregoing it is clear that some of the terms proposed describe only one component of a more complex defect.

True ptosis exists only rarely in patients with baggy eyelids. As early as 1844 Sichel demonstrated that if one supports the skin fold with a forceps, the movement of the lids usually becomes normal again. Loose eyelid skin is due, most often, to age alone. Although it rarely interferes with sight, it may encroach on the superior portion of the visual field in its extreme degrees. Nevertheless, many patients claim a sense of improved vision after surgery.

The term "fat hernia" appears to be a misnomer. Although the periorbital fat may be excessive in amount and may bulge against the orbital septum and orbicularis oculi muscle, it is more likely a pseudohernia than an actual one. The septum and muscle are frequently attenuated, but herniation of the fat into the subcutaneous tissue rearely occurs.

The word "blepharochalasis" ($\beta\lambda\epsilon\phi\alpha\rho o\sigma$ = eyelid, $\chi\alpha\lambda\alpha\sigma\iota\sigma$ = relaxation) means, in itself, no more than the sum total of its parts, namely, relaxation of the eyelids. Likewise, "dermachalasis" signifies only relaxation of the skin.

True blepharochalasis and ptosis atonica are found only rarely. The deformity of "baggy" eyelids is, however, much more common and causes the same symptoms of heaviness and fullness of the eyelids.

Modern variations in the evolution of the technique of blepharoplasty were provided by Holden (1951), Bames (1951, 1958), Fox (1952), Dufourmentel and Mouly (1958), Reidy (1960), Erich (1961), Ginester, et al. (1967), González-Ulloa and Stevens (1961, 1967), Smith and Fasano (1962), Converse (1964), Castanares (1951, 1964a, 1967), Johnson and Hadley (1964), Beare (1967), Rees and Ristow (1968), Rees and Dupuis (1969), Rees (1969 a and b), Lewis (1969), Silver (1969), and others. These techniques are generally similar and vary only in detail.

The techniques of González-Ulloa (1961) and Lewis (1969) differ significantly in the design of the skin incision and, therefore, bear comment. The "racquet" incision of González-Ulloa which joins the incision of the upper with the lower eyelids on the temporal side of the lateral canthus seems to produce satisfactory results in his hands. Some surgeons have criticized this design because hypertrophy of the lateral limb can occur, edema of the skin "trapped" by the scar is conceivable, and secondary operations are more difficult.

The Z-plasty technique of Lewis also differs significantly from other techniques. He utilizes the Z-plasty principle as an interpolation flap at the lateral commissure to elevate the corner of the eye and to eliminate overhang of the upper incision. Further experience by other surgeons is necessary before this procedure can be adequately evaluated.

The operational procedure recently published by Silver (1969) is sensible and would seem well adapted to certain cases in the older age group.

Etiology of Baggy Eyelids

Blepharoplasty, or repair of the eyelids, is performed to correct deformities of inheritance or increasing age. It is perhaps the most exacting and demanding operation in the field of cosmetic plastic surgery. Probably in no other procedure are even minor errors in surgical judgment or technique more apparent. The surgeon must constantly strive for perfection, yet maintain a conservative attitude in his operative approach.

The eyes form the very basis of individual recognition and account for a large part of the expressiveness of the human face. It is the eyes that first establish contact when people meet. The eyes project sorrow, happiness, elation — the gamut of human emotions. It is interesting to consider what actually provides expression to the eyes. Certainly the globes themselves are entirely expressionless structures, unless one considers constriction and dilatation of the pupil as a form of expression. It is, in fact, the shape of the skin, the subcutaneous tissue, the fat, the hair and the lashes around the eyes that convey expression.

We think of lines of expression about the eyes as being "earned" with age. Thus, the eyes of a child or baby are relatively free of wrinkles or bulges and are therefore thought to have a much "clearer" expression than those of an adult. With the passage of time, the presence of wrinkles and deep lines of expression, as well as the gradual formation of puffs or bags of the lids due to relaxing skin or underlying pseudohernias of fat, begins to occur.

Some of these signs of advancing age are thought to be attractive in certain individuals, usually men, but they are generally the cause of constant worry and anguish in women. For example, "laugh lines" radiating laterally from the outer canthus of the eye convey much of the expression of the eyes of the adult and are not generally regarded as unattractive. However, the situation assumes quite a different dimension when these lines are accompanied by deep furrows, creases of the skin of the upper and lower eyelids, overhanging skin folds and bulging fat pockets.

Baggy eyelids can actually occur at any age from a wide variety of causes. In young children they may be the result of edema which accumulates during sleep, or they may be caused by such widely diverse conditions as local allergy or chronic renal disease. In older children, adolescents or young adults they are usually the result of an overabundance or pseudoherniation of orbital fat, and they are generally hereditary in nature. Recurrent swelling in this age group can also be caused by allergy, the menstrual cycle, overindulgence in alcohol, too little or too much sleep, and edema of thyroid, cardiac or renal etiology. During the middle years and beyond, characteristic changes of aging occur in the eyelid and brow region. Extra skin folds, wrinkles, ptosis of the brows and degenerative changes of the skin may herald the onset of baggy eyelids or may compound the fat bags of youth. Again, chronic or intermittent edema from a wide variety of causes will accentuate these changes. Because these changes of age have been considered, until recently, to be part of the normal course of events, it is understandable why most older people accepted their occurrence with little overt complaint and did little to remedy the situation.

Today, however, blepharoplasty has become a commonplace operation which is sought by the lay public and sanctioned by the general physician. A number of operative techniques for the procedure have been described. No one technique is suitable for all patients. Each operation must be highly individualized to meet the needs of the patient at hand. Appropriate teaching of these techniques and their variations is a necessary part of the training program for all plastic surgeons.

Perhaps in no other form of corrective surgery, with the possible exception of nasal plasty, is careful preoperative evaluation of each and every detail of the morphologic defect of more importance. Such objective and meticulous study is essential in planning a personalized operative procedure. It is inexcusable for any surgeon to use only one blepharoplasty technique for all patients. He must be reasonably imaginative and inventive, even in minor details, to achieve the naturalness of expression that marks a good as contrasted to a mediocre result.

Morphologic and Histologic Considerations

The morphologic and histologic changes attending the aging process of the skin and subcutaneous tissue are many. Microscopic findings are reflected in the obvious, visible changes that become increasingly apparent with age. These changes are frequently first manifested in the eyelid area and are often more severe and progressive there than they are in other parts of the face. Many of these changes are thought to be the result of a progressive dehydration of the skin.

In addition to senile changes in the skin of the eyelids, there frequently is bulging of the periorbital fat, often erroneously referred to as "herniated fat." In most patients the offending fat pockets are found in the medial portions of the upper eyelids, and the medial, middle and, less often, the lateral compartments of the lower lids. The bulge of the pseudohernia is caused by an overabundance of normal periorbital fat which exerts pressure on the orbital septum. This occurs in baggy eyelids of both the familial and senile type, although in older people the fat bags are often accentuated by excess skin which may hang in loose folds. The amount, distribution and type of this excess skin should be carefully noted. The thin skin usually found in the older patient tears easily and will have to be handled with great care. Thickened skin contracts more following surgery and is also more likely to retain edema for a longer period of time.

The position of the eyebrows should be observed in order to determine if it will be necessary to elevate these structures during the procedure.

It is important to inform the patient beforehand of the limitations of the procedure. For example, bulges, depressions or bags of cheek skin below the eyelid itself cannot be eliminated. Marked skin bags of the eyelids themselves may require a two-stage procedure with an interval of several months between operations to permit accurate determination of the exact amount of excess skin remaining. Wrinkled skin, whether caused by actinic exposure or age may be improved, but will not be completely smoothed out. Wrinkles that occur in animation will likewise not be eradicated.

47

Systemic and Ophthalmologic Aspects

The surgeon must not allow all his interest to be focused on the eyelids when considering blepharoplasty for a patient with palpebral bags. A number of systemic conditions can directly affect the eyes and the eyelids and should be kept in mind. A thorough history and physical examination are needed to rule out any systemic contribution to the baggy lids. If the plastic surgeon is not inclined toward such a time-consuming examination, he should request a complete work-up from an internist or the family doctor.

Several systemic conditions may be reflected in the tissues about the eye, particularly as laxity or premature aging of the skin, edema of the lids, or vascular changes such as telangiectases. These include chronic renal disease, hypo- or hyperthyroidism, diabetes, chronic liver cirrhosis, cardiac decompensation, allergies, and other disorders of lesser importance. Hypothyroidism, particularly, can mimic the classic appearance of puffiness and palpebral bags. Such bags can miraculously disappear with the administration of thyroid extract or synthetics, thus sparing the patient unnecessary surgery. Hyperthyroidism can, of course, be associated with exophthalmos and excessive drying of the skin. Any condition which predisposes toward or promotes generalized edema can be reflected in the orbital tissues. In the adolescent and the young adult baggy eyelids may be a clue to the presence of such rare conditions as elephantiasis, pachydermoperiostosis and intra-orbital lipoidosis.

Certain localized conditions can also result in hypertrophy of the lids and therefore also have to be considered in the differential diagnosis. These include lymphangiomas, hemangiomas, mixed lymphohemangiomas, neurofibromatoses, lipomatoses, foreign body reactions (from paraffin or silicone injections), and low-grade inflammatory processes. Careful and detailed local examination will often shed light on such pathologic entities.

Clearly, a careful and reasonably thorough ophthalmologic examination is required to rule out associated disease in the eye or adnexa. Although such detailed examinations are best done by a competent ophthalmologist, this is not always practical or possible. The plastic surgeon undertaking such surgery should be able to perform routine eye examinations for visual acuity, peripheral fields, funduscopic evaluation and intra-ocular tension. Measurement of tension can be postponed until the patient is anesthetized at surgery unless there is a history of glaucoma or symptoms of the disease. It should be noted here that chronic glaucoma is not necessarily a contraindication to blepharoplasty.

If slit lamp examination or corroborative funduscopic testing seems indicated, or if disease is suspected, consultation with an ophthalmologist, preferably one who is surgically oriented, should be sought. Any question of muscular imbalance is of particular importance and should be clarified.

Suffice it to say, then, that in elective surgery of any sort, especially of a cosmetic nature, the consultation of a specialist colleague should be sought whenever there is any question of doubt. This is true not only because it helps to ensure the safety of the patient, but because, in the case of blepharoplasty, so many factors can have a direct bearing on the results of surgery.

Anesthetic Technique

Anesthetic techniques vary according to the personal preferences of each surgeon. Blepharoplasty can be done under general or local anesthesia. Either technique, however, is facilitated by the injection of a local anesthetic such as 0.5 per cent procaine (Novocain) or lidocaine (Xylocaine) containing epinephrine 1:200,000 to help to delineate tissue planes and promote hemostasis.

Since adequate removal of intra-orbital fat does require considerable traction on deep structures, which causes pain difficult to block with local anesthesia alone, we prefer a basal narcosis supplemented by local infiltration. This combination of sedation and analgesia is administered under the direction of a competent anesthesiologist. The details of anesthesia for facial surgery are described in Chapter 4.

Operative Technique

The design of incisions to correct palpebral defects must take into account all the different and distinct morphologic factors which comprise the composite deformity. It is the *total* defect that camouflages the natural beauty and shape of the eye, so important to individual expression. The most important factors to consider are: (1) the degree of ptosis of the brow, (2) the amount of excess skin of the upper lid, (3) the amount of protruding orbital fat in the upper eyelid, particularly at the medial angle, (4) the amount and type of excess skin of the lower eyelid, (5) the amount and distribution of the palpebral fat of the lower eyelid, and (6) various associated factors including dislocation of the lacrimal gland and the amount and degree of actinic dermatitis. Each patient has various combinations of these defects in varying degrees of severity. It is important to analyze this combination and to define the role of each factor in order to vary the operative approach appropriately.

UPPER EYELIDS

The upper lids should be repaired first. In many patients a simple elliptical excision of the excess skin will suffice, although in those with marked ptosis of the brows due to senility or paralysis of the frontal branch of the facial nerve, this may be insufficient. In the latter group of patients, excision of the excess skin folds of the upper eyelids by standardized techniques should be augmented by excision of an ellipse of skin superior and adjacent to the brow. The net result of this is not only removal of excess skin, but elevation of the brow (p. 180). It is important that the skin excision above the brow be wider in the lateral two thirds than the medial third. The final suture line is planned to lie just within the upper hair follicle line of the brow.

The placement of the suture line of the standard upper lid excision is also of paramount importance. The lowermost line of the ellipse, which becomes the final suture line, should lie no farther than 5 to 7 mm. above the ciliary margin so that the final scar will fall naturally into the supratarsal folds. The lateral extension should lie in a "crow's foot." Because the final suture line tends to ride upward, it should be drawn at a level lower than its intended destination. A careful and thorough removal of the medial fat pockets through a stab wound in the orbital septum is important to prevent a secondary postoperative bulging of the fat in this region.

The upper eyelid wound is best sutured with a subcuticular suture of fine nylon which can be left in place four or five days. This type of suture is most helpful in preventing troublesome epithelial tunnels or inclusion cysts which easily form around interrupted sutures after 48 hours.

LOWER EYELIDS

Correction of the lower eyelid is the most challenging part of cosmetic blepharoplasty. It is here that the operative technique varies most considerably, and an analysis of anatomic problems is most necessary to achieve the desired correction without such postoperative problems as epiphora, ectropion and secondary fat herniation. Absolute hemostasis with fine needle-tipped forceps and cautery is mandatory throughout the procedure to prevent hematoma, which may prolong convalescence and contribute to other complications.

In those patients with only *moderate protrusion* of the periorbital fat and *minimal skin excess*, the lower eyelid is opened by an incision placed approximately 3 mm. below the ciliary margin. This incision is carried through the skin and orbicularis muscle, thereby creating a skin muscle flap as described by McIndoe, and subsequently by Beare (1967) and by Rees and Dupuis (1969). The orbital septum can then be incised and excess fat removed from the appropriate compartments. The amount of fat removal is determined by the degree of protrusion of fat when pressure is gently applied to the globe. If necessary, a small strip of muscle and skin may be trimmed, although this must be done with caution, as these are generally young patients with tight structures and little tissue to spare. The flap is then replaced and sutured with interrupted sutures of fine black silk.

If a *moderate amount of excess skin* exists in addition to *excessive fat*, a conservative skin excision is done after fat removal. Excess fat is removed through an incision splitting the orbicularis muscle or by making multiple stab wounds through the muscle and orbital septum. In most operations on the lower lids, the majority of excess fat is found in the medial fat compartment. *Fat removal from the lateral pocket should always be conservative to prevent an unsightly postoperative contour depression.*

The amount of skin to be removed can be marked prior to the incision, as recommended by Converse (p. 63), or subsequent to undermining. It is usually necessary to extend the markings for the lower eyelid incision laterally into a so-called crow's-foot. According to the Converse technique, the excess skin is then held with forceps in a manner similar to the method used for the upper lids, and the skin pattern is excised along the lines drawn.

According to Converse (1964), when only a moderate amount of excess skin is the problem, little or no undermining of the skin is necessary, except to make minute final adjustments to allow the skin flap to fit naturally without tension to the upper margin of the wound. Usually the author prefers to make the standard subciliary incision and then undermine the skin conservatively, attempting to estimate the amount of excision required. These two minor variations in skin technique accomplish the same result.

Accurate determination of the exact amount of skin to be trimmed is imperative in surgery of the lower lid in order to avoid an ectropion resulting from an overambitious resection. If the operation is being performed under local anesthesia and the patient can cooperate, two maneuvers can help to avoid the removal of too much skin. The patient is asked to rotate the eyes upward to elevate the lid margin to a "safe" position. The undermined skin can then be draped over the wound edge and the excess removed. Safety is further facilitated by having the patient open the mouth widely to duplicate the forces of an extrinsic ectropion of the type often seen in burns of the face.

If the patient is under general anesthesia or is unable to cooperate, gentle downward pressure applied to the globe results in an upward elevation of the lower lid so the skin may be safely draped over it and excised while the lid is in an elevated position.

Patients with *considerable excess of skin* of the lower eyelids sometimes have skin folds extending to the cheeks. This requires wide undermining, which may extend to the infraorbital margin itself. As noted previously, true cheek pads cannot be corrected by blepharoplasty.

When wide undermining is indicated, it should be done prior to excision of fat. Then, after fat removal, the skin flap is draped over the upper margin of the wound and drawn laterally and superiorly. A slight sling effect is the result of this rotation. The excess skin is then trimmed, mostly from the lateral triangle.

Care must be taken to avoid undue tension on the skin flap because horizontal or vertical foreshortening of the lower lid margin can result in buckling of the tarsus, with epiphora or ectropion.

To avoid tenting of the skin flap, care must be taken to see that the entire skin flap is in approximation with all crevices and contours of the wound bed. Wound edges are then stitched with interrupted sutures of fine silk. A temporary tarsorrhaphy suture is placed in each eye and a moderate compression dressing is usually applied.

The technique of Silver (1969) (pp. 70, 71) is also most useful in correction of marked skin excess in the senile lid.

Postoperative Care

Bandaging of the eyes following operation is not essential. The authors have vacillated about bandaging during the past several years. Theoretically, at least, a moderate pressure dressing for the first few hours following surgery would seem beneficial to help to control oozing, edema and hematoma.

Certainly, if bandages are not used, it is important to make sure that the cornea is covered and that the eyes are well lubricated during recovery from anesthesia. For this purpose, liberal instillation of a bland ophthalmic ointment is recommended. Application of iced sterile compresses as soon as possible, preferably commencing in the recovery room, is important for the same reasons that pressure bandages are used.

If bandages are used, only moderate pressure is necessary. It is highly important to assure that the lids which were operated on are in proper position under such dressings. This is especially true for the lower lids, which must be maintained in the "normal" position and not depressed in a caudal direction by the upper lid or by the bandage. Such depression of the lower lid can result in adherence of the skin flap to the wound in the orbital septum or to a lower-than-normal level on the muscle bed. Either can result in ectropion and eversion and must be treated by immediate reoperation and adjustment of the skin flap. Proper positioning of the skin flaps and lids can be provided by the temporary tarsorrhaphy suture, which is placed through the gray line of the lid, and by the careful application of a wrap-around dressing over two eye pads placed on each eye (p. 69).

If dressings are applied, they are removed the following morning, along with the tarsorrhaphy sutures. The application of continuous ice compresses is then commenced and continued for the next two days.

Eye dressings may cause some patients to experience severe claustrophobia. When this is the case, sedatives or tranquilizers may be helpful in alleviating the patient's anxiety. The dressings are removed at once, however, if the patient cannot be controlled by these medications.

Perhaps the main value of dressings is to

provide an added insurance against reactive bleeding during the immediate recovery phase. Every surgeon has experienced, to his consternation, the development of a hematoma or active bleeding from the wound edges in patients in the recovery room who vomited or retched following general anesthesia, despite the excellence of the anesthetic technique, and sometimes even following local anesthesia.

Most interrupted sutures, including the subcuticular suture, are removed on the fourth postoperative day. Sutures left longer than this often result in the formation of epithelial tunnels or sinuses, which can be most troublesome. Wound agglutination can be ensured even when sutures are removed at this early time by the application of small sterile strips of paper adhesive across the tension lines of the incision. Paper adhesive has proved to be virtually nonreactive in most patients and is extremely effective in maintaining apposition of the wound edges during the period of maximum weakness.

All crusts and scabs are gently cleansed away from the wound at the end of the first week. A bland eyewash is sometimes beneficial if the patient complains of irritation, scratchiness or marked itching. Some patients find the intermittent application of ice compresses to be soothing even several days after the operation, and they are encouraged to continue them if they feel they are helpful.

Exercising of the orbicularis muscles by "squeezing" the eyelids closed at intermittent time intervals is helpful in reducing edema and regaining mobility after the first week. The use of oral or parenteral enzymes has not generally been proved effective in the control of postoperative wound edema.

Women may apply eye make-up on about the tenth postoperative day, but it is advisable to remove it thoroughly and carefully after each use. Oiled eye pads are recommended for this purpose.

The management of minor complications such as inclusion cysts, hematomas and scar thickening are described in the following section on complications.

Complications of Blepharoplasty

The complications of cosmetic blepharoplasty may be divided into two groups: those that are relatively temporary and those that are persistent or even permanent. The latter group often require subsequent surgical intervention

to attempt correction. Temporary complications are usually self-limiting and generally appear almost immediately after surgery.

RETROBULBAR HEMATOMA

Retrobulbar hematoma can occur during the operation as the result of deep injection of anesthetic, with rupture of small vessels, or it may be caused by bleeding from retracted vessels during fat removal. Such bleeding can be sudden and most dramatic. The first sign is sudden and progressive proptosis of the eye during infiltration or surgery. Every reasonable attempt should be made to identify the bleeding vessel and to coagulate it. However, this may not always be possible because such a bleeding point may have retracted deeply into the orbit following fat removal. The application of *gentle* pressure for several minutes may control the problem and the operation may then be completed. If, however, the retrobulbar bleeding is severe and the proptosis pronounced, it may be necessary to delay the remainder of the operation. It is particularly important in such patients to protect the cornea from exposure during the postoperative period. A simple occlusive eyelid suture may be used for this purpose. Some surgeons advocate a pressure dressing for retrobulbar hematoma. Others advise against it, arguing that such pressure may compromise the retinal artery or nerve. The authors prefer not to use pressure dressings for this complication, but do advocate immediate postoperative application of ice packs. Alarming as it is at the time, a retrobulbar hematoma is surprisingly innocuous. It creates a minimum of difficulty, and there is usually prompt resolution.

HEMATOMAS UNDER SKIN FLAPS

Hematomas under the skin flaps are not uncommon following primary blepharoplasty. They can be easily recognized by the marked bulging of the lid and the severe ecchymotic discoloration. Conceivably the immediate postoperative recognition of such a hematoma would lead the surgeon to reopen the wound and remove the hematoma. This approach is rarely indicated except when bleeding continues unchecked. At any rate, hematomas beneath the skin flap are usually not noticed until at

51

least several hours after surgery, and they are rarely massive enough to tempt the surgeon to drain them immediately.

Localized hematomas beneath the eyelid skin flaps can often be evacuated when they become liquefied, usually about seven to 10 days after operation. Incision with a No. 11 blade and drainage permit "squeezing out" of the semiliquid clot (p. 117). By such action, prolonged nodularity can be lessened.

Spontaneous resolution of skin-flap hematomas does occur, but the process is often slow and lengthy, causing mental distress to both patient and surgeon. The firm nodules that develop beneath the skin flaps during the later stages of resolution are sometimes visible as well as papable. During this period the entire eyelid may feel plaquelike. Occasionally a distortion of the lid margin, such as a mild ectropion, may be caused by the process and may persist until organization of the clot has occurred. Injection of steroids such as triamcinolone directly into the organizing blood clot seems to accelerate resolution. Such injections should be of low dosage (2 mg. per injection) and should not be given more often than every two weeks. These precautions are necessary to avoid the subcutaneous atrophy which can occur following overambitious dosage. Such atrophy, should it occur, usually disappears within six months, but is unsightly while present. Fortunately, permanent deformities or serious problems resulting from hematomas are unusual.

EPIPHORA

Epiphora—excessive tearing from the eyes—is common during the first 48 hours after surgery and may persist for longer periods. It is usually caused by the immediate postoperative reaction—edema of the skin, distortion of the canaliculus or tear-drainage mechanism, or distortion of the lid margins. With subsidence of the wound reaction, epiphora usually disappears. Rarely, intermittent epiphora, occurring nocturnally or with sudden changes of the weather, can persist for several weeks or months. Permanent epiphora may occur, but is extremely rare. It is most likely related to stenosis of the canaliculus or lacrimal sac resulting from injury at the time of surgery, or from surgery aggravating a pre-existing problem. For these reasons it is very unwise to extend the incision of the lower eyelid into the extreme medial corner of the lid, particularly

in the skin-muscle flap (McIndoe) operation. If injury to the lacrimal apparatus does occur at surgery and is recognized at that time, immediate repair should be done.

INFECTION

Infection following eyelid surgery is rare because of the superb blood supply of this region. When it does occur, it should be treated with full doses of the antibiotic indicated by sensitivity cultures. Broad-spectrum antibiotics are used until the culture reports are available.

DIPLOPIA

Temporary diplopia during the first few hours or even days following surgery may occur because of wound reaction, edema of the conjunctiva or temporary muscle disturbances. Permanent diplopia can occur, in very rare instances, when the extraocular eye muscles are damaged during surgery. The author has seen one such patient in whom the inferior oblique was damaged. A secondary muscle repair was necessary to correct the diplopia. It is worth noting that the inferior oblique is most subject to injury during blepharoplasty because it straddles the medial and middle fat compartments of the lower lids. This muscle should be directly examined during surgery to make sure that it has not been injured by knife or cautery.

LAGOPHTHALMOS

Lagophthalmos—the inability to completely close the eyes—is a common complaint during the immediate postoperative period. This can result in drying of the cornea and general desiccation and irritation of the conjunctiva and lid margins. A bland eye ointment is prescribed at night for patients with this problem. The use of methylcellulose or other protective solution eyedrops on retiring also provides protection until the condition has corrected itself. Daytime irrigation of the eyes with saline solution or any of the bland proprietary eyewashes is also helpful. Occasionally, temporary lagophthalmos will continue for several weeks or months. The problem is rarely serious but can be a considerable nuisance.

Lagophthalmos may result from excision of too much skin from the upper eyelids. Careful preincision marking of the ellipse to be removed from the upper lids, using the

Green forceps (p. 61 B), will help to avoid this mistake. The upper lid should not remain open more than 3 mm. at the end of the procedure.

If the skin shortage causing lagophthalmos is severe, a serious situation exists, for the cornea is no longer covered and protected by the upper lid. This results in desiccation, exposure keratitis, and eventual ulceration of the anterior chamber, with possible perforation—a set of circumstances frequently seen following thermal burns of the eyelids. This severe degree of what is really ectropion of the upper lid requires emergency consideration, with release of the lid and immediate skin grafting. Such a problem must be exceedingly rare in cosmetic blepharoplasty; the authors are aware of only one case.

ECTROPION

Ectropion is one of the more distressing complications following blepharoplasty. It can be slight, moderate or severe, with marked contracture and eversion of the lids. Following cosmetic blepharoplasty, a very slight downward pull of the lower lids is reasonably common because of scar contraction and wound reaction. It usually subsides within the first two or three weeks, although in unusual circumstances it can persist for several months, with a small amount of white sclera showing beneath the pupil. Such a condition is most likely to occur following removal of very large fat pockets or when the skin is slightly thicker than normal. The surgeon should always be very conservative in excising the skin in such cases. Temporary chemosis or a small hematoma of the wound can also cause a temporary ectropion or even eversion of the lid margin. This subsides with resolution of the chemosis or hematoma.

Ectropion that is the result of excessive skin excision of the lower lids requires reconstruction with full-thickness grafts as described on pages 120–122. The proper timing of such reconstruction is sometimes difficult to define. If the surgeon recognizes that the skin excision is excessive at the operating table, the skin should be replaced then and there. The resulting deformity is surprisingly minimal and may even be unnoticed. If the problem is recognized one or two days postoperatively, and the surgeon is sure that a skin shortage exists, he has up to 48 hours after the operation to perform a graft. From that point on, however, and for the next several weeks, the amount of wound reaction, edema, and subsequent scar contracture precludes the application of a skin graft. Following this, a period of four to six months is needed for wound maturity and softening of the scars before corrections can be made safely. As pointed out elsewhere in the text (p. 122), the choice donor sites for full-thickness skin are: (1) the upper lids, (2) the retroauricular skin, and (3) the supraclavicular areas.

ECCHYMOSIS

Severe ecchymosis, such as may occur after conjunctival operations, is most unusual following cosmetic blepharoplasty. When it does occur, it is highly upsetting to both patient and surgeon. Hypertonic saline packs applied to the eyes after topical anesthesia are useful in reducing edema.

INCISION COMPLICATIONS

Minor complications of the skin incisions or subcutaneous tissue when undermining was done are not uncommon, but they are rarely significant, except as minor disturbances in the immediate postoperative period. Small inclusion cysts or "whiteheads" along the scar line are frequent and respond to enucleation with the tip of a No. 11 blade. Large inclusion cysts also frequently occur and can easily be incised by sharp dissection after a drop or two of topical anesthesia. The formation of epithelium-lined tunnels along interrupted sutures will occur if the sutures are not removed within three or four days following surgery, but it is not necessary to leave sutures in longer now that paper tape is available for wound splinting. Should such epithelial tunnels be encountered, it is best to unroof them or to marsupialize them by snipping away the roof of the tunnel (Converse, 1964).

SCAR THICKENING

Very small areas of thickening in the scars can occur, particularly when extensive undermining of the lid skin has been done. These usually resolve after varying periods of time. Resolution can be hastened in some patients by localized injection of steroid compounds in very small amounts. A 30-gauge needle or a 1-cc. tuberculin syringe is best for this purpose. The treatment is similar to that for localized hematoma.

CHRONIC BLEPHARITIS

Chronic blepharitis of a nonspecific nature has been seen following blepharoplasty. In our opinion it is surprising that this problem is not more common than it is. It is, in fact, so rare as to lead one to the conclusion that its occurrence may be coincidental. Obvious deformities of the lids such as lagophthalmos or ectropion can obviously lead to blepharitis. Treatment by a competent ophthalmologist is recommended. Recurrent chalazions or styes have also been seen following blepharoplasty, but are usually considered coincidental since there is frequently a history of prior occurrence.

LOSS OF EYELASHES

Spontaneous loss of eyelashes has occurred twice in the author's experience. In both patients the process proved to be reversible, however, and the lashes grew in again.

OPTIC ATROPHY AND BLINDNESS

Optic atrophy and blindness following cosmetic blepharoplasty was reported by Hartman et al. (1962), presumedly the result of vascular spasms from pulling on the orbital fat. Such a tragedy could, of course, be completely coincidental to the surgery in view of the thousands of blepharoplasties being performed each year and the paucity of reports of similar incidents. It seems more likely to the authors that such a complication would result from retrobulbar hematoma than from traction on fat, although retrobulbar hematomas occur often enough not to be considered a medical curiosity; serious sequelae are extremely rare.

Secondary Operations

Secondary blepharoplasty is one of the most challenging and hazardous operations in the field of cosmetic surgery. It even ranks ahead of secondary rhinoplasty in technical difficulties and pitfalls awaiting the unwary surgeon. Such surgery should be undertaken only if, after careful assessment, the surgeon is certain that he can achieve a reasonable correction without creating further deformity. It is particularly perilous to undertake correction of minor secondary deformities in patients who have been operated on by another surgeon. Unfortunately, minor degrees of improvement are not always appreciated by the patient, even though the surgeon may feel he has accomplished a virtual miracle.

The most common deformities requiring secondary surgery after a primary eyelid repair are: (1) bulging of the medial fat pockets of the upper eyelids; (2) recurrence of a skin fold of the upper eyelid; (3) ptosis of the brow, often with a marked lateral skin fold; (4) residual herniated fat pockets of the lower eyelids, usually medial and middle and less often lateral; (5) elevated, irregular or uneven scars, or scar contractures such as webbing near the lateral canthus; (6) varying degrees of ectropion because of excessive resection of the skin of the lower eyelids; (7) inability to close the upper lids, with corneal exposure; (8) excessive skin of the lower eyelids because of inadequate excision at the primary operation, best demonstrated on facial animation or squinting; (9) excessive pigmentation of the skin, more common after secondary blepharoplasty; and (10) the appearance of many fine wrinkles not visible before the original surgery and thought to be the result of the release of skin tension after fat removal.

Of prime importance in such surgery is the fact that there is rarely sufficient skin to spare at a secondary operation, particularly on the lower lids. This is of utmost importance in planning the operation. It is *never* advisable to pre-estimate the amount of skin to be resected prior to a secondary procedure. Such advance planning will most often lead to the embarrassing situation of a serious skin shortage. Removal of secondary fat pseudohernias in patients in whom there is no skin to spare can also cause an acute shortage of skin, similar to that in the patient who, at the time of primary surgery, had very large fat bags and little or no excess skin.

In removing skin folds of the upper eyelids during a secondary operation, it is advisable to first mark the estimated amount of skin to be removed by using a marking forceps, and then to excise *less* than this estimated amount. A further strip of skin can be excised should this conservative excision prove insufficient. If too much skin is excised, however, an immediate free graft may be necessary. Should the skin excision of the upper eyelids prove to have been overestimated, it is sometimes possible to narrow the defect by undermining the skin edges of the superior wound margin so that closure can be accomplished without a graft.

Even slight excess skin removal from the lower eyelids can result in a minor degree of ectropion. Lower lid ectropion is the most serious of the secondary complications requiring correction. It is rarely possible to repair a minor ectropion or minimal "scleral show." In fact, this situation is usually made worse by attempts to correct it. Only when significant ectropion exists should operative correction be considered. In rare instances wide undermining of the lower eyelid skin and incisional release of the orbital septum can improve ectropion by giving vertical length to the lid. However, the addition of a full-thickness skin graft is usually necessary. The best possible skin graft for reconstruction of lower eyelid ectropion is full-thickness skin from the upper eyelids. Unfortunately such skin is rarely available. It has usually been removed during the primary operation, thus depleting this skin bank.

When scarring of the wound bed is extensive, with accompanying avascularity, it is not always possible to use full-thickness grafts, although these are usually the grafts of choice for eyelid reconstruction. Under such circumstances it becomes necessary to use thin split-thickness grafts to ensure a "take." In men the hairless areas of the neck provide the best donor site for split-thickness grafts to the eyelids, as skin from this site provides a superior color and texture match (Edgerton, 1960). In women, however, even the minimal scarring of this donor site may prove a disadvantage. The next best alternative for a donor area of split-thickness skin grafts is the medial surface of the arms or buttocks.

The disadvantages of split-thickness grafts include their well known tendency to contract and to become hyperpigmented. Grafts from the neck do seem to pigment less than others. Their advantages, however, are that split-thickness skin is more likely to preserve the natural expression lines occurring on animation than is a full-thickness graft, and that split-thickness grafts are more likely to survive on a heavily scarred base. For these reasons split-thickness skin was preferred by McIndoe for eyelid reconstruction in the treatment of World War II burn casualties.

Among the more common problems requiring a second operation are residual fat pockets in the medial corners of the upper or lower lids. Occasionally the lateral fat compartments also require attention. If the skin excision was adequate, the surgeon need only incise the original wounds, separate the fibers of the orbicularis muscle, locate the bulging orbital septum over the offending fat pocket and tease out the fat. It is then excised. A wide incision and

exposure of the orbital septum is rarely necessary and should be avoided when possible.

If the opposite condition exists, that of excessive removal of orbital fat, a "sunken" lid can give a hollow appearance to the eyes. This distressing deformity is most often seen in patients with deep set eyes and very prominent bony orbital margins. There is no effective method of correction.

The presence of many fine wrinkles or rhytides about the eye may be accentuated by primary blepharoplasty, and these may thus not even be noted by the patient until after surgery. The removal of bulging fat releases tension that tends to stretch the eyelid skin. When such tension is released, the natural elastic forces within the skin, interplaying with the underlying orbicularis muscle action, can result in visibility of previously unnoticed wrinkles. These fine rhytides can often be significantly improved by dermabrasion or chemabrasion. The chemabrasion technique described by Baker (1962) (with taping) is preferred by the author and has proved to be effective in several such patients.

Increase in pigmentation of the skin, particularly of the lower eyelids, can also occur after surgery, especially following severe or prolonged ecchymosis. It is often seen in patients of Mediterranean heritage. Such discoloration is also seen occasionally after rhinoplasty. Sometimes the pigmentation seems to be in the superficial layers of the skin where the breakdown products of hemoglobin may be deposited. Chemabrasion has proved to be of help in several such patients, but time is the best healer even though several months may be required for spontaneous fading to occur. Such pigmentation rarely is permanent.

Superficial pigmentation of the eyelid skin may sometimes respond to chemabrasion (p. 228).

Ptosis, or drooping of the eyelids, may appear more pronounced after blepharoplasty. Removal of large skin folds from the upper lids may seem to bring the brows closer to the lid margins. Ptosis of the brows presents a difficult problem. Correction by excision of skin ellipses above the brows or by extensive temporal lifts with wide undermining of the temporal and forehead skin can be done. These techniques are sometimes disappointing, however. A serious problem with surgical elevation by excision of a skin ellipse above the brow is that the resulting scar may be quite visible in certain patients, particularly those with few or no horizontal forehead lines. Such scars may be obvious even though every effort has been made to place them within the hair follicle line. If the surgeon elects to perform a surgical brow elevation, it is important that he discuss this technique in considerable detail with the patient beforehand so that the patient is aware of the possibility of a visible scar.

Blepharoplasty of the Oriental Eye

Since World War II, operations designed to construct a superior palpebral fold in the Oriental eyelid have become increasingly popular. According to Boo-Chai (1963), such operations have been performed for many decades by ophthalmologists in China and Japan, but have only recently been documented in the English language. In many cities of the Orient, as well as in areas containing large Oriental populations such as Hawaii, this surgery has become commonplace. Except for Hawaii, however, these operations are infrequently performed in the United States.

In the typical mongoloid type of upper eyelid, the superior palpebral fold is absent. This condition occurs in about 50 per cent of Orientals and is apparently caused by a dominant gene. Fernandez (1960) points out that some Orientals refer to the eye without a palpebral fold as the "single eye," and the eye with the fold as the "double eye." Just why many Orientals prefer to "Westernize" their eyes is not known, although it is thought to stem from the influence of motion pictures and the increasing intermarriage of Asian women and Caucasian men, particularly since the Second World War.

The Oriental or "slit" eye differs from the Western eye in several important anatomic ways. There is more fat in the loose subcutaneous tissue than there is around the Caucasian eye. There is also an encapsulated, canary yellow fat pad just beneath the orbicularis muscle and above the levator expansion.

Undoubtedly the most important anatomical difference between the Oriental and Occidental eyelid is the absence of the cutaneous insertion of the levator palpebral superioris in the mongoloid lid. Sayoc (1954) described the double insertion of the levator into the skin and the superior border of the tarsal plate in the Caucasian eye. He pointed out that when the muscle belly of the levator contracts, the entire transverse aponeurosis is "swung backward over the glove like a visor of a helmet, pulling with it the skin of the lid, into which its terminal fibers are inserted, thus deepening and forming the superior folds." This fold formation is not caused solely by the insertion of the aponeurosis into the skin, but is aided by its main attachment along the superior border of the tarsal plate which causes the tarsus to be elevated upon contraction of the muscle.

In the Oriental, however, the absence of the cutaneous insertion is sufficient to cause the absence of the orbital palpebral sulcus and the palpebral fold. The cutaneous extension of the levator expansion ends as a ridge of thickened fascia in the Oriental. The typical Mongoloid eyelid also contains a medial epicanthal fold which hides most of the caruncle.

Valuable contributions to the techniques of operating on Oriental eyelids have been made by Sayoc (1954, 1956), Millard (1955), Fernandez (1960), Boo-Chai (1963a and b), Uchida (1962) and others. They have devised varying ways to construct the supratarsal fold. The simplest of these procedures has been widely advertised as the "20 minute eye operation" and is done in outpatient clinics and offices throughout the Orient. Boo-Chai (1963b) advocates this simpler technique in most cases of the younger age group in whom there is a minimum of excess fat and skin. He places three mattress sutures transconjunctivally which fix the levator to the skin at a level 5 to 8 mm. from the ciliary margin (p. 132). These sutures are of fine nylon and are carefully placed to construct a normal shape and curve to the fold. He excises excess fat through a small stab wound in the supratarsal fold, unless there is a considerable amount of fat, in which case a larger incision is required for removal. Boo-Chai claims this simple technique is effective in most patients and has the additional advantages of minimal scarring and distortion of lids and lashes. He further claims the method is not irreversible in that adjustments can be made if the sutures are not placed in exactly the right position.

Although Boo-Chai states that this simple technique can provide natural results of a permanent nature, other surgeons prefer a more radical approach via a long supratarsal incision with extensive reattachment of the levator expansion to the skin, as well as removal of all excess fat. In patients with more advanced deformities, i.e., more fat and skin, Boo-Chai also does the more radical procedure of the type advocated by Millard (1955), Fernandez (1960) and others.

The extensive and complete procedure described by Fernandez is preferred by the author and has proved successful in his hands. In this procedure the excess skin of the upper eyelid is grasped with a marking forceps very much as in a routine blepharoplasty in a Caucasian, and the excess skin is marked and excised. The incision is planned to lie about 6 mm. above the lid margin. The orbicularis muscle is then split transversely along almost the entire length of the upper eyelid. Immediately beneath the orbicularis muscle a fusiform pad of yellow fat will usually be found lying transversely from medial to lateral. This fat is removed. If separate medial fat pockets exist, a stab wound is made in the orbital septum and this fat is extruded and excised. The levator expansion is found deep to the muscle and supraorbital fat. This structure is carefully dissected and cleared. The inferior thickened edge is carefully freed across its entire width. All bleeding points are coagulated. The inferior edge of the levator expansion is then sutured to the dermis (which is very thin) at the edge of the lower incision. Fine suture material such as 6–0 white nylon, Mersilene or catgut is used. The skin incision is closed with interrupted or subcuticular sutures.

Should correction of the epicanthal fold be desired, a Z-plasty may be done at the same time or at a future date. Operations to correct the epicanthal fold can be fraught with problems and may result in unsightly scarring of the eyelids. These operations are not usually performed even in the Orient and hardly ever in the United States. If excess skin and fat also exist in the lower lids, this is corrected at the same time as upper lid repair.

Uchida (1962), Koonvisal (1969) and others advocate a similar approach with certain technical variations, including anchoring the lower skin margin to the tarsus with nonabsorbable sutures in a manner similar to the original Sayoc (1954) technique. This method of creating a fold by anchoring the skin to the tarsus results in a permanent fold which is present when the eye is open and when it is closed. This technique has been referred to as the "static" method.

The "dynamic" technique, championed by Fernandez (1960), produces a fold in the eye only when the eye is open. It also has the advantage of not disturbing the tarsus or the levator muscle insertion into it.

The type of fold that is acceptable in Japan and other parts of Asia is apparently somewhat different from that accepted in Hawaii or the Western Pacific. A slight crease created in the upper eyelid, which opens the eye somewhat, is considered satisfactory in Japan, whereas in Hawaii and on the mainland of the United States, the fold desired is deeper and is not rounded just above the ciliary border. In eyelids, as in so many other things, the standards of acceptability and beauty are quite different in different parts of the world.

REFERENCES

Alibert, J.-L.: Monographie des Dermatoses ou Précis Théorique et Pratique des Maladies de la Peau. Paris, Daynac, 1832, p. 795.
Arruga, H.: Ocular Surgery. New York, McGraw-Hill Book Co., 1952, p. 171.
Baker, T. J.: Chemical face peeling and rhytidectomy. Plast. Reconstr. Surg. 29:199, 1962.
Bames, H.: (Letter to the Editor) Bags under the eyes. J.A.M.A. 146:692, 1951.
Bames, H.: Baggy eyelids. Plast. Reconstr. Surg. 22:264, 1968.
Barsky, A. J.: Plastic Surgery. Philadelphia, W. B. Saunders Company, 1938, p. 124.
Beare, R.: Surgical treatment of senile changes in the eyelids. The McIndoe-Beare technique. Proceedings of the 2nd. International Symposium on Plastic and Reconstructive Surgery of the Eye and Adnexa, edited by Smith and Converse. St. Louis, The C. V. Mosby Co., 1967, pp. 362–366.
Beer, G. J.: Lehre der Augenkrankheiten. Vienna, C. F. Wappler, 1792.
Beer, G. J.: Lehre von den Augenkrankheiten als Leitfaden Zuseinen Offentlichen Vorlesungen Entworsen. Vol. II, pp. 109–111. Vienna, Lamesina, Heubner & Volke, 1817.
Berens, C.: Aging process in eye and adnexa. Arch. Ophthal. 29:171, 1943.
Bettman, A. G.: Plastic surgery about the eyes. Ann. Surg. 88:994, 1928.
Boo-Chai, K.: Plastic construction of the superior palpebral fold. Plast. Reconstr. Surg. 31:74, 1963a.
Boo-Chai, K.: Further experience with cosmetic surgery of the upper eyelid. Excerpta Med. Int. Cong. Series No. 66. Proceedings of the 3rd International Congress of Plastic Surgery, Washington, D.C., 1963b, pp. 518–524.
Bourguet, J.: La chirurgie esthétique de la face. Le Concours Médical, 1921, pp. 1657–1670.
Bourguet, J.: La chirurgie esthétique de l'oeil et des paupières. Monde Médical, 1929, pp. 725–731.
Callahan, A.: Surgery of the Eye: Diseases. Springfield, Ill., Charles C Thomas, 1956, p. 102.
Castanares, S.: Blepharoplasty for herniated intra-orbital fat. Anatomical basis for a new approach. Plast. Reconstr. Surg. 8:46, 1951.
Castanares, S.: Baggy eyelids. Physiological considerations and surgical technique. Transactions of the 3rd International Congress of Plastic Surgery. Amsterdam, Excerpta Medica Foundation, 1964, pp. 499–506.
Castanares, S.: Correction of the baggy eyelids deformity produced by herniation of orbital fat. Proceedings of the 2nd International Symposium on Plastic and Reconstructive Surgery of the Eye and Adnexa, edited by Smith and Converse. St. Louis, The C. V. Mosby Co., 1967, pp. 346–353.
Caloué, C.: Documents de Chirurgie Plastique et Esthétique. Compte Rendu des Séances de la Société Scientifique Française de Chirurgie Plastique et Esthétique. Paris, Maloine, 1931, pp. 344–353.
Converse, J. M.: The Converse technique of the corrective eyelid plastic operation. In Converse, J. M. (ed.): Reconstructive Plastic Surgery. Philadelphia, W. B. Saunders Company, 1964, pp. 1333–1336.
Converse, J. M.: Treatment of epithelized suture tracts of eyelids by marsupialization. Plast. Reconstr. Surg. 48:477, 1966.
Dufourmentel, C., and Mouly, R.: Traitement operatoire des rides et pochés palpébrales. Ann. Chir. Plast. 3:229, 1958.
Dupuytren, G.: De l'oedéme chronique et des tumeurs enkystées des paupières. Leçons Orales de Clinique Chirurgicale. 2nd ed. Vol. III, pp. 377–378. Paris, Germer-Ballière, 1839.
Edgerton, M. T., and Hansen, F. C.: Matching facial color

with split thickness skin grafts from adjacent areas. Plast. Reconstr. Surg. *21*:455, 1960.

Edgerton, M. T., Webb, W. L., Slaughter, R., and Meyer, E.: Surgical results and psychosocial changes following rhytidectomy. Plast. Reconstr. Surg. *33*:503, 1964.

Elschnig, A.: Fetthernien, Sog. "Tränensacke" der Unterlieder. Klin. Mbl. Augenheilk. *84*:763, 1930.

Erich, J. B.: Surgical elimination of wrinkles, redundant skin and pouches about the eyelids. Proc. Mayo Clin. *36*:101, 1961.

Duverger, C., and Velter, E.: Thérapeutique Chirurgicale Ophtalmologique. Paris, Masson et Cie, 1926, p. 79.

Fernandez, L. R.: The double-eyelid operation in the Oriental in Hawaii. Plast. Reconstr. Surg. *25*:257, 1960.

Fomon, S.: Surgery of Injury and Plastic Repair. Baltimore, The Williams & Wilkins Co., 1939, pp. 135–137.

Fomon, S.: Cosmetic Surgery, Principles and Practice. Philadelphia, J. B. Lippincott Company, 1960.

Fox, S. A.: Ophthalmic Plastic Surgery. New York, Grune & Stratton, 1952.

François, J.: Heredity in Ophthalmology. St. Louis, The C. V. Mosby Co., 1961, pp. 272–275.

Fuchs, E.: Ueber Blepharochalasis (Erschlaffung der Lidhaut). Wien. Klin. Wschr. *9*:109, 1896.

Fuchs, E.: Textbook of Ophthalmology, New York, Appleton, 1899, p. 553.

Ginester, G., Frézières, H., Dupuis, A., and Pons, J.: Chirurgie Plastique et Reconstructrice de la Face. Paris, Flammarion et Cie, 1967, pp. 184–187.

González-Ulloa, M., and Stevens, E. F.: The treatment of palpebral bags. Plast. Reconstr. Surg. *27*:381, 1961.

González-Ulloa, M., and Stevens, E. F.: Senile eyelid esthetic correction. Proceedings of the 2nd International Symposium on Plastic and Reconstructive Surgery of the Eye and Adnexa, edited by Smith and Converse. St. Louis, The C. V. Mosby Co., 1967, pp. 354–361.

Graf, D.: Oertliche erbliche erschlaffung der Haut. Wschr. Ges. Heilk., 1836, pp. 225–227.

Hadley, H. G.: Dermatolysis palpebrarum (blepharochalasis). Rocky Mt. Med. J. *37*:517, 1940.

Hartman, E., Morax, P. V., and Vergez, A.: Complications visuelles graves de la chirurgie des pochés palpébrales. Ann. Oculist *195*:142, 1962.

Holden, H. M.: (Letter to the Editor) Bags under the eyes. J.A.M.A. *146*:692, 1951.

Hotz, F. C.: Ueber das Wesen und die Operation der Sogenannten Ptosis atonica. Arch. Augenheilk. *9*:95, 1880.

Hotz, F. C.: Eine neue Operation für Entropium und Trichiasis. Arch. Augenheilk. *9*:68, 1880.

Hunt, H. L.: Plastic Surgery of the Head, Face and Neck. Philadelphia, Lea & Febiger, 1926, p. 198.

Johnson, J. B., and Hadley, R. C.: The aging face. *In* Converse, J. M. (ed.): Reconstructive Plastic Surgery. Philadelphia, W. B. Sunders Company, 1964, pp. 1306–1342.

Jones, L. T.: An anatomical approach to problems of the eyelids and lacrimal apparatus. Arch. Ophthal. *66*:111, 1961.

Joseph, J.: Plastic operation on protruding cheek. Deutsch. Med. Wschr. *47*:287, 1921.

Joseph, J.: Verbesserung meiner Hängemangenplastik (Melomioplastik). Deutsch. Med. Wschr. *54*:567, 1928.

Journal Universel et Hebdomadaire de Médecine et de Chirurgie Pratiques et des Institutions Médicales, Vol. 1–13, Oct. 1830–Dec. 1833.

Kahn, K.: Plastic surgery in the removal of excessive cutaneous tissues obstructing vision. New York J. Med. *34*:781, 1934.

Kapp, J. F. S.: Die Technik du kosmetischen Encheiresen. Beih. Med. Klin. *3*:65, 1913.

Kapp, J. F. S.: Premature Old Age in Women: A Study in the Tragedy of the Middle Aged. New York, P. L. Baruch, 1925.

Kolle, F. S.: Plastic and Cosmetic Surgery. New York, Appleton, 1911, pp. 116–117.

Koonvisal, L.: Panel on oriental eyelids. Pan-Pacific Surgical Association Congress, Oct., 1969.

Kreiker, A.: Operation der Blepharochalasis mit Hilfe der v. blaskoviesschen Lidfalten Bildenden Nähte. Klin. Mbl. Augenheilk. *83*:302, 1929.

Lewis, J. B., Jr.: The Z-blepharoplasty. Plast. Reconstr. Surg. *44*:331, 1969.

Mackenzie, W.: A Practical Treatise of the Diseases of the Eye. London, Longmans, 1830, pp. 170–171.

May, H.: Reconstructive and Reparative Surgery. Philadelphia, F. A. Davis Co., 1947, pp. 325–326.

McIndoe, A.: Personal communication, 1955.

Millard, D. R.: Oriental peregrinations. Plast. Reconstr. Surg. *16*:319, 1955.

Miller, C. C.: Cosmetic Surgery. The Correction of Featural Imperfections. Chicago, Oak Printing Co., 1908, pp. 40–42.

Miller, C. C.: Cosmetic Surgery. Philadelphia, F. A. Davis Co., 1924, pp. 30–32.

Miller, C. C., and Miller, F.: Folds, bags and wrinkles of the skin about the eyes and their eradication by simple surgical methods. Med. Briefs. *35*:540, 1907.

Noël, A.: La Chirurgie Esthétique. Son Role Sociale. Paris, Masson et Cie., 1926, pp. 62–66.

Noël, A.: La Chirurgie Esthétique. Clermont (Oise), Thiron et Cie, 1928.

Padgett, E. C., and Stephenson, K. L.: Plastic and Reconstruction Surgery. Springfield, Ill., Charles C Thomas, 1948, p. 514.

Panneton, P.: Le blepharochalazis. A propos de 51 cas dans la même famille. Arch. Ophthal. *53*:724, 1936a.

Panneton, P.: Mémoire sur le blepharochalazis. 51 cas dans la même famille. Un. Med. Canada *65*:725, 1936b.

Passot, R.: La chirurgie esthétique des rides du visage. Presse Méd. *27*:258, 1919.

Passot, R.: La correction chirurgicale des ride du visage. Bull. Acad. Méd. Paris *82*:112, 1919.

Passot, R.: La Chirurgie Esthétique Pure (Technique et Résultats). Paris, Gaston Doin et Cie, 1931, pp. 176–180.

Personal correspondence regarding panel discussion on Oriental eyelid surgery. Pan-Pacific Surgical Association Congress, Oct., 1969.

Rees, T. D.: In panel discussion on the cosmetic eyelid plastic operation. Proceedings of the 2nd International Symposium on Plastic and Reconstructive Surgery of the Eye and Adnexa, edited by Smith and Converse. St. Louis, The C. V. Mosby Co., 1967, p. 376.

Rees, T. D.: Technical aid in blepharoplasty. Plast. Reconstr. Surg. *41*:497, 1968.

Rees, T. D.: Technical considerations in blepharoplasty. Transactions of the 4th International Congress of Plastic and Reconstructive Surgery. Amsterdam, Excerpta Medica Foundation, 1969a, p. 1084.

Rees, T. D.: Selection of appropriate technical variations in blepharoplasty. *In* Rycroft, P. V. (ed.): Corneo-Plastic Surgery. New York, Pergamon Press, 1969b, pp. 55–69.

Rees, T. D., and Dupuis, C.: Baggy eyelids in young adults. Plast. Reconstr. Surg. *43*:381, 1969.

Rees, T. D., and Dupuis, C.: Cosmetic blepharoplasty in the older age group. Ophthal. Surg. *1*:30, 1970.

Rees, T. D., and Ristow, B.: Blefaroplastia consideracoes gerais sobre tecnica, pos-operatorio e complicacoes. J. Brasil. Med. *15*:307, 1968.

Reidy, J. P.: Swelling of eyelids. Brit. J. Plast. Surg. *13*:256, 1960.

Sakler, B. R.: Plastic repair of lid hernia with fascia lata. Amer. J. Ophthal. *20*:936, 1937.

Sayoc, B. T.: Plastic construction of the superior palpebral fold. Amer. J. Ophthal. *38*:556, 1954.

Sayoc, B. T.: Absence of superior palpebral fold in slit-eyes; an anatomic and physiologic explanation. Amer. J. Ophthal. *42*:298, 1956.

Sayoc, B. T.: Blepharochalasis in upper eyelids, including its classification. Amer. J. Ophthal. *43*:970, 1957.

Schmidt-Rimpler, H.: Fett-Hernien der oberen Augenlider. Zbl. Prak. Augenheilk. *23*:297, 1899.

Sheehan, J. E.: Plastic Surgery of the Orbit. New York, The Macmillan Company, 1927.

Sichel, J.: Aphorismes pratiques sur divers points d'ophtalmologie. Ann. Oculist *12*:187, 1844.

Silver, H.: A new approach to the operation of blepharoplasty. Brit. J. Plast. Surg. *22*:253, 1969.

Smith, B., and Fasano, C. V.: The diagnosis and treatment of baggy eyelids. Bull. New York Acad. Med. *38*:163, 1962.

Smith, F.: Multiple excision and Z-plasties in surface reconstruction. Plast. Reconstr. Surg. *1*:170, 1946.

Smith, F.: Plastic and Reconstructive Surgery. Philadelphia, W. B. Saunders Company, 1950.

Spaeth, E. B.: The Principles and Practice of Ophthalmic Surgery. 4th ed Philadelphia, Lea & Febiger, 1948.

Steckler, M. I.: Baggy eyelids. Amer. J. Ophthal. *37*:113, 1954.

Stein, B.: Blepharochalasis des Unterlides. Klin. Mbl. Augenheilk. *84*:846, 1930.

Stieren, E.: Blepharochalasis. Report of 2 cases. Trans. Amer. Ophthal. Soc. *13*:713, 1914.

Uchida, J. I.: A surgical procedure for blepharoptosis vera and for pseudo-blepharoptosis orientalis. Brit. J. Plast. Surg. *15*:271, 1962.

von Graefe, C. F.: De Rhinoplastice. Berlin, Dietrich Reimer, 1818, p. 13.

Weidler, W. B.: Blepharochalasis. Report of 2 cases with the microscopic examination. J.A.M.A. *61*:1128, 1913.

Weinstein, A.: Ueber zwei eigenartige Formen des Herabhängens der Haut der Oberlider: Ptosis atrophica und Ptosis adiposa. Klin. Mbl. Augenheilk. *47*: 190, 1909.

Excess skin folds of the upper eyelids are removed by designing an ellipse with a dart that extends as far laterally as necessary and is best slanted slightly upward (B). The marking forceps are used to estimate the skin incision, which is planned so that when the wound is sutured the eye will be open approximately 3 or 4 mm.

Skin excision from the upper eyelids can always be quite generous (C), but overly enthusiastic removal can result in lagophthalmos. This complication can be troublesome, particularly if the eyes remain slightly open during sleep. The cornea then will not be properly lubricated, and desiccation of the cornea can progress to abrasion or ulceration.

The lower limb of the elliptical excision is located approximately 5 to 7 mm. above the ciliary margin, not exactly in the supratarsal fold (B). The final suture line tends to be drawn superiorly, and the scar should end up in the supratarsal fold.

Excess fat at the medial angle of the upper eyelid is teased out through a stab wound in the orbicularis muscle (D). If the horizontal fat compartment bulges, it too can be teased out through a similar stab wound.

The base of the fat herniation is clamped and cauterized. The wound can then be closed with a subcuticular suture of fine nylon (E). Several interrupted sutures can be used at the lateral angle of the wound, where tension is greatest. All sutures are removed on the third or fourth postoperative day. The subcuticular suture is helpful in preventing epithelialized suture tunnels, which are difficult to eradicate, although a technique for removing them has been described by Converse (1966).

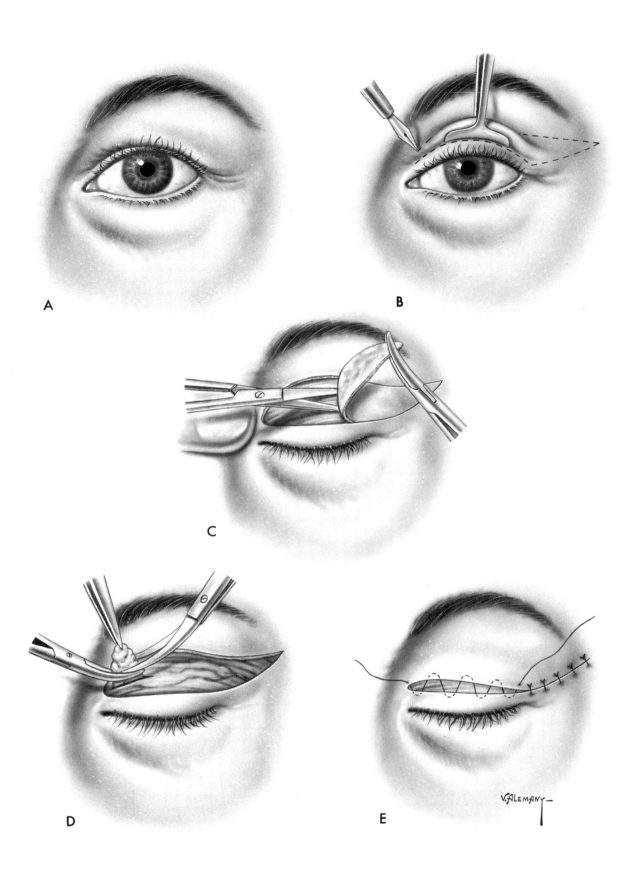

A

B

C

D

E

61

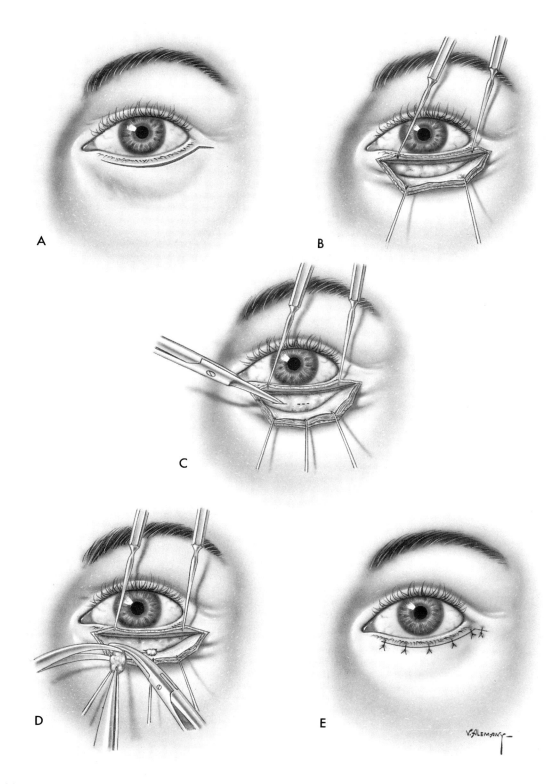

The skin-muscle flap technique is ideally suited for removal of excess periorbital fat in the young patient with familial fat bags and minimal or no excess skin to be removed. An incision is made approximately 2 mm. below the ciliary margin and extending slightly into a lateral crow's foot (A). The incision is carried through skin and muscle, forming a skin-muscle flap (B) exposing the conjunctiva. Excess periorbital fat is removed through stab wounds in the orbital septum (C and D), and the wound is sutured with several interrupted sutures of fine silk or Dermalon (E).

The technique has the distinct advantage of causing minimal trauma to the lid structures. The skin is not undermined, and therefore subsequent procedures to remove excess skin are facilitated.

In some patients a small cuff of skin or skin and muscle can be excised from the skin-muscle flap if redundancy exists after removal of the fat. (From Rees, T. D., and Dupuis, C. C.: Plast. Reconstr. Surg., *43*:381, 1969.)

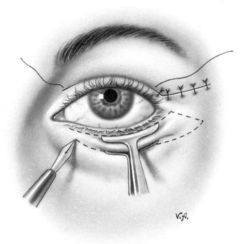

This illustrates Converse's method of preoperative estimation of the amount of skin to be excised from the lower eyelids with marking forceps. The patient should be in a sitting or semisitting position for marking. Care is taken not to drag the lid margin downward. This technique requires expert judgment and considerable experience, and it should not be attempted by the beginner except as a rough means of estimating the amount of skin to be excised. Just as in the undermining technique, the majority of the skin is excised laterally as a triangle. This Converse technique of preoperative skin marking is best used in those patients with marked skin excess and minimal fat bags. These are, in general, the characteristics of the senile lid.

Technique for limited undermining and excision of excess skin of the lower lids in a patient who requires moderate skin excision is shown. The skin-muscle flap is no longer suitable to correct such a deformity, which is usually seen in early middle age. In this more advanced degree of degenerative lid change, the upper eyelids almost always require correction also. It is preferable to correct both upper and lower lids at the same operation, the upper ones first because the lateral extension of the upper eyelid design alters the skin tension lateral to the eye (in the region of the "laugh lines") and thus affects the lower lids.

The lower eyelid incision is usually located 2 to 3 mm. below the ciliary margin, as in the skin-muscle flap operation (A and B). Usually there is a natural skin crease at about that point, which can be used as a guide. The lower eyelid skin is undermined as far as necessary to reach below the redundancy. It should be separated from the orbicularis muscle and, thus, constitutes almost a full-thickness skin graft.

Absolute hemostasis is necessary (B). Each small vessel is coagulated with pinpoint jewelers' forceps.

Excess periorbital fat is removed from the offending compartments of the lower lid through stab wounds in the muscle and orbital septum (C and D). The medial and middle fat pockets are most commonly entered.

The authors' method of judging how much skin is to be excised from the lower eyelid is shown in E. After the skin is undermined and the fat is removed, the redundant skin is draped over the lid margin with traction lightly applied in a superior and lateral direction. The eyeball is depressed by finger pressure from above. This displacement of the globe elevates the lower lid margin, which must be freely mobile. The maneuver is similar to having the patient look upward during local anesthesia. Excess skin is carefully excised, being sure that too much traction is not exerted on the skin so that overcorrection will result. Pressure on the eyeball must be applied with the upper lid open. This technique has the advantage of allowing safe skin removal under general anesthesia or in the heavily sedated patient. It is generally a safer method for the inexperienced surgeon.

The wound is sutured with interrupted 6–0 black silk sutures (F). (From Rees, T. D.: Plast. Reconstr. Surg., 41:497, 1968.)

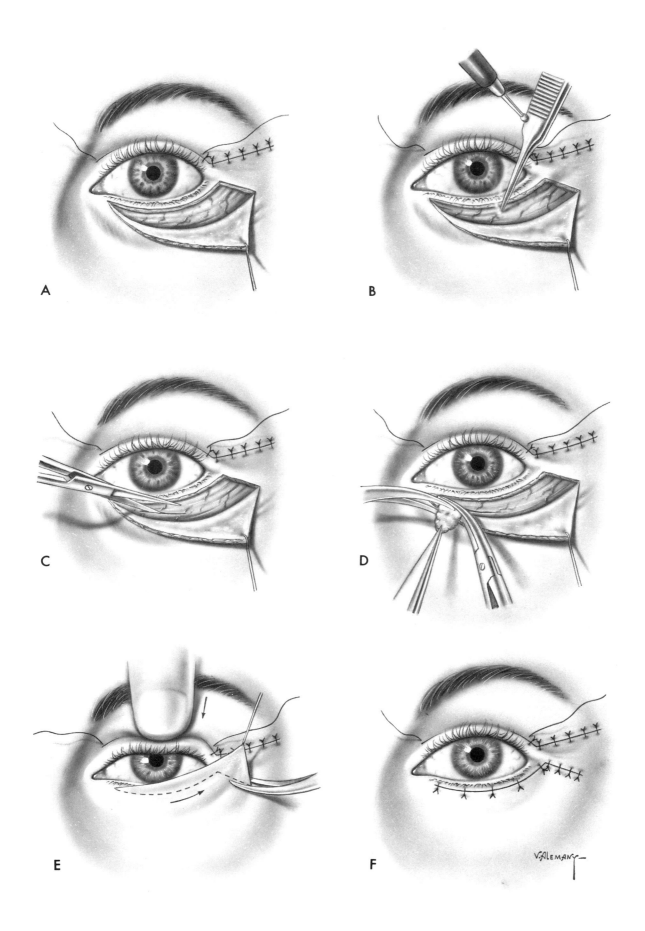

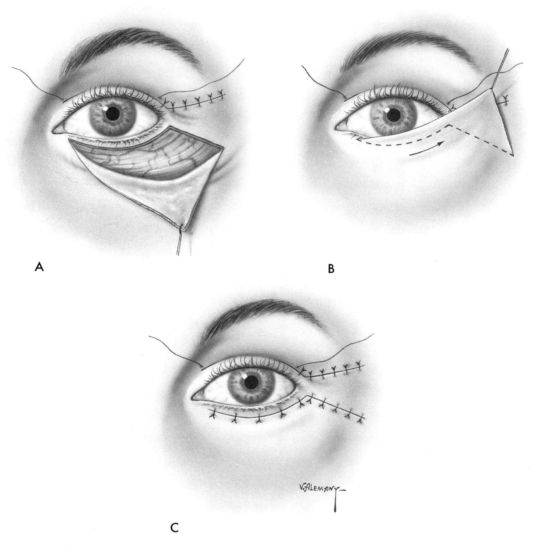

A

B

C

As senile degenerative changes in the eyelids progress, the skin becomes more and more thinned and wrinkled. Skin (and sometimes fat) bags of the lower eyelids form and can extend to and even below the infraorbital rims. The fat compartments of the lower lid become more prominent and sometimes seem to herniate through the overlying muscle. The orbital septum becomes increasingly attenuated. Upper eyelid correction remains essentially as depicted on page 61, but is more frequently associated with operative elevation of the brows, which become more ptotic as years and the pull of gravity take effect (see page 180).

Undermining of the skin of the lower eyelids must be quite extensive in the older patient and almost always must extend beyond the lowermost redundant skin fold (A). It may be necessary to open the muscle and orbital septum widely to retrieve the fat, as stab wounds may not suffice.

Extreme caution must be exercised in removing excessive skin in these patients because of the natural tendency toward ectropion with advancing years (B). As in the more moderate operation, the majority of the skin excess is best excised as a lateral triangle. Hemostasis is most important, as well as delicate handling of tissue. Senile skin can be very thin and friable and is, therefore, easily torn with skin hooks or forceps.

The authors prefer a temporary tarsorrhaphy suture for a few hours after surgery until the lower skin flap adheres to the muscle (C). This is another preventive measure against ectropion.

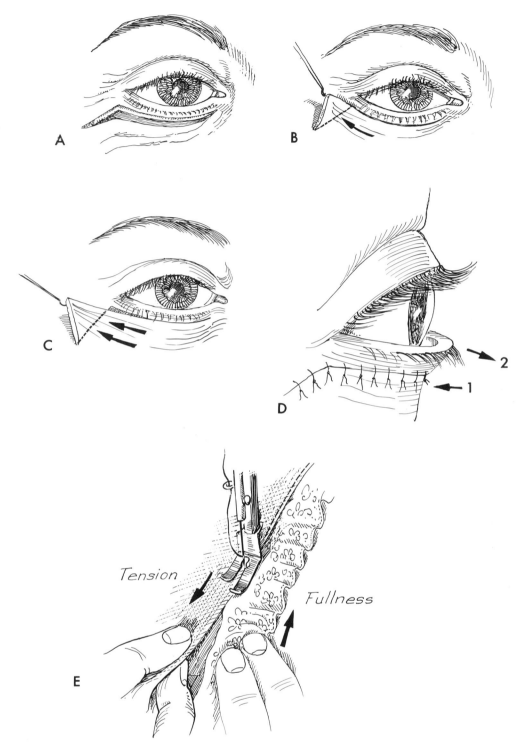

Caution is required in exerting lateral and superior traction on the lower lid skin flap preparatory to excision of the excess. If traction is excessive, and the incision is located just below the tarsal plate, an outward buckling of the plate can occur because of the shortness of the skin and the tightness of the closure. The mechanism can be likened to the dressmaker's trick of making a ruffle (E). The lid will not be in contact with the globe, and tearing can result as well as conjunctival irritation from exposure.

The usual method of trimming excess skin of the lower lids is to exert lateral traction on the skin flap (A and B) and to remove most of the redundancy as a lateral triangle (C) rather than as a horizontal strip along the lower lid, which promotes the possibility of pull down. If too much is excised as a lateral triangle, the lower border of the tarsal plate can buckle forward (D). (Rees, T. D.: Technical Considerations in Blepharoplasty and Rhytidectomy. Transactions of the Fifth International Congress of Plastic and Reconstructive Surgery, Australia, 1971. Sidney, Butterworth & Co. (Australia), Ltd., 1971, p. 1067.)

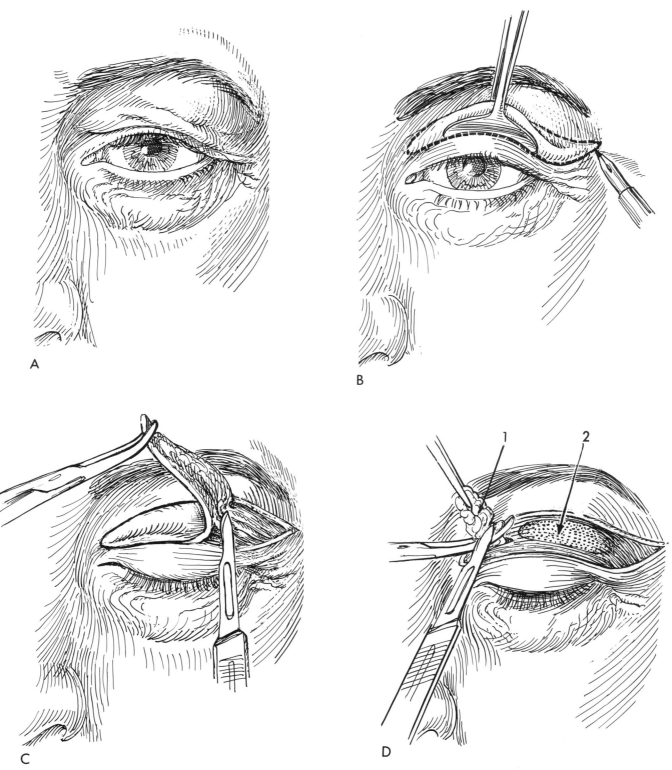

The senile lid, in addition to having considerably more skin excess (blepharochalasis) (*A*) which must be amply removed and tailored laterally (*B* and *C*), also usually contains an extra horizontal sausage-shaped fat collection (*D* 2) which is butter yellow in color. This fat can be removed through the medial lid incision, or by a separate stab wound (*D* 1). It lies between the orbicularis muscle and the levator; therefore, care should be exercised to avoid injuring the levator.

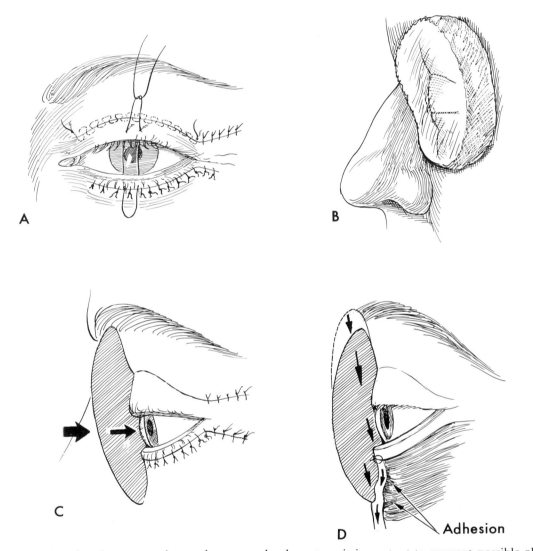

When compression dressings are to be used, a tarsorrhaphy suture is important to prevent possible abrasion of the cornea (A). Even more important, such a temporary suture keeps the dressing (B) from pushing the lower lid downward by shearing force so that it adheres to the muscle at a lower level, resulting in ectropion (C and D).

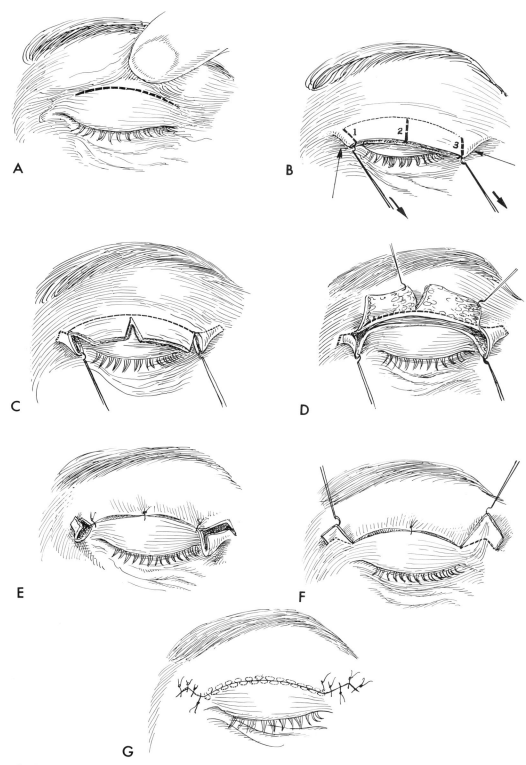

Silver has devised a novel and quite practical approach to the excision of skin folds of the upper eyelids that aids in dealing with the redundancy or "dog-ear" frequently encountered at the medial angle of the wound, where the incision must be terminated before the side wall of the nose is encountered. Instead of marking an ellipse of redundant skin, Silver first makes his incision in the supratarsal fold (A). He then undermines the skin superiorly (toward the brow), creating an apron of skin that is allowed to hang over the lid margin (B). This skin flap is split in three places (C) and pulled laterally (D), which helps to avoid the bunching effect that so often occurs medially.

70

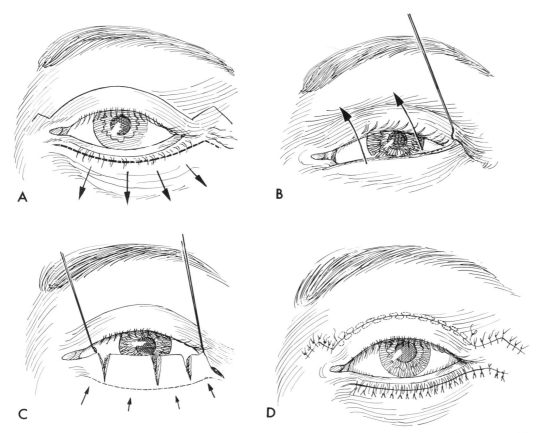

Silver advises a technique similar to that shown in the previous illustration to remove the excess skin of the lower eyelid. The technique is somewhat reminiscent of the multiple incisions and excisions described in early literature on blepharoplasty (Miller, 1908); however, it is unquestionably effective in correcting the presenile or senile lid with marked excess of skin.

The incision is made along the solid line in *A*. The lower flap is undermined as far as necessary and the excess skin is draped over the lid margin (*B*). As in all techniques, it is important that the lid margin be free and lie in a natural position before skin is excised. Depression of the globe to raise the lid margin (p. 65, *E*) might be helpful at this juncture. Multiple cuts are then made in the skin flap (*C*) and the excess is excised. The vertical incisions have the advantage of preventing too much skin from being removed in one cutting. Another considerable advantage of the technique is that by suturing from lateral to medial (*D*), a dog-ear at the lateral edge of the wound is avoided.

Silver's techniques have merit for removing markedly redundant skin, but they should be used only with great care by the beginner and are of doubtful value in the young patient with only a small amount of skin excess.

The flap is trimmed along a complex line (dotted in *C*), paying special attention to the trimming of the excess skin at the medial aspect (*E*). Laterally, too, Silver undermines the skin to connect with his lower eyelid incisions and to help to iron out the crow's feet (*F* and *G*). This technique for the upper lids helps to solve the problem of excess skin at the inner or medial angle of the wound and seems to help in tailoring the outer angle as well. It is most applicable in the older patient with very marked skin excess.

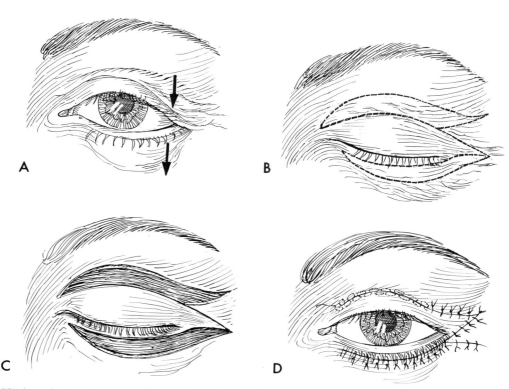

Lewis (1969) has designed an operative variation based on the Z-plasty or interpolated flap principle which he advocates, particularly to elevate the lateral canthal region in those patients with senile ptosis and marked skin excess (A). The skin excisions of the upper and lower lids are marked in the usual fashion, but connected with an oblique limb from the upper to the lower lid to convert the design to a Z-plasty (B). The skin excision is demonstrated in the shaded areas (C). The flaps are then switched (interpolated) and sutured (D), elevating the skin strip extending laterally from the lateral canthus.

This technique has not been used by the authors, but is intriguing. It should be remembered that the fewer incisions the better is the rule to follow, and that one should always plan for future secondary operations and skin trims, which may be made more complicated by the presence of connecting incisions.

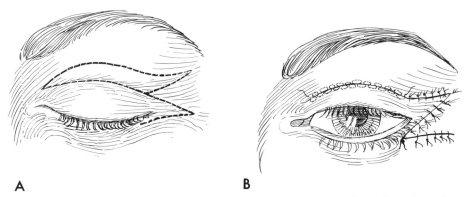

A   **B**

An alternate procedure recommended by Lewis to elevate the lateral canthus when there is no redundancy of lower eyelid skin, but excision of upper lid skin is required. A small interpolation flap is designed from the upper lid in the form of a Z-plasty (*A*). The flap is let into the lower lid and sutured (*B*).

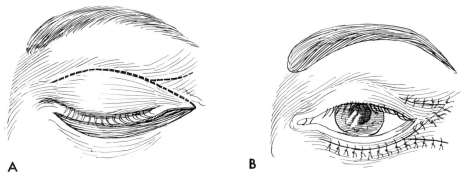

A   **B**

Lewis's variation for a complete lower blepharoplasty and Z-blepharoplasty in the external canthal area and lateral portions of the upper lids only (*A* and *B*). In this case the interpolation flap is from the upper to the lower lid, which helps to elevate the lateral canthus. It is useful only when little or no redundancy of the upper lid skin is present.

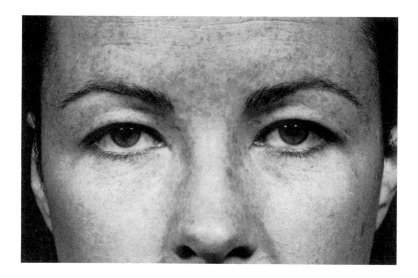

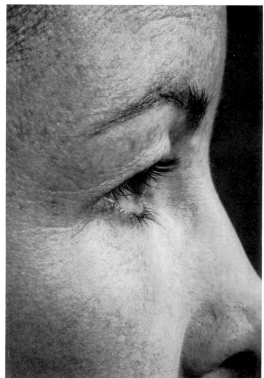

This shows a skin fold of the upper eyelids in a 22 year old girl. Such a fold is easily removed by the technique shown on page 61. In the young patient, care should be exercised in measuring the skin with the marking forceps so that not too much skin is excised. The young eyelid is less forgiving than the senile lid, and lagophthalmos can result more easily. Very early reports in the literature described excess upper lid skin folds that were probably similar to this example. The fold may resemble the so-called mongoloid fold seen in Asians, in spite of a lack of Asian heritage.

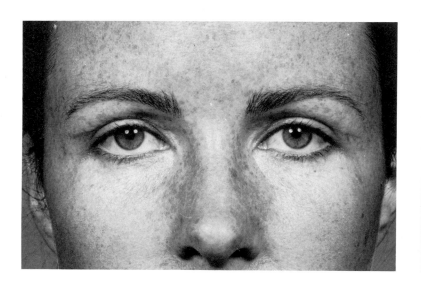

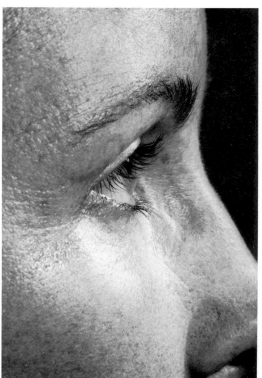

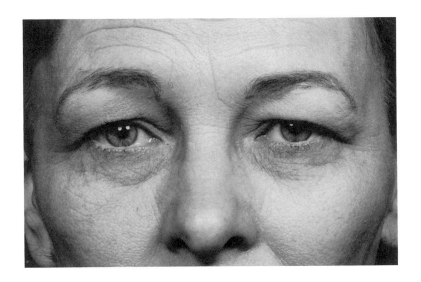

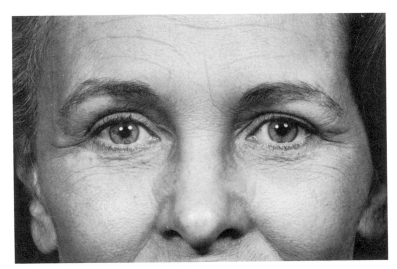

Another example of marked redundancy of the skin of the upper eyelids is shown. The surgical result was satisfactory, but only part of the patient's problem has been corrected. There is, in addition, a degree of ptosis of the eyebrows which gives the effect of a slight downward slant to the eyes. The forehead has few horizontal wrinkles (which usually appear later in life); this makes elevation of the brows difficult because the scar resulting from such a procedure would very likely be noticeable.

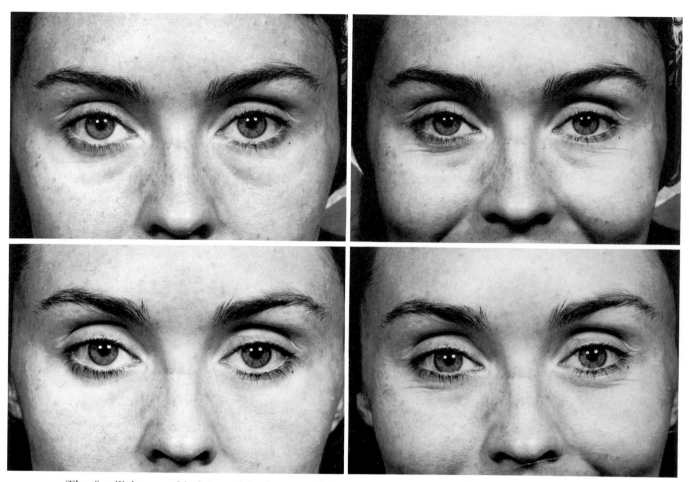

The familial type of bulging of the lower eyelids caused by excessive (or pseudoherniated) periorbital fat usually occurs in the second or third decade of life. It is easily corrected by the skin-muscle flap technique of McIndoe and Beare (page 62), which produces minimal trauma and rarely requires any excision of skin in these young patients.

The incision is placed 2 to 3 mm. below the ciliary margin. The offending fat compartments are usually found to be the medial and middle ones, as described by Castanares (1951). Fat is removed through stab wounds in the orbicularis muscle and the orbital septum. Four to six sutures suffice to close the wound. On occasion, a small strip of skin and muscle can be trimmed if these tissues are redundant. Sutures are removed in 48 hours.

Preoperative views are at the top; postoperative views are below. In the two photographs on the right, the patient is smiling. Comparison with the left-hand views will demonstrate that, on animation of the facial muscles, even in such a young adult, fine lines or rhytides remain after surgery, though they are usually improved by the procedure. Patients should be advised that these "laugh lines" will not be eradicated by the operation. (From Rees, T. D., and Dupuis, C. C.: Plast. Reconstr. Surg., 43:381, 1969.)

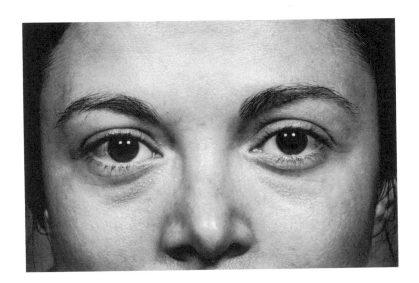

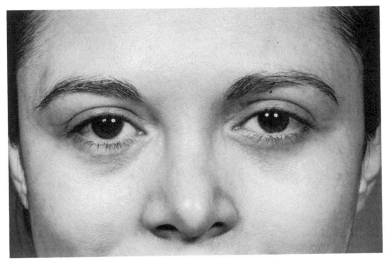

A similar problem of familial palpebral bags is shown in a young patient in whom the condition is slightly more advanced. Familial fat bulges are progressive and should be removed early in their development. The upper eyelids may or may not be involved in a similar manner.

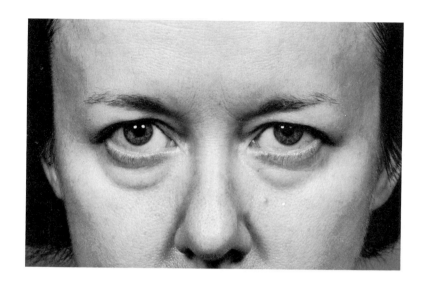

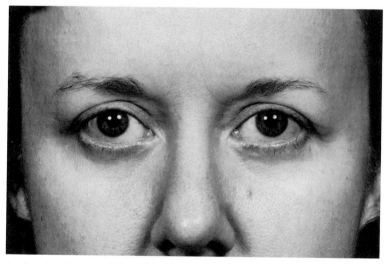

This patient had marked redundancy of fat of the lower eyelids with minimal skin excess. The skin-muscle flap technique sufficed in this patient without removal of skin. Such a patient demonstrates the upper limit of fat abundance that can be removed without skin excision.

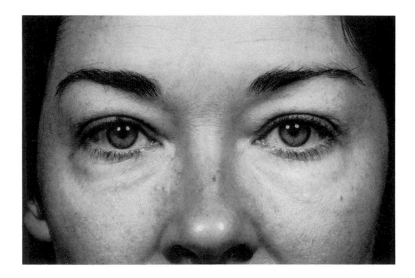

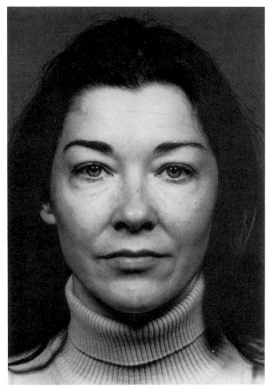

This attractive young woman represents an ideal patient for blepharoplasty. She had been aware of her "puffy" eyes since childhood, for the condition was transmitted through the maternal side of her family. With age, the patient began to notice a definite sense of heaviness in her eyes and complained that her eyes fatigued easily. A standard skin-muscle flap blepharoplasty was done, with removal of a small strip of skin and of medial fat from the upper eyelids. Note the dramatic effect of this surgery on the patient's facial expression: the "dissipated" look has vanished.

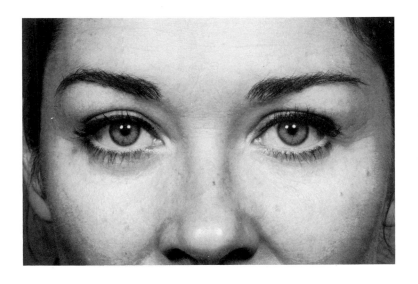

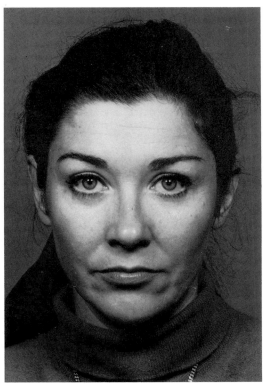

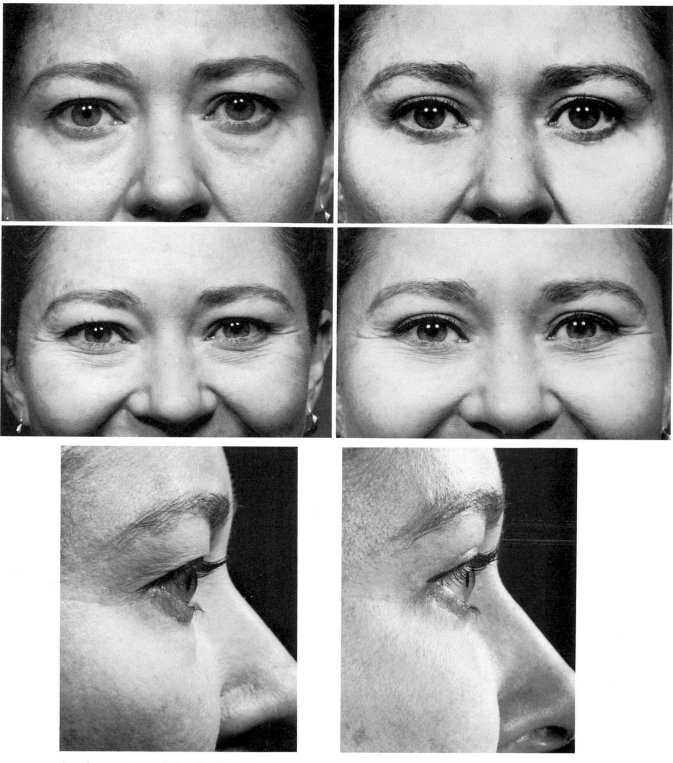

Another variant of the familial condition of pseudoherniation of orbital fat, but in a slightly more advanced state, is demonstrated by this patient, whose upper lids are involved as well as the lower lids. The fat pockets of the upper lid in such patients consist of a medial collection of whitish "fibro-fat" as well as a sausage-shaped horizontal fat pad that is butter-yellow in color and lies between the orbicularis oculis muscle and the levator expansion.

The operative procedure is slightly more complicated. It is necessary to remove an ellipse of excess skin from the upper lids and take out the offending fat from the upper lid compartments. The lower eyelids will also require removal of a small strip of skin, but the skin-muscle flap operation can be used, after which a small amount of undermining is done to provide a skin cuff for excision.

Again, note that the fine wrinkles of facial expression are *not* eliminated by the surgery. The lateral views show how the appearance of the eye is "cleared" by this technique.

80

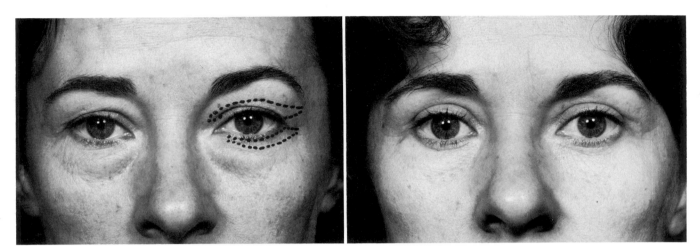

Upper and lower palpebral bags were corrected by the technique described and illustrated on page 65. Dotted lines in *A* indicate the approximate skin incisions required; note the small amount of skin to be removed from the lower lids in spite of the relatively large visible swellings. Lid bulges in this area are primarily due to fat, and the actual skin excess is minimal to moderate.

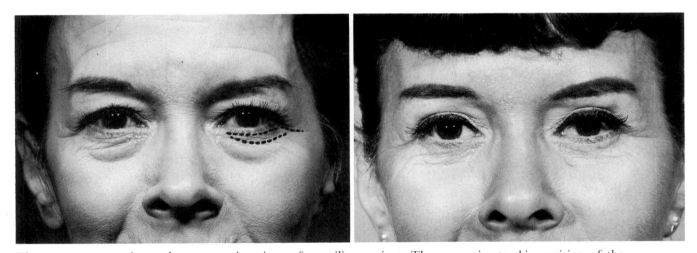

These are preoperative and postoperative views of a smiling patient. The approximate skin excision of the lower lids is marked in the preoperative photograph. Note that the fine rhytides that appear when the facial muscles are animated are still present after surgery. Patients such as this, with particularly deep wrinkles, complain that the wrinkles are even more noticeable after blepharoplasty. The reason is that the underlying fat formerly present smoothed the skin and ironed out some of the wrinkles. If wrinkling is marked after primary surgery, deep chemical peel should be considered to improve the wrinkles and possibly even to obliterate them.

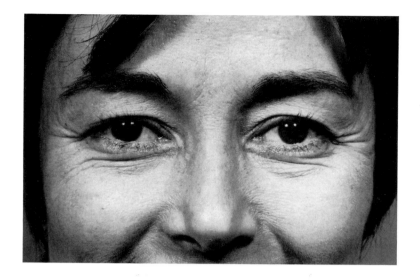

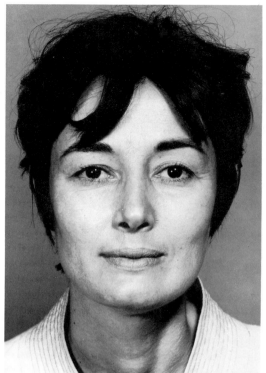

(See opposite page for legend.)

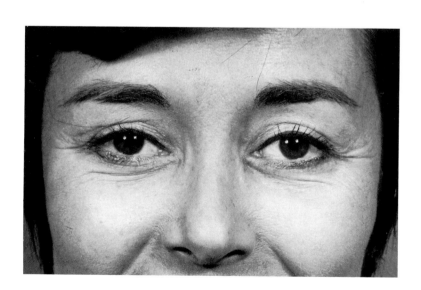

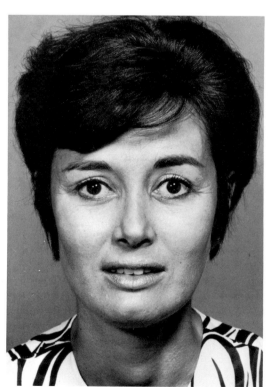

82

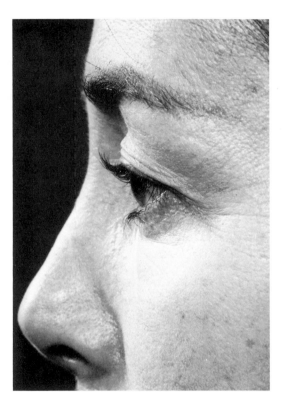 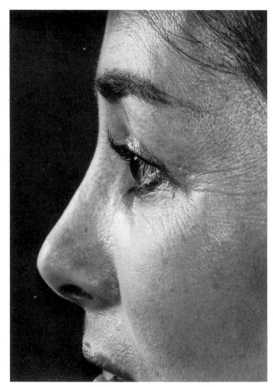

This patient was in her early thirties and had a typical familial skin fold of the upper lid, the type that was described in the early literature on the subject and that has been termed "blepharochalasis." In such patients it is sometimes wise to plan an operation in two stages several months apart in order to avoid excess skin removal in the first stage, which may result in lagophthalmos.

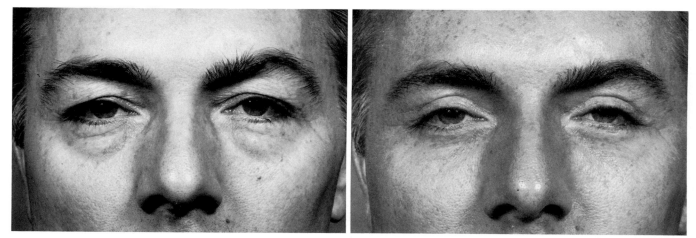

This is a 38 year old man with moderately advanced blepharochalasis, or excess skin folds of the upper lids, and palpebral bags of the lower lids, consisting mainly of pseudohernias of periorbital fat. Correction was achieved by the technique shown on page 65.

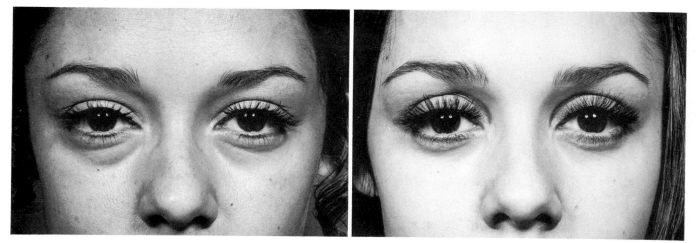

This young woman had palpebral bags of fat and skin. In such a patient skin and fat are equally at fault, and the deformity cannot be corrected with a skin-muscle flap. The skin must be undermined and redraped; the procedure for limited undermining as required in this case is shown on page 65.

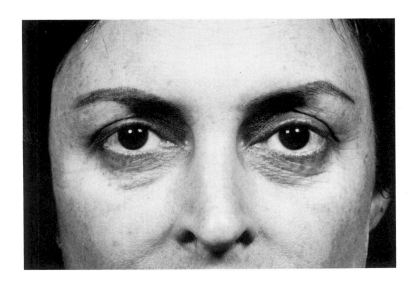

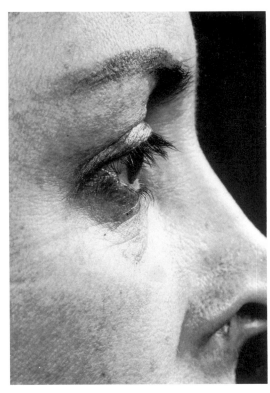

The essential problem in this woman, who is approaching middle age, is excess skin of the lower eyelids as well as increased pigmentation of the skin. Such pigmentation is common in some families and in some peoples, particularly those of Mediterranean origin. The dark coloration cannot be changed by blepharoplasty, but often it will seem to be lightened by the operation because many wrinkles are removed or smoothed out. If the fat pockets are prominent, tangential lighting will cast a shadow, further accentuating the dark circles. Patients without such dark pigmentation may occasionally show discoloration below the eyes for many months if ecchymosis following surgery was unusually severe. This results from hematoma and the accumulation of breakdown products of blood, particularly pigments; there is no known method of hastening its removal. Increased pigmentation can be improved by deep chemabrasion after blepharoplasty.

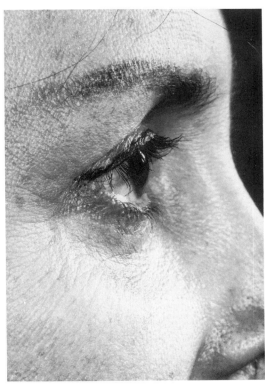

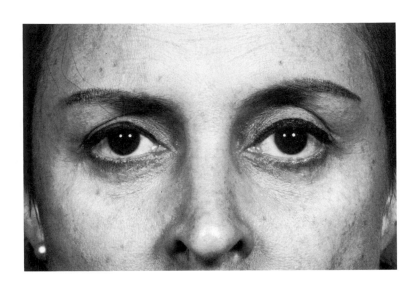

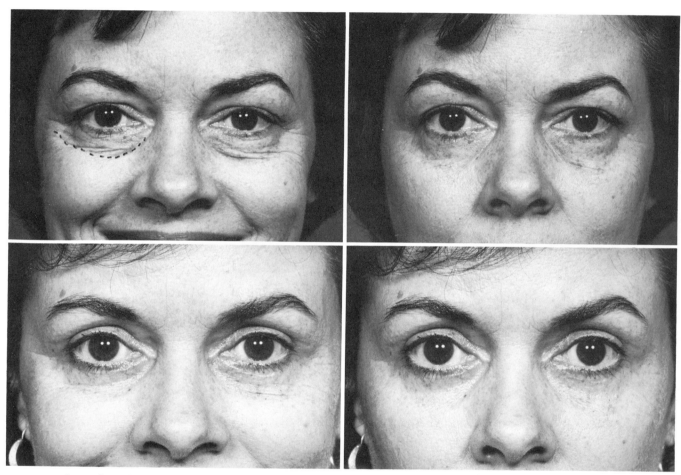

Sometimes in patients approaching or in middle age the excess of skin of the lower lids is more apparent in animation than when the face is in repose. The excess becomes apparent on animation because of the interaction of the underlying orbicularis oculis muscle fibers and the flaccid skin on top. This is often the chief complaint of a patient in this age group and may be associated with little or no excess fat.

Blepharoplasty in such patients does not eliminate these expression wrinkles, but with very wide undermining, as indicated by the dotted line in the preoperative animated (smiling) photo, the postoperative result can be quite an improvement. This degree of change cannot be expected in all patients, a fact that is best pointed out to the patient before surgery.

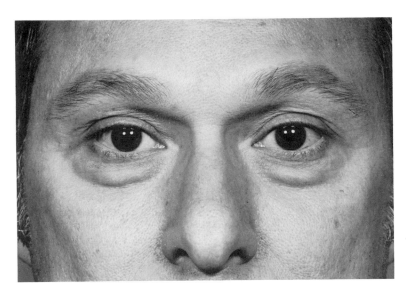

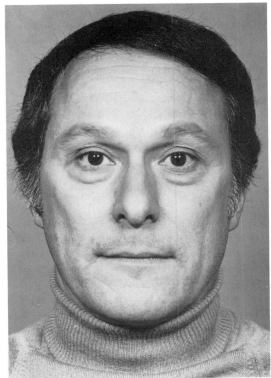

Excess fat with some redundancy of skin in a young man is shown. This problem requires excision of skin as well as fat, although the skin excision is minimal. Limited skin undermining is needed, as shown on page 65. The skin-muscle flap can still be used; however, the fat can also be removed through stab wounds in the orbital septum. Note that the amount of sclera visible is only slightly increased after the operation, provided the amount of skin excised is conservative. The operation results in a brighter and clearer expression that is particularly noticeable in the full-face photographs. The facies also appears more rested.

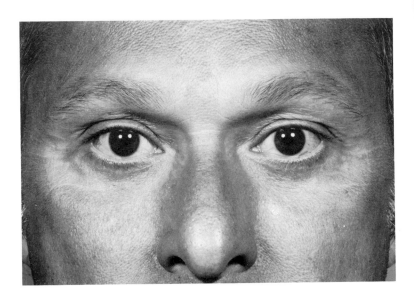

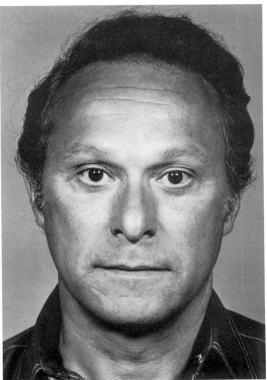

87

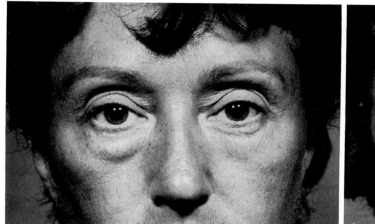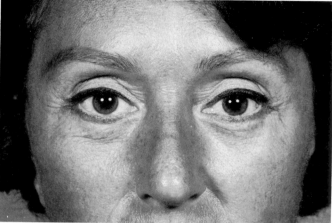

Note that in the preoperative photograph of this patient there is a marked discrepancy between the size of the bulges caused by the orbital fat pockets of the lower lids. The right lower lid contains considerably more fat than the left. Expert professional photographs such as this (by Don Allen) are particularly important to guide the surgeon during blepharoplasty. Each detail, including asymmetrical problems such as this one, becomes apparent in the photograph, yet may not be obvious during physical examination of the patient.

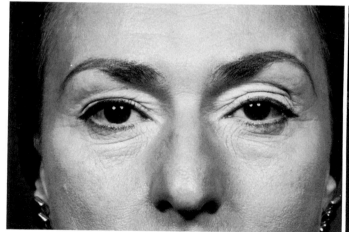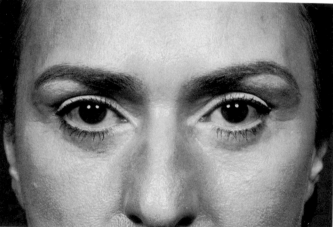

As middle age advances, certain changes occur in the eyelid skin as well as the pseudoherniations of fat, which tend to increase. The skin changes may be accentuated by exposure to the wind and sun, by diminution of the effects of female hormones, by recurrent edema and by other factors. The skin becomes thinner and therefore more wrinkled. The sebaceous glands may increase in number, and sometimes many small adenomas appear. Xantholasma patches develop in some patients. These pictures show a typical set of changes in a patient in her fourth decade of life, and the improvement obtained by blepharoplasty. (From Rees, T. D., and Guy, C. L.: Surg. Clin. N. Amer. *51*:353, 1971.)

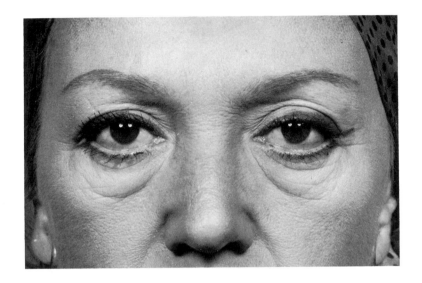

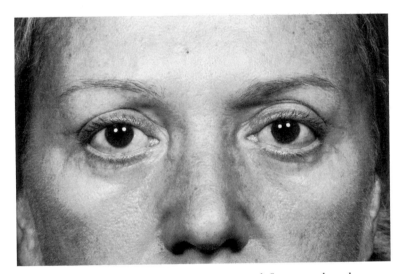

The preoperative photograph of this patient shows two unusual features that the surgeon needs to observe and discuss with a prospective patient: the moderate degree of scleral "show" and the slight exophthalmos. The scleral show cannot be improved by surgery, but it also should not be increased unless too much skin is excised. Often, however, a slight exophthalmos can be ameliorated by removal of orbital fat.

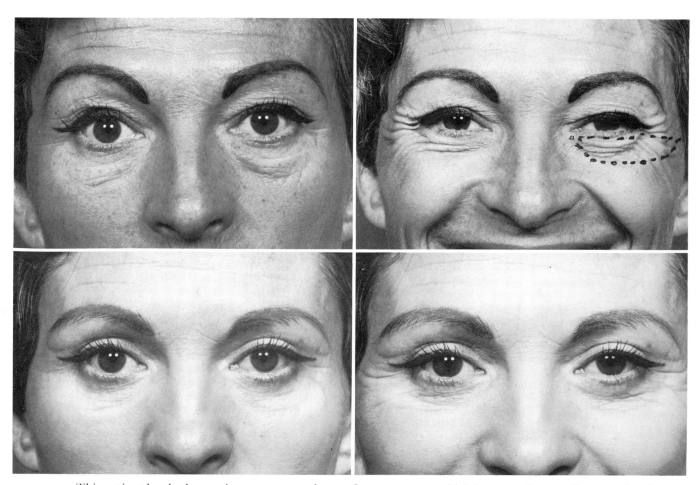

This patient has had excessive exposure to the sun for many years, which has caused severe degenerative changes in the skin. There are many deep lines and wrinkles, which are markedly aggravated by any kind of facial animation. Definite but somewhat limited correction can be achieved by wide undermining of the affected skin. Fat removal, on the other hand, was conservative in this patient. Undermining must extend far enough laterally to include the "laugh lines," as has been pointed out by Gurdin (dotted lines in the preoperative "animated" photo). Wide wedges of skin are also removed from the lateral extensions of the incisions. The postoperative view showing the patient smiling demonstrates the amount of correction possible with this technique. Before surgery it should be made clear to patients with weatherbeaten skin and rhytidosis that blepharoplasty will not eliminate the deeper lines.

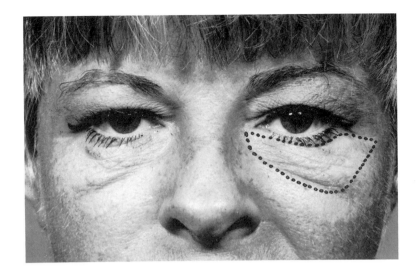

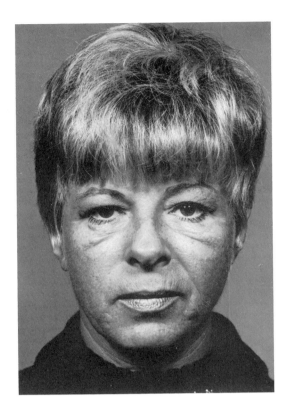

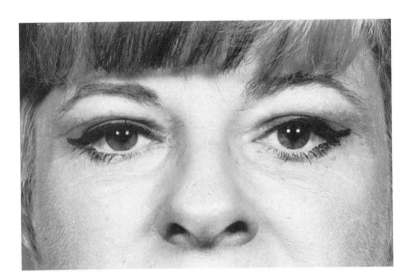

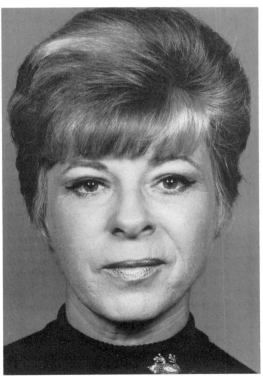

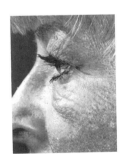 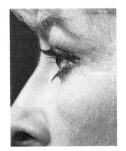

A woman aged 40 who shows marked premature aging of the skin of the eyelids in the preoperative photographs. The skin is wrinkled and thickened, and the "bags" extend well down into the cheeks. This condition is partly the result of a hereditary predisposition, but it has been hastened considerably in this patient by excessive exposure to actinic rays. The dotted line in the preoperative close-up indicates the area that must be undermined in order to achieve correction of the loose skin. Note that the undermining extends down to the cheek. Skin like this is quite leathery and thick. There is considerable inherent support, so that ectropion is unlikely; nevertheless, great care must be exercised as usual in the resection. The technique shown on page 66 is particularly useful in this type of patient. The marked change in the patient's entire facial appearance from blepharoplasty alone is most noticeable. (From Rees, T. D.: Technical Considerations in Blepharoplasty. Transactions of the Fourth International Congress of Plastic and Reconstructive Surgery. Excerpta Medica Foundation, Amsterdam. 1969, p. 1084.)

One of the pitfalls of blepharoplasty is to be found in the patient with large fat bags of the lower lids, but with virtually no excess skin (A). In fact, the skin is stretched tight by the bulging fat, and removal of the fat may produce a slight concavity (C 2). No skin is excised in such patients. Instead, the undermined skin is looked upon as a full-thickness skin graft (B) and is draped over every contour of the wound exactly as a graft would be applied. Bridging over pockets or concavities can create a dead space (D 3), where fluid or blood can accumulate; subsequent contracture of the flap (E 5) can cause ectropion (E 4). The surgeon must always be cognizant of the fact that under anesthesia (even local anesthesia), the lower eyelid is relaxed and tends to sag. Failure to take this into account can result in too much skin being excised. Pressure on the globe elevates the lower lid skin into true position (H), and this maneuver can safely be exaggerated somewhat in many patients.

The skin flap (which is actually more of a full-thickness graft) must be applied exactly to the somewhat concave surface beneath (F and G). This usually leaves little excess to be resected in such patients.

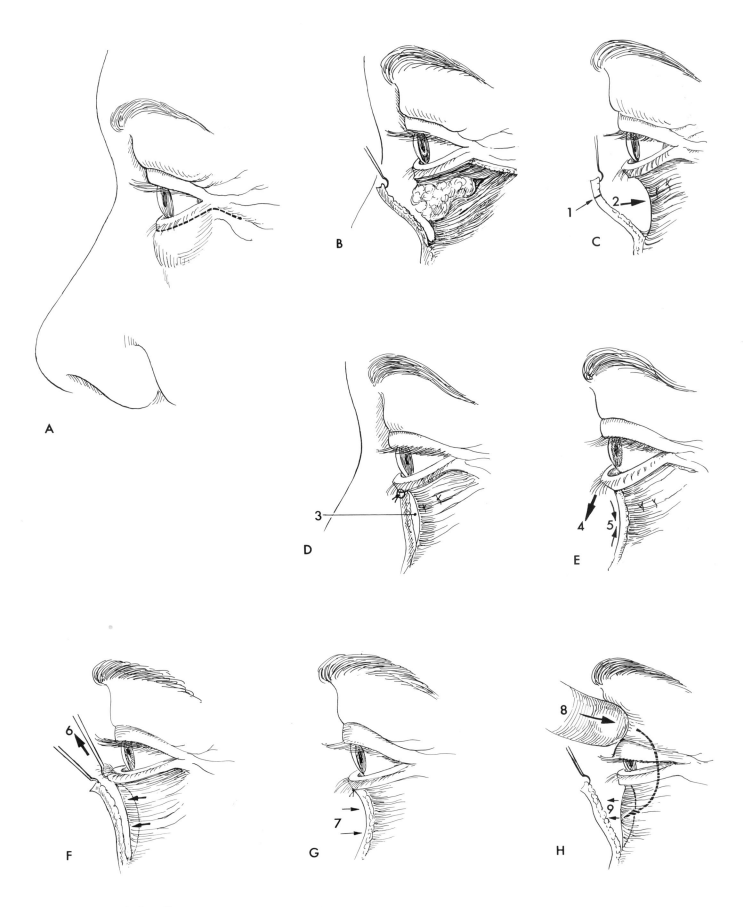

(See opposite page for legend.)

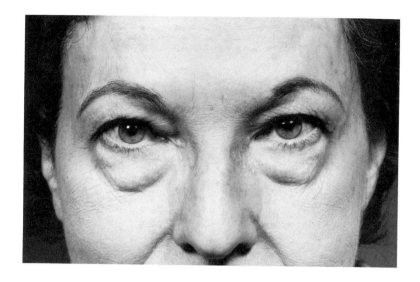

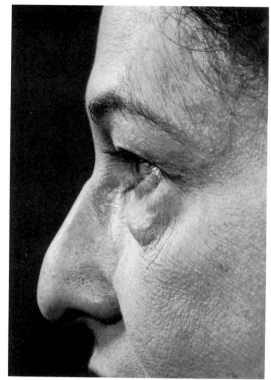

The authors have been impressed by several patients with very large fat pockets of the lower eyelids who had some degree of scleral show or even mild ectropion after surgery, even when minimal skin was excised. The mechanism for this is possibly explained in the drawings on page 93. Preoperative estimates of the skin excision in patients such as this are obviously valueless and even dangerous.

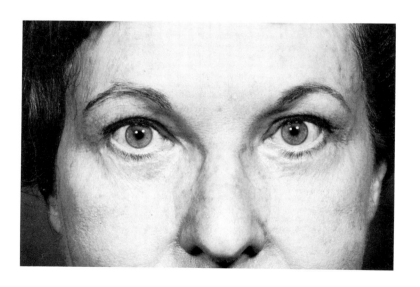

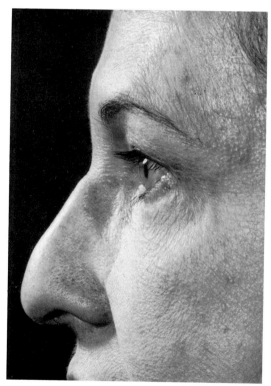

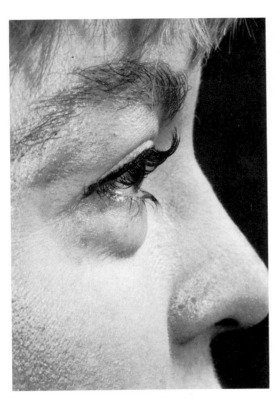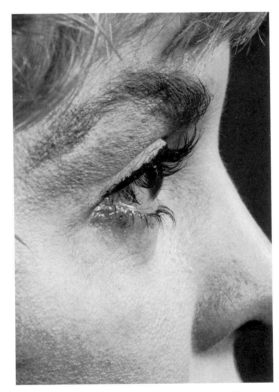

A 24 year old patient had marked bulging of the lower eyelids caused by pseudoherniation of fat. The condition was present in her mother and grandmother as well. Correction was obtained by the skin-muscle flap technique, but it was also necessary to remove a 3-mm. strip of muscle from the upper margin of the orbicularis because a localized ridge of muscle was present. Many patients have such a ridge lying horizontally just at the level of the tarsal plate, which becomes activated on facial animation. These ridges can be trimmed, but this should be done with great care to prevent a drag on the lower lid.

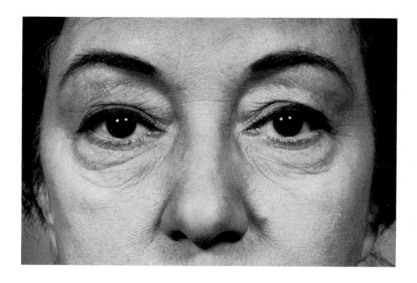

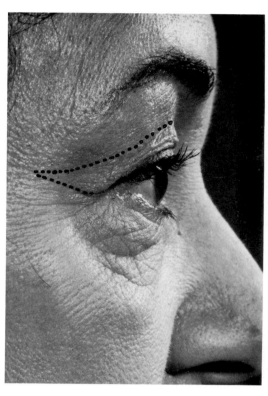

An attractive woman of middle age had marked palpebral bags of the upper and lower eyelids caused by a combination of overabundant periorbital fat and progressive degenerative changes in the skin. Correction of such a condition requires generous excision of both skin and fat. The elliptical excision of the upper eyelid skin must be carried well laterally, to or beyond the lateral corner of the eyebrow (p. 97); otherwise, a small dog-ear can appear at this angle of the wound. These extreme lateral extensions of the incision, which are carried at a slight upward angle, are quite worrisome to most patients until the scars have settled in. Their presence should be explained to the patient before the operation. The lateral dog-ear, if left, can result in a pleat or overhang as shown on page 97. The lower lids of this patient were dealt with as shown on page 97.

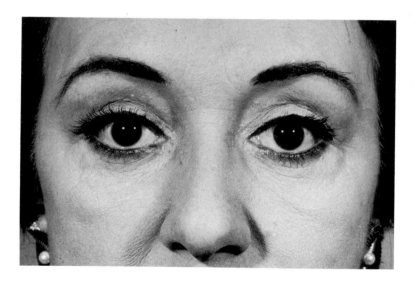

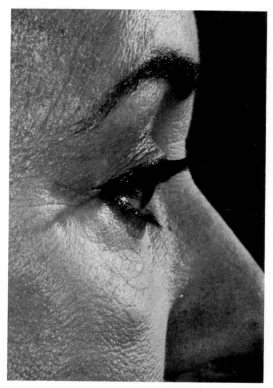

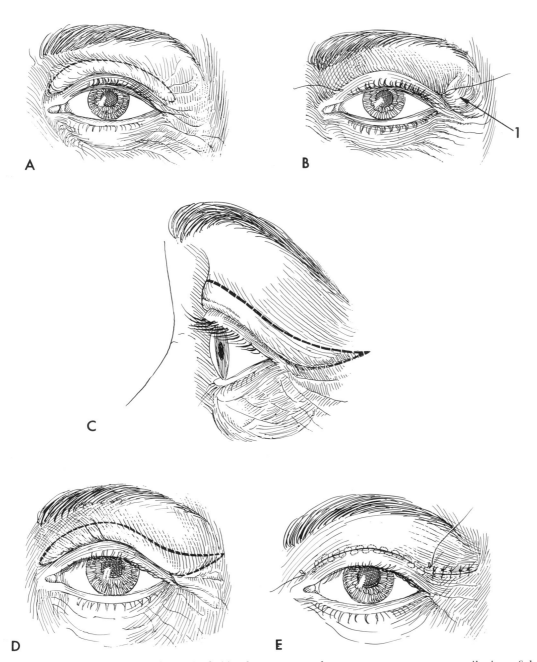

In the senile patient or in those with marked skin changes secondary to exposure, accurate tailoring of the upper lid excision is most important. Ending the lateral extent of the incision at the lateral canthus (*A*), as can be done in the young patient, results in a "dog-ear" or pucker of the skin laterally (*B* 1). In such patients it is best to extend the lateral incision quite far laterally in natural skin creases and slanted slightly superiorly (*C* and *D*). This eliminates the skin fold and tailors the incision to prevent a dog-ear while at the same time tightening the skin lateral to the canthus, which aids in the lower eyelid surgery (*E*).

One disadvantage is that the eyebrow may end closer to the lid margin after such trimming. It may be necessary to simultaneously elevate the brow, or to advise the patient to pluck the eyebrows of the lateral two thirds of the brow and create a new line with makeup pencil. (Rees, T. D.: Technical Considerations in Blepharoplasty and Rhytidectomy. Transactions of the Fifth International Congress of Plastic and Reconstructive Surgery, Australia, 1971. Sidney, Butterworth & Co. (Australia), Ltd., 1971, p. 1067.)

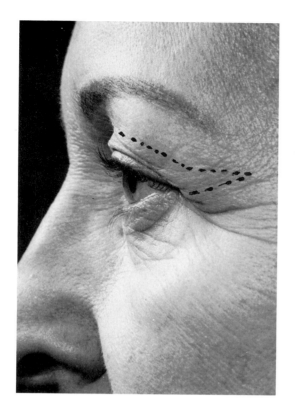

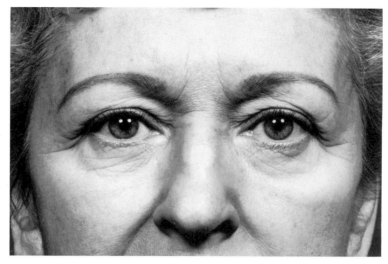

Despite very generous excision of redundant skin from the upper eyelids, in which the line of incision is carried far laterally even beyond the farthest extent of the eyebrow, there can be a persistent skin fold after surgery. It will appear at the point where the brow is fullest in patients with ptosis of the brows. When the maximum amount of skin has been removed from the upper lids, and lagophthalmos would occur if any more were taken, the operative result can be improved only by a brow lift (an elliptical skin excision above the brow) or sometimes by a temporal lift as shown on page 97. The temporal lift, to be effective in such a patient, must achieve upward rotation, which requires extensive undermining of the temporal skin medially as far as the brow and almost to the upper canthus. This procedure can be somewhat hazardous, and the temporal branch of the facial nerve must be carefully protected.

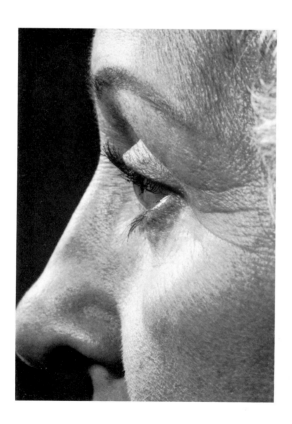

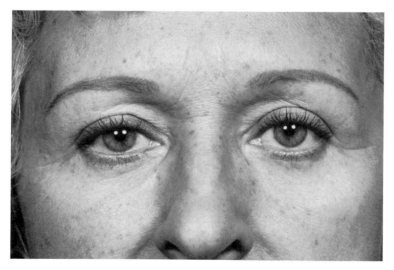

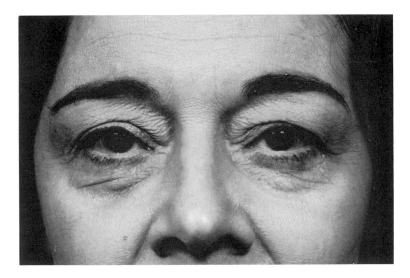

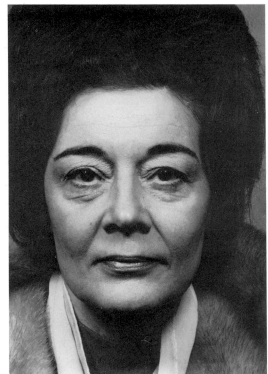

A thorough and quite extensive blepharoplasty with generous skin excision can often result in a remarkable improvement in the entire facial appearance, particularly when the rest of the face is much younger looking than the eyelids. In this respect blepharoplasty can have a much more profound effect on the facial appearance than a face lift, because the eyes are the real focal point of facial expression. It is the eyes, too, that are first noticed when one meets a stranger.

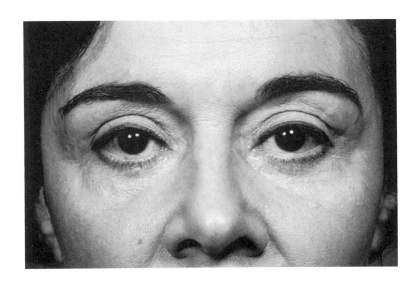

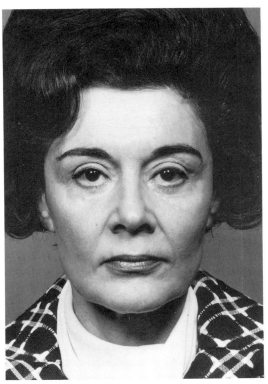

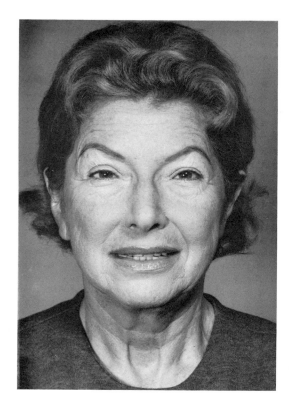

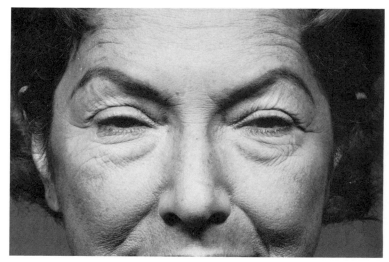

In some older patients, blepharochalasis and marked excess of orbital fat can be of such an extent that vision is interfered with. Symptoms of heaviness, blurring, and easy fatigability are present. Furrowing of the forehead by horizontal frown lines is common in such patients because of the effort required to elevate the brows to improve vision. Note the diminution in the forehead frown lines in the postoperative photographs taken one year after the operation.

Blepharoplasty and facial plastic surgery with wide undermining of the neck and jawline achieved a good result in this patient. But the blepharoplasty result stands out as giving the greatest improvement in the appearance of the face.

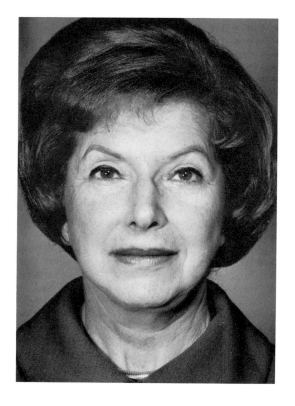

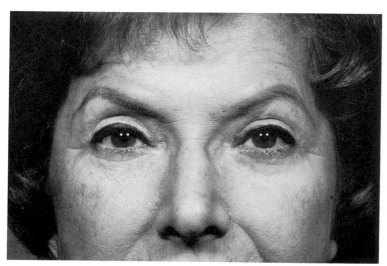

100

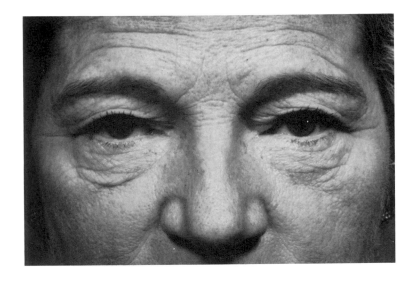

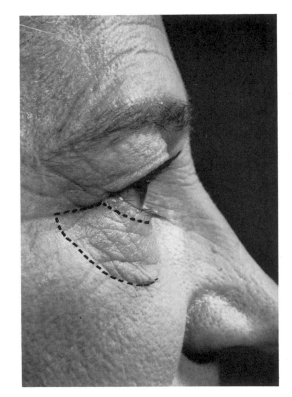

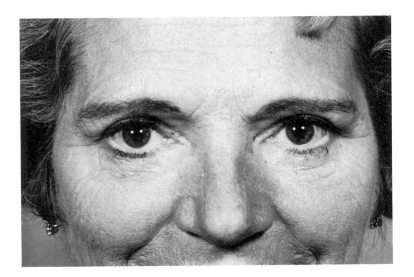

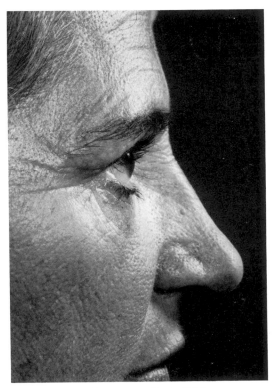

Blepharoplasty can sometimes produce alterations in facial appearance that are almost startling. Wide undermining, as indicated by the dotted lines on the preoperative lateral view, is mandatory. In this patient, excess skin was the principal problem, and very little fat was excised. Note that excision of the heavy skin fold of the upper lid (variously called dermochalasis or blepharochalasis) has apparently lowered the eyebrows. This in itself is not particularly objectionable, but it does limit the number of operations that can be done on the upper lids; elevation of the brows by a suprabrow excision must eventually be resorted to.

101

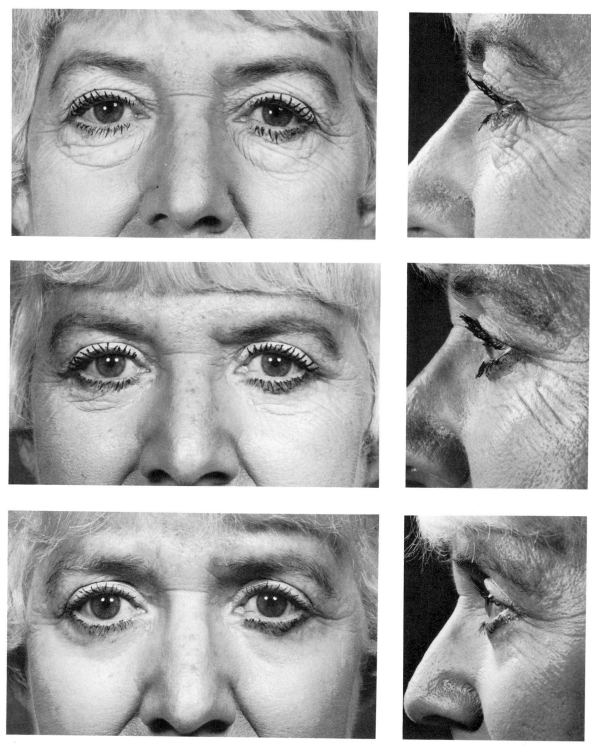

This patient shows marked rhytidosis of the face and eyelids. Improvement in such a patient can be obtained only by blepharoplasty with wide undermining, followed in several weeks by a deep skin peel that can be done selectively to the eyelids and not necessarily to the entire face. This patient's peel followed her blepharoplasty by six weeks.

The preoperative condition is shown in the upper views, the postoperative in the center, and the final result after chemical peel at the bottom. Note the smoothness in skin texture obtained from peeling.

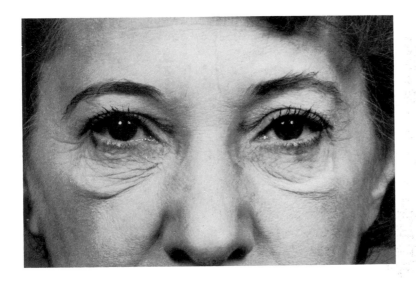

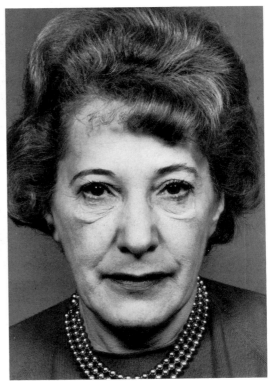

A patient had marked skin bags but little periorbital fat. Skin folds that extend to the cheeks or even lower can be very difficult to eradicate. Improvement will be obtained only by extensive undermining. Small bags or depressions of the cheeks themselves cannot be greatly improved by operation, even with wide undermining. These cheek bags, or "malar bags," should be spotted by the surgeon preoperatively and pointed out to the patient. (From Rees, T. D., and Guy, C. L.: Surg. Clin. N. Amer. *51*:353, 1971.)

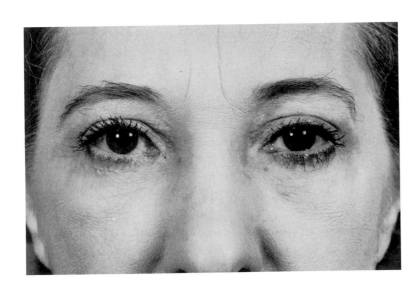

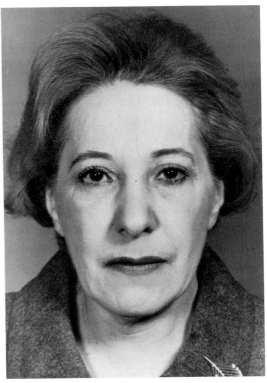

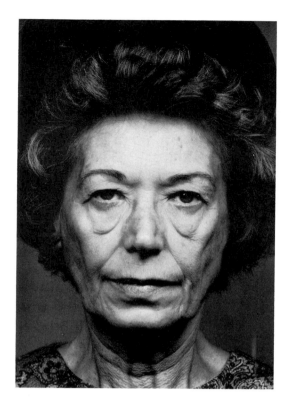

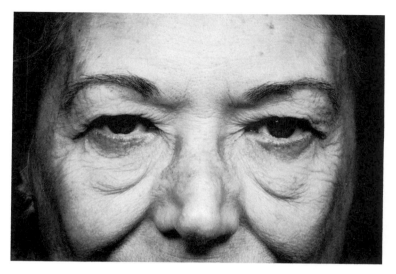

Blepharoplasty may be performed for advanced senile type eyelids. Undermining must be extensive but tempered by conservative skin excision; the danger of inducing ectropion is great in the older patient. Lid structures are apt to be attenuated and weakened, particularly the orbicularis oculis muscle. The aim of surgery is to "clean up" the facial expression, not to change it, and certainly not to produce an illusion of youth. Certain limitations of a morphological nature exist in older people, and they must be accepted as part of the postoperative appearance too. Skin wrinkles will still be present, and in spite of extensive removal of upper eyelid skin folds, these cannot be completely obliterated. Ptosis of the brows is almost always a strong factor in the older patient, who also usually has considerable horizontal wrinkling of the forehead skin. These wrinkles facilitate elevation of the brows, inasmuch as the resulting scar is more easily camouflaged. When a face lift is done in conjunction with blepharoplasty, a strong temporal lift also helps to raise the brow, but the final result of direct brow elevation and temporal lift is still less than optimal.

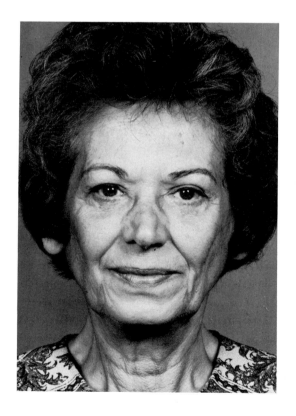

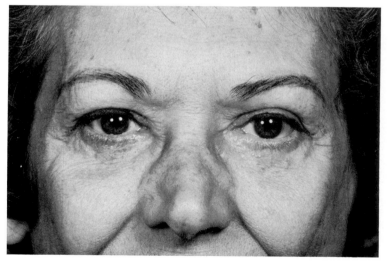

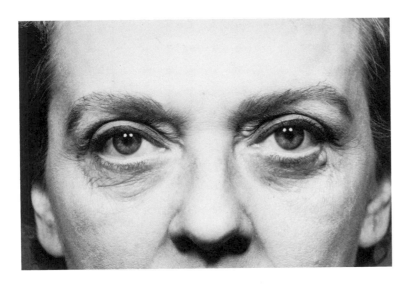

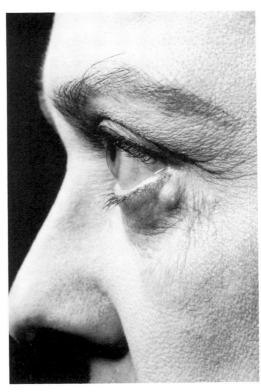

This patient was operated on at another institution, and a good result was achieved by blepharoplasty. However, she complained of the small bulge in the lateral aspect of the left lower lid (quite obvious in the lateral close-up) and also of residual wrinkling of the skin of the lower lids, which she believed was due primarily to the blepharoplasty done to correct large fat bags. The latter complaint is not uncommon in this situation, because the skin over large pseudohernias of fat is stretched tightly and will sag when the fat is removed.

A secondary operation in this patient permitted wide undermining of the skin, a lateral pull as shown on page 65, and excision of the excess. As might be supposed, the bulge seen in the preoperative lateral photograph was a lateral fat pocket that was not removed at the original operation. Note that some improvement in the skin wrinkling was achieved as well with the secondary procedure, but it is not often possible to eliminate these wrinkles. Further improvement might be obtained with a deep skin peel.

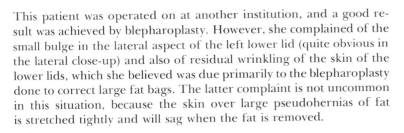

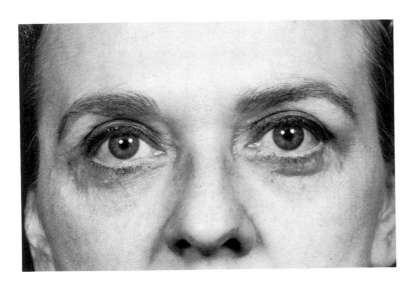

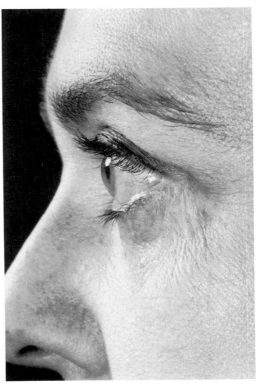

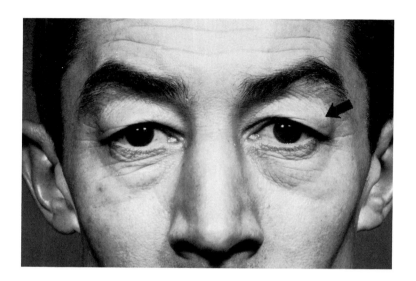

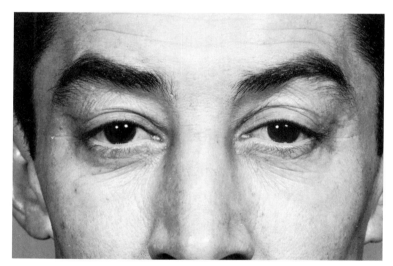

The arrow in the preoperative photograph points to an unusual bulge at the lateral margin of the orbit in the upper eyelid. Ballottement and palpation revealed a rounded, smooth tumor beneath the skin, which protruded farther with pressure on the eye. These masses, one on each side, were ptotic lacrimal glands, which should be suspected and looked for in patients with marked fullness in this region. At operation the glands can be delivered through a small incision placed laterally through the orbicularis muscle and the septum. A major portion of a lacrimal gland can be resected without untoward effects, provided lacrimation is normal. About one half of the gland was resected in this patient.

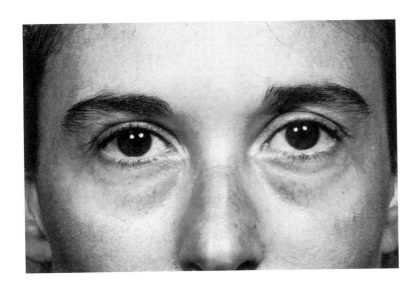

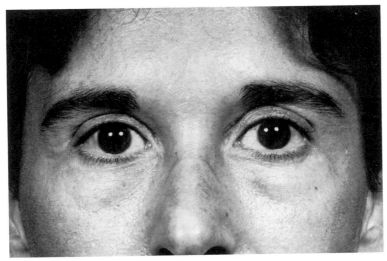

This young woman demonstrates bulging of the lower eyelids from what was thought to be protruding fat. However, as can be seen in the postoperative view, blepharoplasty with removal of the fat pockets did not entirely correct the appearance of swelling in the lower lids. On careful postoperative examination, it was determined that these remaining ridges were caused by prominence of the bony infraorbital rim. It behooves the surgeon to examine each patient carefully before the operation to avoid disappointment with the operative result.

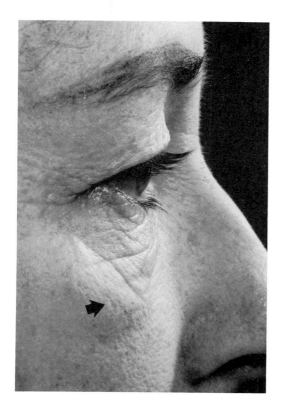

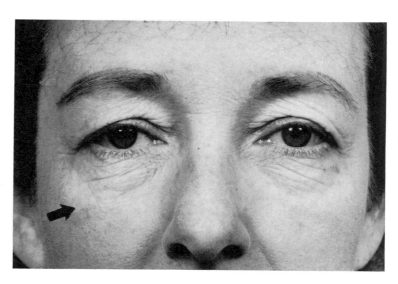

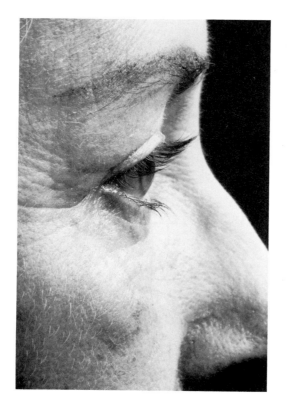

Excision of skin from the upper eyelids produced a slightly less than optimal result in this patient. One of the reasons for the limited improvement is the presence of brow ptosis; elevation of the brows was decided against.

The small cheek pouch or elevation indicated by the arrows in the preoperative photographs was of particular interest. These pouches overlying the malar eminence are often found in association with, but not necessarily related to, palpebral bags. Sometimes they are improved by very wide undermining during blepharoplasty, but the improvement is minimal. It is most important to discover these cheek deformities prior to surgery and to point them out to the patient, for they will not be removed by the operation and some patients expect that they will be.

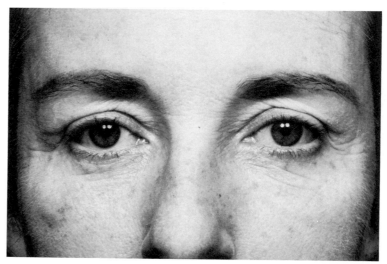

108

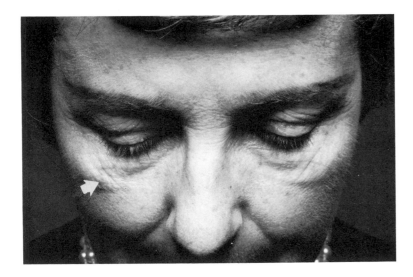

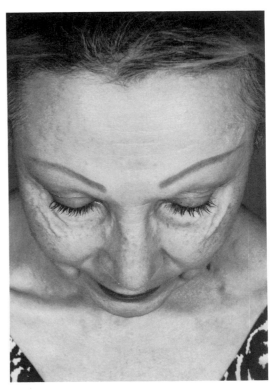

Wrinkling of the skin associated with large, dilated veins presents a problem in blepharoplasty, and such wrinkles usually cannot be obliterated.

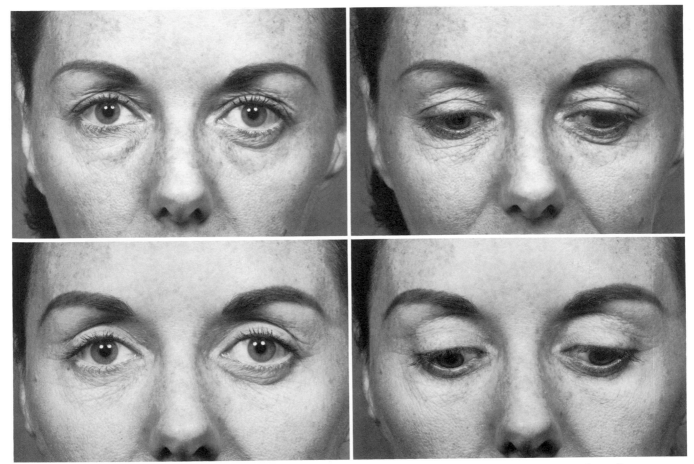

Postoperative problems and dissatisfied patients can often be avoided more easily if the surgeon exercises all his powers of perception in studying each patient preoperatively. Professional photographs such as these are sometimes more revealing than personal examination. This patient underwent a standard blepharoplasty but was not happy with the result; friends said that she looked "peculiar" and that her eyes were different. Because she was a photographers' model, her problem was acute. Examination of the photographs in retrospect clearly showed that the two eyes were indeed quite different, the left appearing much larger than the right—an asymmetry camouflaged preoperatively by excess skin and small fat bags.

109

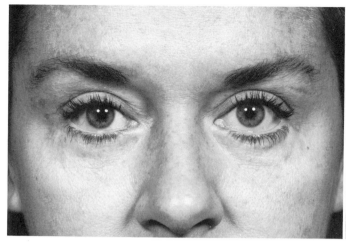
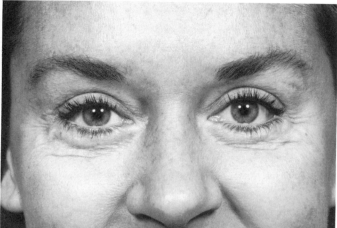

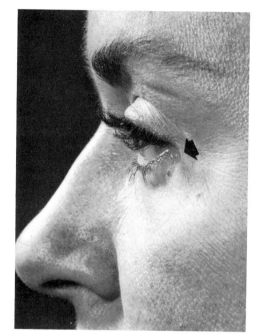

This patient shows some of the typical minor deformities that may prompt a patient to seek secondary correction after a primary blepharoplasty. There is very slight ectropion, residual excess fat in the medial compartments of the lower lids, and a small web at the lateral canthus on the left side (arrow in lateral view). Though slight, these minor irregularities are exceedingly difficult to correct without further compounding the problem, particularly that of skin shortage. Operation must be very conservative.

In this case the old incisions were reopened, the medial fat pockets excised, and the skin redraped in such a way as to eliminate the web and redistribute the skin to eliminate the wrinkling evident on animation—and yet no skin was excised. This is most important, as further excision of skin, particularly in the young patient without significant senile skin changes, will lead to ectropion. The postoperative views show the small but significant improvement achieved in this patient. Despite the fact that no skin was excised, the pull-down of the lower lids was somewhat accentuated for several months. With eventual softening of the scars, the result was satisfactory.

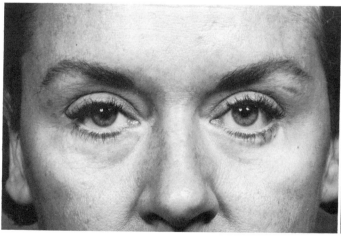
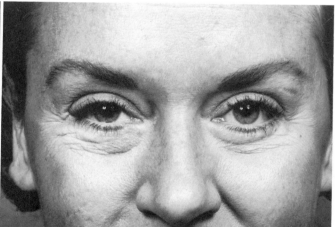

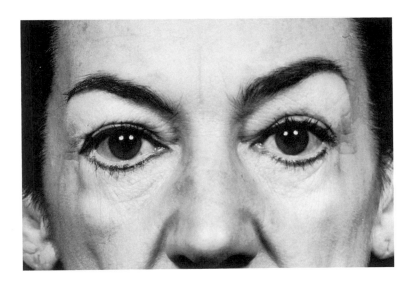

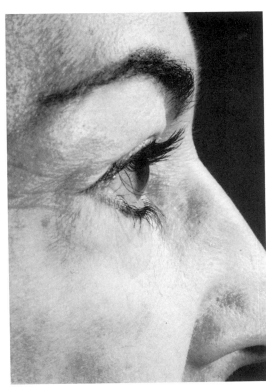

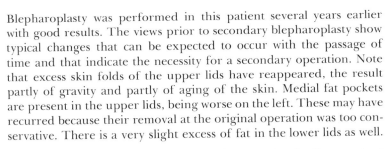

Blepharoplasty was performed in this patient several years earlier with good results. The views prior to secondary blepharoplasty show typical changes that can be expected to occur with the passage of time and that indicate the necessity for a secondary operation. Note that excess skin folds of the upper lids have reappeared, the result partly of gravity and partly of aging of the skin. Medial fat pockets are present in the upper lids, being worse on the left. These may have recurred because their removal at the original operation was too conservative. There is a very slight excess of fat in the lower lids as well.

The secondary procedure in this patient consisted of a standard removal of the upper lid skin fold, vigorous fat removal from the upper lids, and a very conservative fat removal and redraping of the skin of the lower lids after moderate undermining. No skin was excised from the lower lids since a slight shortage of skin already existed.

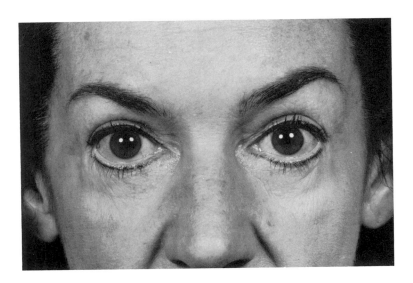

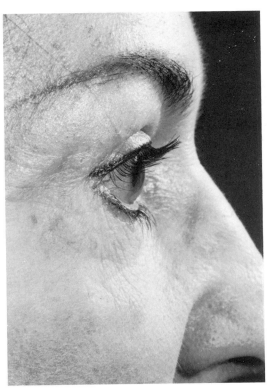

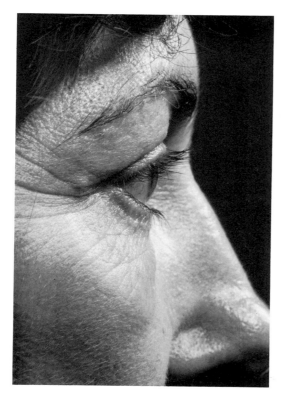

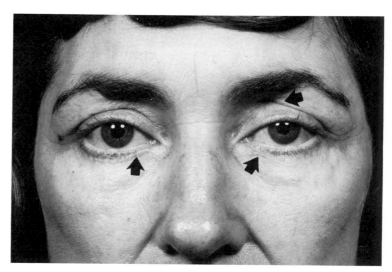

Cosmetic blepharoplasty by another surgeon left this patient unhappy about the deep depression at the medial region of the left upper lid as well as the marked scar ridges with small suture marks still present six months after surgery in the lower lids (arrows in the preoperative photograph). Such persistent suture marks result from allowing sutures to remain in place for more than four days. The previous scars were excised, but no skin was removed, at a secondary operation. Exploration of the left upper eyelid revealed that the medial levator expansion was severed at the first operation, which may have occurred when the surgeon sought the medial fat pocket. The edges of the interrupted levator were located and united with sutures.

The postoperative result was satisfactory to the surgeon except for the small cyst seen in the lower left incision, which had to be removed later. The patient, however, was still unhappy—a not uncommon phenomenon when blepharoplasty must be repeated. There is a slight increase in scleral show in spite of the fact that only the scars of the lower lids were excised, with no removal of additional skin.

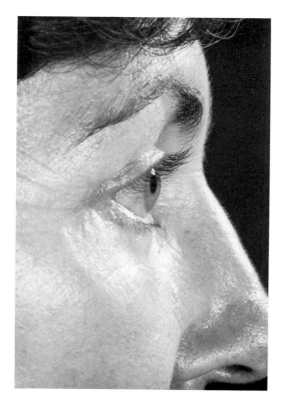

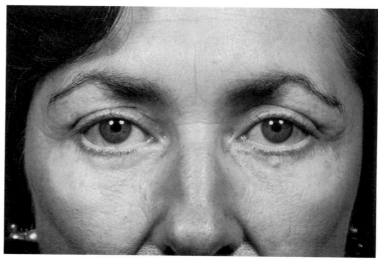

(*Illustration continued on opposite page.*)

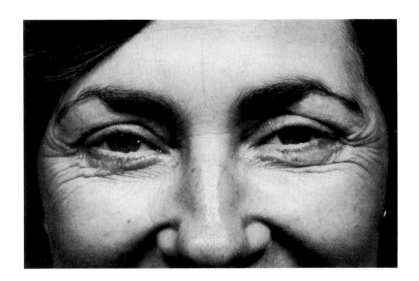

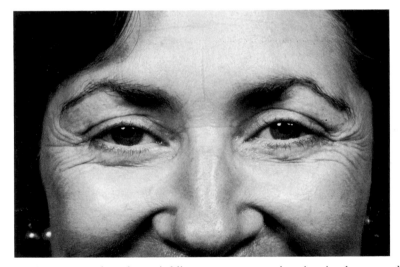

As in primary blepharoplasty, note that the wrinkling present on animation in the secondary case can be improved but by no means eliminated. In the preoperative photograph, wrinkling is accentuated by the scars, which act as contracting bands. Smooth redistribution of the skin at the second operation helps to improve the situation.

These photographs show what can reasonably be accomplished by secondary blepharoplasty performed to correct two of the more common problems that exist after primary surgery: slight ectropion from overly generous skin removal, and insufficient removal of medial fat pockets in the lower lids, resulting in a noticeable bulge.

The secondary correction requires reopening the previous incisions, wide undermining of the lower eyelid skin, and removal of the offending pockets of fat through stab wounds in the orbicularis and septum orbitale. Wide undermining permits some improvement in coverage by the skin, which can also be shifted laterally, as shown on page 65. Except for the old scar, no skin is excised from the upper margin of the lower lid except as a lateral triangle. Ectropion is improved and there is less scleral show postoperatively.

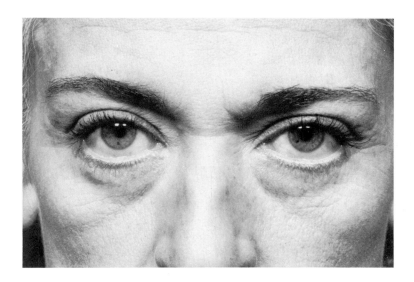

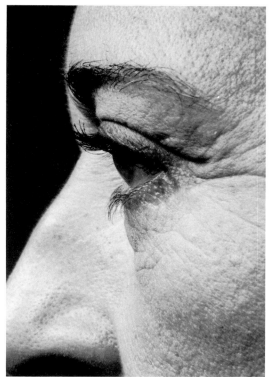

Another patient demonstrating the sort of minor defects that commonly follow blepharoplasty, in this case performed elsewhere. In the preoperative view note a recurrent skin fold of the upper lids, not necessarily because too little skin was removed, but more likely the result of ptosis of the brow. Imperfect results in the upper lids must be expected in such patients unless the brow is elevated. There is also a small residual medial fat pocket of the right lower lid and a small degree of ectropion at the lateral third of the left lower lid.

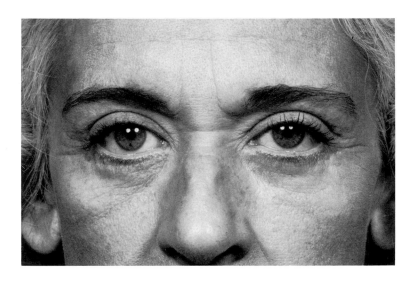

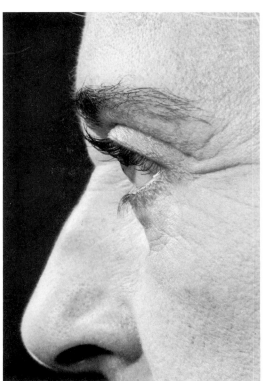

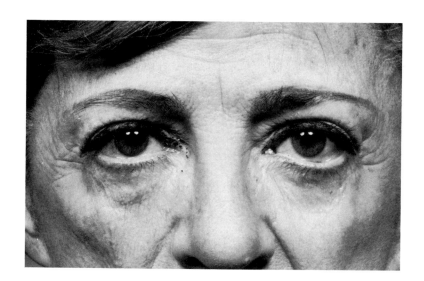

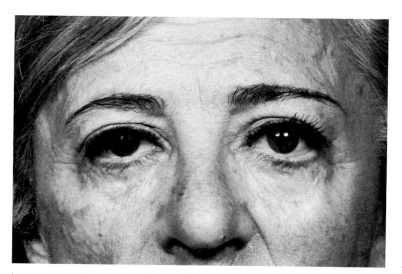

The secondary operation consists of removing the residual fat pocket through a stab wound in the orbital septum, opening the original subciliary incision for the length of the lid, and rather wide undermining and redraping of the skin of the left lower lid to allow the lid to relax and relieve some of the skin pull responsible for the ectropion. No skin is excised.

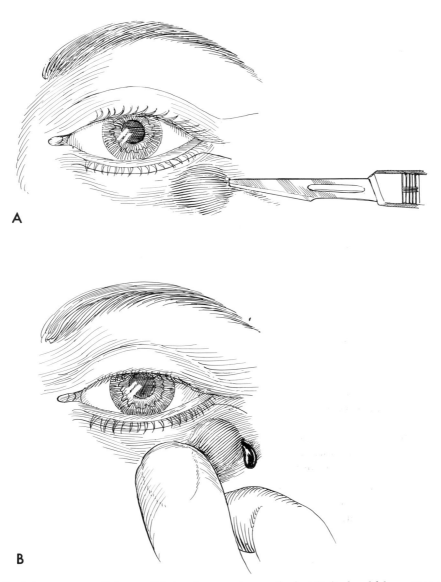

A

B

If a small, localized hematoma of the eyelid develops postoperatively (*A*), it should be removed at about eight days by making a stab wound with a No. 11 blade and pressing out the contents with the thumb (*B*).

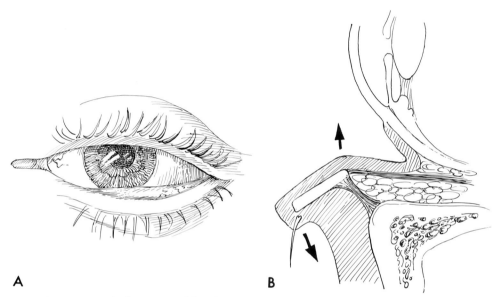

A   **B**

Temporary ectropion can result from a combination of edema and normal wound contraction; however, resolution occurs in a few days when these factors are resolved. Permanent ectropion such as this is the inevitable result of removal of too much skin and sometimes muscle. The lid is everted and held away from the eyeball because of scar contraction and outward and downward buckling of the tarsal plate (*B*). Chronic chemosis of the conjunctiva results (*A*), as well as chronic irritation of the conjunctiva and occasional secondary bacterial infection. Exposure keratitis or corneal ulceration usually does not occur unless excessive skin has also been removed from the upper lid, resulting in lagophthalmos.

If the lower lid is sufficiently pulled or everted in correction of permanent ectropion, the tear drainage mechanism is distorted, with the canaliculus pulled away from the globe. This gives rise to chronic epiphora, which is most distressing to the patient.

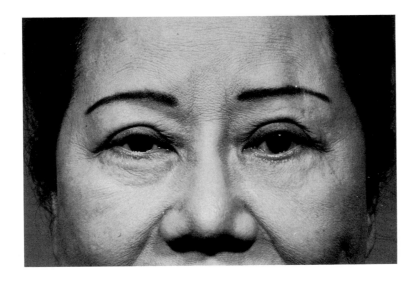

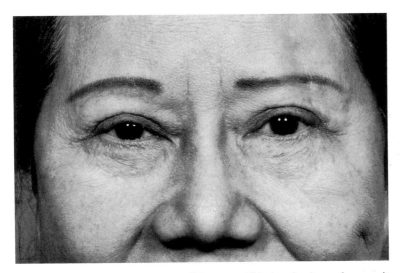

When ectropion follows cosmetic surgery of the eyelids, even if it is of minor degree, it usually is seen at the outer third of the lids. Sometimes, however, overambitious removal of skin at the medial third of the skin flap can result in a slight pull-down of this portion of the lid. Even slight degrees of buckling of the lid in this area can result in epiphora by forcing the canaliculus away from the globe and interfering with the drainage mechanism. In this patient, ectropion of the left medial lower lid was causing such a problem. Correction was achieved by a small full-thickness graft of upper eyelid skin, which was abundant.

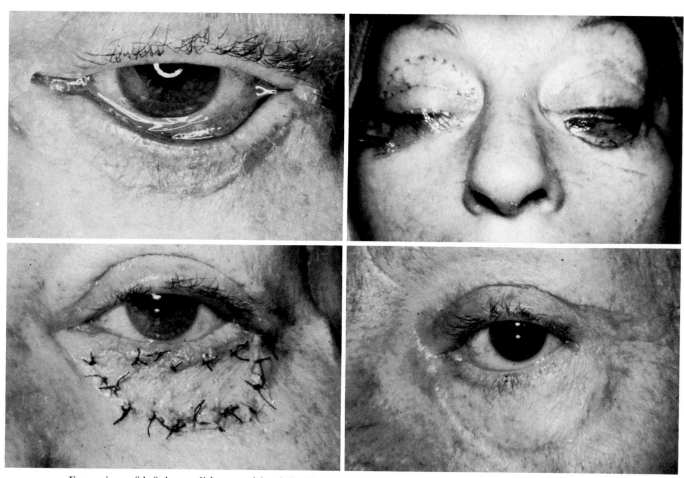

Ectropion of left lower lid treated by full-thickness skin graft according to the technique shown on page 121.

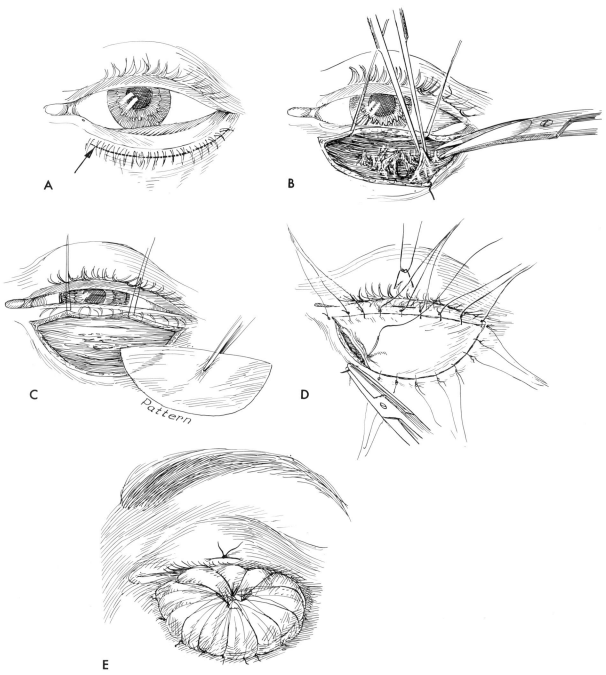

Correction of ectropion requires replacement of the missing skin. The old wound is opened widely and all scar tissue is excised (A, B). The wound edges should not be undermined, because dead spaces beneath the skin can be the site of fluid accumulation or hematoma formation, which mitigates against graft survival. A pattern of the defect is then constructed with a thin sheet of plastic (C), and a full-thickness skin graft of the exact size is cut from the upper lid—provided a sufficient amount of skin is available. The graft is trimmed of all subcutaneous fat and sutured into place (D). A tie-over dressing is left in place for seven to ten days (E). The lids are closed during this period with a temporary tarsorrhaphy suture. A certain amount of contraction of the graft must be expected in the few weeks following surgery, but this is minimal with full-thickness grafts. If there is not enough skin on the upper lid to provide a graft of proper size, the graft should come from the retroauricular region, or, as a last resort, the supraclavicular area. The scar that results will probably be unsightly in this area, especially in a woman.

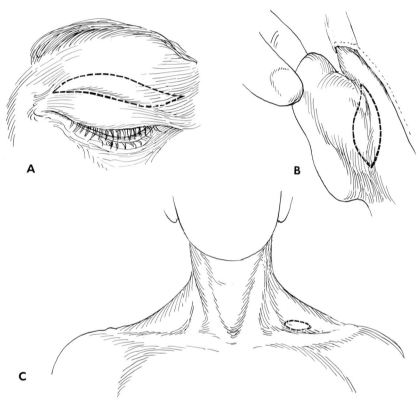

The preferred donor sites for full-thickness skin grafts in eyelid reconstruction are shown in order of their preference for color match, texture, and donor site scarring; these are skin from the upper eyelid (*A*), retro-auricular skin (*B*), and supraclavicular skin (*C*).

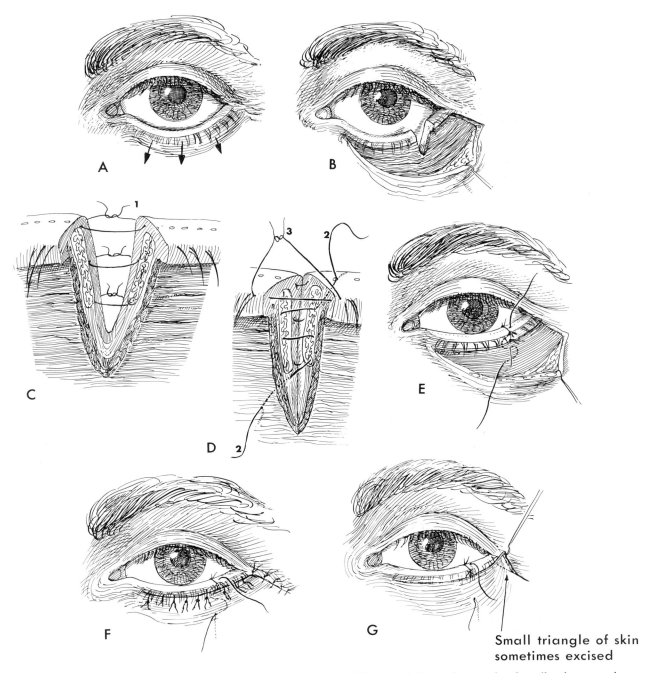

A

B

C

D 2

E

F

G

Small triangle of skin sometimes excised

In patients with atonicity of the lower lid, which can be familial in origin or the result of senile changes, the tendency toward ectropion can be aggravated by blepharoplasty. This is particularly true in males for some unknown reason. If ectropion develops after cosmetic blepharoplasty, and atonicity seems the primary cause (A), correction can be achieved by incising along the old blepharoplasty incision, undermining the skin flap, excising a suitably sized full-thickness wedge lateral to the lumbus (B), and repairing the defect according to Mustardé's technique, with layer closure and a pull-out as shown in C, D, E, F, and G.

123

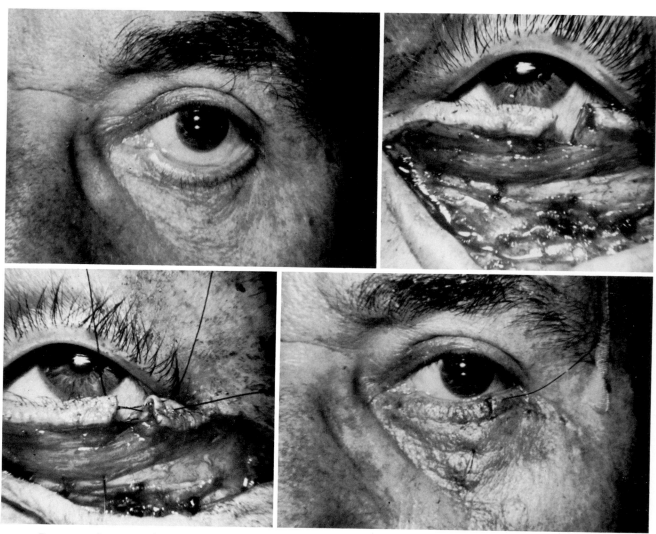

Postoperative ectropion related to atonicity and not to excessive tissue removal is shown at the upper left. The defect was re-created and a wedge excised (upper right). A Mustardé repair was then accomplished (lower left). The immediate and permanent postoperative correction is shown at the lower right.

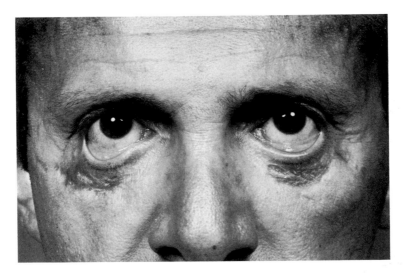

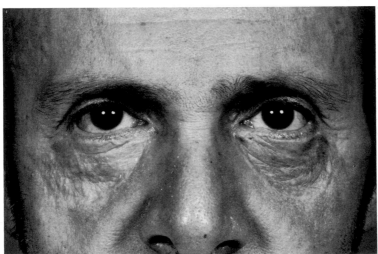

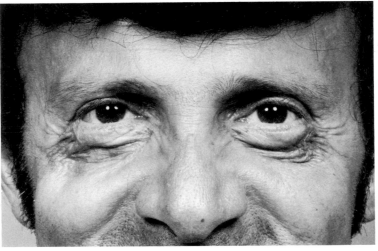

Severe ectropion can result from excessive skin removal and poor timing of operations aimed at correcting the initial problem, as shown in this patient. Several attempts had already been made to correct bilateral ectropion that resulted from cosmetic blepharoplasty performed by another surgeon. Each of these procedures consisted of split-thickness skin grafting, and they were performed within several weeks of each other, during the period of maximum wound reaction and scar contracture. The final result consisted not only of severe ectropion but also of extensive scarring of surrounding skin and underlying muscle. The patient was not able to close his eyes.

The postoperative photographs of this patient demonstrate correction of the ectropion, but the large skin grafts are permanent cosmetic defects that cannot be eradicated.

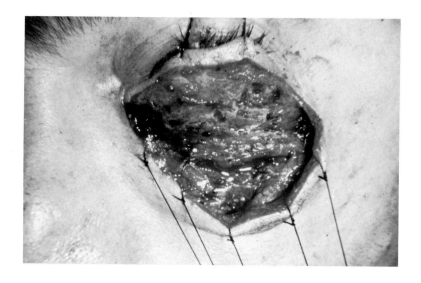

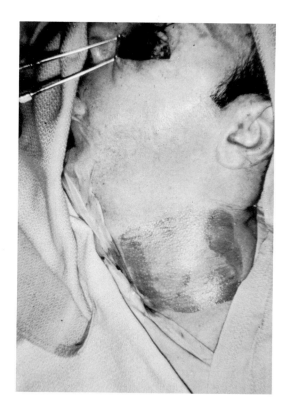

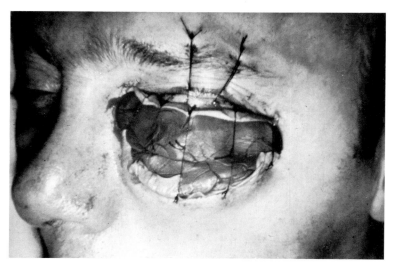

Correction of the difficult problem shown on the previous page was undertaken by first re-creating the original defect. The remnants of the split grafts were excised, one side at a time. All scar tissue was dissected from the orbicularis muscle, and the septum orbitale was released along its entire attachment to the infraorbital rim (upper left). This was necessary in order to increase the vertical length of the lower lid, which had been firmly bound to the orbital rim by scar tissue. The skin edges of the inferior margin of the wound at the junction of the skin of the cheek were undermined to create a pocket after the method of McIndoe (pages 127 and 128).

The neck was chosen as the donor site for a skin graft because a superior color match could be obtained (right). A thick split graft was used because of the size of the defect and because the scarring was so extensive that a full-thickness graft would have less of a chance of obtaining an adequate blood supply for survival. It is possible to obtain a rather large graft from the neck with a dermatome. The technique is facilitated by extending the skin by means of subcutaneous injections of large volumes of saline solution. Thus "blown up," the skin presents a sufficiently large and flat surface for the dermatome to be operated.

The graft is carefully draped into the pocket-like defect so that it is in contact with all raw surfaces and has a cuff of excess skin (lower left). Dental wax is then used to make an exact impression of the defect, taking care to fill all of its ramifications. The skin graft is applied to this stent with the raw surface up, and the stent is held in place by tie-over sutures. Note that the lower lid margin is elevated in a cephalad direction and maintained in an exaggerated position by sutures fixed to the forehead skin. This technique of overcorrection allows for subsequent contraction of the split-thickness graft.

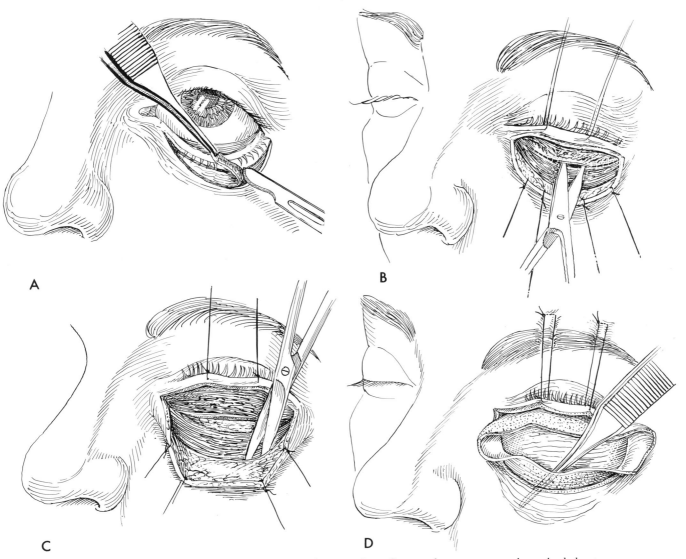

A

B

C

D

Severe cicatricial ectropion of the lower lids with extensive scarring of normal structures and marked shortage of skin may simulate the deformity seen following burn injury. Such deformities may not be correctable with full-thickness skin grafts when circulation is in question because of thick scar tissue. Repair demands excision of all scar tissue (*A*) and dissection of a large pocket (*B* and *C*) into which a split-thickness skin graft molded around dental compound or similar material can be fitted (*D*).

One eye should be treated at a time. The stent is left in place for about 10 days. The immediate postoperative result is somewhat unpleasant, even with the ectropion corrected. The deep groove or pocket that is created is unsightly, but with the passage of several weeks, during which the graft contracts, the pocket will be greatly reduced in size. After contraction is complete and the scar tissue is sufficiently softened and matured, a secondary trim and correction of the junction between graft and skin can be undertaken.

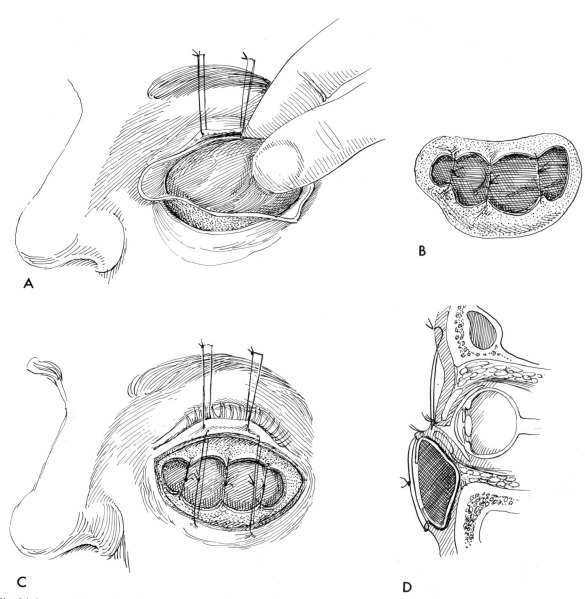

A

B

C

D

Split-thickness skin grafts for correction of ectropion are sometimes favored over full-thickness grafts in the repair of very large defects of the lids (p. 125) when thick scar tissue precludes early vascularization of full-thickness grafts. Such split grafts can be taken from the neck skin if donor scarring is of secondary importance; otherwise, they are taken from the buttocks or thighs. The graft is applied to the stent mold of dental compound with the raw surface out (A). Dermatome glue can be applied to the mold for fixation, or sutures may be used to bridge across the mold (B and C). The lower lid is sutured to the brow for several days (C and D). Subsequent trimming of the raised edges of the recipient pocket may be necessary after contraction has occurred.

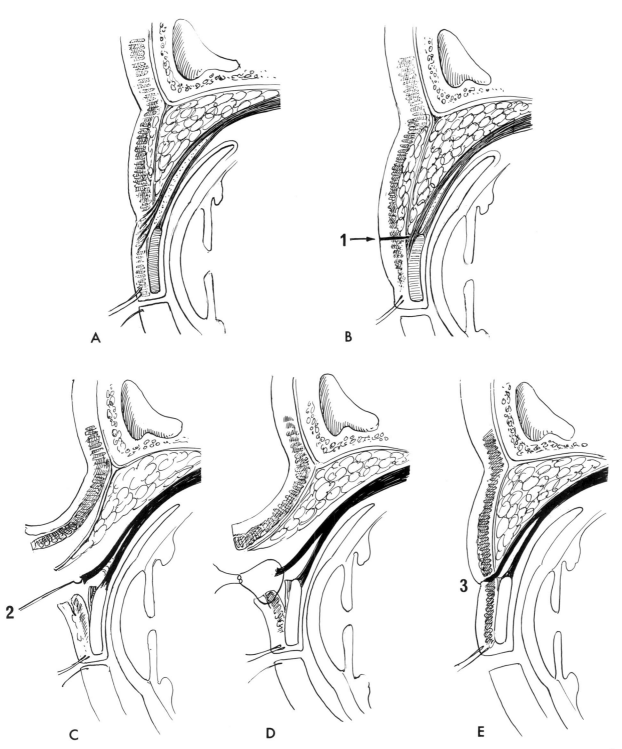

The Caucasian eyelid (*A*) shows a dual insertion of the levator muscle into the superior border of the tarsus and a slip inserting into the dermis at the site of the supratarsal fold. The typical Oriental lid (*B*) lacks the dermal insertion of the levator aponeurosis.

The Fernandez operation in sagittal section shows the superficial layer of the levator aponeurosis dissected and held with a hook (*C*). This thin aponeurotic sheet is sutured into the dermis at the skin incision with a buried nonabsorbable suture (*D*). The desired fold is created by this insertion (*E*).

129

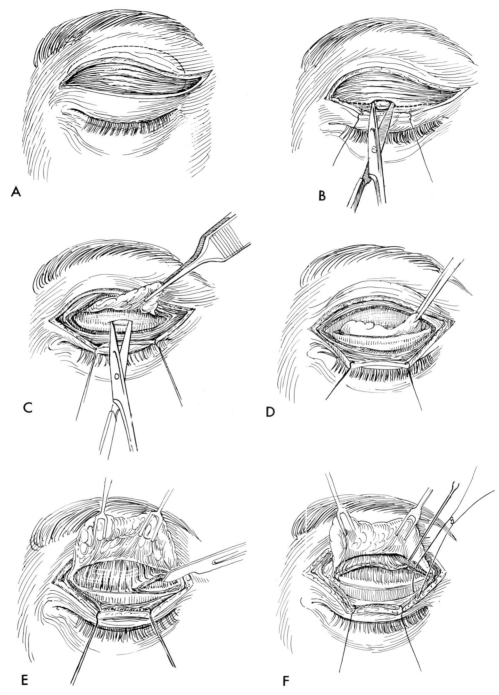

The radical Fernandez procedure for alteration of the Oriental eyelid. A strip of redundant skin is excised from the upper lid, as in cosmetic blepharoplasty; the lower limb of the incision is 7 to 8 mm. from the ciliary margin (*A*). The orbicularis muscle and orbital septum are dissected along the lower edge of the incision; a small strip of muscle can be excised (*B*). The supraorbital fat is dissected free and the excess is excised (*C* and *D*). The levator aponeurosis is dissected as a thin sheet and sutured into the dermal edge of the lower wound margin, establishing a supratarsal fold (*E* and *F*). The skin margins are sutured with interrupted sutures.

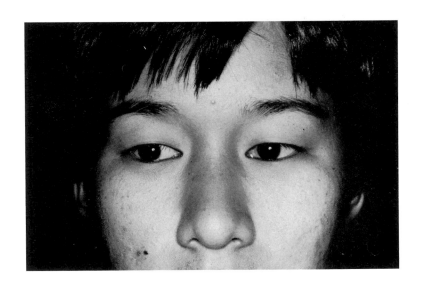

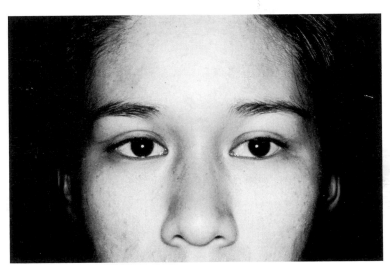

Preoperative and postoperative photographs showing typical results from the operative procedure described by Fernandez. (Courtesy of Dr. Leabert Fernandez.)

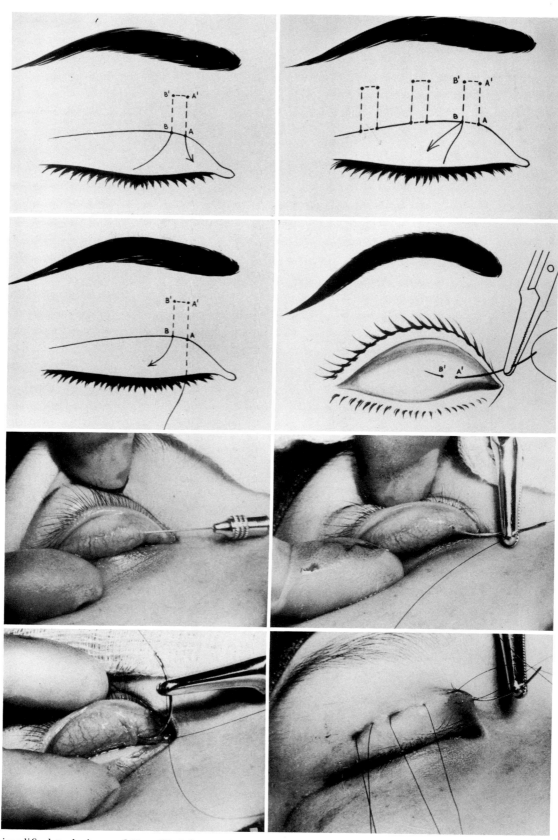

The simplified technique of Boo-Chai for establishing a supratarsal fold in an Oriental eyelid with three mattress sutures. These sutures are passed subconjunctivally through needle puncture wounds, and they affix the levator to the skin. The knots are buried and allowed to retract through the suture holes in the skin wound. This technique is often satisfactory in younger patients who have a minimum of fat and skin. Boo-Chai advocates a more radical approach similar to that of Fernandez in more advanced deformities.

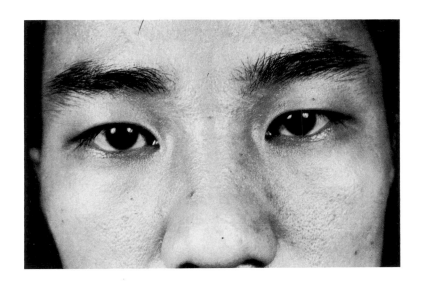

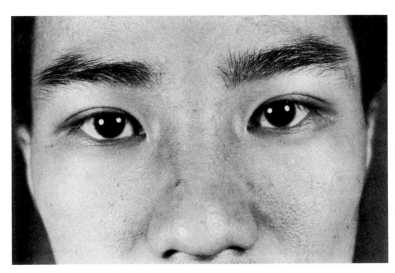

The result shown in the postoperative photograph is typical of those achieved with the Boo-Chai procedure in young patients with Oriental eyelids (Drawings on the previous page and photographs courtesy of Dr. Khoo Boo-Chai.)

Chapter 6

FACE LIFT

Tʜᴏᴍᴀs D. Rᴇᴇs, M.D.

"C'était pendant l'horreur d'une profonde nuit.
Ma mère Jézabel devant moi s'est montrée,
Comme au jour de sa mort pompeusement parée.
Ses malheurs n'avaient point abattu sa fierté;
Même elle avait encore cet éclat emprunté
Dont elle eut soin de peindre et d'orner sa visage,
Pour réparer des ans l'irréparable outrage."
"It was during the horror of a dark night.
My mother Jezabel appeared before me,
As on the day of her death pompously adorned.
Her misfortunes had not humbled her pride;
She still had that assumed luster
With which she carefully composed and embellished her face,
So as to repair the years' irreparable outrage."
                                    Jᴇᴀɴ Rᴀᴄɪɴᴇ
                       Athalie, Act II, Scene V (1960).

History

It is not known exactly who attempted the first face lift, but there is little doubt that the operation was being done in the early 1900's by many surgeons in Europe and by a few in America. Most of these early efforts were mainly in the nature of a "mini-lift," that is, excision of strips of skin in front of and behind the ears. Extensive undermining of the facial and cervical skin flaps was not done until later, probably not until the 1920's.

Stephenson (1970) credits von Hollanden with publishing the first paper on the correction of the sagging face in "Handbuch von Kosmetick" by Max Joseph in 1912. At about this time, there was considerable interest in facial surgery by such eminent surgeons as Lexer (1910) and Joseph (1921, 1928a and b) in Germany, and Passot (1919a and b, 1931), Morestin (1915),

DeMartel, Bourguet (1921) and Lagarde (1928) in France. Madame Noël (1926, 1928), a Parisian physician and student of DeMartel, devoted most of her professional life to such cosmetic surgery.

In early 20th century Europe the performance of such operations was often shrouded in secrecy. Individual techniques were jealously guarded by many of their originators, causing Passot to complain in the literature about such tactics, especially among the "German surgeons." Unquestionably this secretive attitude is the reason that not more is known about the early history and development of face lifting. Much more is known about the development of blepharoplasty, probably because the early cases were reported as being performed to correct true pathologic entities which could in some way affect vision and which were frequently familial in nature, as reported by Panneton (1936a and b). This made operations designed to correct eyelids somehow more "respectable" than face lifting, which could only be construed by most people at the turn of the century as a catering to excessive vanity, and vanity was generally frowned upon in post-Victorian Europe.

Secrecy surrounded face lifting for several reasons. As just noted, public disdain for surgery catering to vanity undoubtedly forced both surgeons and patients to seek anonymity by "going underground." Much of this surgery, therefore, was done as an office procedure or in small private nursing homes. This in its own way discouraged extensive procedures, such as wide undermining, and prolonged the age of the mini-lift. Madame Noël was especially noted for her minor office surgery and, by description, her surgery was minimal indeed. Certainly the facial operation published by Passot (1931) in his "Chirurgie Esthétique du Visage" was limited in the extent of undermining, as shown on page 151.

Another reason for secrecy was the low esteem in which such operations were held by many of the leading surgeons of the day. Their attitude was that no surgery, except that which was necessary to save life or to alleviate severe suffering or crippling deformity, was indicated. Many considered cosmetic surgery trivial, unnecessarily risky and downright against the laws of nature. This attitude undoubtedly kept many talented and eminent surgeons from developing the techniques further.

Unfortunately this unfavorable attitude by the medical profession toward facial cosmetic surgery, and face lifting in particular, persisted, although lessening in intensity, until recently. Advances in anesthesia have done much to minimize risk as well as to encourage more extensive undermining, which yields more dramatic improvements. The present widespread social demand for such surgery, as well as the improvements in results and safety of the procedure, has done much to dispel the older misguided attitude. The face lift is finally gaining wide acceptance. Indeed, many of the patients are even members of doctors' families. Nevertheless, the condemnation or implied unacceptability of face lifting by men in powerful positions in hospitals, universities and other institutions had a strong inhibiting effect on face lift surgery. Many prominent plastic surgeons were forced to "hide" their face lift patients in small private hospitals or to purposely misname the procedure on the operating schedule of major hospitals. Such shenanigans still sadly persist in some medical centers.

Paradoxically many of the most prominent plastic surgery pioneers of this century have perpetrated the secrecy and implied taint associated with cosmetic surgery. These are men who have pushed ahead the frontiers of reconstruction, yet have publicly shunned "cosmetic" surgery while practicing it at the same time, often extensively. Fortunately the present young generation of plastic surgeons, as well as doctors in other disciplines, are recognizing the increasing role of cosmetic facial surgery as an integral part of modern life. Teaching in this field is now emphasized, for the livelihood of many young surgeons depends on their cosmetic surgical skill.

Still another reason for secrecy was greed, man's constant companion. The early cosmetic surgeons were well aware of the potential growth of cosmetic surgery and its financial implications. They were not eager to share their knowledge, and perhaps their profits, with others. New techniques were closely guarded by their developers, and imparted only grudgingly to younger colleagues. This attitude persisted among many surgeons until very recently. In fact, it has been only in the past decade or so that many of the "tricks" or "secrets" of cosmetic surgical technique have been freely exchanged.

Even less is known about the early development of cosmetic face lifting in America or the British Isles—the Anglo-Saxon world. Very little on the subject was published, most likely because of a reticence on the part of most surgeons to be identified with "vanity surgery" by their colleagues. At the turn of the century the Anglo-Saxon world was still very much under the influence of the post-Victorian era, more so even than continental Europe, and vanity was considered almost sinful. Miller, of Chicago, was perhaps the earliest American surgeon to publish extensively on the subject, starting in 1907 and continuing until his textbook on cosmetic surgery was published in 1924. Hunt (1926), of Scotland, also openly practiced face lifting and published on the subject in his book "Plastic Surgery of the Head, Face and Neck."

Many of the giants of plastic surgery who emerged after World Wars I and II practiced face lifting to some degree. Some of these surgeons did a great deal of "cosmetic" surgery, yet curiously wrote very little on the subject although they were most prolific on other topics. Gillies, Blair, Davis, Pierce, McIndoe, Mowlem, Conway and many others did face lifts, yet were hesitant to publish on the subject. Many of the greatest reconstructive plastic surgeons relied on face lifting and other cosmetic operations for their livelihood, enabling them to pursue their interest in reconstruction. This same financial state of affairs is still present in many of our major cities where reconstructive surgery alone simply cannot pay the bills.

As anesthesia became safer and techniques improved, the extent of the face lift operation became more radical. That is, the amount of skin undermining became more extensive, reaching well down into the neck and toward the corners of the mouth. The early operations, as noted, were essentially mini-lifts in which a strip of redundant skin in front of the ear was removed and the wound edges undermined just enough to achieve closure, usually only 1 to 2 cm. The mastoid skin was also sometimes undermined for a short distance and a small segment removed. The temporal lift consisted of excision of a strip of skin behind the hair at the temples. Many unique and imaginative designs, particularly in regard to the incisions in the scalp, were put forth. These very conservative techniques were as ineffective then as they are today, making it difficult to understand the current resurgence of the mini-lift vogue. The very ineffectiveness of such operations and their limited period of benefit were what caused surgeons to undertake more extensive undermining in the first place in order to achieve the more lasting results now available.

Miller's (1924) textbook shows many interesting designs for excision of facial skin. It is to his credit that the basic operation performed by most surgeons today is essentially similar. As pointed out by Stephenson (1970), a review of the early literature on face lifting, limited as it is, shows that surprisingly little has been thought of since the early part of the century. Her quotation of Miller in this regard is cogent: "Operations a century old are refaced as original contributions with the slightest modifications and put forward with emphatic seriousness. Even our best surgeons, when they write upon subjects in which their experience is extensive and their understanding great, are often given to the hasty practice of crediting originality to those writers who in the previous few years have written upon similar subjects. Masterpieces of description in older literature are thus lost, and men who have made inessential changes in detail of technique are frequently credited with being originators of operations which they have really had nothing to do with developing." These words by Miller are as true today as when he wrote them.

Although the face lift operation has been practiced for at least the past 70 years, there is no question that the demand for this type of surgery has risen very sharply over the past dec-

ade. This is not only because the present techniques yield consistently satisfactory results, but also because the operation is rapidly loosing the social stigma attached to it. People in all walks of life, in big cities and small and of all economic strata, are increasingly aware of the benefits of this surgery and are seeking it in ever-increasing numbers. In some communities, having a face lift has almost become a status symbol.

It is interesting to note that more and more requests for face lift surgery are coming from men. Although they make up a very small segment of the overall number of rhytidectomy patients, some plastic surgeons state that up to 15 to 20 per cent of their requests for facial cosmetic surgery are now coming from males. The typical man who seeks facial plasty is no longer a stage or screen star, but rather a successful executive who feels a more youthful appearance will help his career, or a widower or divorcé in his 40's or 50's who is dating a younger woman. Having observed the emphasis on youth all around him—and perhaps the excellent results of face lifting on women acquaintances—the male of the species is adding to the unprecedented growth in cosmetic facial repair. In fact, the progressive rise in demand is so great that there is a considerable shortage of trained surgeons, thus making it imperative to increase the availability of training in the techniques of cosmetic facial surgery.

Selection of Patients

In selecting patients for rhytidectomy, the face lift operation, both physical and psychological criteria must be kept in mind.

PHYSICAL CONSIDERATIONS

The ideal face lift candidate is usually a woman in the middle forties who is slightly on the thin side and who has prominent or strong malar eminences and mandibular angles. The chin, without being prominent, should be strong, and the natural cervicomental angle should approach 90 degrees when the head is held erect. Further, the skin should not be markedly degenerated from excessive actinic exposure or aging, for multiple rhytidoses, or "prune wrinkles," are not helped by the basic face lift procedure.

It is also helpful for the patient to have a full head of hair, styled in such a manner as to cover the ears, so that incisions can better be camouflaged. It is sometimes necessary for the patient whose hair style exposes the ears to temporarily change the hair-do following rhytidectomy for a period of several weeks until the scars have faded.

Unfortunately this type of "ideal" physical candidate is not always the one who arrives at the surgeon's office in search of a face lift. Therefore, it is important to recognize what variations of these criteria may or may not lead to good surgical results.

A strong bony framework of the face is particularly important in obtaining a good result from a face lift. This is not necessarily a racial characteristic, although it is more frequently encountered in Slavs, Scandinavians and Asians, than, for example, in people of Mediterranean origin. The high cheekbones which characterize the faces of many personalities of motion picture fame typify this skeletal criterion. Well developed mandibular angles, often associated with prominent cheekbones, are also most helpful in providing a bony framework over which undermined skin can be drawn and redistributed. A well formed mandibular body is particularly important in eliminating loose folds of skin or "jowls." If there is retrusion of the mentum or flattening along the body of the mandible on either side, it becomes difficult to eradicate jowls despite the extent of skin undermining.

In those patients with mandibular retrusion, microgenia or retrognathia, it is sometimes desirable to insert a chin implant at the same time as rhytidectomy. Such a subtle alteration in the standard face lift technique can make a remarkable difference in the final result, particularly the profile line. If these conditions exist, it behooves the surgeon to point them out to the patient preoperatively and to indicate tactfully that a chin implant may spell the difference between an indifferent and a superior result in surgery.

If the line of the neck is more or less straight from the tip of the symphysis to the hyoid bone, complete redistribution of the skin, even with total undermining across the midline of the neck, may not be sufficient to restore an esthetically pleasing angle. This is so because a loss of the cervicomental angle may result from accumulation of subcutaneous fat, which exists much as a lipoma, as well as from excess skin. Should this be the case, a marked improvement can be obtained by auxiliary excision of fat accumulations. These are usually found beneath the strap muscles and can be removed by opening the superficial musculature layer and excising the underlying fat. Sometimes the subcutaneous fat can be removed from beneath the undermined skin without resorting to a submental incision; however, a separate submental incision in the natural skin fold beneath the chin greatly facilitates the exposure. When using a short submental incision to remove fat accumulations, it is possible to utilize the same incision for the insertion of a chin implant, if needed. Robertson (1965) and Pitanguy (1970) suggest augmenting the chin by using the submental fat pad as a turn-over flap—a most useful concept.

When submental fat is removed, it is important to leave a small adipose layer attached to the skin in order to prevent adherence of the skin to the underlying strap muscles. Removal of all fat may result in adhesions, with fixation of skin to muscle causing unsightly contour irregularities which are emphasized during motion of the neck musculature as in swallowing.

When an obtuse cervicomental angle exists, correction by standard rhytidectomy is often disappointing. An obtuse angle—often referred to as a "turkey gobbler" deformity—can result from an excess of skin with or without a submental fat pad. Marino et al. (1963) reported that such an increase in the cervicomental angle can also occur because of an anatomically low placement of the hyoid bone in respect to the inferior border of the chin and the fifth cervical vertebral body. The latter anatomical variation from the norm was described by Marino's group after studying several patients with "double chins." Their radiographic studies indicated that when the condition is due to a low placement of the hyoid bone, the deformity cannot be corrected by conventional operations. In general, when the hyoid bone is located higher than the inferior border of the chin, the cervicomental angle is sufficiently acute to be amenable to surgical correction by removal of submental fat and/or excess skin. If, on the other hand, the hyoid bone lies lower than the chin, the angle becomes obliterated by the geniohyoid strap muscle and is therefore not surgically correctable. Such patients should be informed of this anatomic limitation prior to operation and told that in all probability the result will be modified.

Pangman and Wallace (1961) suggested removal of excess submental fat using scissors or curettage. Maliniac (1932) and Davis (1955) stressed the need for local excisions of excessive chin and neck skin, along with the removal of submental fat pads or lipomas through submental incisions. Millard, Pigott, and Hedo (1968), on the other hand, advocated dissection and removal of excessive submental fat from beneath the skin flaps through standard rhytidectomy incisions when possible.

137

Adamson, Horton and Crawford (1964) studied the necks of 12 cadavers and discovered that the submental fat pad in older individuals varied between 15 and 25 gm. in weight and between 15 and 27 ml. in volume. They suggested a rather aggressive technique for correction of the cervicomental angle. This method required a long transverse incision made across the neck at approximately the level of the apex of the cervicomental angle, through which the excess fat could be removed and the platysma muscle plicated. They recommended this procedure as an adjunct to standard rhytidectomy and emphasized the importance of placing the skin incision in the transverse neck crease. The author suggests a cautious approach to this somewhat radical technique.

If the skin hangs in loose folds inferior to the level of the hyoid, it becomes necessary to undermine it above the level of the platysma muscle as far inferiorly as the thyroid gland, in order to redistribute the skin and to excise the redundancy. When marked folds or depressions extend from the lateral commissures of the mouth downward to the chin or superiorly to the alae nasi (labiomental or nasolabial folds), extensive undermining may be required to achieve improvement. Such undermining, medially to the corner of the mouth, may result in some difficulty in the postoperative period, as localized hematoma formations are commonly encountered. There is also the possibility of damage to the buccal and mandibular branches of the facial nerve, since they are quite superficial this far medially.

Correction of deep nasolabial folds is one of the most disappointing aspects in current face lift technique. Although extensive undermining can result in some softening of these deep grooves (p. 190), the improvement is still limited. Patients should be advised during the preoperative evaluation that correction will be minimal in this area.

Isolated deep lines or furrows of the face, such as glabellar frown lines or the aforementioned nasolabial or labiomental creases, may be helped by liquid silicone injections. Some such lines may be ablated by this experimental technique. Injections of silicone fluid are best carried out *following* rhytidectomy, except those for the ablation of glabellar frown lines. Injections in this region may be done at the same time as the operative procedure. Indications for and techniques of silicone fluid injection will be discussed in Chapter 8.

Extensive undermining of the skin over the malar prominences is also fraught with hazard. The buccal, ophthalmic and zygomatic branches of the facial nerve become very superficial in this region and can easily be damaged during dissection. The amount of redistribution of skin that can be accomplished in this area is also limited. Therefore, undermining over the cheeks should be curtailed.

The course of the frontal branch of the facial nerve, where it emerges from the parotid gland and courses superiorly and medially to the orbicularis and frontalis muscles, was well described by Pitanguy and Ramos (1966). The nerve becomes superficial at a point midway between the anterior hairline and the lateral canthus of the eye. Extreme caution should therefore be exercised in undermining the temporal skin in order to preserve and protect these branches of the seventh nerve. A nerve stimulator should be employed whenever such undermining is indicated, as in the case of ptosis of the eyebrows, in order to identify the course of the nerve branches so they will not be destroyed.

Patients in whom the angles of the mandible are prominent and in whom the distance between the angles of the mandible is foreshortened, or those in whom the mandibular body assumes a more direct or flat course, are most apt to demonstrate a strong jowl formation from excess skin in this region. Extensive undermining and upward traction on the skin flaps is doubly important in such patients. Even then, correction of the jowls may be limited. Patients whose facial configurations are least amenable to surgical correction by rhytidectomy are those without strong malar eminences or with actual flattening of the cheekbone.

As mentioned previously, patients with marked rhytidosis from extensive senile changes of the skin or from atrophy of the skin because of prolonged actinic or wind exposure can also be expected to obtain only limited improvement from a standard rhytidectomy. Such patients, however, can often benefit from a deep skin peel (chemabrasion) subsequent to operation. When ancillary procedures such as chemabrasion are thought to be necessary by the surgeon, the complete surgical program should be discussed in detail with the patient prior to the rhytidectomy.

Certain inherited or acquired conditions of the skin, while not constituting an absolute contraindication to face lift surgery, may contribute to troublesome sequelae or prolonged healing time. These conditions should be recognized prior to surgery and the patient should be advised of their potential influence on the results of the operation. For example, patients with very thin, transparent skin with hypopigmentation are prone to severe ecchymosis which may be prolonged for many weeks or months post-operatively, particularly in the thin skin of the eyelids.

Patients with telangiectasia may experience an exacerbation of the small lesions following rhytidectomy. These may be particularly noticeable in the neck region. In some cases these multiple telangiectases become permanent, with a resulting reddish discoloration of the neck skin and, sometimes, the cheeks. Patients with small telangiectases should be advised prior to surgery that new lesions may appear. Such disturbances in skin color can usually be camouflaged by appropriate face make-up.

A keloid diathesis does not necessarily mean that keloids will develop in the face lift scars. However, thickening or hypertrophy of the scars behind the ears is more apt to occur in such patients. They should be advised of this possibility. True keloids following face lifting are extremely rare, even in patients who exhibit true keloids of scars elsewhere on the body.

As mentioned previously, the thin patient is a better candidate than the obese patient, not only because the immediate operative result is better, but also because the obese patient has a tendency to gain and lose weight intermittently, a habit which can have disastrous effects on even the best performed rhytidectomy by causing recurrent stretching of the skin. Some obese patients can be induced to lose weight preoperatively by being made to understand that the facial plastic operation will then be more successful. The obese patient who loses significant weight and maintains the weight reduction for some time prior to surgery is often an excellent face lift candidate, for the weight loss and its maintenance indicate good motivation for the procedure. Obese patients who do not lose weight can still be helped by rhytidectomy and submental lipectomy when jowls or a double chin are the prominent factors.

Most surgeons now agree that the best time for the first facial plastic operation is whenever it is needed. In most instances this is between the ages of 45 and 55, when the tell-tale signs of age usually first appear. In the authors' opinion, it is unnecessary and unwise to wait for advanced signs of aging before advising surgery. When the decision to operate is postponed until the changes assume the characteristics of senility in the sixth or seventh decade, the immediate results are highly satisfying, but the improvement lasts for a shorter period than in the younger patient, and a second operation may be required sooner than if surgery was first performed in the fourth or fifth decade of life.

Uncommonly a face lift may be required by a patient in her middle or late thirties. Early cessation of hormonal function resulting from hysterectomy or premature menopause may bring about skin changes that require surgery at an early age. Facial surgery in such patients should, however, be supplemented by hormone replacement therapy, proper skin hygiene, and related measures which will aid in maintaining the result.

Preoperative Preparation for Rhytidectomy

The use of moulages, plaster casts and similar three-dimensional preparations is of limited or no value in planning the face lift operation, except perhaps to impress the patient. Accurate, standardized and realistic photographs can, however, be of immense value to the surgeon both in his preoperative planning and in the operating room. Such photographs are best taken by a professional medical photographer using standardized lighting and techniques so that every detail of the facial structure is clearly shown. Full-face, both profiles and three quarter views showing the face in repose and in animation can be most helpful in deciding the amount of undermining to be done and in delineating those facial configurations which can be only slightly or not at all improved by surgery. It is important that such defects be pointed out to the patient on the photographs prior to surgery.

Because adequate hemostasis is so essential to a successful operative result, it is important for the surgeon to be aware of any potential bleeding problems. Patient who are on "the pill" or other forms of hormone treatment such as estrogen-replacement therapy are more apt to ooze than others. It is therefore advisable to discontinue hormone medication in female patients 10 days to two weeks before surgery. It is also thought to be unwise to operate on patients just prior to or immediately following the onset of menses since bleeding of the oozing type is more apt to occur at this time.

Blood dyscrasias can often be discovered prior to surgery, and a history of easy bruising, and most particularly a history of prolonged bruising following minor injury, should be thoroughly investigated. Although true hemophilia does not occur in the female, certain bleeding disorders do occur. A carefully taken history should disclose if there is or ever has been any prolonged bruising, spontaneous bleeding, excessive bleeding during any previous operative procedures or any bleeding problems in the family.

Preoperative antisepsis techniques are indicated in all patients to lessen the likelihood of postoperative infection, although surgical infection in rhytidectomy wounds is extremely uncommon, unquestionably because of the rich blood supply to this region which enables the body to mobilize its natural defenses to ward off bacterial infiltration. Thorough facial washings with pHisoHex for three days preceding surgery are recommended. A 15-minute pHiso-Hex shampoo of the hair on the night prior to operation has proved to be highly beneficial in promoting an antiseptic field in which to work. Because of the small chance of infection of the skin in this region, it is rarely necessary to shave the margins of the hair before rhytidectomy, and the authors have not, in fact, employed shaving for the past 10 years, during which time not a single case of postoperative infection has been encountered. Limited clipping of the hair with sharp scissors at the sites of the surgical incisions is done just prior to operation (p. 154). Usually only the areas where the excision will be accomplished are clipped, so that the eventual suture line lies virtually within the hair, particularly in the temporal scalp. Just before surgery an aqueous solution such as Zephiran is employed as a final skin preparation of the operative field.

The patient should be placed on the table in such a way that the head can be elevated during the operative procedure. Elevation of the head is helpful in (1) control of bleeding, (2) demonstration of areas of loose or ptotic skin folds, and (3) giving the surgeon greater access to the operative field. A cerebellar head rest or similar attachment has been found to be most useful in providing access to the operative area without the interference caused by the conventional, cumbersome headpiece found on most operating tables. The access provided by the cerebellar head rest also permits suturing both sides at the same time during final closure of the wound.

The headrest should be elevated so that the head lies in a natural position in relationship to the rest of the body. The head should also be slightly flexed at the neck to permit redraping and trimming of the skin flaps at the most advantageous angle.

Postoperative Care

Dressings are removed 48 hours after surgery. If soft rubber or suction drains were used, these may also be removed at the same time, or they may be left in place for an addi-

tional 24 hours. No additional dressings are required unless the patient wishes to cover the incisions in front of the ears.

After the dressings are removed, the patient's hair is usually matted and snarled. It may be gently combed out, using a comb with large teeth dipped in soapy water. The skin should also be gently cleansed of all caked blood, adhesive and other debris. This cleansing, in combination with combing of the hair, tends to lift the patient's spirits at a time when they are apt to be at a low ebb. The initial response of the patient to her image in the mirror at this time is likely to be shock. Despite extensive preoperative discussion of the postoperative course, most patients are somewhat overcome by what they see, as ecchymosis and edema tend to be maximal at this time. Therefore, if it is at all possible, patients should be kept away from mirrors for a few days. This is obviously not always feasible, so patients should be cautioned as the dressings are being removed that what they see may be upsetting. If ecchymosis is minimal, however, patients may be pleasantly surprised. These immediate reactions, as well as the need to see what is going on, vary with the personality of the patient more than any other factor.

Patients should be kept in bed until the dressings have been removed. During this crucial two-day period, the possibility of hematoma formation is greatest, and it is therefore best for the patient to remain relatively quiet. Excessive talking should be discouraged. It is often best to have the telephone disconnected. The upper body and head should be kept elevated at least 30 degrees in order to lower venous pressure and to decrease the likelihood of hematoma. A soft or liquid diet should also be prescribed until the dressings are removed. Some surgeons prefer giving liquids through a straw only.

If suction drains are used, it is essential to maintain their patency. Attention must be paid to see that the suction is functioning and that the drains are not plugged. Gentle irrigation with a large-bore needle and saline solution at regular intervals is useful in keeping drains open. It is also worth noting that suction must be discontinued prior to removal of the drains. If this is not done, bleeding may be provoked by pulling away clots that are adherent to the holes in the tubing.

The author does not employ drains unless there is difficulty in obtaining hemostasis during operation. Drains will not prevent hematoma formation. They are merely useful in siphoning off small collections of pooled blood. In fact, stiff drains, such as the polyethylene type used in suction drainage, may even promote postoperative bleeding in that their innate stiffness may act as a shearing force when the head moves.

Postoperative medications are usually minimal. Appropriate drugs may be used to control pain, although pain per se is not a significant factor following facial plastic surgery. Routine prophylactic antibiotic therapy is preferred by most surgeons, but this is not essential since the rich blood supply of the facial and cervical tissues mitigates against infection. In apprehensive patients, diazepam (Valium) or other suitable tranquilizers may be helpful in allaying apprehension and in maintaining a relative degree of quiet during the immediate postoperative period. These are particularly helpful in high strung, exceedingly active individuals.

Following removal of dressings, the patient's activities need not be restricted, providing no hematoma is present. Bleeding after this initial 48-hour period is unusual. Patients may be discharged from the hospital on the second or third postoperative day and subsequently may be treated on an outpatient basis.

Suture removal begins on the fifth postoperative day with removal of all sutures in the preauricular incisions. These are normally the only incisions which are visible, and therefore it is important to prevent suture marks. The post-auricular or temporal sutures are removed alternately from the seventh to the tenth or twelfth postoperative days. Those sutures which support the most tension in the temporal scalp and across the mastoid skin are removed last.

The hair may be shampooed with a bland soap as soon as all sutures have been removed. The patient may also set her hair, but it should be dried under warm not hot air. A hair drier set on "hot" may burn the ears, which may still be "anesthetized" at this time. Other routine postoperative instructions are provided in the "Letter to Patients" on pages 20 to 22. Patients should be encouraged to massage the final scars lightly with moisturizing creams or bland ointments to promote early softening and maturation of the scars.

Considering the highly emotional aspects of face lift surgery, the surgeon performing these operations should not be too surprised to find a high incidence of complaining and "niggling" from his patients in the immediate postoperative period. He should not be unduly distressed when a patient upon whom he has operated seems disappointed with what appears to be a superb result. No matter how completely the limitations and realities of surgical intervention are explained, the patient still dreams of regaining youth. Anything short of complete restoration of youth by surgery engenders a degree of resentment against the surgeon (whose job it was to restore it), no matter how much he may have tried to make clear the limits of surgical reconstruction. This is not to say that the majority of patients undergoing rhytidectomy are not eventually pleased with the results. For the most part they are satisfied. This satisfaction increases as the months pass after operation, but it would be expecting too much of human emotions to anticipate immediate satisfaction with an imperfect result (which surgery is when compared to a fantasied self-image of restored youth).

A certain amount of minor complaining following facial cosmetic surgery must therefore be expected in most patients. The surgeon should not take personal offense at this, but rather should attempt to understand the complicated motivations that give rise to these complaints so he can discuss them frankly, one by one, as they arise. Careful and thorough preoperative discussions with accurate appraisal and frank opinions freely aired help to alleviate postoperative disappointments. However, the education of the patient must be carried through the postoperative period as well. Unpleasant facts or pieces of information that the patient does not want to hear may be psychologically blocked out during initial discussions. Apparent lapses of memory in reference to facts that were painstakingly imparted by the surgeon should not surprise him, nor should they try his patience. The pertinent information should be reiterated and re-emphasized. This type of continuous calm outlook on the part of the surgeon and his staff often results in the transformation of what appeared at first to be a dissatisfied patient into a satisfied one. It is important that the surgeon's staff—nurses, assistants, secretaries and others—have insights into those mechanisms at work in the patient undergoing cosmetic surgery so that they, too, can understand and deal with the myriad details of psychological management as they arise during the course of treatment.

The authors have found it useful to provide a letter of information to patients who are candidates for facial cosmetic surgery. Such a document can be read and reread before and after surgery. It reinforces the verbal information and instructions provided by the surgeon and his staff. Although it has not completely eliminated misunderstandings between patient and surgeon, it has been of great value in minimizing them. The letter is reproduced in Chapter 2. It can provide a guide for others who wish to prepare a similar document.

The doctor-patient relationship between the cosmetic patient and the surgeon is a unique one and differs greatly from that between most patients and other surgical specialists. It is more in the nature of that between psychiatrist and patient, particularly in that a strong transference is often established. The cosmetic patient frequently expects, or hopes, that the surgeon is going to be a prime force in providing the means for success, in recapturing lost youth, in gaining job opportunities, in rekindling love life, and on and on. These attitudes are, of course, unrealistic, yet they do exist, particularly in the emotionally dependent patient. The relationship, even if of relatively short exposure and duration, can become strong during the course of most cosmetic operations. The patient may actually transfer to the surgeon the responsibility for opening the way to complete success or happiness—an impossible goal. When the impossible dream is not realized, the disappointment is then, quite logically in the patient's eyes, the fault of the surgeon. He is blamed for his inability to be a "miracle worker."

In certain severe mental disorders such as paranoia, this moment in the relationship between surgeon and patient can become a dangerous one for the surgeon. These episodes have been well documented, but fortunately have rarely resulted in violence. All surgeons experienced in the practice of cosmetic surgery have encountered patients they recognize as being potentially dangerous. Such patients should be guided away from surgery into competent psychiatric hands.

In considering the average person, however, and not the psychotic or borderline psychotic, it is still not clear why many patients experience a period of depression following what appears to be highly successful cosmetic surgery. Such postoperative depressions do frequently occur, however, and should therefore be anticipated by the surgeon. Unless the depression appears to be unduly severe, it can usually be handled by the surgeon on a day-to-day basis with tact, understanding and discussion. It is natural for the surgeon to feel somewhat hostile toward that patient who complains about a result that the surgeon considers excellent. Such hostility obviously stems from a wounded ego. The clear realization that such feelings on the part of the patient, particularly the middle-aged patient, are frequently to be expected, and the knowledge that they will usually pass with time and patience and understanding, should help the surgeon to survive in his relationship with the patient at this trying

time. More importantly, it may prevent his precipitating a crisis or even permanent breach in the relationship by keeping his hostility from getting out of hand. Unresolved "transference" at this stage results in a permanently unhappy patient and possible legal trouble for the surgeon, much of which can be avoided by an understanding attitude.

Although the foregoing is true, it is not to be inferred that the cosmetic surgeon should not, at times, be quite firm and authoritative, particularly with the patient who appears to be getting aggressively out of hand. The patient who disrupts the surgeon's waiting room, patients and office staff and who is generally a nuisance need not be tolerated. If communication on a meaningful level with such a patient cannot be established by gentle persuasion, the surgeon has every right to adopt a firm attitude.

Patients undergoing blepharoplasty are often less troublesome, in this regard, than other cosmetic patients such as those undergoing facial plastic or nasal plastic procedures. Usually the results of blepharoplasty are more immediately pleasing to the patient. Also, this operation is the most effective operation for actually restoring a "youthful look." It is usually the expression around the eyes which ages first, and it is, of course, the eyes which are the center of expression of the face.

Patients undergoing rhytidectomy fall into three broad groups in regard to their postoperative reactions: (1) those who are exuberant and completely delighted with the results; (2) those who are initially somewhat disappointed that not all signs of age were removed, but who are generally pleased and become more so with the passage of time; and (3) those who are moderately to severely disappointed with the results and remain so. Fortunately this last group is small in number, and most often patients in this category are there because of improper selection of candidates by the surgeon. However, such patients cannot always be weeded out, no matter how careful the selection process. Those patients who are immediately pleased, even thrilled, with the results are usually people who are "up" and prone to look on the positive side of life anyway. Such patients are usually externalized types who easily overcome the minor setbacks of life without much difficulty. Their inner feelings, however, may sometimes be another matter, and if they are in any way disappointed in the results of surgery, they are careful not to show it. Sometimes, if such patients are followed over a long period of time, the surgeon may gain an inkling that all is not what it seems. However, it is often best not to probe too deeply.

Common causes for disappointment in the results of rhytidectomy are early recurrence of the so-called double chin and failure to ablate it at the time of the initial operation.

Complications

Complications following rhytidectomy can be divided into two distinct groups: true complications, such as hematoma or infection, and untoward results, such as dissatisfaction on the part of the patient with the operative outcome.

HEMATOMA

Hematoma is the most significant and troublesome complication which can occur in facial cosmetic surgery. Hematomas may be very small or massive. They occur in 10 to 15 per cent of all patients undergoing face lifting. However, minute hematomas are often ignored and thus not included in the general statistics.

Prevention is, of course, the best cure for hematoma. Every effort should be made to obtain adequate hemostasis at the time of operation. Vessels of large caliber should be ligated or coagulated with fine-pointed forceps and cautery. Drains, which are of questionable value in the prevention of hematoma, may be used if the surgeon questions the degree of hemostasis. Delayed bleeding under the skin flaps, resulting in hematoma, may occur for many reasons, ranging from rebound bleeding following loss of epinephrine effect to blood dyscrasias.

Massive hematoma requiring immediate attention is usually the result of bleeding from one or more vessels of significant size which have slipped their ties or sloughed their cauterized ends. This form of bleeding usually occurs within the first 48 hours after operation, although it may develop as late as 10 days to two weeks postoperatively. In late developing hematomas, bleeding is usually caused by some form of trauma as simple as pulling the hair or bumping the cheek. Massive hematoma is almost always heralded by sudden and acute discomfort. Unilateral swelling and ecchymosis are frequently associated with the pain. Rarely, the patient may experience a feeling of dyspnea and the apprehension associated with this symptom. The complaint of pain, particularly unilateral

pain, in the immediate postoperative period requires that the possibility of hematoma be carefully ruled out. The dressing should be removed if the slightest doubt exists and careful observation maintained.

It is important to recognize significant hematoma formation in its earliest possible stages, since progressive pressure and separation of the skin flap from its underlying bed may result in compromise of circulation and sloughing of the skin. In the author's experience the largest skin slough seen following rhytidectomy occurred following hematoma formation that was unrecognized for only a few hours.

Whereas smaller and more localized hematomas can be treated more conservatively, large hematomas must be promptly evacuated. This may necessitate taking down all sutures on the affected side to permit a careful exploration of the wound bed. This should be carried out without hesitation in order to locate the source of bleeding. General anesthesia is preferred for such hematoma evacuation for two reasons: First, the patient is usually extremely apprehensive, and secondly, it is often difficult to obtain good anesthesia by local infiltration under such circumstances.

It should be noted that when a hematoma is being sought on one side of the face or neck, the surgeon and anesthesiologist should treat the opposite side with extreme care. It is not uncommon for a hematoma to develop on the opposite side during or shortly after exploration, probably as a result of manipulation. Massive hematomas which result from bleeding due to occult blood dyscrasias are usually bilateral and associated with bleeding in the eyelid wounds and into other areas of the skin with extensive ecchymosis. Bleeding of this type is extremely rare and is difficult to diagnose by even the most sophisticated coagulation studies. A hematologist should be consulted at the slightest suggestion of such a problem, since control of the bleeding may require fresh whole blood or plasma transfusion.

Smaller localized hematomas are often not recognized until the postoperative edema has subsided. Small collections of blood are frequently found over the body of the mandible, far down the neck, or at the medial extremity of the cheek flap where the accessability and the surgeon's vision are limited during operation. These small hematomas are quite common, occurring in approximately 15 per cent of all patients. Ordinarily they are not troublesome and are spontaneously absorbed within a few weeks. However, some patients are distressed by them, and in these instances, every effort should be made to aspirate them. Between the seventh and fourteenth days small hematomas can often be aspirated with a large 15- or 16-gauge needle since the clot is then liquefied.

There are two other methods for removing small hematomas after they liquefy, at about one week. If a small hematoma is located near a suture line, one or two sutures may be removed and the clot "milked" out. If it is located some distance from the nearest incision line, it is sometimes possible to incise it with a No. 11 blade and then "milk" out the clot. Such an incision should be placed in a natural skin crease. After the fourteenth day, the clot becomes firm. Sometimes during the period of organization of the clot considerable dermal contracture can occur, causing a puckering or minor contour deformity of the skin over the site. Intralesional steroid injections during the organizational phase of clot formation tend to accelerate absorption.

SKIN SLOUGH

Skin slough is the most feared complication of face lifting. In experienced hands it is quite rare. Minor degrees of slough occur most often in the mastoid skin flap where the tension is the greatest and where the blood supply is farthest from the tip of the flap. Fortunately these sloughs are rarely extensive, and the resulting scar is behind the ear where it can easily be hidden by appropriate hair styling. During the phase of necrosis, a black eschar forms. This should be treated conservatively. It should be debrided at intervals, but only when separation of the edge occurs. Aggressive debridement has no place here, for the eschar is acting as a biological dressing. If infection occurs beneath the slough, however, debridement is, of course, necessary.

Major skin sloughs are exceedingly rare. They are usually the result of massive hematoma which has been neglected. Occasionally a large slough occurs for undetermined reasons. Such sloughs are undoubtedly the result of marginal circulation in the skin flap or localized thrombosis or ischemia. It is actually somewhat surprising that such problems are not encountered more often in face lifting, since the skin flaps are very thin and the undercutting often extensive.

When these sloughs occur in the preauricular area, the resulting scar can be unsightly and may require secondary excision and repair as soon as the elasticity of the skin permits. As with

the treatment of hematoma, the best treatment of skin slough is prevention. Flaps should be handled gently and hematomas evacuated promptly.

INFECTION

Infection is very rare following face lifting. This is undoubtedly because of the superb blood supply in the region. Even with the presence of hair follicles in the hair-bearing portion of the wound, infection is uncommon. Localized pustules are sometimes found around sutures or hair follicles. These are treated by evacuation. More extensive infections should be treated with appropriate antibiotic regimens and the local application of heat.

HAIR LOSS

Hair loss can occur in the temporal skin flap or adjacent to the incisions in the hair-bearing scalp. Such loss is most often found in patients with thinning hair and a tendency toward alopecia. It is most likely to occur following a second operation performed in the same area within a few weeks after the first procedure. Temporary hair loss is more common than permanent loss. Patients with healthy hair and scalp can be reasonably certain that the hair will grow back within a few weeks. However, this may take up to six months.

When hair loss appears unusually extensive, a dermatologic consultation should be obtained. Often suitable medication, such as topical or injectable steroids, can reverse the trend. Localized hair loss adjacent to incisions or from spreading of scars can occasionally be improved by scar excision and revision. An obvious hair loss may be noticed in the postauricular scalp if the hairline has not been accurately approximated, resulting in a "stair step" effect.

SCARS

Scar hypertrophy and keloid formation can occur in face lift scars, but these complications are actually quite rare. As might be expected, scar hypertrophy is usually found in the postauricular scar where the greatest tension exists. Hypertrophy is exceedingly rare in the preauricular scar and is almost never found in the scalp. True keloids are very rare in face lift scars, but when they do occur they are extremely difficult to control. Keloids are more common in patients with darkly pigmented skin such as Indians or Negroes.

Hypertrophic scars must be treated with patience, time and, occasionally, intralesional steroid therapy. Such scars may itch and burn and be the source of considerable discomfort. This irritation can be controlled with local steroids and often with superficial x-ray therapy in doses of from 1200 to 1500 R.

Keloids are difficult, unpredictable and stubborn to treat. Intralesional steroid injections, x-ray therapy and serial excisions may be employed. Escharotics and other locally destructive techniques, such as cryosurgery, have produced improvement in isolated incidents but should be reserved for use in patients who are refractory to more conservative modalities of treatment.

FACIAL NERVE INJURY

Facial nerve injury is exceedingly rare. Here, as in all complications, prevention is again the best cure. The dissection level is almost always superficial to the level of the branches of the facial nerve. The danger points, as indicated on page 179, are (1) over the mandibular body at the point where the facial artery crosses and the mandibular branch of the facial nerve becomes superficial, (2) over the malar eminence, and (3) at the midpoint of the patch of temporal skin between the outer canthus of the eye and the superior auricular angle. Extensive dissection in these regions should be avoided, although injury to one of these most peripheral branches of the nerve results in only temporary loss of function in most instances. Conceivably, injury to the nerve branches could occur quite easily to nerves with aberrant courses; however, aberrations of the seventh nerve and its branches are usually in favor of the surgeon, there often being more additional branches and anastomoses than fewer. The classic report of Dingman and Grabb (1962) on the course of the facial nerve and its branches is well worth reviewing.

Temporary weakness or paralysis of a branch may occur following local anesthesia in which the nerve branch is injected accidentally or when the anesthetic agent is carried down to the branch by hyaluronidase (Wydase), which is routinely used by some surgeons. Such paresis normally lasts only a few hours. Branch paresis or paralysis which persists usually means that the branch has been injured during the operative procedure. Such injury may be the result of overheating by the cautery or actual section of the nerve. Attempts to repair the nerve, unless a major trunk has been cut, are unwarranted and generally unsuccessful. If the frontal or mandibular branches are not completely cut, return of function often occurs. If complete sectioning has occurred, some function may return in the form of muscle twitching, which can be most distressing.

A word of warning is in order. A careful preoperative examination of all patients for potential nerve weakness is mandatory. This is particularly important in those patients seeking secondary facial plastic surgery. The patient shown on page 181 is an example of a patient with nerve weakness.

Facial paresis or segmental paralysis following facial plasty is extremely rare.

Temporary paresthesias or hypoesthesia of the skin flaps around the ears and the ear lobes is quite common following face lift operations. This is unquestionably the result of section of small sensory nerves during operation. Full sensation is usually restored within a few weeks following surgery unless the great auricular nerve has been severed, in which case a permanent anesthesia of the lower portion of the ear will result. Sectioning of this nerve during operation should be recognized and the nerve ends repaired with 7-0 or 8-0 silk sutures whenever possible.

PAIN

Intractable pain of the skin of the post-auricular and preauricular areas, and sometimes the ear, occurs but is quite rare. The explanation for this rare phenomenon is usually never discovered. In the author's experience, two cases have occurred. Both patients were classified as being disappointed with the cosmetic result of the operation, although the physicians concerned found the results excellent. No neuromas, excessive scar tissue, or other reasonable explanation could be found. The pain disappeared within six months in both cases.

Conway (1969) reported a similar case and offered trauma or surgical resection of the branches of the cervical sensory nerves as a possible explanation. These branches emerge from the posterior border of the sternocleidomastoid muscle and are theoretically encountered in the operative field.

When such prolonged pain occurs, the patient should be reassured that it is of a temporary nature. Regional sensory nerve blocks at weekly intervals may be of help as well as other supportive measures such as local applications of heat and ultrasound therapy.

Careful palpation of the wound and a sensory nerve examination should be carried out in an effort to delineate localized neuromas. However, such examinations have rarely pinpointed such a lesion.

Secondary Rhytidectomy

It is not possible to predict with any reliable degree of accuracy just when a secondary face lift operation will be required in any individual patient. This question is frequently posed by patients during the initial consultation. Certain generalities apply in guessing when a second operation may be required, but these are only generalities. The patient who shows marked premature aging of the skin with dehydration, loss of elasticity, rhytidosis, and so forth, will probably require a second operation sooner than the patient with more youthful skin who may, for example, have only some excess skin of the neck or jaw line as a complaint. Older patients with degenerative skin changes who have their first rhytidectomy in the sixth or seventh decade of life will require secondary surgery sooner than the patient in the 40 to 45 year old age group with early evidence of skin aging. Weight fluctuation is the most common cause of hastening the date for secondary face lifts. For example, the patient who is slightly heavy before surgery, and who loses weight after primary rhytidectomy, will quite obviously require a secondary operation sooner because of the skin sag resulting from loss of the subcutaneous adipose tissue.

Any changes in the patient's general health that would promote rapid or premature degeneration of the skin can also accelerate the need for secondary surgery. These include: excess alcoholic intake, loss of hormonal effect, certain systemic diseases, especially chronic cardiac and renal disorders, and severe emotional upsets. Heredity certainly plays a prominent role in the aging process in some families. Everyone knows of families in which people live to a ripe old age without a wrinkle in the facial skin, thus maintaining a surprisingly youthful appearance. Cessation of ovarian function after menopause or following oophorectomy can also rapidly and sometimes dramatically accentuate aging of the skin. This effect can often be offset by the administration of conjugated estrogens.

Prolonged and repeated exposure to the elements, especially the wind and sun, accelerates skin aging more than any other environmental factor. This is particularly noticeable in fair-skinned blonds or red heads of Northern European descent. People with darkly pigmented skin can be remarkably deceptive about their age. For example, it is often very difficult to estimate the age of a black African. Maybe this is an explanation of why so many Caucasians spend so much time basking in the sun to darken their skin. Perhaps if they were aware of how much this practice hastened the aging process they would give it up, but, instead, sun bathing flourishes because "everyone looks better with a tan."

It is unwise to make any predictions to patients as to when a second operation may be required, except under certain conditions. The patient with very marked sagging and skin folds might well require a second operation in six months to one year if a maximum operative result is to be obtained. The author advises such patients of this possibility. Likewise if there is considerable skin and fat in the submental cervical area ("turkey gobbler" neck), it is often wise to do a second procedure within six months using direct incisions in the submental region as shown on pages 194 to 196. These patients, too, are advised of the probable need for two operations within a relatively short time.

Most patients should simply be told that a second operation can be done when and if it becomes necessary or desirable to them, usually somewhere within five to ten years. However, they can also be advised with reasonable assuredness that the results of the second operation will be more lasting than those of the first. Some patients may require a third or even a fourth operation.

The typical face lift patient today has her first operation in the early or mid-forties, the second in the fifties, and perhaps a third in her sixties. It could be conjectured that, with the increasing life span and the growing popularity of face lift surgery, these rules will no longer apply and that rehabilitative facial surgery will be continued for one or two decades past the sixties.

Many patients are of the opinion that once a face lift has been done, the second is a necessity because some sort of sudden collapse occurs requiring another operation. This is totally without fact, of course, and the patient should be so advised. It is interesting how such a rumor can create undue fear of a primary face lift in highly intelligent and otherwise well informed individuals.

Exactly when to do a second operation depends on the subjective feelings of the patient and the objective findings of the surgeon, just as

146

the first one does. In general, the first indication that the aging process has again caught up and made itself evident is slight relaxation of the skin under the chin at the cervicomental angle and along the jaw line (jowl). Surgery can then be undertaken for the second time, or the situation can be allowed to progress further until the patient desires correction.

A word is in order about the patient who becomes obsessed with the idea that a second operation is indicated before objective evidence is present. The surgeon must tactfully prolong the waiting period and provide moral support to the patient. Often a divorce, death or other personal tragedy will hasten the request for a second operation in a way similar to that in which such emotional traumas cause people to seek surgery in the first place. The patient hopes the operation will change her life or give her morale a boost. If such a patient was exceedingly happy with the first operation, it may be difficult to get her to wait. Even under such highly charged circumstances, however, the surgeon should not be coerced into operating again before he feels something can be accomplished, because at best the results of a secondary face lift are never so dramatic as the first, and the satisfied face lift patient may be turned into a disillusioned one. Such problems can be avoided by operating only when the objective evidence necessary to indicate a second operation is present.

There is no doubt but that repeated facial operations associated with wide undermining and a certain amount of tension have an effect on the skin itself. Recent work has shown that repeated stretching under tension eventually elicits great and definite changes in the architecture of the skin, principally in the dermal collagen. Stretching of the skin, particularly repeated stretching, unquestionably causes a certain amount of ischemia because the tension is bound to have an effect on skin biology. This effect is probably less extensive following flap surgery on the face and neck skin than elsewhere because of the rich blood supply of this region.

Tension per se is apparently not so significant a fact as tension in the presence of wide undercutting. Myers (1964) utilized fluorescein dye injections to demonstrate the vascularity of wound edges in skin closures following radical mastectomy. His studies showed that tension was less a factor in postoperative skin slough than devascularization due to extensive undermining or undercutting of the skin.

Many studies on the biomechanical properties of skin have been conducted in both animals and man in recent years. These studies have shed light on the relationship between the structure of the skin; its thickness; the effects of edema, obesity and other disease conditions; and, especially, the aging process which is thought to be essentially a process of atrophy and progressive dehydration. Interesting and provocative studies have been carried out along these lines by Rollhäuser (1950), Kirk and Chieffi (1962), Fry, Harkness and Harkness (1964), Ridge and Wright (1959, 1966), Tregear (1966), Parot and Bourlière (1967), Graham and Holt (1969), and Gibson and Kenedi (1969). These studies, particularly those of Gibson and Kenedi, indicate that the skin owes much of its tensile properties to its dermal collagen and possibly its interstitial fluid. The physical relationship of the dermal collagen fibers is particularly of interest when considering repeated stretching of the skin such as occurs in face lifting. It has been shown that the collagen fibers tend to orient themselves perpendicularly to the stretch force when tension or a certain stretch load is applied to the skin.

The formation of natural wrinkles of the skin is unquestionably also a result of skin tension, as well as of anchorage of the underlying muscles of facial expression to the integument. Most such creases are congenital and indicate the attachment of the skin to the tela subcutanea by connective tissue strands which extend from the epidermis through the dermis to the superficial aponeurosis. These wrinkles are often unrelated to the lines of Langer, making the Langer's lines of limited value to the surgeon in planning the effects of facial surgery. Cox (1941) and later Kraissl and Conway (1949) showed the discrepancies which exist between the classic Langer's lines and the normal skin folds and wrinkles in the face and neck which limit the value of the former in planning the incisions and scars.

Montandon (1967) carried out a series of very interesting experiments on the biomechanics of the thoracic esophagus of puppies, particularly on the effects of stretching the esophagus under tension. He did multiple excisions of esophageal segments with successive reanastomoses. He found that the esophagus not only stretched after each excision, but that a certain amount of tissue growth apparently took place so that the normal thickness and texture of the esophagus were restored. There was, however, a limit above which regeneration did not take place. Relating this experiment to stretching of the skin is not apropos, however,

147

because of the anatomical differences of these two structures. Undoubtedly the esophagus "gives" more easily because of its muscularis layer.

As the skin increases in age, its capacity to extend, or stretch, decreases. This same decrease in elasticity is observed in the presence of edema or obesity. It is well known that the skin of the younger patient will withstand repeated stretching with less effect than will that of the elderly or aged patient. This is probably true because the elastic fiber meshwork is more highly developed in the young and the collagen fibers are in a more active state of metabolism, so they are more easily able to adapt themselves to repeated stretch loads. More stretching is therefore needed in youthful skin (when stretching is desired) to overcome the natural resiliency of the elastic fibers or to cause perpendicular reorientation of the collagen bundles. An example of this is in the well known technique of serial excision of benign lesions such as hemangiomas, hairy nevi or wide scars in the young.

The multiple-stage excision technique was first described by Morestin, who, in 1915, used this technique to remove a large benign lesion. He proposed and advised serial excisions for many types of lesions, including nevi, hemangiomas and scar tissue, but cautioned against such excisions if they would produce pull on vital cosmetic areas such as the eyelids or the commissures of the mouth. In his early experimentations with this technique, he advised repetition of the serial excision every three to four days. However, in subsequent publications (1916), he allowed at least a month's interval between operations. Morestin's excisions were not accompanied by undermining or undercutting of the flaps, which was later recommended by Smith (1946, 1950, 1958), who was a strong advocate of the staged excision technique for the ablation of facial lesions.

The multiple-stage principle is applicable to both children and adults. However, it is noted that with repeated undercutting and stretching of the skin in adults, such as also occurs in several face lifts, the skin does seem to lose its natural elastic properties and can at times assume an unnatural appearance. This can result in a "mask look" which is considered most undesirable by both patient and surgeon. This most often occurs in patients who have repeated face lift operations at too frequent intervals. Such patients often travel from surgeon to surgeon until they find one who will accommodate their desires. It rarely occurs after judicious surgery, properly timed by a competent surgeon who varies his operative technique at each operation to meet the demands at that time.

Secondary operation is almost invariably technically easier to perform than the first. The original incisions are used, sometimes with added innovations such as the horizontal temporal hair line incision (p. 167) or variations in the postauricular hair line incision. Such variations allow for changes in the direction of pull that may be required to correct secondary jowls or progressive loosening of the skin of the neck. All scar tissue at the previous incision site is excised. However, this should not be done until the undermining is completed, as it is frequently astonishing just how little skin margin can also be excised. In fact, the surgeon is usually surprised to find that despite extensive undermining of the skin, an unexpectedly small amount of tissue can be resected in secondary operations. Often it is possible to excise no more than the previous scar itself. The improvement in results at secondary surgery is, therefore, probably more likely the result of redistribution of skin and whatever physical changes occur from undermining than from actual excision of excess skin, for, as just noted, there often is little or no excess. This may well be the result of the loss of the ability of the skin to stretch following previous surgery, which is probably related to the natural atrophy of the elastic fibers which occurs with age, dehydration of the skin (also a phenomenon of aging), and application of tension to the skin which has caused a realignment of collagen fibers perpendicular to the direction of pull.

The undermining should proceed from the clearly visible scar plane left over from the primary surgery and should extend beyond the edge of this plane anteriorly over the jaw well into the neck. It is more often necessary in secondary than primary surgery to undermine completely across the midline of the neck and to join up with the undermining of the opposite side. Contrary to what occurs in scar tissue planes elsewhere, as in the peritoneal cavity, bleeding from face lift scar planes is usually minimal or greatly reduced at secondary rhytidectomy. This significantly diminishes the operative time.

Secondary surgery may change the hair line by raising it or drawing the temporal hair line farther back. The patient should be advised of this, although it is rarely a significant problem.

The recovery period from secondary face lifting is also usually shorter than with the first, and the incidence of skin slough is also less, as would be expected. The primary operation acts as a "delay."

148

REFERENCES

Adamson, J. E., Horton, C. E., and Crawford, H. H.: The surgical correction of "turkey gobbler" deformity. Plast. Reconstr. Surg. *34*:598, 1964.

Alibert, J.-L.: Monographie des Dermatoses ou Précis Théorique et Pratique des Maladies de la Peau. Paris, Daynac, 1832, p. 795.

Aufricht, G.: Surgery for excess skin of the face and neck. Transactions of the 2nd Congress of the International Society of Plastic Surgeons, edited by Wallace. Baltimore, The Williams & Wilkins Co., 1960, pp. 495–502.

Baker, T. J.: Chemical face peeling and rhytidectomy. Plast. Reconstr. Surg. *29*:199, 1962.

Baker, T. J., and Gordon, H. L.: Complications of rhytidectomy. Plast. Reconstr. Surg. *40*:31, 1967.

Baker, T. J., and Gordon, H. L.: Rhytidectomy in males. Plast. Reconstr. Surg. *44*:219, 1969.

Bames, H.: Truth and fallacies of face peeling and face lifting. Med. J. & Rec. *126*:86, 1927.

Bames, H.: Frown disfigurement and ptosis of the eyebrows. Plast. Reconstr. Surg. *19*:337, 1957.

Barsky, A. J.: Plastic Surgery. Philadelphia, W. B. Saunders Company, 1938, p. 124.

Bourguet, J.: La chirurgie esthétique de la face. Le Concours Médical, 1921, pp. 1657–1670.

Bourguet, J.: La chirurgie esthétique de l'oeil et des paupières. Monde Médical, 1929, pp. 725–731.

Castanares, S.: Forehead wrinkles, glabellar frown and ptosis of the eybrows. Plast. Reconstr. Surg. *34*:406, 1964.

Claoué, C.: Documents de Chirurgie Plastique et Esthétique. Compte Rendu des Séances de la Société Scientifique Française de Chirurgie Plastique et Esthétiques. Paris, Maloine, 1931, pp. 344–353.

Claoué, C.: La ridectomie cervico-faciale. Correction de la ptose cutanée cervico-faciale par accrochage parieto-temporo-occipital et résection cutanée. Acad. Nat. Méd. Bull. *109*:257, 1933.

Conley, J.: Face-lift Operation. Springfield, Ill., Charles C Thomas, 1968.

Conway, H.: Factors underlying prolonged pain following rhytidectomy. Transactions of the 4th International Congress of Plastic and Reconstructive Surgery. Amsterdam, Excerpta Medica Foundation, 1969, pp. 1120–1122.

Conway, H.: The surgical face lift—rhytidectomy. Plast. Reconstr. Surg. *45*:124, 1970.

Cox, H. T.: The cleavage lines of the skin. Brit. J. Surg. *29*:234, 1941.

Cronin, T. D., and Biggs, T. M.: The T-Z-plasty for the male "turkey gobbler" neck. Plast. Reconstr. Surg. *47*:534, 1971.

Davis, A. D.: Obligations in the consideration of meloplasties. J. Internat. Coll. Surg. *24*:568, 1955.

Dingman, R. O., and Grabb, W. C.: Surgical anatomy of the mandibular ramus of the facial nerve based on the dissection of 100 facial halves. Plast. Reconstr. Surg. *20*:266, 1962.

Dupuytren, G.: De l'oedéme chronique et des tumeurs enkystées des paupières. Lecons Orales de Clinique Chirurgicale. 2nd ed. Vol. III, pp. 377–378. Paris, Germer-Ballière, 1839.

Duverger, C., and Velter, E.: Thérapeutique Chirurgicale Ophthalmologique. Paris, Masson et Cie, 1926, p. 79.

Edgerton, M. T., Webb, W. L., Slaughter, R., and Meyer, E.: Surgical results and psychosocial changes following rhytidectomy. Plast. Reconstr. Surg. *33*:503, 1964.

Edwards, B. F.: Bilateral temporal neurotomy for frontalis hypermotility: Case report. Plast. Reconstr. Surg. *19*:341, 1957.

Elschnig, A.: Fetthernien, Sog. "Tränensacke" der Unterlieder. Klin. Mbl. Augenheilk. *84*:763, 1930.

Erich, J. B.: Surgical elimination of wrinkles, redundant skin and pouches about the eyelids. Proc. Mayo Clinic *36*:101, 1961.

Fomon, S.: Surgery of Injury and Plastic Repair. Baltimore, The Williams & Wilkins Co., 1939, pp. 135–137.

Fomon, S.: Cosmetic Surgery, Principles and Practice. Philadelphia, J. B. Lippincott Company, 1960.

Fry, P., Harkness, M. L., and Harkness, R. D.: Mechanical properties of the collagenous framework of skin in rats of different ages. Amer. J. Physiol. *206*:1425, 1964.

Gibson, T., and Kenedi, R. M.: The significance and measurement of skin tensions in man. Transactions of the 3rd International Congress of Plastic Surgery. Amsterdam, Excerpta Medica Foundation, 1964, pp. 387–395.

Gibson, T., and Kenedi, R. M.: Biomechanical properties of skin. Surg. Clin. N. Amer. *47*:279, 1967.

Gibson, T., and Kenedi, R. M.: Factors affecting the mechanical characteristics of human skin. *In* Dunphy, J. E., and Van Winkle, W., Jr. (ed.): Repair and Regeneration. New York, McGraw-Hill Book Co., 1969, p. 87.

Gillies, H., and Millard, D. R.: Principles and Art of Pastic Surgery. Boston, Little, Brown and Company, 1957.

Ginester, G., Frézières, H., Dupuis, A., and Pons, J.: Chirurgie Plastique et Reconstructrice de la Face. Paris, Flammarion et Cie, 1967, pp. 184–187.

González-Ulloa, M.: Facial wrinkles. Plast. Reconstr. Surg. *29*:658, 1962.

González-Ulloa, M., and Stevens, E. F.: Senility of the face. Basic study to understand its causes and effects. Plast. Reconstr. Surg. *36*:239, 1965.

Graft, D.: Oertliche erbliche erschlaffung der Haut. Wschr. Ges. Heilk., 1836, pp. 225–227.

Grahame, R., and Holt, P. J.: The influence of ageing on the in vivo elasticity of human skin. Gerontologia *15*:121, 1969.

Hollander, M. M.: Rhytidectomy: Anatomical, physiological and surgical considerations. Plast. Reconstr. Surg. *20*:218, 1957.

Hunt, H. L.: Plastic Surgery of the Head, Face and Neck. Philadelphia, Lea & Febiger, 1926, p. 198.

Johnson, J. B., and Hadley, R. C.: The aging face. *In* Converse, J. M. (ed.): Reconstructive Plastic Surgery. Philadelphia, W. B. Saunders Company, 1964, pp. 1306–1342.

Joseph, J.: Plastic operation on protruding cheek. Deutsch. Med. Wschr. *47*:287, 1921.

Joseph, J.: Nasenplastik und Sonstige Gesichtsplastik nebst einen Anhang über Mammaplastik. Leipzig, Curt Kabitzsch, 1928, pp. 525–527.

Joseph, J.: Verbesserung meiner Hängemangenplastik (Melomioplastik). Deutsch. Med. Wschr. *54*:567, 1928.

Journal Universel et Hebdomadaire de Médecine et de Chirurgie Pratiques et des Institutions Médicales, Vol. 1–13, Oct. 1830–Dec. 1833.

Kapp, J. F. S.: Die Technik du kosmetischen Encheiresen. Beih. Med. Klin. *3*:65, 1913.

Kapp, J. F. S.: Premature Old Age in Women; A Study in the Tragedy of the Middle Aged. New York, P. L. Baruch, 1925.

Kirk, J. E., and Chieffi, M.: Variation with age in elasticity of skin and subcutaneous tissue in human individuals. J. Geront. *17*:373, 1962.

Knorr, N. J., Edgerton, M. T., and Hoopes, J. E.: The "insatiable" cosmetic surgery patient. Plast. Reconstr. Surg. *40*:285, 1967.

Kolle, F. S.: Plastic and Cosmetic Surgery. New York, Appleton, 1911, pp. 116–117.

Kraissl, C. J., and Conway, H.: Excision of small tumors of skin and face. Surgery *25*:592, 1949.

Lagarde, M.: Nouvelles techniques pour le traitement des rides de la face et du cou. Arch. Franco-Belges. Chir. *31*:154, 1928.

Lewis, G. K.: Surgical treatment of wrinkles. A.M.A. Arch Otolaryng. *60*:334, 1954.

Lexer, E.: Zur Gesichtsplastik. Arch. Klin. Chir. *92*:749, 1910.

Litton, C.: Chemical face lifting. Plast. Reconstr. Surg. *29*:371, 1962.

Macgregor, F. C.: Some psychological hazards of plastic surgery of the face. Plast. Reconstr. Surg. *12*:123, 1953.

Macgregor, F. C.: Selection of cosmetic surgery patients: Social and psychological considerations. Surg. Clin. N. Amer. *51*:289, 1970.

Macgregor, F. C., and Schaffner, B.: Screening patients for

149

nasal plastic operations: Sociologic and psychiatric considerations. Psychosomat. Med. *12*:277, 1950.

Maliniac, J. W.: Is the surgical restoration of the aging face justified? Med. J. & Rec. *135*:321, 1932.

Marino, H.: Frontal rhytidectomy. Bol. Soc. Cirug. B. Aires *47*:93, 1963.

Marino, H., Galeano, E. J., and Gandolfo, E. A.: Plastic correction of double chin. Plast. Reconstr. Surg. *31*:45, 1963.

May, H.: Reconstructive and Reparative Surgery. Philadelphia, F. A. Davis Co., 1947, pp. 325–326.

Mayer, D. M., and Swanker, W. A.: Rhytidoplasty. Plast. Reconstr. Surg. *6*:255, 1950.

Millard, D. R., Pigott, R. W., and Hedo, A.: Submandibular lipectomy. Plast. Reconstr. Surg. *41*:513, 1968.

Miller, C. C.: Semilunar excision of the skin at the outer canthus for the eradication of crow's feet. Amer. J. Derm. *11*:483, 1907a.

Miller, C. C.: Subcutaneous section of local muscles to eradicate expression lines. Amer. J. Surg. *21*:235, 1907b.

Miller, C. C.: The eradication by surgical means of the nasolabial line. Therap. Gaz. *23*:676, 1907c.

Miller, C. C.: Cosmetic Surgery. The Correction of Featural Imperfections. Chicago, Oak Printing Co., 1908, pp. 40–42.

Miller, C. C.: Cosmetic Surgery. Philadelphia, F. A. Davis Co., 1924, pp. 30–32.

Miller, C. C.: Facial bands as supports to relaxed facial tissue. Ann. Surg. *82*:603, 1925.

Montandon, D.: Quelques aspects des techniques du traitement chirurgical de l'atréside de l'oesophage. Thèse No. 3079. Geneva, Editions Médecine et Hygiène, 1967.

Montandon, D.: Personal communication, 1970.

Morel-Fatio, D.: Cosmetic surgery of the face. *In* Gibson, T. (ed.): Modern Trends in Plastic Surgery. London, Butterworth & Co., Ltd., 1964, pp. 221–222.

Morestin, H.: La réduction graduelle des déformités tégumentaires. Bull. Mém. Soc. Chir. Paris. *41*:1233, 1915.

Morestin, H.: Cicatrice très étendue du crâne réduite par des excisions successives. Bull. Mém. Soc. Chir. Paris *42*:2052, 1916.

Myers, M. B.: Wound tension and vascularity in the etiology and prevention of skin sloughs. Surgery *56*:945, 1964.

Noël, A.: La Chirurgie Esthétique. Son Role Social. Paris, Masson et Cie, 1926, pp. 62–66.

Noël, A.: La Chirurgie Esthétique. Clermont (Oise), Thiron et Cie, 1928.

Padgett, E. C., and Stevenson, K. C.: Plastic and Reconstructive Surgery. Springfield, Ill., Charles C Thomas, 1948, p. 514.

Pangman, W. J., II, and Wallace, R. M.: Cosmetic surgery of the face and neck. Plast. Reconstr. Surg. *27*:544, 1961.

Panneton, P.: Mémoire sur le blepharochalazis. 51 cas dans la même famille. Un. Med. Canada *65*:725, 1936b.

Parot, S., and Bourlière, F.: Une nouvelle technique de mesure de la compressibilité de la peau et du tissu sous-cutané. Influence du sexe, de l'âge et du site de mesure sur les résultats. Gerontologia *13*:95, 1967.

Passot, R.: La chirurgie esthétique des rides du visage. Presse Méd. *27*:258, 1919.

Passot, R.: La correction chirurgicale des rides du visage. Bull. Acad. Méd. Paris *82*:112, 1919.

Passot, R.: La Chirurgie Esthétique Pure (Technique et Résultats). Paris, Gaston Doin et Cie, 1931, pp. 176–180.

Pitanguy, I.: Personal communication, 1970.

Pitanguy, I., and Ramos, A. S.: The frontal branch of the facial nerve: The importance of its variations in face lifting. Plast. Reconstr. Surg. *38*:352, 1966.

Ridge, M. D., and Wright, V.: The rheology of skin: A bio-engineering study of the mechanical properties of human skin in relation to its structure. Brit. J. Derm. *77*:639, 1965.

Robertson, J. G.: Chin augmentation by means of rotation of double chin fat flap. Plast. Reconstr. Surg. *36*:471, 1965.

Rollhäuser, H.: Die Zugfestigheit der menschlichen Haut. Gegenbaur. Morph. Jahrb. *90*:249, 1950.

Sheehan, J. E.: *In* McIndoe, A. H.: Personal communication, 1955.

Smith, F.: Multiple excision and Z-plasties in surface reconstruction. Plast. Reconstr. Surg. *1*:170, 1946.

Smith, F.: Plastic and Reconstructive Surgery. Philadelphia, W. B. Saunders Company, 1950.

Smith, F.: Multiple excision with occasional Z-plasty for correction of disabilities of exposed surfaces. Amer. J. Surg. *95*:173, 1958.

Spira, M., Gerow, F. J., and Hardy, S. B.: Cervicofacial rhytidectomy. Plast. Reconstr. Surg. *40*:551, 1967.

Stark, R. B.: Plastic Surgery. New York, Paul B Hoeber, 1962, p. 229.

Stephenson, K. L.: The "mini-lift," an old wrinkle in face lifting. Plast. Reconst. Surg. *46*:226, 1970.

Tregear, R. T.: Physical Functions of Skin. New York, Academic Press, Inc., 1966.

Uchida, J. I.: A method of frontal rhytidectomy. Plast. Reconstr. Surg. *35*:218, 1965.

Vogt, A.: Die senile determination des Keimplasmas, bedbachtet an eineigen Zwillinges des 55–81 jahres. Schweiz. Med. Wschr. *16*:576, 1935.

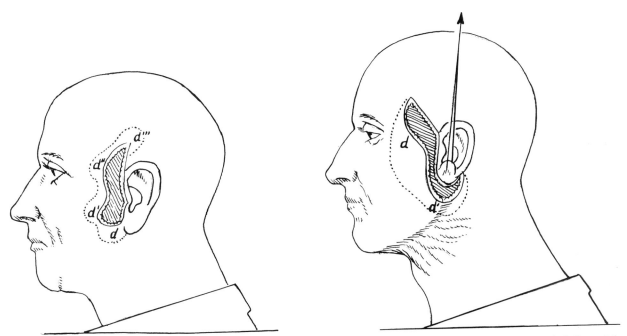

Perhaps the first description of the "minilift" was provided by Passot; this drawing has been copied from his book on the subject, published in 1917. Preauricular skin excision accompanied by little or no skin undermining was abandoned by most surgeons because the results were short-lived. The procedure has recently regained a certain vogue, but it should be relegated to history.

Patients inquiring about the possible results of facial plastic surgery often indicate the desired improvement by pulling the skin of the face and neck taut with their fingers (*B*). Although this maneuver gives a general idea of what may happen, it is not an accurate picture, as the correction tends to be exaggerated, particularly around the mouth and nasolabial folds. This point has to be emphasized to the patient seeking cosmetic surgery. On the other hand, the tautness of the jawline and the visible improvement of the neck will approach this simulated result. Fine rhytides in the facial skin will be improved somewhat, but not nearly to the degree that this manual tightening maneuver implies.

Immediately after surgery, particularly while postoperative edema persists, the results most often equal the patient's expectations. As time passes and edema subsides, folds and wrinkles will recur, particularly in severe cases. These shortcomings of the operative procedure must be emphasized before the operation.

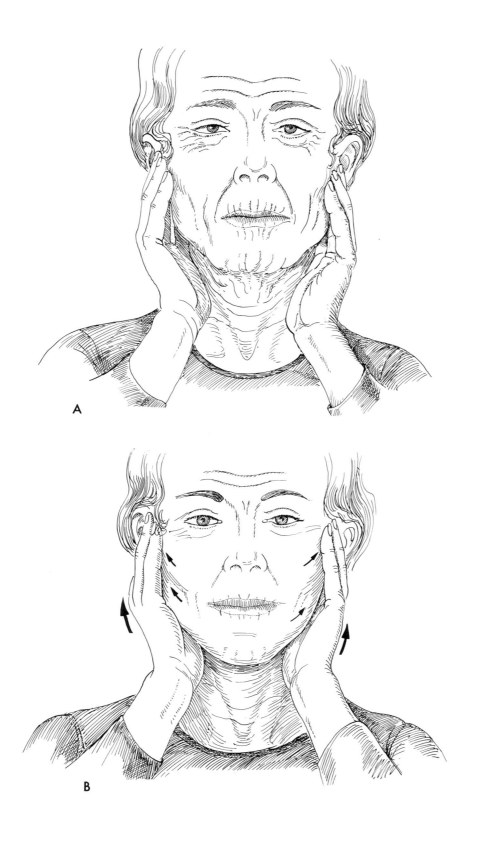

A

B

153

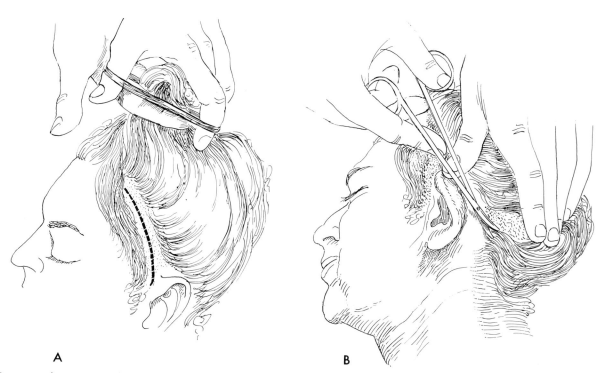

A   **B**

Preoperative preparation for the usual face lift operation begins by combing the hair upward and fixing it with a rubber band as a top knot or "pony tail" (*A*). Sharp barber's scissors can be used to cut tracks in the temporal scalp and behind the ear to coincide with the planned incisions (*B*). These trimmed areas should be only as large as the amount of skin to be excised, so that the final suture lines lie virtually within the hair. Because preoperative preparation with pHisoHex shampoo has practically eliminated wound infections, shaving of the hair is not necessary.

154

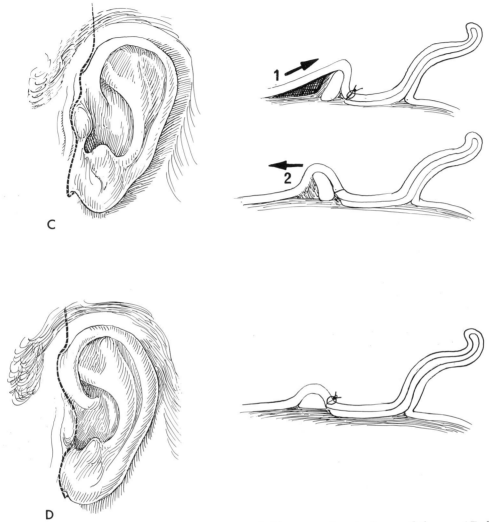

C

D

The preauricular incision is usually placed in the normal skin crease just in front of the ear (*C*), but in some patients the incision can be carried behind the tragus so that most of the scar will be virtually invisible (*D*). This is done only in patients who have no natural line in front of the ear and who do not have a prominent or sharp tragal cartilage; otherwise, normal wound contraction may result in distortion of the tragus and an unnatural look (*C*, 1 and 2).

The usual preauricular incision heals surprisingly well and with minimal scarring, provided the sutures are removed within six days. The incision should form a slight angle at the superior edge of the tragus in order to follow the natural line of the ear.

(Illustration continued on following page.)

The skin is marked with dye or a marking pen, the exact design of the planned incisions varying with each patient according to the amount of skin excision intended, the direction of pull, and so forth (E). An educated guess at the amount of skin to be removed from the temporal and preauricular regions can be arrived at by gently pushing the skin of the face in the direction of pull (upward and backward), so that a fold is formed in front of the ear (F). The excess is then marked, and the excision is shaped to allow later rotation of the skin flap. For example, if marked upward rotation of the upper face is required in a patient with considerable ptosis of the lateral brow, the temporal incision is angled posteriorly to allow this greater rotation. It is wise to occlude the external auditory canal with cotton or earplugs to prevent accumulation of blood that can be difficult to remove postoperatively (G).

In making such a preoperative estimation of the amount of skin to be excised, it is very important that the surgeon (particularly the beginning surgeon) underestimate markedly. It is not difficult to excise additional skin later in the operation, but it may be impossible to stretch skin adequately if too much has been removed. The wound may possibly be closed under great tension, but the resulting scar will testify to the drastic measure employed. It will probably spread, and it may hypertrophy.

Tension on the skin flaps should exist only in the temporal scalp and behind the ear in the mastoid skin and posterior scalp. Skin flaps in front of the ear should lie exactly in place (gently "kissing"), with no tension whatsoever. Excellent scars will result in most patients if this technique is used. Always be conservative with the preauricular incision; allow for final adjustments at the end of the operation. (From Rees, T. D.: Technical considerations in blepharoplasty and rhytidectomy. Transactions of the Fifth International Congress of Plastic Reconstructive Surgery, Australia, 1971. London, Butterworth & Co. Ltd., 1971, p. 1067.)

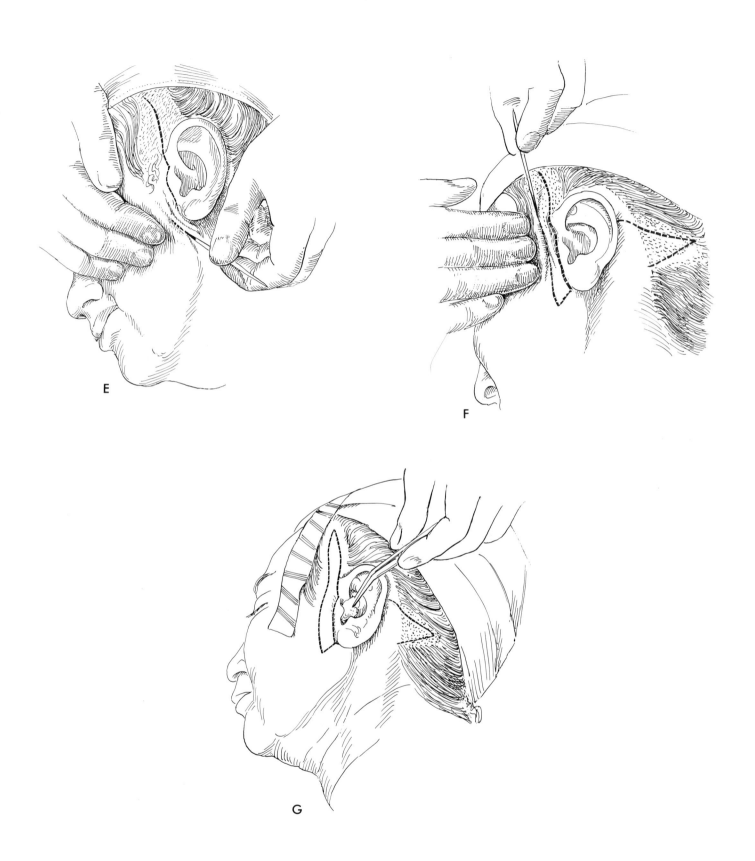

E

F

G

(Illustration continued on following page.)

As the skin incision is continued around the earlobe (*H*), it should hug the anterior lobe crease exactly and then be carried slightly posterior to the posterior crease, creating a small flange or flap (*I*, line 2). This incision will help to avoid breakdown of the suture line later on. If line 1 (*I*) is used, anterior and posterior suture lines will be so close together that dehiscence can occur, resulting in a detached lobe.

The authors rarely attempt to create an earlobe if one does not exist, unless the patient strongly requests it.

When the incision line is being marked around the earlobe, no traction may be put on the lobe in a misguided attempt to facilitate the marking (*J*). Such traction distorts the natural lines and creases in this region and can make a great deal of difference in the position and, hence, in the appearance of the final scar. Moreover, traction can cause accidental detachment of the earlobe if it is applied while the incision is being made (*K*).

Once past the lobe, the incision marking is placed in the depth of the cephalo-auricular groove (*I* 2) and then turned onto the conchal convexity. Such far forward placement of the incision, actually on the posterior surface of the concha, produces a suture line in the auricular crease and not several millimeters back on the mastoid skin. Subsequent placement of an anchoring suture in the conchal cartilage is also made much easier.

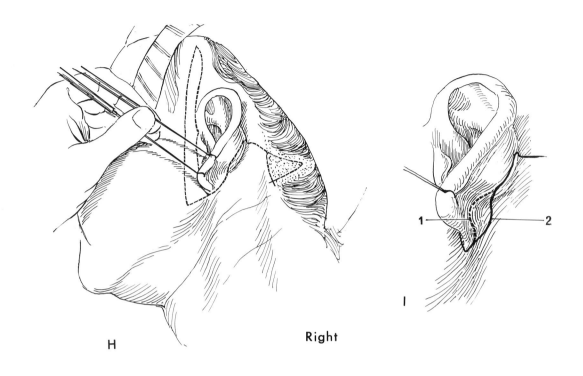

H

Right

I

1 2

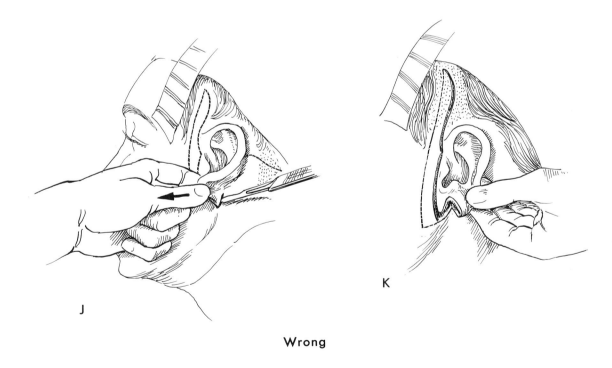

J

Wrong

K

(Illustration continued on following page.)

The incision line then sweeps backward over the mastoid skin at about the level of the superior edge of the external auditory canal, or slightly higher. It is quite unnecessary to place the line any higher than that. Where the line meets the hairline is another matter for individual decision. Whether the incision is carried posteriorly directly into the hair or follows the hairline downward depends on the configuration of the skin of the neck, the width of the skin over the mastoid process between the ear and the hairline, and the amount of rotation of the skin flap that will be required. A further consideration, though not a matter of major importance, is the patient's hair style. If the hair is worn swept back, every effort should be made to place the incision well within the hair so that there will not be a scar extending down the neck.

In the patient with early jowl formation and some loose skin under the chin, it is usually possible to extend the posterior part of the incision directly back into the hairline so that rotation is possible and a scar that follows the hairline is avoided (M 3). But if the neck is very loose, and particularly when there is excessive skin as far down as the suprasternal notch, it is almost impossible to achieve sufficient tightening except by following the hairline with the posterior incision. At times it may even be necessary to continue it back as far as the midline, but the authors have done this extremely rarely.

When the isthmus of skin between the ear and the hairline is quite narrow (L 1), following the hairline with the skin incision would create a correspondingly narrow skin flap, which would be prone to circulatory troubles when placed under tension. Thus, it is safer to design a flap that extends back into the hair (M). Following the hairline is safer when there is a wide band of skin behind the ear (N 2).

(From Rees, T. D.: Technical Considerations in Blepharoplasty and Rhytidectomy, Transactions of the Fifth International Congress of Plastic and Reconstructive Surgery, London, Butterworth and Co., Ltd., 1971, p. 1067.

160

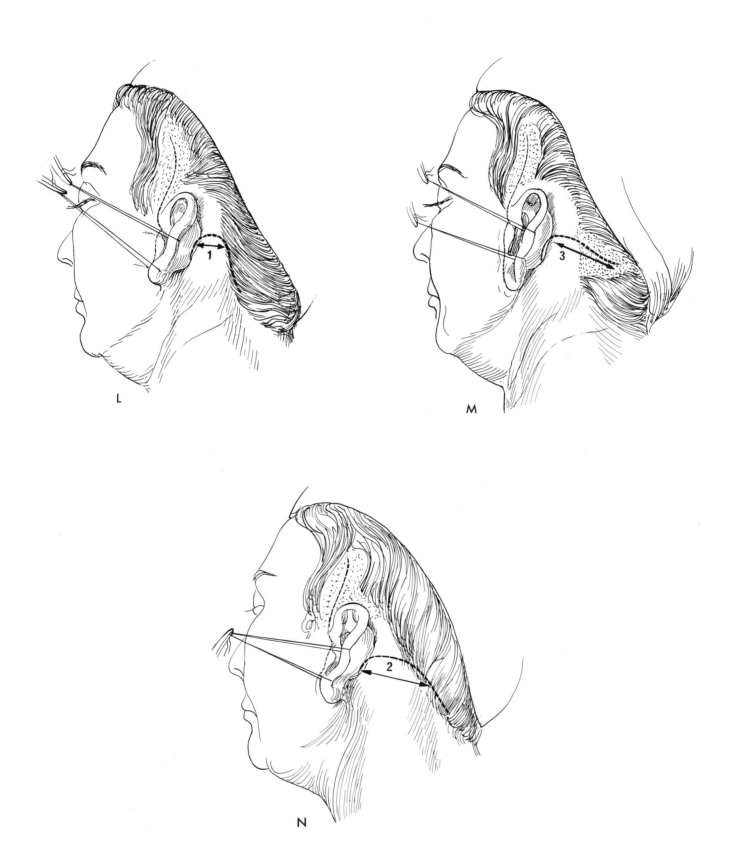

The first steps in the face lift operation for the average patient. The dotted line in *A* shows the *minimal* amount of undermining; more is usually needed, particularly in the neck. The skin incision is preplanned, on the conservative side, as indicated in *A* by the shaded area in front of the ear (and as described in the preceding pages). *B,* The strip of skin is excised. *C,* Undermining is best accomplished with double-edged scissors that have been sharpened on both sides of both blades. The mastoid skin and that overlying the sternocleidomastoid muscle is usually lifted by sharp dissection with a scalpel, as it is adherent. *D,* A key traction suture is placed in the temporal scalp and rotates the cheek flap superiorly, as indicated by the arrows.

The amount of undermining naturally varies from patient to patient. In the younger subject with small jowls over the body of the mandible, it is necessary to undermine only to the anterior extent of this skin fold and as much of the neck as seems necessary. Slackness of the skin over the jaw is almost inevitable in face lift patients, so that undermining is almost always required, whereas the extent of undermining on the neck depends on the configuration of the soft tissues of the neck. It may be minimal or it may cross the midline so that the skin of the neck is completely lifted. Such undermining is best kept to a superficial level to avoid damage to the seventh cranial nerve and to blood vessels, particularly the jugular vein.

The skin flap is raised with a very thin layer of fat, almost as in a full-thickness graft. When such a flap is retracted and seen from beneath, it is almost transparent. It is so thin that extreme care must be taken to preserve the blood supply and to avoid injuring the vessels. Traction is exerted only with skin hooks or traction sutures, and the flaps are not handled manually. Squeezing or excessive traction during the dissection can result in irreversible damage to the blood vessels, causing embarrassment of circulation, thrombosis, and sloughing of the skin. Minor skin sloughing is most frequently encountered over the mastoid process, where the maximum stretch is exerted, and it is also in this area that skin flaps are most likely to be abused between the thumb and the forefinger during surgery.

Dissection in the loose subcutaneous and supraplatysmal tissue plane of the neck and face is best accomplished by the "spread and cut" scissor technique. Scalpel dissection serves best over the mastoid process and down the neck above the sternocleidomastoid muscle, where the skin is intimately associated with the underlying fascia. Take care to avoid injury to the postauricular nerve during these procedures. Severing this nerve produces permanent numbness of the lower part of the ear and the earlobe. If the nerve is accidentally cut and the damage is recognized during surgery, repair using 7–0 or 8–0 silk sutures in the epineurium should be carried out immediately.

Hemostasis should be meticulously carried out with fine pointed forceps and cautery. Larger vessels are ligated; if the jugular vein is cut, it is divided between clamps and tied. Pinpoint electrocoagulation of bleeding vessels is called for, without offense to the surrounding normal tissue. Excessive cauterization, especially on the underside of the skin flap, will cause focal necrosis and sometimes small perforations; scarring will mar the final result. Larger vessels, again particularly those on the flap, should be protected from the cautery when possible to avoid segmental infarction.

The facial nerve will not be endangered if the dissection can be maintained at a superficial level. Where the ramus mandibularis becomes superficial (penetrating the platysma near the external maxillary artery over the body of the mandible), particular care is required. Another dangerous area is the temporal region, and caution must be exercised to avoid injuring the temporal branch of the facial nerve. Dissection should be superficial to the temporal fascia; as it proceeds anteriorly, a nerve stimulator can be used if doubt exists as to the location of this branch. Pitanguy has recommended dissection beneath the temporal fascia on this account, but this procedure seems hazardous to the authors in spite of his anatomical evidence.

We do not recommend dissecting as far anteriorly as the corner of the mouth, or the nasolabial fold. The terminal branches of the facial nerve become extremely superficial at these places and can be easily injured, resulting in partial or complete paralysis of the muscles they innervate. It is quite true that these terminal branches may regenerate, but regeneration is not always complete, and in some instances disassociated muscle fasciculations persist indefinitely.

Dissection over the malar eminence is rarely necessary and should be undertaken with care to avoid damaging the buccal or ophthalmic branches of the facial nerve. Dissection medial to the lateral wall of the zygoma is practically never indicated.

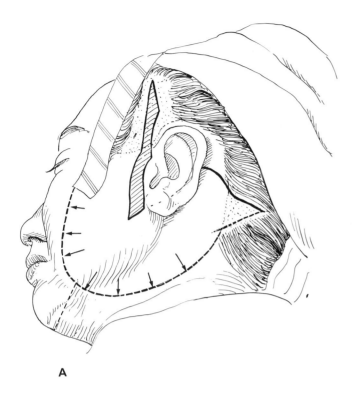

A

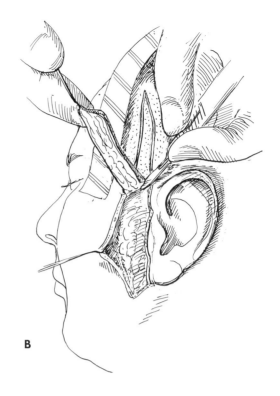

B

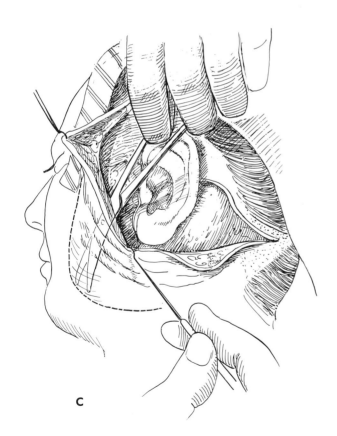

C

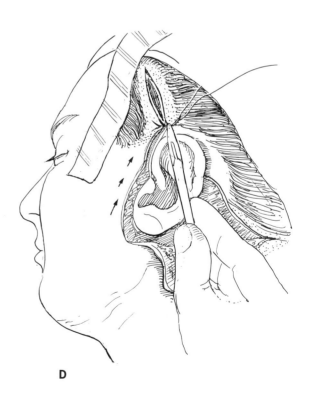

D

(Illustration continued on following page.)

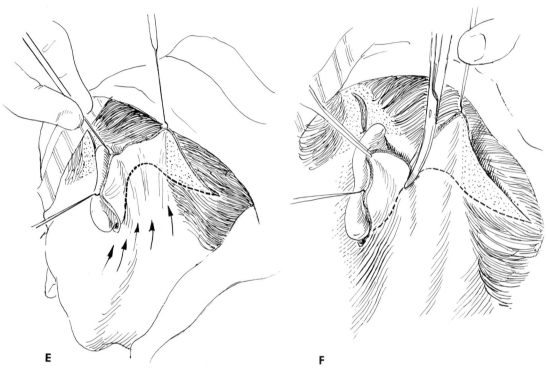

E   F

When undermining has been completed and hemostasis secured, the skin flaps are redraped over the bony framework of the face and excess skin is removed. The direction of pull depends on the deformity that is to be corrected in the individual patient. Excess skin may exist along the jaw, in the neck, or in the upper part of the face. Excess skin is most easily correctable in the neck; skin folds that deepen the nasolabial crease are the most difficult to erase.

Redraping is done by rotating the cheek flap superiorly by traction with a skin hook. A point of fixation is then secured with a suture. The mastoid skin is pulled with a skin hook (E), which places traction on the whole posterior neck flap. A fixation point is located at the peak of the postauricular incision (F), the skin flap is cut to this point, and the point is secured with a suture (G, H). The excess skin of the temporal and postauricular flaps is cut out with scissors, leaving the excess or overlapping skin around the ear to be trimmed last. It is helpful to fix the flap with one deep suture taken through the conchal cartilage (I). Skin suturing is done with 4–0 and 5–0 Dermalon sutures. Some surgeons prefer to add a row of buried dermis sutures, particularly in the postauricular and hairline regions, to reduce the tension on the skin sutures and to permit their early removal. The authors find such sutures more troublesome than necessary and rarely use them, except in men.

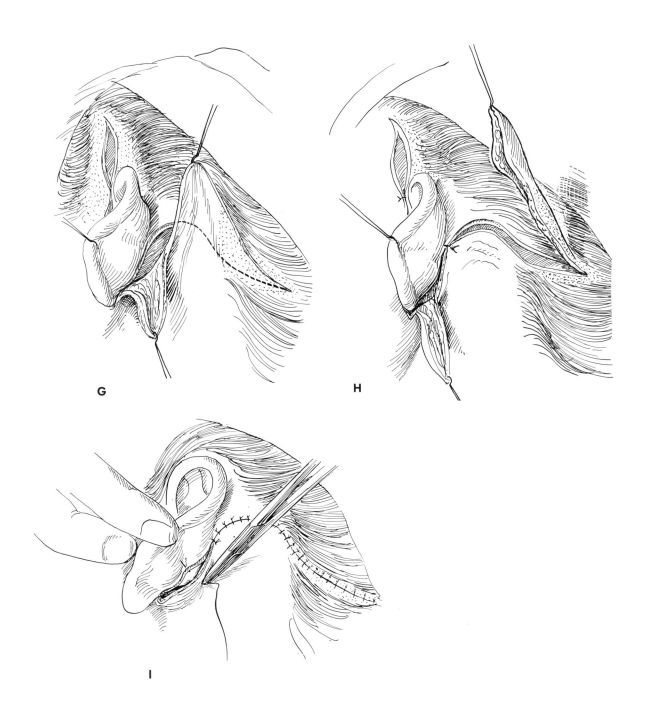

G

H

I

(Illustration continued on following page.)

165

When the fold of excess skin is quite marked along the mandible, the upward rotation that can be achieved with the standard preauricular and temporal incision may be insufficient. A horizontal incision at the lower border of the hairline, usually at the level of the superior end of the cephalo-auricular groove, constitutes a suitable modification of the standard technique in such cases (*J*). The incision is made through the skin flap. The point of the small flap thus created is grasped with forceps or a skin hook and traction is applied cephalad, thus achieving greater upward rotation of the entire cheek flap (*K*). The triangle of this small flap is then excised (*L*). The horizontal incision made for this purpose should not extend any farther forward than the anterior hairline, except in patients with deep wrinkling of the temporal skin ("crow's feet"). There will sometimes be a small dog-ear left at the point of the flap, but it can be corrected by undermining in all directions. The wound is then sutured along with the key traction suture, pinning the point of the flap to the more stable scalp (*M*). Precise additional tailoring of the preauricular skin flap is usually required when such a horizontal incision is made.

(From Rees, T. D., and Guy, C. L.: Surg. Clin. N. Amer., *51*:353, 1971.)

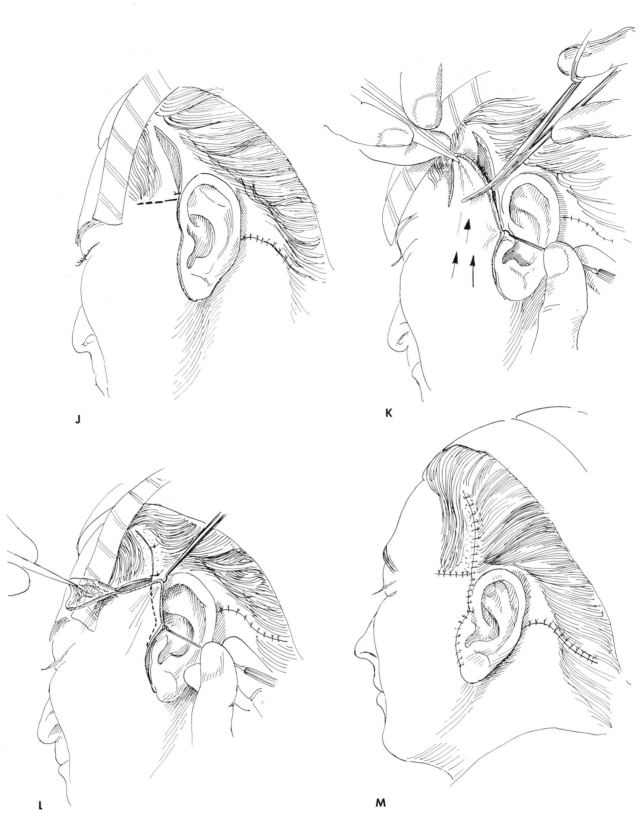

J

K

L

M

(Illustration continued on following page.)

167

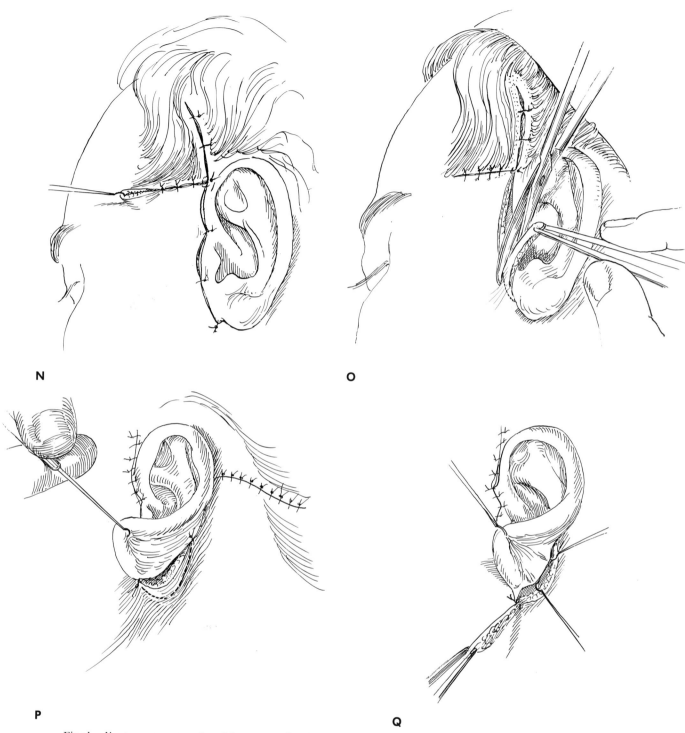

N

O

P

Q

Final adjustments to excise skin are made after key sutures have been placed. A small dog-ear may present at the anterior angle of the horizontal incision (if any); it is trimmed by the conventional method of elevating it with a skin hook and removing a triangle (N). These small dog-ears should not be pursued farther forward than the limit of the hairline, in order to avoid visible scars. In some patients a small redundancy here may be necessary for this reason, but these usually smooth out with time.

Any excess of preauricular skin is trimmed as a final step (O). Trimming here should be conservative, so that there is absolutely no tension on the preauricular closure; otherwise, spreading of the final scar will result. The preauricular scar must be as inconspicuous as possible, for it is the only part of the incision that is likely to be visible.

A very small strip of skin behind the earlobe is removed to allow accurate tailoring of the wound (P and Q). This is semicircular in design, conforming to the slight flange effect of the original preoperative plan.

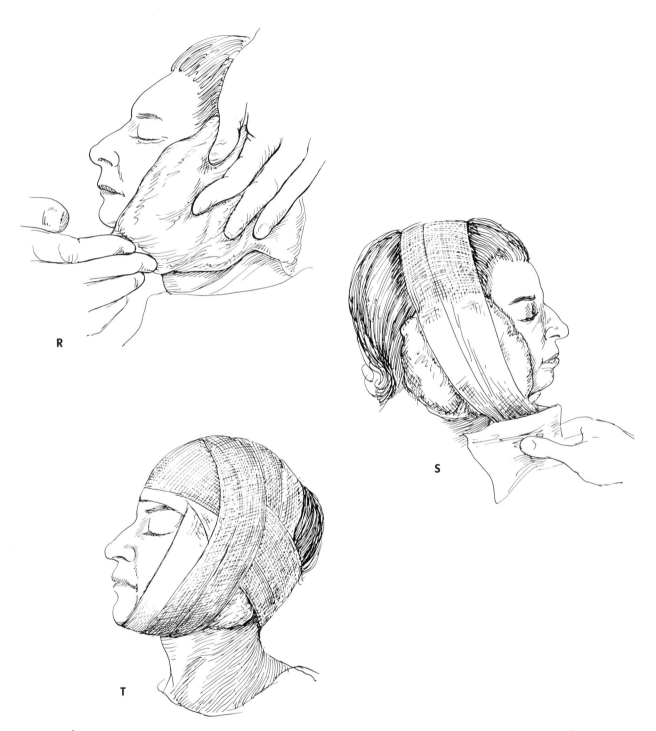

A wraparound compression bandage is applied (*R*), with or without drains. This bandage should be secure, but as comfortable as possible (*S*). The ears should be well padded fore and aft (*T*), as the major cause of pain and discomfort in the immediate postoperative period is pressure on the ears. The bandage remains in place for 48 hours. Some surgeons use suction drainage, but drains of any sort are reserved by the authors for patients in whom complete hemostasis could not be achieved during surgery.

Plication of the superficial fascia is thought by some to be beneficial in maintaining and prolonging the result of a face lift. This is, of course, impossible to prove. But in patients with marked laxity of the soft tissues and ptosis of the jaw line, the technique makes sense.

A and *B*, The fascia is grasped with fine forceps or a skin hook and overlapped so that it can be sutured along a line that begins in front of the ear at the lower margin of the zygomatic arch and extends downward around the ear to end over the mastoid. Chromic catgut sutures or synthetic materials (Dermalon or Mersilene) are used, preferably clear or colorless, because colored sutures may show through the final skin flap in patients with particularly translucent skin. Tie the sutures so that the knots are buried; sharp Dermalon suture ends, even if cut off very short, have been known to perforate the skin, requiring subsequent removal. In some patients, using chromic catgut sutures in fascial plication has resulted in the formation of local sterile abscesses that required incision and drainage.

The suture line is often palpable as a ridge beneath the skin for several weeks postoperatively, and in some patients this ridge may even be visible when the skin of the face moves over it. However, these effects are always temporary and do not detract from the applicability of plication in the patient with flaccid tissues.

(Rees, T. D.: Technical Considerations in Blepharoplasty and Rhytidectomy, Transactions of the Fifth International Congress of Plastic and Reconstructive Surgery, Australia, 1971. London, Butterworth & Co., Ltd., 1971, p. 1067.)

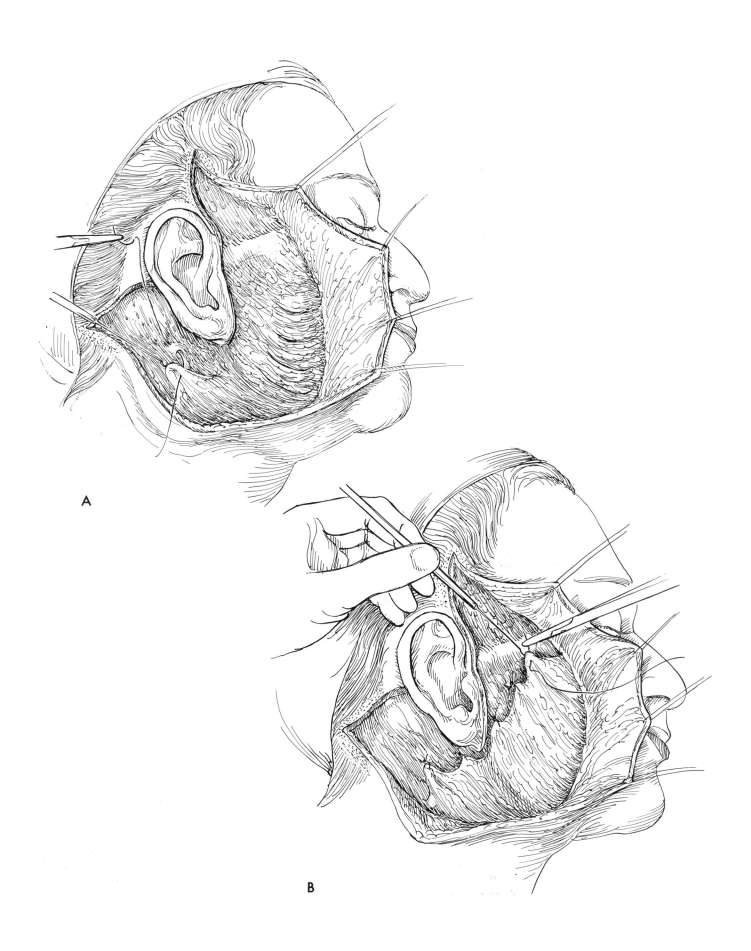

A

B

171

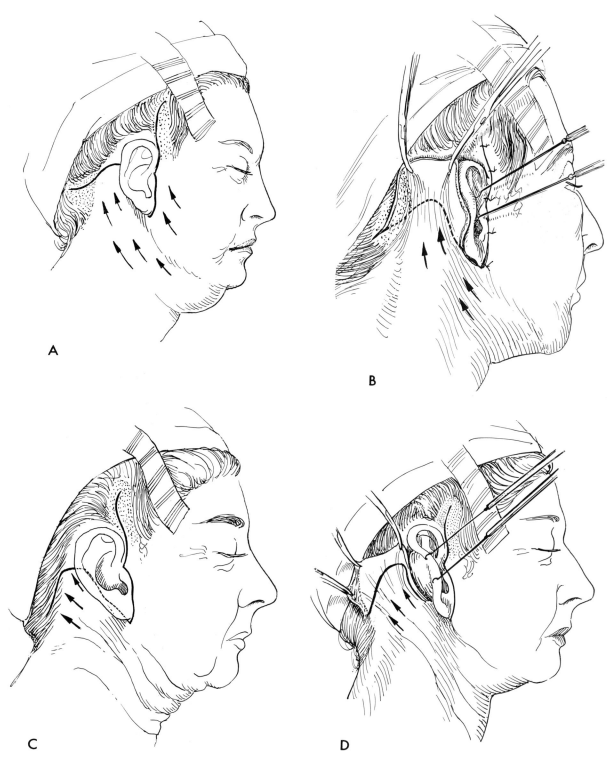

A

B

C

D

Judgment must be employed in the final draping of the skin flaps after undermining has been completed. The flaps are pulled more superiorly than posteriorly in patients whose redundant tissue is mostly in the submental area and along the jaw (*A* and *B*). If tightening of the neck is the foremost consideration, the direction of pull is more posterior than cephalad (*C* and *D*).

172

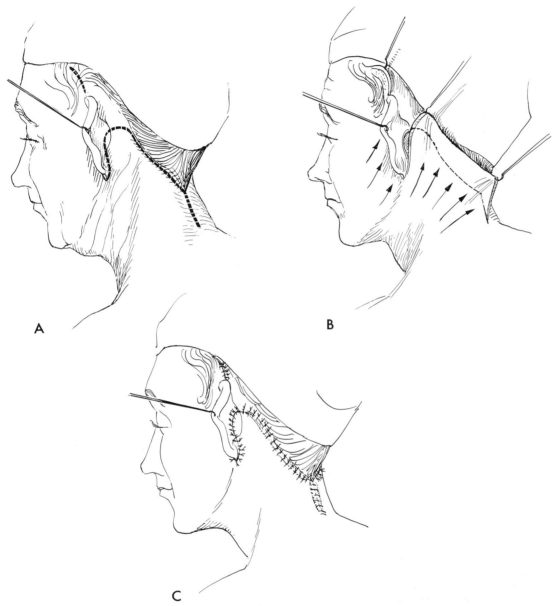

A

B

C

When the skin of the mid and lower neck is loose and redundant, traction is applied in a more posterior direction than usual, toward the midline of the back of the neck (*A*). The incision into the posterior scalp must be continued downward along the hairline. It is occasionally tempting to extend the incision and the undermining around to the midline of the neck posteriorly, where a redundant wedge is removed as in these drawings (*B* and *C*). In the experience of the authors, however, this more radical procedure (advocated especially by Gonzalez-Ulloa and Edgerton) has not been necessary. Our main objection is to the unsightly scars so often left in the posterior nuchal region. Our approach to redundant neck skin is a secondary operation several months after the first procedure to take up the slack, reopening standard incisions.

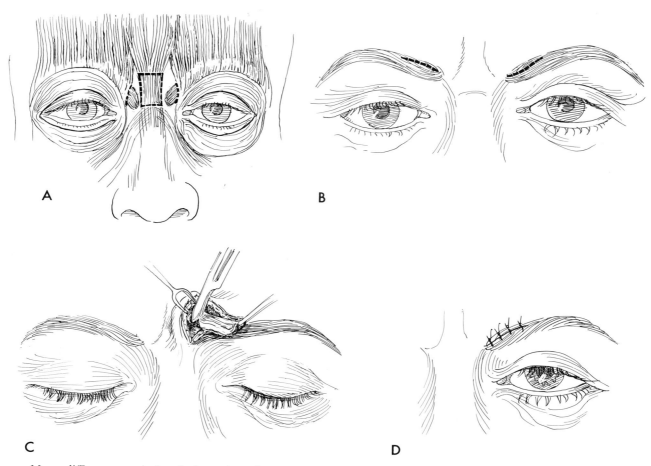

A

B

C

D

Many different surgical techniques have been proposed for the correction of horizontal forehead wrinkles and vertical frown lines. None has been successful to the extent that it has been widely accepted and used. Temporary benefits may be achieved, but the cause of such wrinkles is the strong pull of the underlying muscles, which cannot be lessened without producing sequelae even less desirable than the original deformity. This illustration and the one that follows show two methods in wide use for resecting portions of the procerus and corrugator muscles (A, C) to diminish muscle action as a cause of frown lines, whereby the muscles are resected through a small incision in the medial brow (B, D) as here or through a vertical incision in the natural frown line (next page). A multiple Z- or W-plasty closure of this vertical line is advocated by some.

174

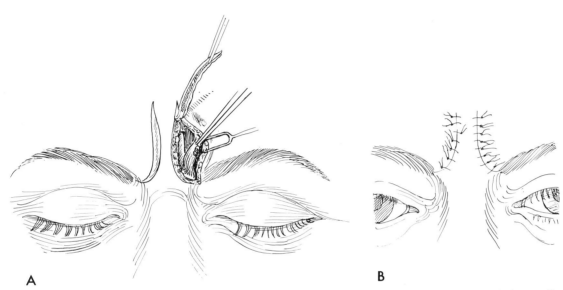

A   **B**

Partial resection of the procerus and corrugator muscles (*A* and *B*) is sometimes thought to help to eliminate vertical frown lines. but the procedure affords only limited improvement, which is usually short-lived.

Purposeful paralysis of the temporal branches of the facial nerve to cause total relaxation of the forehead was advocated by Edwards. This is a rather drastic technique that the authors consider rarely justified because it cannot be reversed and ultimately leads to marked ptosis of the brows.

Various implants of dermis and fat or of alloplastic sheet materials have been used to permanently separate the skin in the glabellar region from the underlying muscles, but this approach has also been largely unsuccessful, most of the alloplastic implants eventually requiring removal.

Unquestionably the most promising technique to appear thus far has been the injection of silicone fluid, which has been under investigation in this country for several years but is readily available abroad. There seems to be little doubt that correction of vertical frown lines is one of the valid uses for this material in plastic surgery. Several injections are required, the silicone fluid being placed immediately beneath the dermis along the full length of the frown line. No more than 0.25 ml. can be injected at a single site in one injection. Deep furrows are often eliminated entirely by this technique, and fine lines or creases are usually improved.

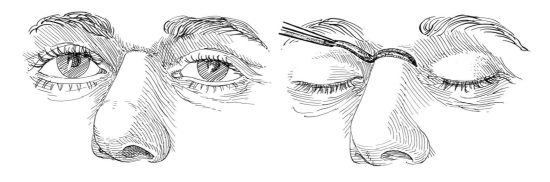

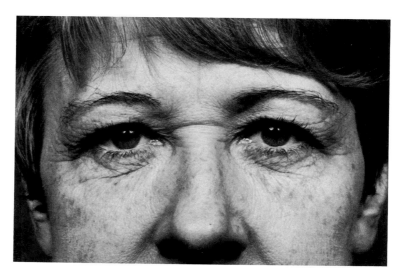

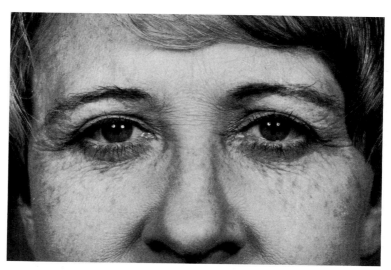

A deep wrinkle across the root of the nose, a very common problem, can be distressing to the patient. These are extremely difficult to eradicate. The only really effective method requires that the wrinkle be traded for a scar, a somewhat drastic technique that should obviously be used only when the patient fully understands the consequences. Simple excision and careful closure with fine sutures is the technique used. (Courtesy of Dr. Cary L. Guy.)

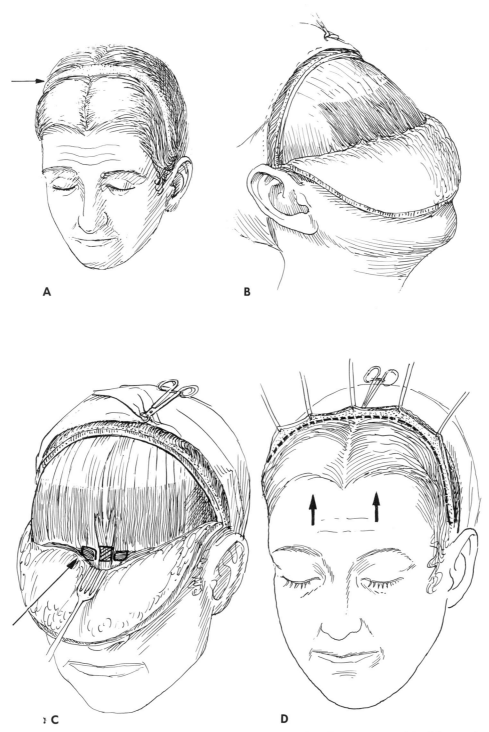

Still another way to improve forehead wrinkles is to turn down a flap from a coronal incision and separate the muscles from the skin. *A* and *B*, Incising and turning the flap. The level of dissection is superficial to the frontalis muscle, which in itself is sometimes hazardous to the blood supply. *C*, An optional step is resection of segments of the procerus, frontalis, and corrugator muscles. *D*, The flap is replaced and a margin of excess skin is excised under tension; the wound is then sutured.

The authors do not favor this technique but include it here because it is advocated by some responsible surgeons. It has not been found permanently effective and it carries a significantly high incidence of complications, including baldness, wound slough, anesthesia of the forehead skin, and unsightly scars, which may appear as the result of natural recession of the hairline in men or as the result of baldness induced by the operation in women.

A so-called upper face lift or temporal lift may be requested by a patient with an erroneous idea of what such a procedure can accomplish. Much publicity has been given to this procedure in the popular press, where it is explained as a method of lifting the outer canthus of the eye, elevating the brow to produce an almond-eyed or slightly Oriental effect. The desired outcome will be demonstrated by the patient pulling the temporal skin upward and backward to stretch the eyelids. Some actresses simulate this effect by binding their temporal hair in tight twists, which tightens the temporal scalp and lifts the lids.

There is no doubt that the temporal lift can raise the corner of a ptotic eyebrow or modify the advanced wrinkling of the temporal skin ("laugh lines"). But as a sole technique for a patient requesting facial plastic surgery, it is rarely justifiable.

The incisions are essentially similar to the design shown on page 157 for the temporal and preauricular area.

To do a proper temporal lift, extensive undermining is needed (A and B). It must extend medially as far as the brow and almost to the outer canthus of the eye, and the operation is therefore anything but a "minilift." In fact, it is hazardous, because the temporal branch of the facial nerve is quite superficial in this region, coursing generally along a line drawn from the outer canthus to the external auditory canal. It is almost mandatory to use a nerve stimulator in order to avoid damage to this branch when doing a proper temporal lift.

Hemostasis can also be difficult because of the profusion of small blood vessels in the area. Excessive electro-coagulation of such vessels requires that the surgeon identify and protect the facial nerve so as not to injure its branches with the heat of the cautery. We do not subscribe to Pitanguy's advice that undermining above the theoretical transfacial course of the temporal branch can be deep to the temporal fascia while that below is superficial. On the other hand, all undermining in the temporal region should be superficial, with injury to the temporal branch of the facial nerve carefully avoided by positively identifying it.

After wide undercutting, the skin flap is rotated posteriorly with considerable posterior and cephalad traction applied (C and D). Excess skin is removed, and the wound is sutured (E). Most of the tension will be taken up in the posterior scalp, well behind the hairline; therefore, the scar in this region tends to stretch and widen with time, leaving a strip of hairless scalp.

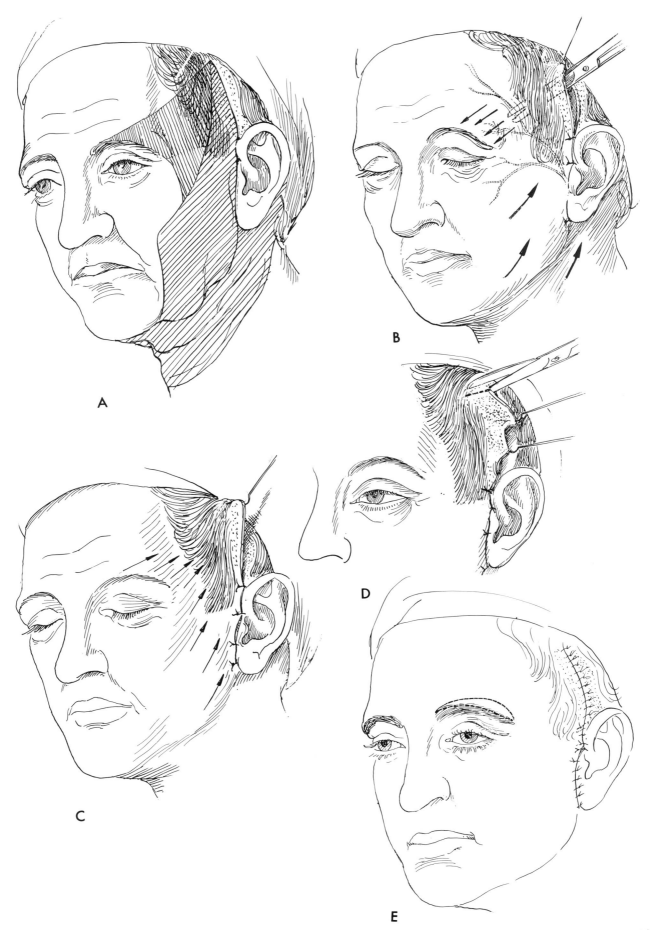

A

B

C

D

E

179

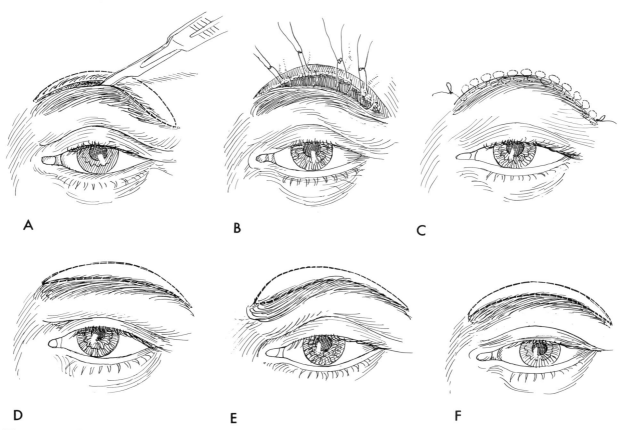

A   B   C

D   E   F

The temporal lift is most often done to correct (or to help to correct) ptosis of the brows and sagging of the upper face, Brow ptosis may be a prominent familial characteristic, in which case elevation can be achieved only by direct excision of a strip of skin immediately above the brow. This technique has been described by Castanares and others.

The design of the ellipse to be removed differs according to where the greatest amount of elevation is desired (*D*, *E*, and *F*). In most patients the lateral third of the brow has dropped and cannot be corrected by upper eyelid plasty alone. In fact, repeated excision of excess skin from the upper eyelid can eventually result in bringing the brow closer to the lid margin, thereby increasing the brow deformity.

The principal objection to skin excisions over the eyebrows is the resulting scar, which can be obvious in the patient with few or no horizontal forehead wrinkles. When the surgeon decides that such excision would be helpful, he must advise the patient that after surgery it may be necessary to pluck and shape the brows, using an eyebrow pencil to create a new shape corresponding to the scar formed by the surgery.

It is important to place the incision just inside the superior row of hair follicles, as the final scar tends to migrate above the brow line (*A*). After the ellipse of skin is excised, it is not advisable to undermine the edges. The dermis should be approximated by several buried sutures of nonabsorbable material (*B*): the skin is closed with a subcuticular suture (*C*) and can be further sealed with sterile tape strips or interrupted sutures. Such sutures should be removed by the fourth or fifth postoperative day in order to prevent "cross hatches" on these incisions. The subcuticular suture is removed on the seventh day, after which the wound is supported by sterile tape strips for several more days.

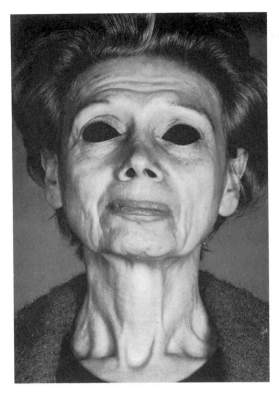

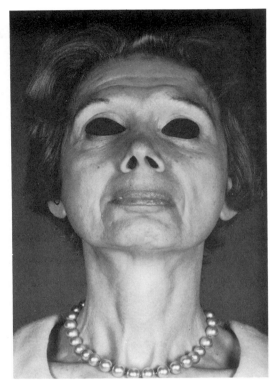

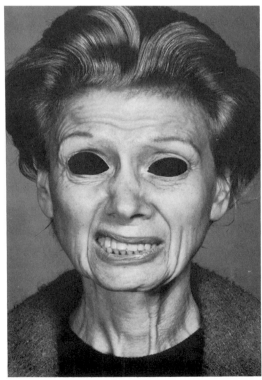

Preoperative examination of every patient who is a candidate for facial plastic surgery should include a careful inspection of the facial musculature for evidence of unilateral weakness or paralysis. If such a condition can be shown to exist preoperatively, it cannot later be ascribed to the surgery performed. This patient exhibited a left partial hemiparesis, the residual of an old Bell's palsy, that was hardly noticeable except with extreme animation. The same principle applies to facial asymmetry, which can be accentuated by surgery. Minor degrees of asymmetry or even paralysis can be missed in the initial examination unless the patient is instructed to display marked facial animation. Such minor deformities must obviously be pointed out to the patient before surgery in order to avoid postoperative repercussions.

This patient demonstrated the degree of skin laxity and ptosis of the lower face that are present in an "ideal candidate" for primary rhytidectomy (face lift) in the opinion of the authors. The skin is slightly loose, there is early jowl formation, and there is minimal loose skin in the upper neck and submental region, with little subcutaneous fat. Deep nasolabial grooves are absent, and malar bone formation is strong. The texture of the skin is soft and its elasticity of good tension. There are few fine rhytides, a further promise of a good result as opposed to what can be expected in the "sunbaked" patient with dry, leathery, and wrinkled skin.

Age is less important than the factors described in obtaining an excellent result. There is no need to wait for the further passage of time and corresponding increases in laxity and ptosis before advising surgery. A second operation can always be done if it becomes necessary. Early changes such as those shown here characteristically occur in patients between 40 and 50 years of age, but there is wide variation. Heredity plays a major role in the aging process of the skin, accounting for some of the variability.

Plication of the superficial fascia is rarely necessary at this stage, as the operation will consist primarily of a readjustment of the skin envelope and removal of the excess.

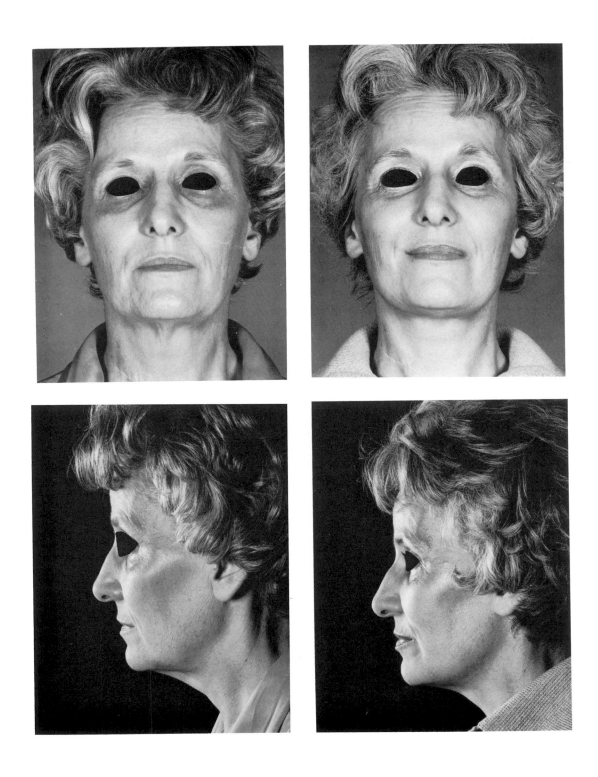

183

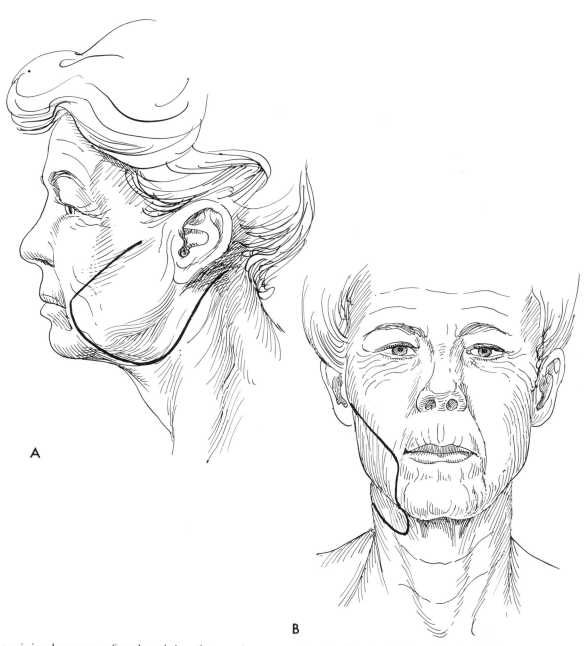

A

B

The minimal amount of undermining that can be expected to be effective is shown by the heavy line drawn over the jaw and upper neck (*A* and *B*). The earliest indications for face lifting include small jowl formation, for which the undermining must extend to the edge of the redundant skin over the jaw. Complete undermining of the neck skin is not necessary in early cases.

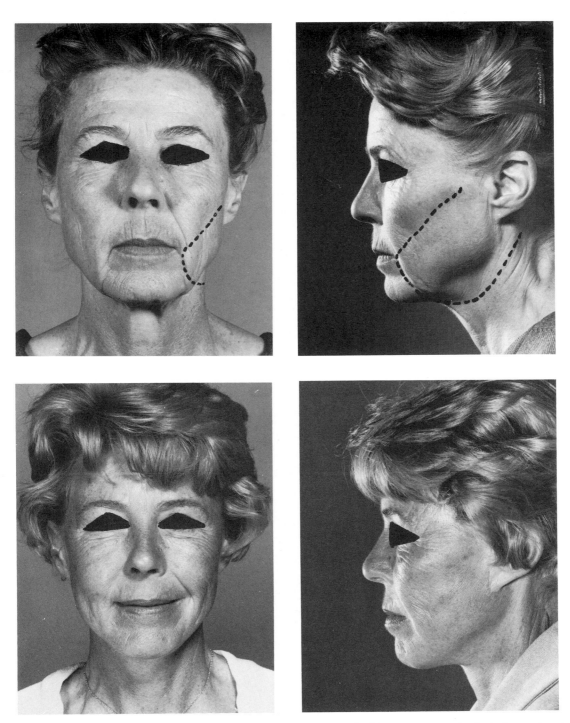

This patient was managed as shown on the opposite page. Her neck skin was not particularly loose, but it was tightened as an incidental part of the face lift procedure. The neck need not be widely undermined in such a patient, but it has been our experience that we are now undermining more extensively than used to be the case in almost all patients. The rhytides of the upper lip were improved by deep chemical abrasion. Their presence, however, limits the result somewhat in comparison with the previous patient.

(From Rees, T. D., and Guy, C. L.: Surg. Clin. N. Amer. *51*:353, 1971.)

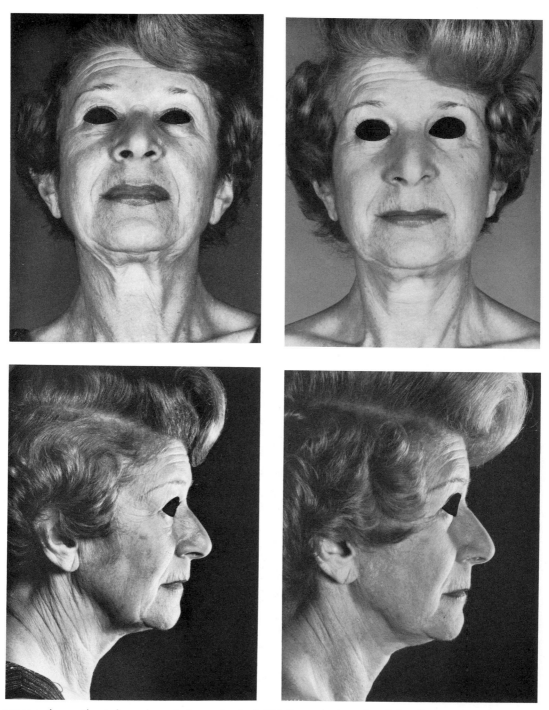

Many prospective patients have heard about the "minilift," a technique involving little or no undermining that goes back to the earliest days of face lifting. This patient, while not an early case, had limited undermining. The postoperative result was a definite improvement up to six months after surgery, but there is little doubt that the results would have been better if there had been wide undermining over the border of the mandible and extending well toward the midline of the neck. The patient was disappointed with the result.

186

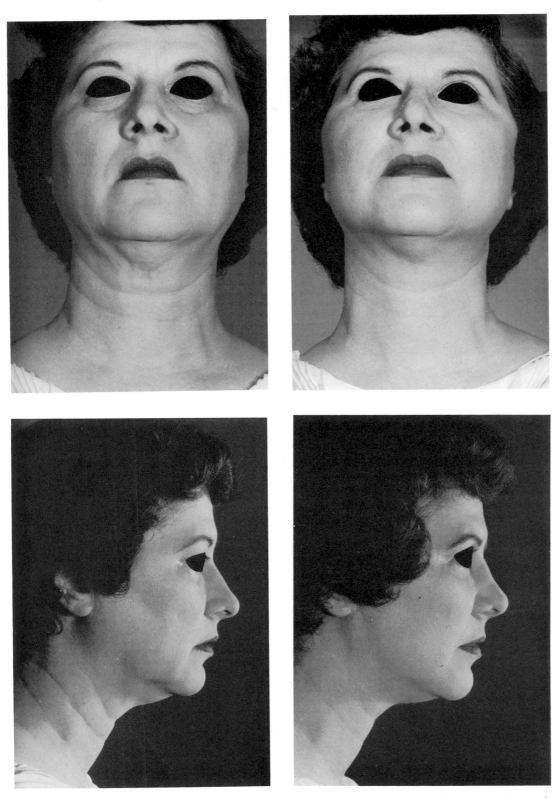

Although obesity sharply limits the results that can be achieved in face lift surgery, there are patients who have ample cushions of subcutaneous tissue by virtue of their general body habitus or heredity. These patients are not truly obese, and the chance that they will lose weight to improve the operative result is a small one. Surgery can benefit them considerably, as this patient demonstrates. In general, however, patients who are overweight or obese should lose weight before surgery to achieve the best results. They should be advised that a marked weight gain or any significant shifting of weight after surgery will most likely have an adverse effect on the longevity of the results, because of stretching of the skin.

187

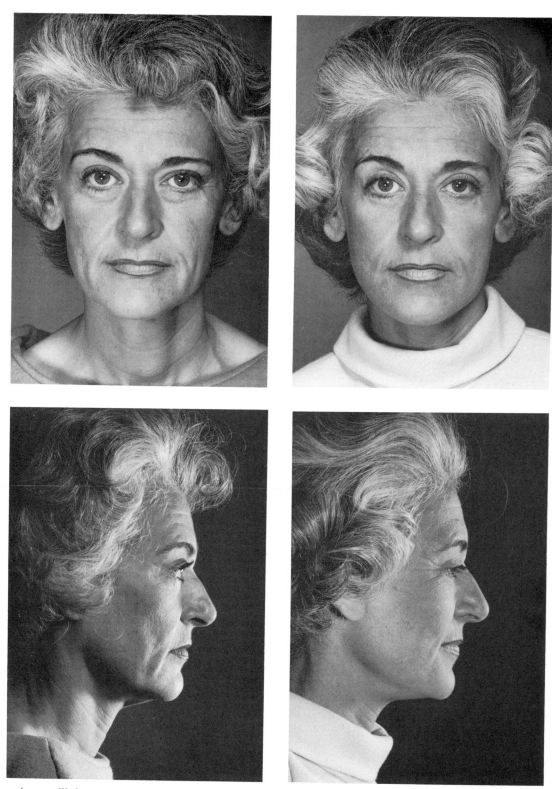

Some patients will demonstrate slight redundancy of skin along the jaw line and on the neck as their only sign of aging. The other tissues of the face are quite healthy and relatively youthful in appearance, which is aided by a characteristic rounding of the facial outline. Even though the excess skin is not overly loose, a good result from a cervicofacial rhytidectomy requires wide undermining and redraping of the skin. It is tempting to do limited undermining in such a patient, but the result will last only for weeks or a few months at the most. This patient was an ideal candidate for the operation.

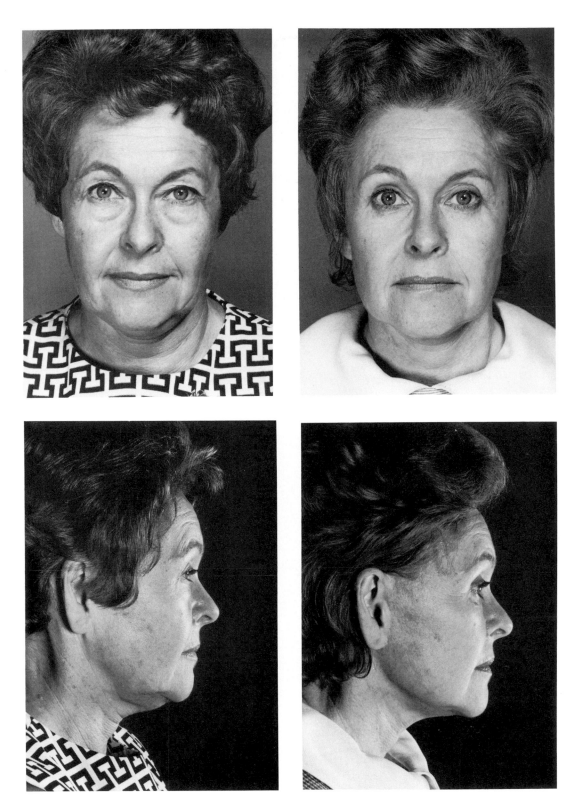

Certain anatomical features impose built-in limitations to the results that can be achieved in facial plastic surgery. This patient, for example, has a wide or squared lower jaw and fullness of the submental tissues which is not the result of excess fat. Jowl formation takes place relatively early in such patients. Surgery must include undermining that extends to the medial edge of the jowl or beyond. The postoperative result is acceptable, as seen here; however, a slight fullness along the line of the jaw must be accepted and mars the result to a slight degree, even though it is a natural contour in this patient.

189

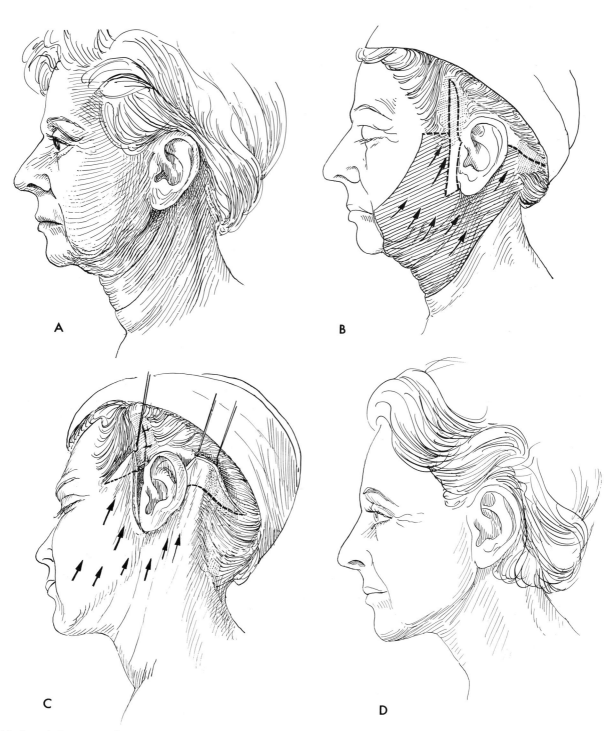

Undermining must always extend beyond the most peripheral limit of the deformity. When marked redundancy of the skin of the neck is the main problem (*A*), the undercutting must extend completely around the anterior circumference of the neck (*B*). The excess is then pulled slightly posteriorly, but mostly in a cephalad direction (*C*), where it is excised in large triangles in front of and behind the ear, leaving a pleasing result (*D*).

190

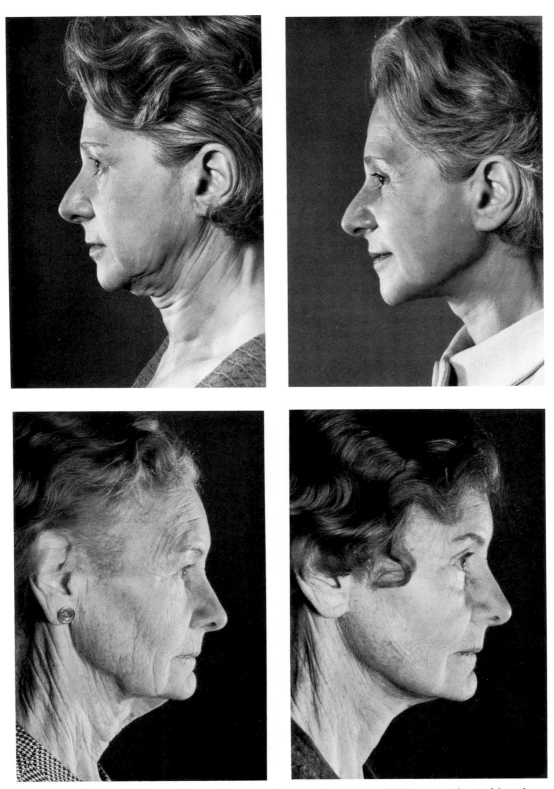

Two patients with the problem shown on the opposite page, and the correction achieved.

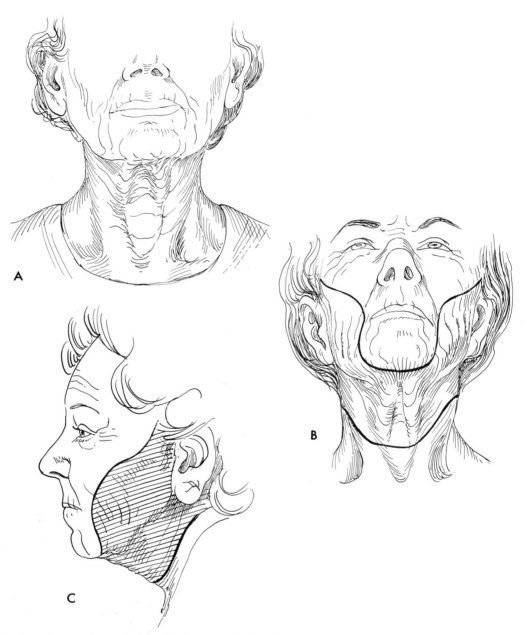

In the elderly patient with marked senile changes of the skin (*A*), undermining must be very extensive, and a certain limitation in the result is inevitable. The extent of undermining is indicated by the heavy lines in *B* and *C*.

192

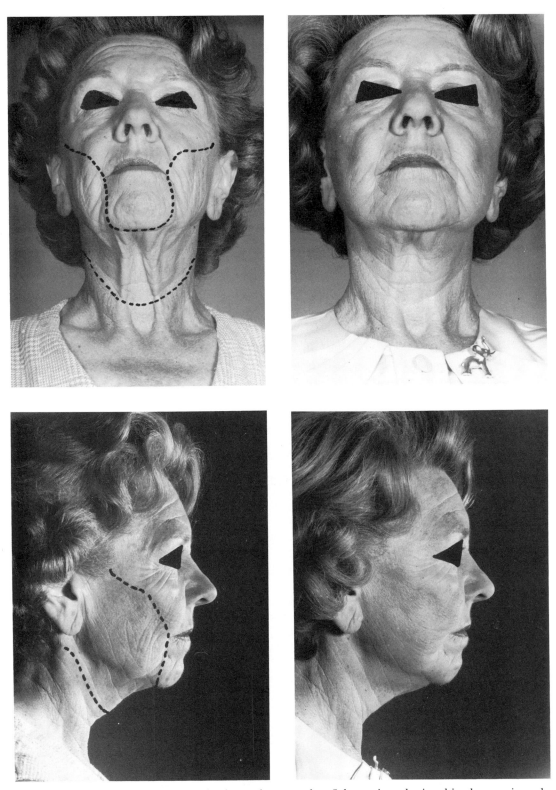

The result of wide undermining is shown in these photographs of the patient depicted in the previous drawing. The many fine rhytides are improved but not eliminated by the face lift procedure; further improvement might be anticipated with chemical abrasion.

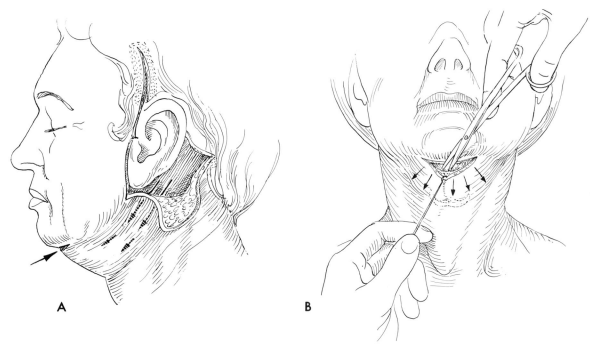

An operation to correct a double chin may be done at the same time as a face lift, but in the opinion of the authors it is better delayed until healing from the facial plastic surgery procedure is more or less complete (about six weeks). Large submental fat deposits may be removed at the time of facial plastic surgery through an incision in the natural crease behind the symphysis (A), but vertical incisions in the midline of the neck should not be done at this time. Their scars may hypertrophy because tension will be applied from both sides when the skin is redraped following a face lift. Furthermore, during the course of a facial plastic procedure, it is difficult to be sure that the incision is being placed just at the midline of the neck, as tension on one side of the facial skin may be greater than on the other.

In making the submental transverse incision, it is important to leave a cushion of fat beneath the skin (B) so that the replaced skin flap does not adhere directly to the underlying hyoid muscles, which will cause an unsightly depression or puckering. Remove submental fat as far laterally as possible (C), and join the undermining with that from each side (in the face lift procedure) (C). After the facial incisions are sutured, the excess submental fat is pulled forward with skin hooks or forceps to overlap the anterior margin of the wound (D). Two small dog-ears usually remain at the ends of the incision (E), which must be carefully trimmed so as not to extend above the lower mandibular margin where they will be visible (F).

(From Rees, T. D.: Technical Considerations in Blepharoplasty and Rhytidectomy. Transactions of the Fifth International Congress of Plastic and Reconstructive Surgery, Australia, 1971. London, Butterworth & Co., Ltd., 1971, p. 1067.)

194

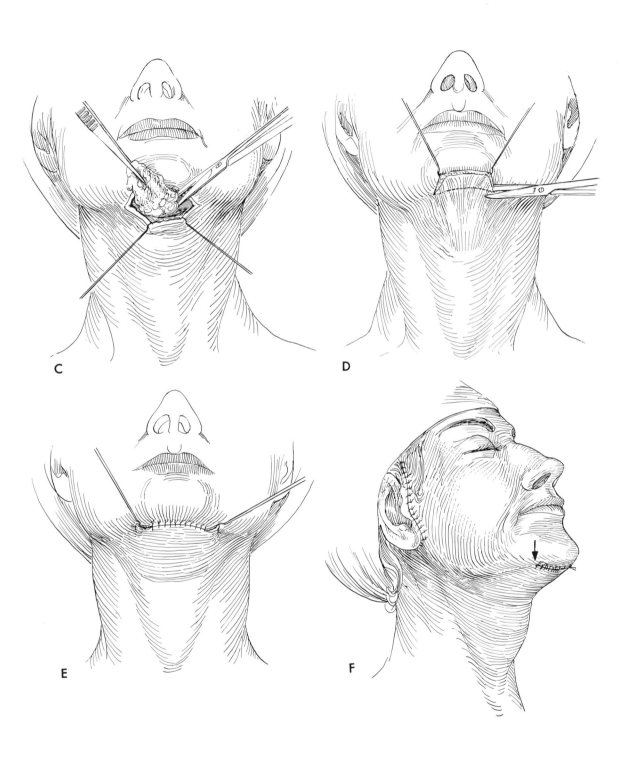

C

D

E

F

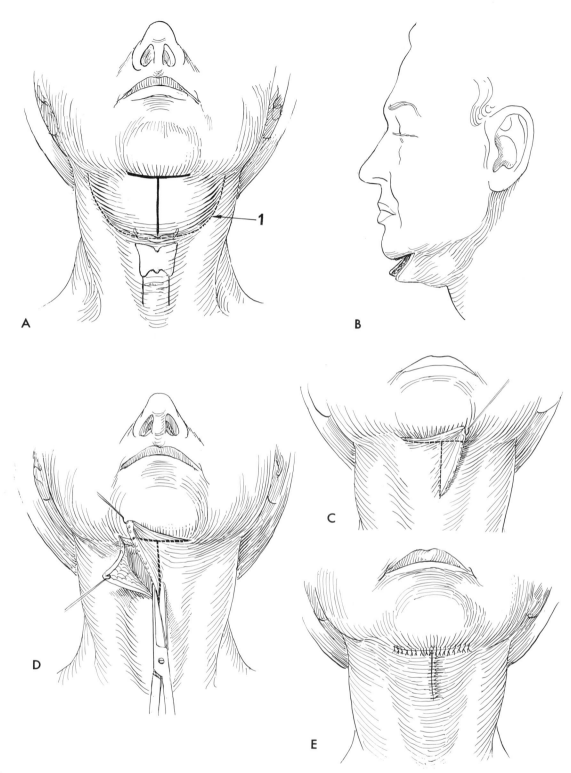

Patients with marked submental fat or very loose necks are told before face lift surgery that a second, relatively minor operation may be required. Even a complete undermining of the neck may not correct a difficult problem, and a secondary neck procedure will then be in order.

Vertical neck incisions heal surprisingly well if they do not extend inferior to the deep fold of skin at the cervicomental angle. Below this line, they are apt to become hypertrophic and may even form keloids. In our hands, the simplest and most effective secondary procedure to correct the double chin has consisted of a single T-shaped incision beneath the mandible (*A* and *B*) with wide undermining of the flaps on each side. This is followed by removal of excess fat (ensuring retention of a sufficient layer), overlapping the skin flaps in the midline (*C*), and

196

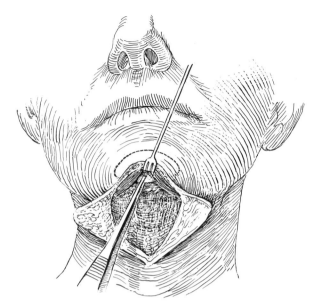

Augmentation mentoplasty is often helpful in enhancing the effect of rhytidectomy and submental lipectomy when microgenia or retrognathia is also a component of the problem. A silicone rubber implant of suitable size can be inserted through a submental incision at the time of rhytidectomy or subsequently with little added trauma. This technique can be combined with a T-shaped incision. Implants, of course, can also be inserted through a simple submental cut.

excising the excess skin (*D*). Operations more elaborate than this effective procedure—including multiple interlocking Z-plasties and other difficult techniques—seem unnecessarily extensive; however, they may have a place in the correction of "turkey neck" deformities, particularly in men.

Vertical neck incision should never extend below the thyroid cartilage (*E*).

(From Rees, T. D.: Technical Considerations in Blepharoplasty and Rhytidectomy. Transactions of the Fifth International Congress of Plastic and Reconstructive Surgery. Australia, 1971. London, Butterworth & Co., Ltd., 1971, p. 1067.)

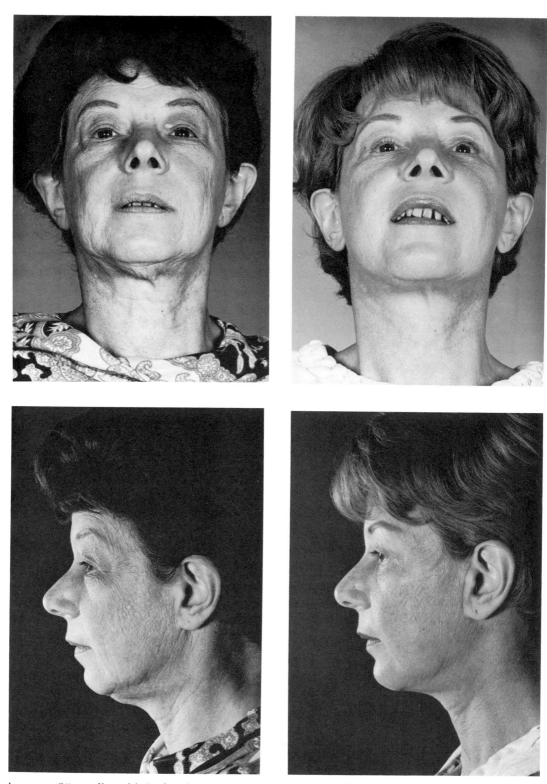

Minor degrees of "receding chin" often become more noticeable with age. Chin implants have a subtle enhancing effect on the face lift operation and are rarely conspicuous. This patient demonstrates such a result.

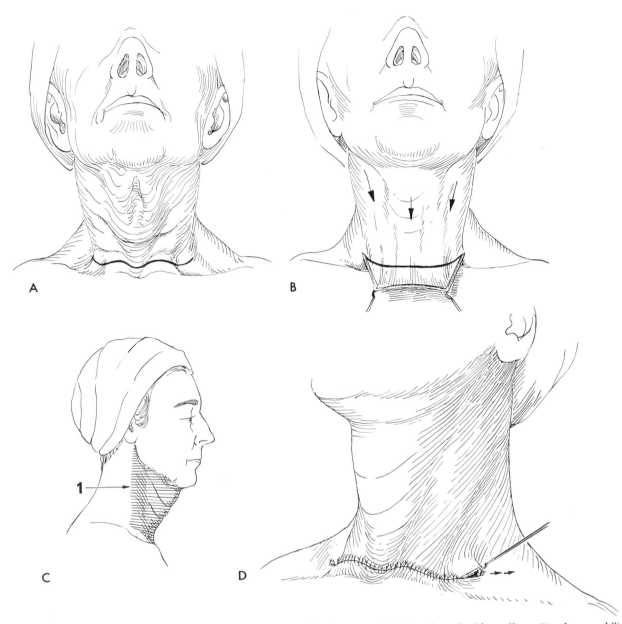

Another approach to marked looseness of the skin of the lower neck below the cricoid cartilage ("turkey neck") that can be used as a secondary procedure when no satisfactory result can be achieved at the primary operation is the use of a thyroid incision (*A*), which permits undermining of the entire lower neck below the level of the larynx in the supraplatysmal plane. This technique was suggested by B. O. Rogers. The skin flap is then pulled inferiorly and the excess skin resected (*B*). Just as with the submental incision, the disparity in length of the upper and lower skin flaps results in small dog-ears at both ends of the closure. These can be trimmed so as to extend the line in a natural neck crease running laterally (*D*).

The lateral extent of the undermining is to the border of the sternocleidomastoid muscle (*C 1*), or further if necessary.

A thyroid incision should never be employed at the time of the primary face lift procedure. It will tend to migrate superiorly because of the upward pull on the face lift flaps. Several weeks should elapse between the two operations.

We do not favor extension of face lift incisions to the posterior neck midline and removal of wedges of skin in this area as a means of improving the appearance of the neck.

Patients who present with extreme ptosis and excess skin folds of the neck or marked submental fat pads should be advised that two operations will probably be necessary. In extreme cases, a second face lift may be needed in as little as six months' time to achieve a satisfactory result, and a submental incision may be required as well.

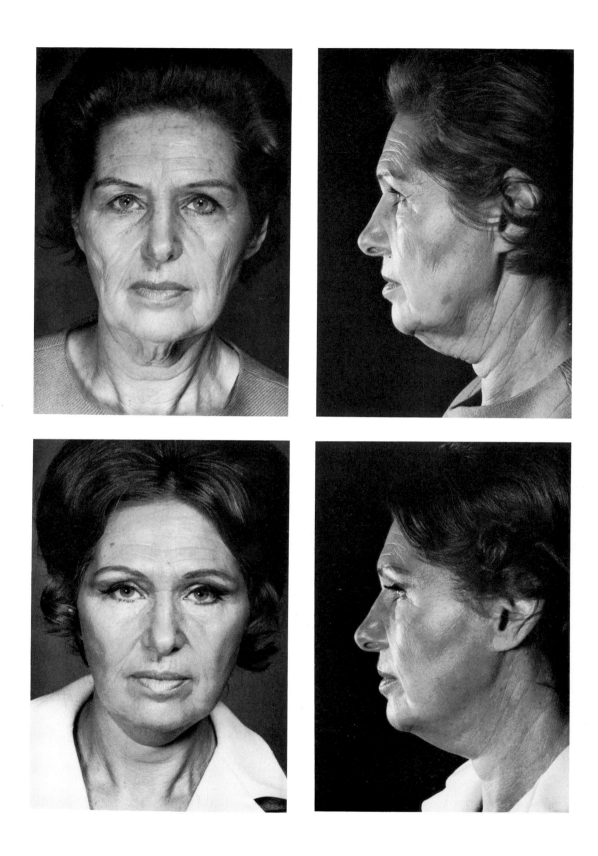

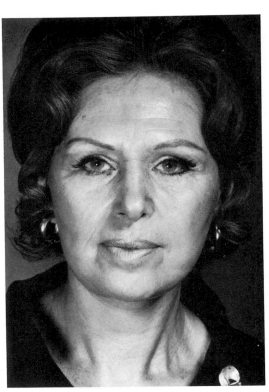 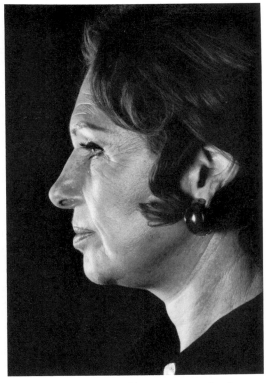

The very marked redundancy of the skin of the neck in this patient was corrected in two stages. In the preoperative pictures note that the skin fold is essentially in the submental region. A thyroid type of incision in such a patient would be useless. The first operation consisted of a standard face lift procedure with complete undermining of the neck and a strong upward lift. The result was considerable improvement; however, as had been anticipated because of the degree of the deformity, it was not perfect. A second operation was done two months later. A submental T-shaped incision (as shown previously) achieved an almost perfect result (see above).

(From Rees, T. D., and Guy, C. L.: Surg. Clin. N. Amer. *51*:353, 1971.)

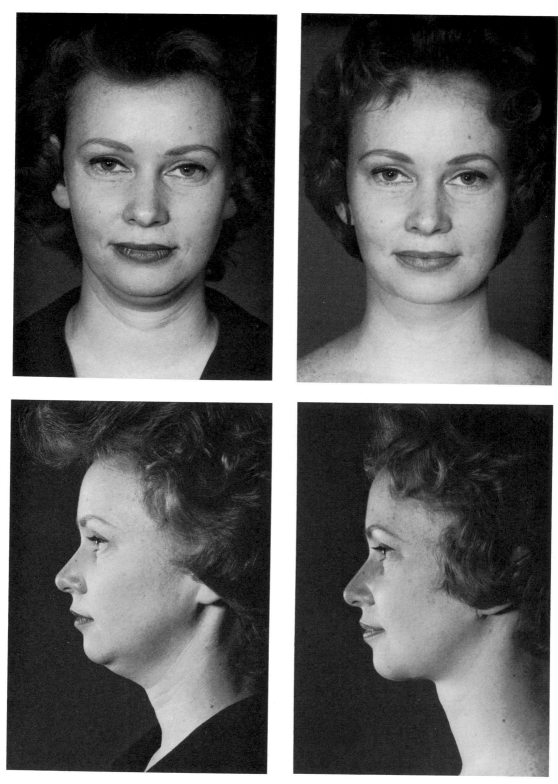

This type of "double chin" is often familial and is a true submental lipoma. It occurs in patients who are not obese, and it may be the only evidence of excess fat accumulation. It is removed through a submental incision, but the patient will also probably need a face lift to take up the slack skin that may result from the incision.

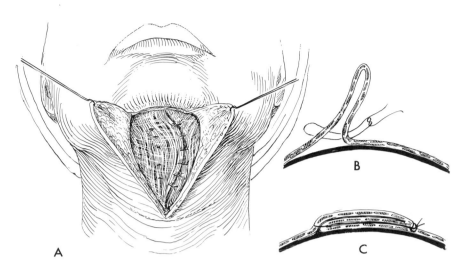

A

B

C

Vertical folds extending down the neck from beneath the chin are common. They are pleats or folds of the platysma accompanied by redundant skin. Wide skin undermining and a thorough face lift do not always correct the muscle deformity. Plication of the muscle under direct vision (*A*) through a horizontal or T-shaped submental incision (as described on previous pages) helps to obliterate such folds. The redundant muscle is folded over and a plication suture is placed (*B*). The row of plication sutures is completed (*C*). Resection of the anterior borders of this muscle is also an effective technique (suggested by Millard).

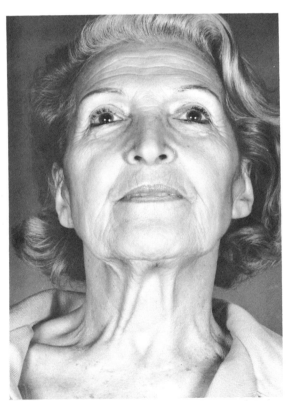 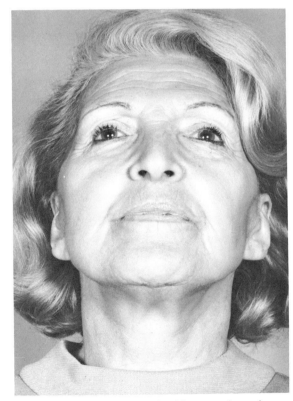

Plication of the platysma muscle was required in this patient along with cervicofacial rhytidectomy in order to correct the vertical neck folds.

203

These photographs portray the development of the aging process in a patient over a seven-year period. In the first row are three views of the patient at age 40; and the pictures in the second row were taken five years later. Slackness of the skin of the lower face, along the jaw line, and on the upper neck had developed; face lift and blepharoplasty were done at this time. The last row of pictures shows the patient two years later. At that time, a slight double chin had re-formed, and the excess was removed with a short submental incision.

In patients with strongly formed mandibular angles, such as this woman has, a slight excess of skin under the chin can often be dealt with by a submental incision, whereas a secondary face lift procedure may be required for less well formed jaws.

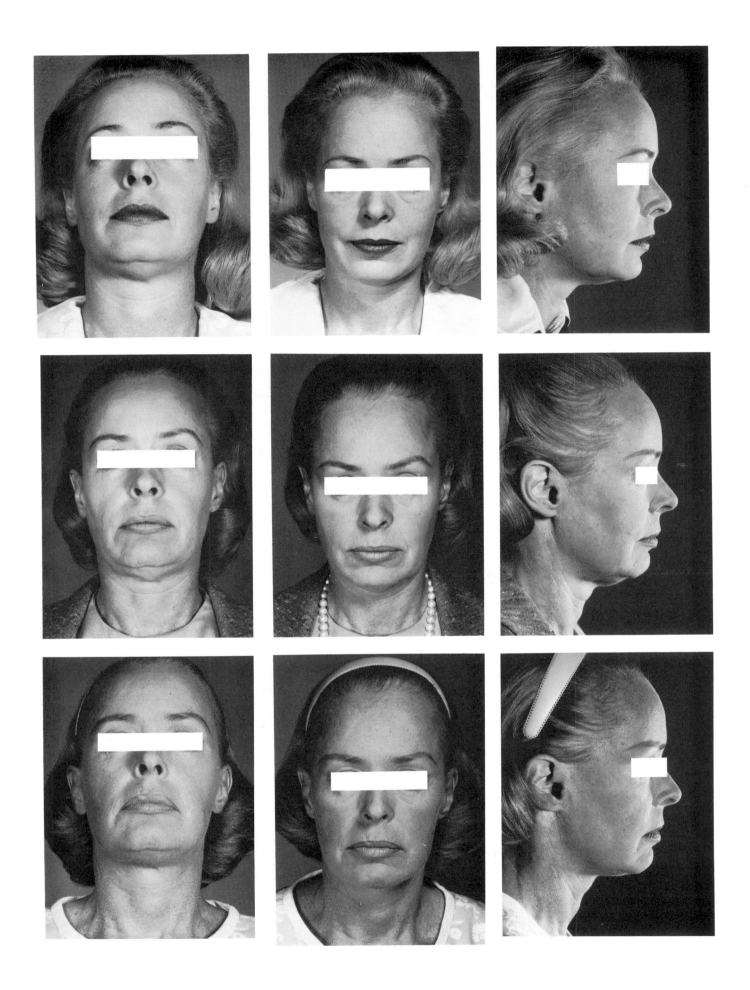

205

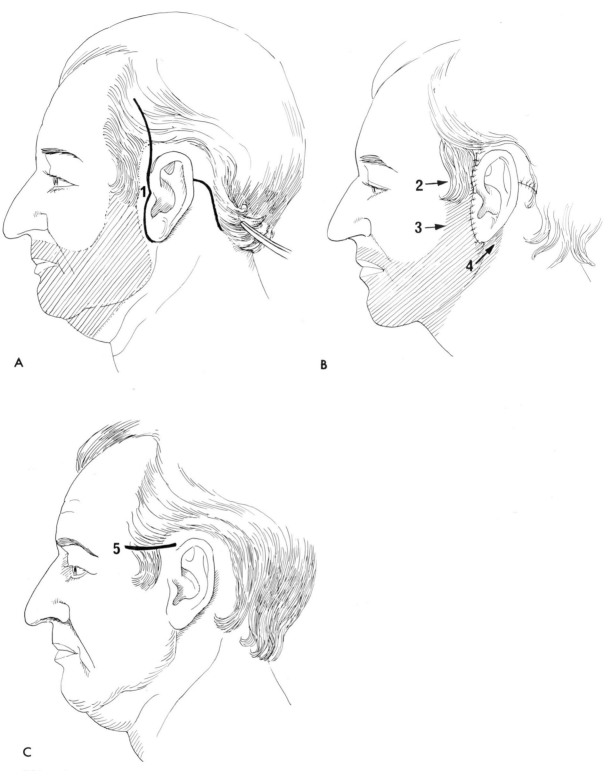

Face lifting for men presents certain unique features. Camouflaging scars behind the ears is more difficult because most men do not wear their hair long enough to comb it over the scars. The preauricular incision is much less of a problem, as most men naturally have rather deep creases in front of their ears in which the incisions can be placed. The sideburns (B 2) must be moved back in face lifting so that the beardless area (A 1) usually present between the posterior limit of the sideburn and the anterior helical and tragal margin will be obliterated. Moreover, the beard itself is moved posteriorly (B 3) and superiorly so as to lie behind the lobule of the ear (B 4), virtually to the mastoid skin, necessitating shaving of this region after surgery. Men should be advised of these eventualities prior to surgery. A horizontal incision through the hairline (C 5) is inadvisable in men. A staggered anterior hairline can result.

206

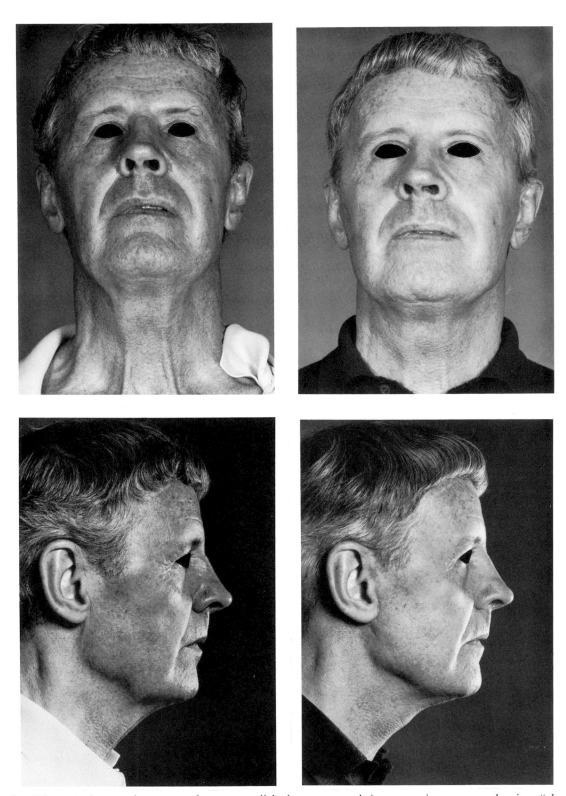

The face lift operation can be expected to accomplish the same result in men as in women—that is, a "cleaning up" of the jawline and upper neck, particularly in the early candidate such as this man. The same deficiencies are inherent in the operative technique too—namely, the nasolabial area is improved little or not at all by the operation. If great care is taken to avoid tension on the preauricular suture line, the resulting scar is virtually invisible. Most men have a deep natural skin crease at the exact site of the preauricular incision. Retrodisplacement of the hairline further camouflages the scar.

207

The most common complaint of men in middle age or older who seek facial plastic surgery is loose neck skin. A "wattle" of neck skin causes discomfort when shirts and ties are worn, is not attractive, and makes it difficult to wear turtle-neck shirts and other items of sportswear. In this patient, the problem was corrected by a two-stage operation. A rhytidectomy with very wide undermining of the skin around the midline of the neck was done first, followed after several weeks by a T-shaped incision of the front of the neck. A slightly longer hair style is helpful after surgery to hide the incisions. A sharp (acute) cervicomental angle could not be obtained in this patient because it had never been there. A hereditary neckline was related to a low position of the hyoid bone (see text).

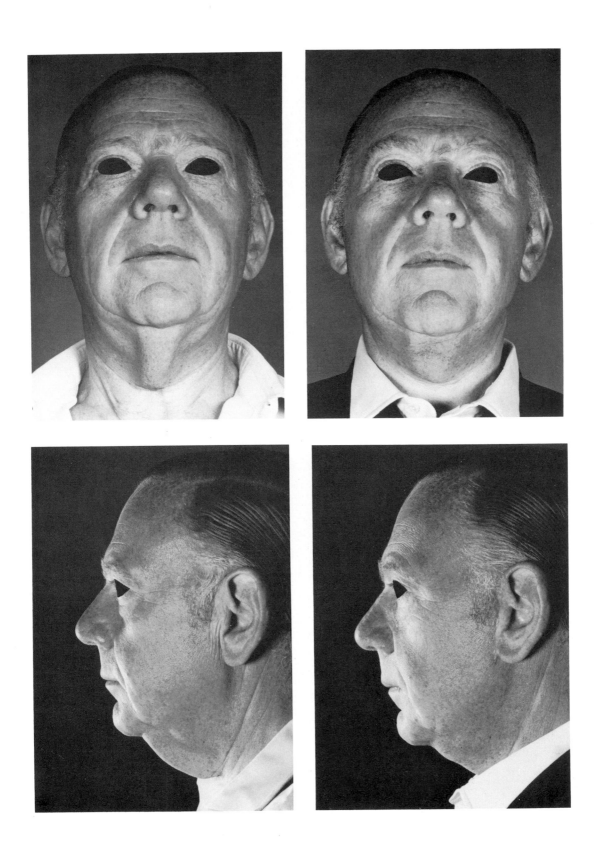

209

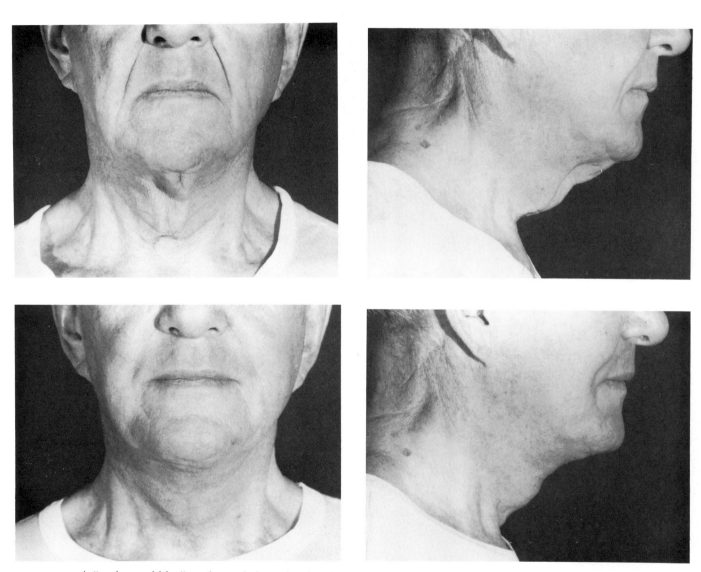

A "turkey gobbler" neck consisting of redundant skin of the upper neck region is apt to be the chief complaint in men. Some men are loath to undergo the standard rhytidectomy because of the difficulty in hiding the circum-auricular incisions. In carefully selected cases, however, a Z-plasty of the lax skin with excision of the redundancy by direct approach to the anterior neck can be considered. This technique has been advocated by Carlin and Gurdin as well as by Cronin and Biggs. The resulting scar usually ages well. It is a necessary price to pay for a clean neckline. Such a "turkey gobbler" neck was corrected by the Z-plasty technique. Such a radical approach is rarely if ever indicated in women. (From Cronin, T. D., and Biggs, T. M.: Plast. Reconstr. Surg. *47*:534, 1971.)

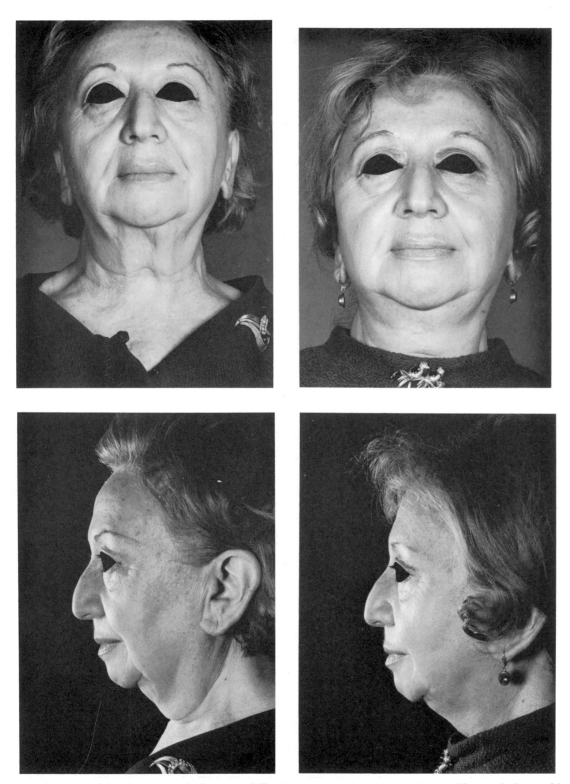

This type of neck and jaw formation is the most difficult to correct, in our experience. The angle formed by the chin and the neck (the cervicomental angle) is obtuse, probably because of a low hyoid arch. When this combination is enveloped by loose skin, it is exceedingly difficult to obtain complete correction; something less than perfection must be settled for. An added horizontal submental incision is sometimes helpful in such corrections, but a perfect result is defeated by the angle of the geniohyoid muscles.

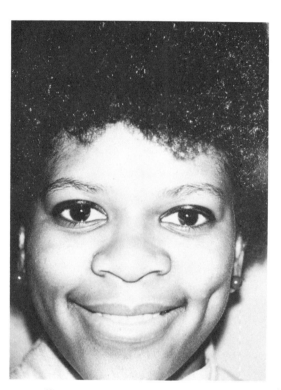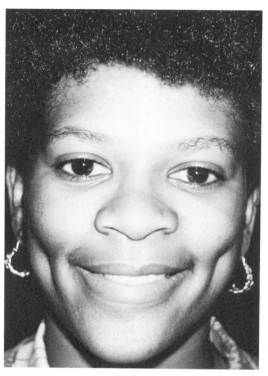

Argamaso utilizes an 8-mm. skin punch to create cheek dimples. The area to be excised is anesthetized, and a core of tissue is cut from the buccal mucosa to the dermis of the overlying cheek by a rotary motion of the punch biopsy from within. The wound is closed with one or two monofilament 4-0 nylon sutures which include a bite of the dermal base. (Courtesy of R. V. Argamaso.)

Chapter 7

CHEMABRASION AND DERMABRASION

Donald Wood-Smith, M.D., and
Thomas D. Rees, M.D.

Chemical Face Peel

The technique of chemical face peeling has a specific place in the armamentarium of the cosmetic surgeon in the eradication of fine wrinkling without gross sagging of facial skin. It is a most useful adjunct to a facial plastic procedure in a patient in whom, in addition to sagging and excess, the skin is involved with fine rhytides, especially in the perioral region (pp. 224 and 225). Further indications for its use are telangiectasia, superficial keratosis, chloasma and areas of irregular pigmentation. First popularized in plastic surgical literature by Brown et al. in 1960, it had, however, enjoyed a somewhat patchy and occasionally notorious popularity among lay operators for many years prior to this time.

Without publishing the method, Sir Harrold Gillies had used the acid painting and taping technique for many years for correction of "slight laxity of lid," using pure carbolic acid as his agent (Gillies and Millard, 1957; Batstone and Millard, 1968). Dermatologists had also frequently employed phenol peeling for removal of superficial skin blemishes, but it fell to the lay beauty operators and subsequently to the followers of Brown et al. (1960) to first popularize and finally refine this technique to its present-day efficiency (Baker and associates 1961, 1962, 1963, 1966; Litton, 1962, 1966; Ayres, 1962, 1964, Sperber, 1963, 1965a and b).

CHEMICAL AGENTS

The basic agent used for the chemical peel is phenol, to which is added, in the most commonly used formula of Baker, distilled water, croton oil and liquid soap. The action of the phenol (C_6H_5OH) is to produce an immediate reaction of keratolysis and coagulation; this is probably accomplished by disruption of the sulfur bridges of keratoprotein, aided by denaturation by virtue of the acidic nature of the phenol. However, the application of too concentrated a solution of phenol (more than 80 per cent) produces so much keratocoagulation that it acts as a barrier to further penetration of phenol into the dermis (Rothman, 1945). Schwartz and Peck (1946) emphasize the importance of the passage of absorbable material via the skin appendages as a prime route to the site of action on dermal collagen.

Both penetration and absorption are modified by the addition of soap which, by increasing surface tension, acts to retard these factors. An increase in phenol concentration will have the opposite effect, bearing in mind, however, that too great a concentration will then begin to form a barrier to further penetration.

The croton oil acts as an additional irritant and functions to speed the destruction of the epidermal layer; it may also facilitate penetration of the phenol to the dermal layers, al-

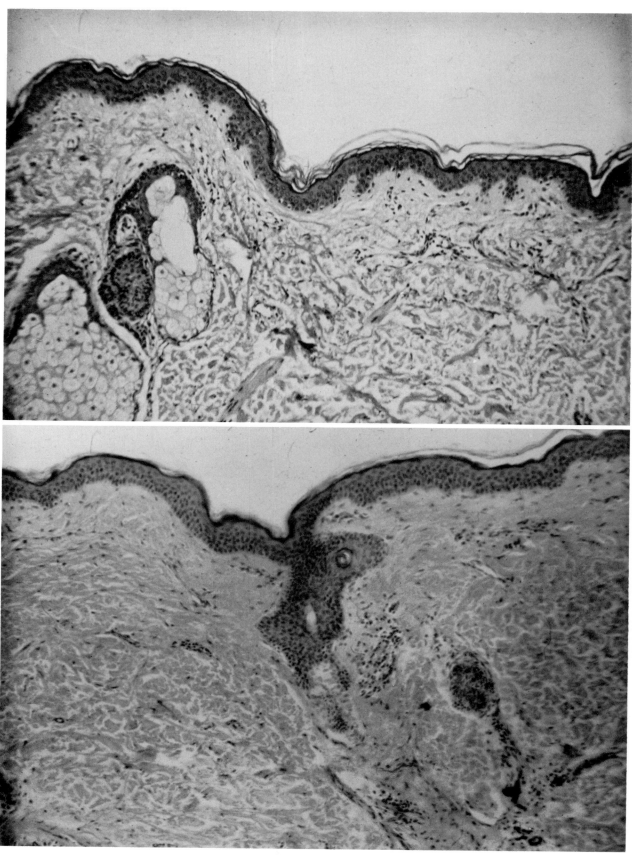

Changes that occur in skin subjected to chemabrasion are shown in these photomicrographs. Normal skin is shown on the left, while the postchemabrasion picture on the right demonstrates a marked increase in collagen, in a lamellar distribution. (Courtesy of Dr. Tom Baker.)

though evidence for this must be inferred rather than proved. Certainly leaving it out of the formula does appear to lower its efficiency as a whole.

The action of the chemical is prolonged by application of a vapor barrier, usually waterproof adhesive tape. Indeed, in patients with thin fair skin, it is often advisable to delay tape application while the solution dries and the phenol, in part, evaporates. The tape acts to confine the active agents to the region and to promote maceration, which will, in turn, aid penetration of the phenol.

TOXICITY

The phenol is absorbed in part into the systemic circulation, with readily determinable blood levels accurately measured by a spectrophotometer. Deaths have been recorded following "peeling" of excessively large areas by lay operators, Brown et al. (1960) reporting such a case. The reason is application of phenol over an extensive area, such as face, neck, and upper thorax, with consequent absorption of a large volume of phenol. Blood levels of phenol as high as 23 mg. per 100 ml. have been reported after phenol ingestion with survival; however, Litton (1962), in a careful study after application of 3 ml. of 50 per cent phenol to an entire face, recorded levels of 0.68 mg. per 100 ml. one hour after application, 0.19 mg. two hours after, and 0.10 mg. four hours after exposure. It is thus demonstrated that, while no true toxic levels of blood phenol have been established, careful application to a restricted area of a reasonable volume of phenol would appear to pose little risk (Litton, 1966).

After absorption, the phenol is conjugated with glycuronic and sulfuric acids and excreted by the kidneys. Another mode of removal is by detoxification to hydroquinones and pyrocatechin; some free phenol is also excreted as such by the kidneys.

PATHOLOGY

Biopsy studies have all demonstrated three basic anatomic changes in the treated skin (Brown et al., 1960; Baker, 1962; Baker et al., 1966; Spira et al., 1970.) First there is a reorientation of dermal collagen, with a change from the usual wavy shape to a straight pattern lying parallel to the skin surface. This is accompanied by an increase in the density of the associated fibroblasts. The changes are of long duration and appear to be the basic factors in the clinical benefits from this procedure. It should be noted that such collagen changes do not occur after a mechanical dermabrasion, and this appears to explain the relative inefficiency of dermabrasion in long-term eradication of fine rhytides. The second observable sequela is a marked diminution of the number of melanin granules that may be demonstrated in the basal layers of the epidermis by the Fontana-Masson silver strain. A third change routinely noted is an increase in the amount of elastic tissue, demonstrable by special stains in the dermis. There is also a transient inflammatory reaction that passes its peak by the third week and is gone by the third month (Litton, 1962).

The immediate inflammatory reaction after application of the phenol solution to the skin is characterized by keratocoagulation and epidermolysis, with a deeper zone of cellular destruction in the upper dermis. A crust of keratin, necrotic epidermis and proteinaceous precipitate forms. Epidermal regeneration begins on the second day and is complete by the seventh day. Dermal thickening occurs at about two weeks, secondary to an inflammatory reaction with intercellular edema (Spira et al., 1970).

INDICATIONS

Chemical peeling is indicated when fine wrinkling forms all or part of the problem. Deeper wrinkles are only partially affected by the technique; if their removal is desired, chemical peel must be used in concert with other techniques (pp. 222 and 226). The upper and lower lips are often involved in a fine, vertically oriented wrinkling, which is unaffected by the usual techniques of face lift. While mechanical abrasion will produce temporary improvement, chemical peel results in a more prolonged effect. Moderate tightening of the forehead skin may also be achieved by this technique without the risks of hair loss or obvious scars so often encountered with the more radical approaches to this problem (pp. 177 and 179).

Often an ideal candidate for this procedure is the younger patient with a minimal facial sag and finely wrinkled skin which has been constantly exposed to the elements, who is not quite a candidate for face lift but desires improvement just the same. However, it must be emphasized that the patient with a fair complexion is the better candidate, as the olive-skinned patient tends to show an obvious line of demarcation between treated and untreated skin and to have a tendency to blotchiness in the final skin color. Negroes or other dark-skinned patients should be accepted for chemabrasion with great caution for similar reasons.

Diffuse patchy pigmentation, such as that observable after some episodes of dermatitis or in chloasma, is removed by the peel, which seems to offer a prolonged, if not permanent, cure to this problem.

In patients with a combination of lax facial skin and fine wrinkling, the first procedure should be an eyelid plasty and facial plastic procedure; after a period of three or more weeks to allow the skin to recover from the operative insult, a full face peel may be done. It is not, however, necessary to defer the peeling if it is to be done only to the lips and/or the forehead.

PRECAUTIONS

A full history and complete physical examination should be obtained, with special attention being given to the hepatorenal system. Routine blood analysis should also be obtained prior to embarking on a chemical peeling procedure.

Attempts to peel the neck skin frequently result in hypertrophic scarring, since the depth of the "burn" is difficult to control in this region. No attempt should be made to do a blepharoplasty and an eyelid peel at the same time, as ectropion may result. Certainly the presence of a tight lower lid after blepharoplasty should caution the operator against an eyelid peel. Additionally, because of the marked reaction, it is unwise to do both upper and lower eyelids at the same time since the swelling will render the patient temporarily without vision. Attempts to peel arms and thorax have been quite unsuccessful.

Although superficial keratoses and telangiectasia are amenable to improvement by this technique, it does not result in any improvement of more extensive malformations such as strawberry hemangioma or nevus flammeus, which continue to present their usual enigmatic challenge.

TECHNIQUE

For all save small areas of the face, the patient is best admitted to the hospital. However, in either instance the previously noted precaution of complete examination must be taken. The procedure with its discomfort and usual sequelae should be carefully explained to the patient since the postoperative appearance is, to say the least, frightening.

A history of drug sensitivity or prior exposure to this treatment by another surgeon deserves a test of a small area of skin; this is usually conveniently done in the preauricular region. Preoperative photographs in both black and white and, ideally, color should also be taken.

The solution should be freshly mixed for each use to the following formula:

> Phenol 88% U.S.P. 3 ml.
> Croton oil 3 drops
> Septisol soap 8 drops
> Distilled water 2 ml.

This volume will suffice for a full face application.

The skin is washed on the evening prior to surgery to remove all cosmetics and again on the morning of surgery. No anesthesia is necessary, but the patient should be well premedicated. We use the following medication schedule with appropriate modification:

> Nembutal 200 mg., p.o., 2 hours preoperative
> Pantopon 20 mg.
> Scopolamine 0.3 mg.
> Sparine 25 mg., I.M., 1 hour preoperative

The patient is placed on the operating table with the head slightly elevated. The skin oils and residual soap are removed with ether.

The solution is applied by means of a cotton-tipped applicator stick with the tip well wrung out so as to avoid any chance of dripping or splashing of the solution. A transient stinging sensation, replaced by anesthesia, is often complained of by the patient during application. The application should be made evenly to produce a smooth white surface; when an area of greater penetration is desired, a more vigorous rubbing of the applicator will achieve this result; however, care is called for in this regard. Gentle stretching of the skin will enable the fluid to coat the depths of the wrinkles evenly, an important point to observe.

The hairline should be slightly encroached on to avoid a visible margin of untreated skin; no permanent damage to the hair will result.

It is necessary to come right to the vermilion border of the lips, and, if in doubt, a margin of vermilion may be included. The vermilion will blister and be somewhat painful, but a thin band of obviously untreated skin is avoided. The ciliary margins should be skirted by 2 mm. to avoid any chance of corneal or conjunctival burns. The treated area should extend just below the mandibular margin but no farther.

In treating the whole face it should be sectioned; in the average type of skin, the tape is applied to each completed area prior to treating the next. Suitably sized regions for treatment are the left cheek (with lower lid, if planned), the right cheek, the nose and upper lip, the chin and lower lip, and the forehead (and upper lids, if planned).

Many varieties of occlusive cover exist, the most elegant of which is a custom made rubber mask. However, for all practical purposes a standard ½-inch zinc oxide adhesive tape applied in two or three layers, with care to avoid producing skin creases below it, is both the easiest and best means of occlusion. In patients with thin, fair and delicate skin, the solution should be allowed to dry, with partial evaporation of the phenol, prior to tape application.

The application of such an adhesive tape "mask" produces a deeper peel with more lasting results. This impression is shared by most surgeons, and was recently confirmed in the study of Spira et al. (1970).

Various authors have described many different methods of tape application. However, the use of short strips with care not to produce underlying skin creases and butting the first layer edge to edge has proved satisfactory in our hands. The second and, if necessary, third layers are laid in any convenient fashion over the first layer, again with care not to produce creases in the underlying skin.

It is occasionally necessary to give further medication during the course of the application. After return to his room, the patient will often complain of a fiery itching sensation, and the narcotics need to be repeated. The patient is best left well sedated for the first 48 hours, with relatively free access to narcotic relief of discomfort.

If the lips have been treated, it is advisable to keep the patient silent and to administer a fluid diet by straw for the first 48 hours. This is necessary to avoid lifting of the adhesive from the skin, which will allow for a corresponding area of lesser effect. Bed rest is usually desirable for at least the first 24 hours (preferably the first 48 hours) when a large area of the face has been treated.

After 48 hours have elapsed, the patient is given another dose of narcotic, and the adhesive mask, with its adherent necrotic superficial skin layers, is gently peeled off the face. A raw, moist area is evident and is dusted with thymol iodide powder, U.S.P., to produce a thin coagulum. Other coagulating powders have been used, particularly antibiotic-based powders, but appear to offer no advantage and indeed may carry a risk of producing hypersensitivity. Use

of the powder two or three times a day on any moist areas is necessary for the first 72 hours, after which time it may be discontinued.

Coincident with the removal of the adhesive mask, the diet may be liberalized, but chewing should still be kept to a minimum, as should talking. General activity is to be encouraged, but overexertion and sweating must be avoided.

On the fifth day after removal of the adhesive, the patient is instructed to apply a liberal coating of bland cold cream, polymyxin B (Neosporin) ointment or petrolatum jel to the coagulum; on the following day the powder mask is usually easily removed to reveal a layer of delicate pink new skin. In patients with a relatively hairy face, it is occasionally advisable to wait another day to remove the coagulum, the added time loosening the hair's grip on the crust. The face is cared for by daily washing with a mild soap and water. The new skin should be kept moist by cold cream or moisturizing creams. After the passage of a week, to allow for maturation of the new skin, a light make-up may be applied. Regular make-up use may commence after two to three weeks.

The intense pink color will fade rapidly, but an excess pink coloration will remain for six to eight weeks. The skin will be somewhat tense and smooth, with the finer rhytides gone and the deeper grooves much less evident. Care should be taken to protect the area from exposure to the sun for a period of three to six months, and a sun screen, such as Uval or A-Fil, should be advised for use in any sunny region.

Milia are frequently seen in the treated areas, but usually disappear in two to three weeks without specific therapy.

COMPLICATIONS

The commonest problem after chemical peeling is a disparity of skin color between the treated and untreated areas. This may be made less troublesome by careful selection of patients on the criteria of dry skin and blond coloration. Careful preoperative explanation of the postpeeling results will also allow the patient to adjust to any minor irregularity of color. Treatment of complete esthetic units of the face, rather than a partial unit, aids greatly in camouflage of any disparity of color or texture. The area of treatment should just cross the mandibular margin to the "shadow area" to prevent a noticeable edge; feathering of the depth of peel at the margins is also valuable.

Hypertrophic scarring and a tight "postburn" appearance is avoided by keeping the peel superficial by careful light application of the solution. In any patient with thin delicate skin, consideration of allowing partial phenol evaporation should be made to lessen the chemical effects. Peeling of the neck and arms not infrequently results in the above noted complication, even when no tape is applied or its application is delayed; hence, treatment of this area is best avoided (Baker, 1962). No specific therapy for the scars or tightness is effective, save passage of time or excision with consequent surgical defects.

Phenol intoxication should not present as a problem if the criteria of area treatment, noted previously, are adhered to by the surgeon. However, Litton as recently as 1966 advised that a two-hour period be allowed before completion of the second section of the face to allow for phenol detoxification, a view not shared by the majority of operators in this field.

Ectropion has been noted after ill advised peeling of the lower lids. If, after an adequate period of softening of the skin, aided by adhesive support, the problem has failed to correct, then surgical intervention is indicated. (See Chapter 5).

Attempts at peeling for acne scars have shown results notably less effective than mechanical abrasion (MacKee and Karp, 1952; Sperber, 1965b).

REPEAT CHEMICAL PEELING

The procedure may be cautiously repeated, but this is rarely indicated (Baker et al., 1962, 1966), and certainly the advice of Litton (1962) that this therapy may be repeated in six weeks to two months is best discarded for a much longer wait of 12 to 18 months.

Surgical Planing of the Skin

Surgical planing or dermabrasion of the skin is the removal of the epidermis and a portion of the superficial layer of the dermis with preservation of sufficient epidermal adnexa to allow for spontaneous re-epithelialization of the abraded surface. Dermabrasion results in a smoothing of surface irregularities produced by scars and acne pits. The effect is similar to chemical peeling; however, dermabrasion has proved more useful in the treatment of acne and other depressed scars, while chemabrasion is more effective in the treatment of wrinkles and certain types of hyperpigmentation. Another indication for abrasion is to aid in the preparation of a re-

cipient site for a skin graft; a layer of deep dermis is left intact and a split-thickness skin graft is placed on this dermal bed—a so-called overgraft (Webster, 1954; Hynes, 1957). By this technique a greater skin thickness results than might be obtained with a single, thick-skin graft. Also, contraction does not occur. The result of overgrafting is frequently a cosmetically and functionally superior skin grafted area. Overgrafts rarely fail.

HISTORY

Kromayer (1905) reported the first efforts at mechanical abrasion of the skin for treatment of dermatologic lesions. His initial efforts were with cylindrical knives, and he later progressed to the use of dental burs on skin made firm and anesthetic by ethyl chloride spray.

The use of the wire brush as an abrading instrument was first reported by Janson (1935), but it remained for Iverson (1947) to spark the modern revival of abrasive therapy. McEvitt (1950) and Curtin (1953) rapidly added to its popularity with the electrically driven, waterproof, carbide abrasive paper cylinders and diamond-impregnated burs. The latter are capable of producing a very fine and easily controlled depth of abrasive therapy and have proved of particular advantage where very superficial abrasion is required.

HEALING OF THE DERMABRADED AREA

Success in dermabrasion therapy is dependent on the ability of the skin to rebuild a new epidermal layer from epithelial elements in the deep skin adnexa. Scarred areas where there is a loss of skin adnexa from either thermal, direct or irradiation injuries heal incompletely or slowly following abrasive therapy. The same, of course, holds true for regions of the body such as the eyelids, the skin of the lower anterior neck, the inner aspect of the arm, the dorsum of the hand and other areas relatively deficient in pilosebaceous adnexa. The risk of delayed healing and/or increased scarring is higher in such regions.

Immediately following dermabrasion the serum from the wound forms a coagulum across the abraded surface, entrapping much cellular detritus within its interstices. This is followed by a period of intense proliferation of squamous epithelium from the adnexal elements as early as three to four days after the operative procedure (Eisen et al., 1955).

In most instances by the fifth day a thin epidermis has regenerated, lacking rete pegs but possessing developing hair follicles and sebaceous glands. On the third day a cell-free layer is noted under the new epidermis which shows evidence by the fifth day of beginning dermal regeneration; by the seventh day some loose attachment of the new epidermis to the dermis may be observed.

During the first two weeks following the operative procedure many young fibroblasts lying with axes in a horizontal plane are noted in the newly regenerated dermis. Luikart and his associates (1959) noted a persistence of this horizontal striated collagenous pattern for at least four years following abrasive therapy. They attribute the smoothness of the skin, at least in part, to the presence of this newly formed collagen.

A further factor in the smoothness and tautness of the abraded skin is the phenomenon of interisland contraction described by Converse and Robb-Smith in 1944. The interisland contraction is probably a significant factor in the smoothing of the skin following abrasion for acne scars and in the collapse and constriction of some of the deeper acne pits.

There is little evidence of pigment formation the first three or four weeks postabrasion, but this appears to progress from that time. It is important during this crucial period of pigment reformation that the skin be protected from actinic radiation, since the complication of hyperpigmentation appears to be directly related to careless exposure to actinic rays. Effective sunscreens and avoidance of direct sun or sunglare exposure is mandatory for two to four months, as for the postchemabrasion skin.

OPERATIVE PROCEDURE

In all but the most minor dermabrasion procedures we prefer general anesthesia. The use of topical sprays and local anesthesia infiltration has proved to be disappointing and will frequently result in a compromise on the part of the surgeon because of patient discomfort.

A useful means of pinpointing deep pits is the application of ink or Bonney's blue to the depths of the pits; this is readily visible following dermabrasion when a complete obliteration of the depths of the sulci has not been achieved. The operator should protect his eyes from both flying cellular debris cast by the abrasion apparatus and from the occasional disintegration of an abrasion wheel. We routinely use a bronchoscopy shield for protection.

The depth of abrasion is best confined to superficial or intermediate thickness. Abrasion to deeper levels may result in hypertrophic scarring and increase the likelihood of irregular pigmentation. We prefer to re-abrade on one or two occasions rather than to attempt to completely obliterate the scar irregularities at a single session.

A rest period between abrasions of three to six months suffices, during which time the skin returns more or less to normal activity and pigmentation approaches normal.

Hemostasis is achieved by the application of gauze sponges soaked in 1:50,000 epinephrine solution or topical thrombin. Final hemostasis is achieved by the use of warm air from a hairdryer, which is played over the dermabraded area and helps with hemostasis and with the formation of a dressing eschar.

A thick paste of topical thrombin mixed with saline also aids in promoting an early firm eschar across the abraded area. We do not routinely employ dressings.

POSTOPERATIVE CARE

Patients are discharged on the day following surgery and is instructed to daily utilize hairdryer to dry all exudate and maintain the eschar. On the sixth or seventh day the patient is to apply a generous layer of cold cream or vegetable oil to the eschar. These applications begin the separation of the coagulum. The patient is instructed not to forcibly peel the coagulum from the abraded area except in hairy regions.

Exposure to direct or reflected sunlight must be avoided, and the patient is instructed in the use of a good quality sunscreen cream for a period of two to four months following treatment. The use of the sunscreen should be even more prolonged in those patients in whom full pigmentary return has not occurred during this time.

In the rare instance in which hyperpigmentation occurs, it usually undergoes spontaneous regression over a period of three to eighteen months. When regression does not occur, secondary chemabrasion may help to establish uniform color match. In our experience, most problems of hyperpigmentation or irregular pigmentation have been associated with excessive exposure to actinic radiation.

REFERENCES

Chemabrasion
Ayres, S., III: Superficial chemosurgery in treating aging skin. Arch. Dermat. 85:385, 1962.

Ayres, S., III: Superficial chemosurgery, its current status and relationship to dermabrasion. Arch. Dermat. *89*: 395, 1964.

Baker, T. J.: Ablation of rhytides by chemical means. J. Florida M.A. *47*:451–454, 1961.

Baker, T. J.: Chemical face peeling and rhytidectomy, a combined approach for facial rejuvenation. Plast. Reconstr. Surg. *29*:199, 1962.

Baker, T. J.: Chemical face peeling: An adjunct to surgical face lifting. South. Med. J. *56*:412, 1963.

Baker, T. J., Gordon, H. L., and Seckinger, D. L.: A second look at chemical face peeling. Plast. Reconstr. Surg. *37*:487–493, 1966.

Batstone, J. H. F., and Millard, D. R., Jr.: An endorsement of facial chemosurgery. Brit. J. Plast. Surg. *21*:193, 1968.

Brown, A. M., Kaplan, L. M., and Brown, M. E.: Phenol-induced histological skin changes: Hazards, technique, and uses. Brit. J. Plast. Surg. *13*:158, 1960.

Combes, F. C., Sperber, P. A., and Reich, M.: Dermal defects treated by chemical agents. N.Y. Phys. & Amer. Med. *56*:36, 1960.

Litton, C.: Chemical face lifting. Plast. Reconstr. Surg. *29*: 371, 1962.

Litton, C.: Followup study of chemosurgery. South. Med. J. *50*:1007, 1966.

MacKee, G. M., and Karp, E. L.: Treatment of acne scars with phenol. Brit. J. Dermat. *64*:456, 1952.

Sperber, P. A.: Chemexfoliation—a new term in cosmetic therapy. J. Amer. Geriat. Surg. *11*:58, 1963.

Rees, T. D.: Rehabilitation of the aging face. Geriatrics *20*:1039, 1965.

Sperber, P. A.: Treatment of aging skin and dermal defects. Springfield, Ill., Charles C Thomas, 1965 a, Ch. 1, p. 3.

Sperber, P. A.: Chemexfoliation for aging skin and acne scarring. Arch. Otolaryng. *81*:278, 1965.

Spira, M., Dahl, G., Freeman, R., Gerow, F. J., and Hardy, S. B.: Chemosurgery—A histological study. Plast. Reconstr. Surg. *45*:247, 1970.

Dermabrasion

Converse, J. M., and Robb-Smith, A. H. T.: The healing of surface cutaneous wounds: Its analogy with the healing of superficial burns. Ann. Surg. *120*:873, 1944.

Eisen, A. Z., Holyoke, J. B., and Lobitz, W. C.: Responses of superficial portion of human pilosebaceous apparatus to controlled injury. J. Invest. Derm. *25*:145, 1955.

Hymes, W.: The treatment of scars by shaving and skin graft. Brit. J. Plast. Surg. *10*:1–10, 1957.

Iverson, P. C.: Surgical removal of traumatic tattoos. Plast. Reconstr. Surg. *2*:427, 1947.

Janson, P.: Eine einfache Methode der Entfernung von Tatauierungen. Dermat. Wschr. *101*:894, 1935.

Kromayer, E.: Rotationinstrumente: Ein neues technisches Verfahren in der dermatologischen Kleinchirugie. Chir. Dermat. Z. (Berlin) *12*:26, 1905.

Kurtin, A.: Corrective surgical planing of skin; New technique for treatment of acne scars and other skin defects. A.M.A. Arch. Derm. *68*:389, 1953.

Luikart, R., Ayres, S., and Wilson, J. W.: Surgical skin planing. N.Y. J. Med. *59*:413, 1959.

McEvitt, W. G.: Treatment of acne pits by abrasion with sandpaper. J.A.M.A. *142*:647, 1950.

Webster, G. V.: Report at the Annual Convention of the American Society of Plastic and Reconstructive Surgeons, Hollywood, Florida, October, 1954.

Steps in chemical abrasion of the face. The patient is heavily sedated and the face thoroughly cleaned with ether to remove all sebaceous material (A). This patient is a young woman who is not yet a candidate for facial surgery, but who has early rhytides of the skin.

First the forehead skin is painted with the phenol mixture as a unit (B). It is then taped with water-repellent adhesive (C). The remaining portions of the face are painted and tape is applied (D and E).

The result six weeks after the procedure is shown in F and G. Note that the skin is quite smooth and that most of the wrinkles have been eradicated. This patient is a brunette and therefore not the best candidate for chemabrasion. Fair-skinned blonds and redheads with dry skin are better, such as the patient shown in H 10 days after the application of the escharotic. Note that the skin is a bright pink color, a condition that persists for several weeks.

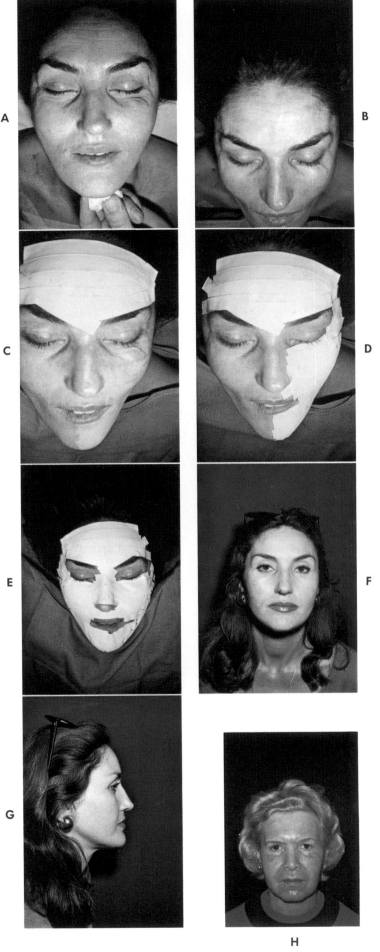

221

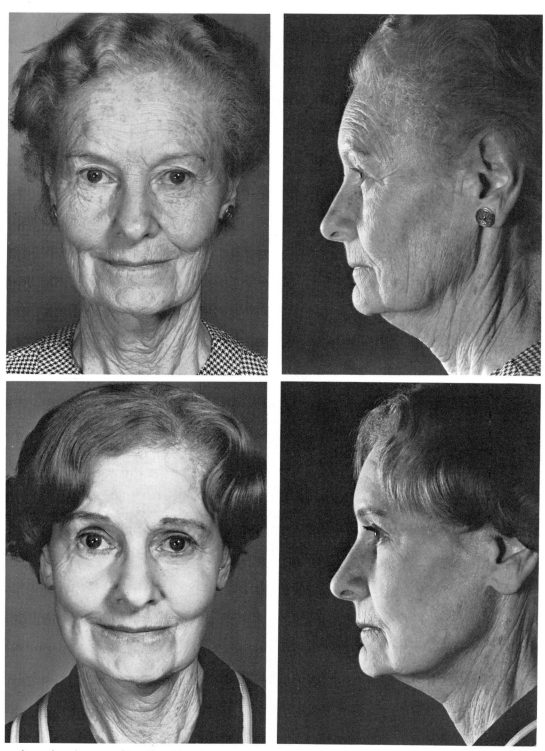

Full-face chemabrasion was done for this patient several weeks after facial plastic surgery. Although the improvement shown here may be regarded as typical, the results of chemical abrasion are not consistent. It is not possible to promise any particular degree of improvement in attempts to ablate fine rhytides. Chemical peel is better done after facial and cervical rhytidectomy, although the sequence can be reversed if necessary. Notice the neck is still wrinkled after peeling because the chemical cannot be applied to this area with safety.

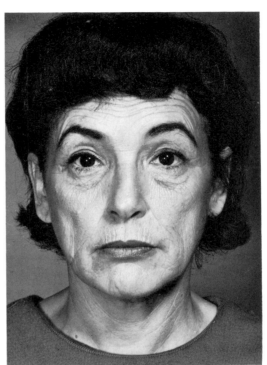

This patient obtained a remarkable improvement from blepharoplasty, rhytidectomy and, finally, full-face chemabrasion using the formula published by Baker (1962). In this instance postoperative photos were taken as 35-mm. transparencies and are not true representations because of overexposure. But the results were, in fact, exceedingly good.

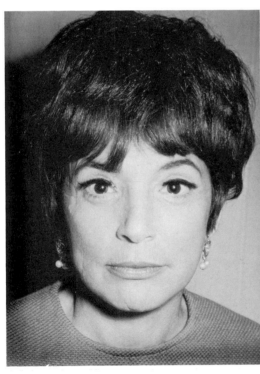

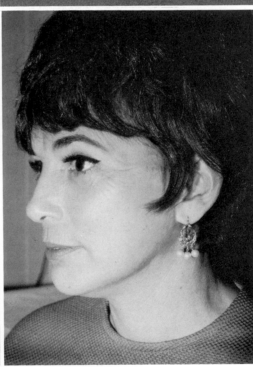

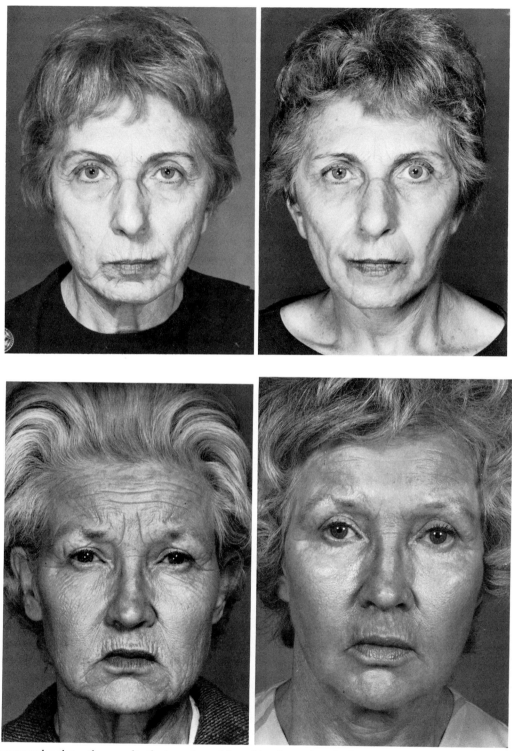

These photographs show the results that can be achieved by deep chemical peel of the rhytides that form around the mouth in many patients. Such lines are often the result of progressive dehydration of the skin, hereditary in nature, and they are thought to occur sometimes from progressive absorption of the alveolar bone. If the lines are very deep, additional improvement may be obtained after chemabrasion by subdermal injection of minute amounts of silicone fluid. (These two sets of photographs depict two different patients.)

224

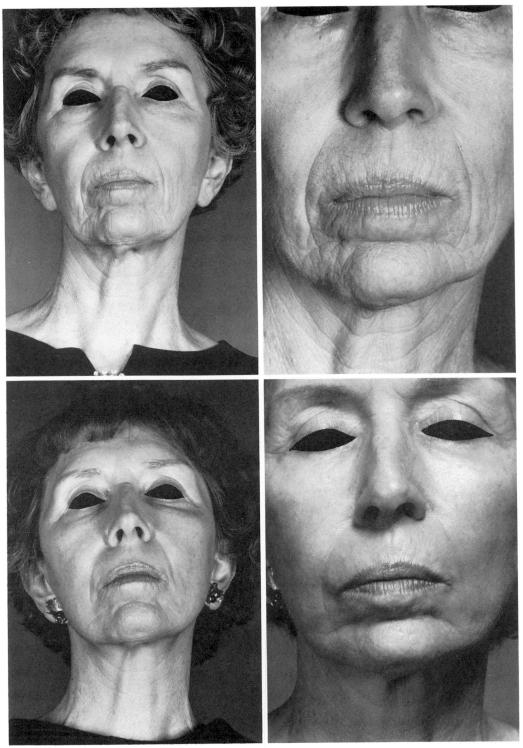

Loose skin along the mandibular border and of the neck is not improved to a significant degree by chemical peel. But chemical abrasion following a standard face lift procedure will aid the final result quite considerably because it will improve the rhytides about the mouth.

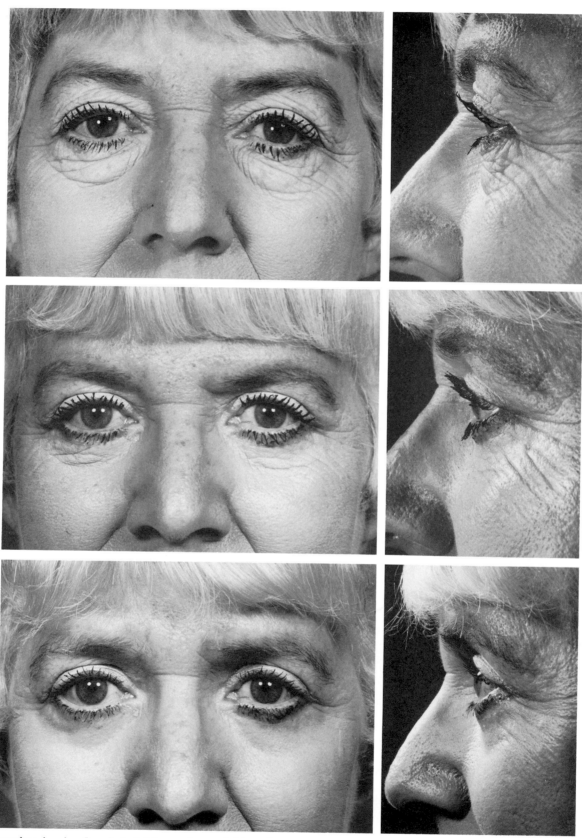

Chemabrasion is often helpful in erasing wrinkles of the eyelid skin which cannot be removed—and which may even be accentuated—by blepharoplasty. The photographs at the top of the page show the preoperative condition; note the unusual thickness of the skin and the deep wrinkling. In the middle set of photos are shown the results after a complete blepharoplasty. The palpebral bags are gone, but much of the wrinkling remains. The final result after deep chemical peeling, shown in the lower photos, is long lasting. Chemabrasion for this purpose is better and safer than dermabrasion.

226

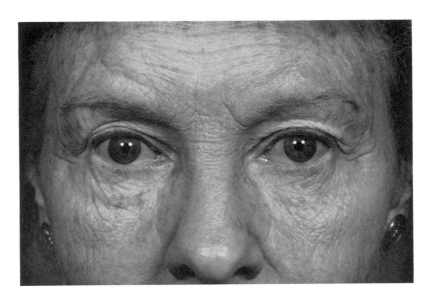

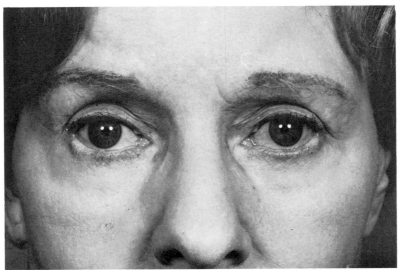

Typical senile changes in the eyelids of a woman with very thin skin. Note that the postoperative photograph, which shows the patient smiling, demonstrates a marked improvement; however, there are many fine rhytides still present which cannot be eliminated by further surgery. These are quite characteristic of such thin skin. Chemical peel can further improve such wrinkles.

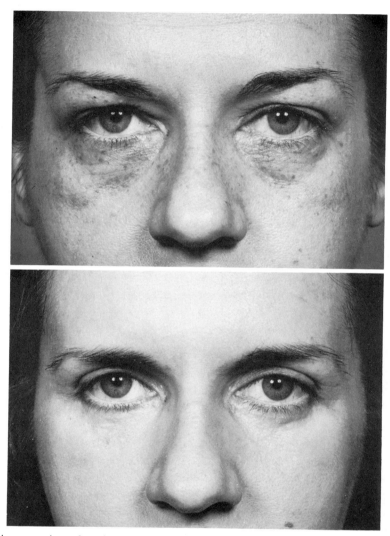

In certain types of pigmentation, the pigment is quite superficial and responds to chemabrasion. The irregular and unsightly pattern of pigmentation seen in this patient had been present since her childhood. Blepharoplasty followed in six weeks by deep chemical peel achieved the result shown in the postoperative view, which has persisted for two years.

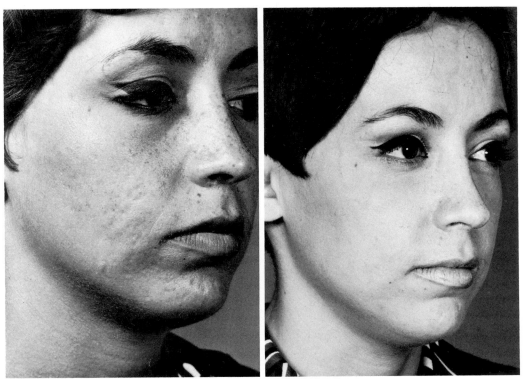

Surgical planing of the face for the treatment of superficial acne pits and chickenpox scars is quite adequate when the pits are shallow and the scarring does not extend deeply into the dermis, as in this patient.

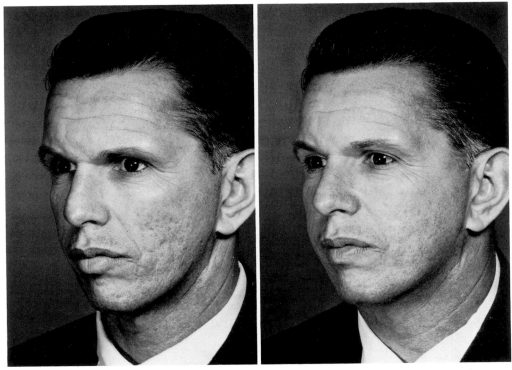

The results of surgical planing when deep dermal scarring is present, as in this patient, are an improvement but are not so dramatic as when scarring is superficial. Such patients should be advised of the limitations of the procedure before surgery.

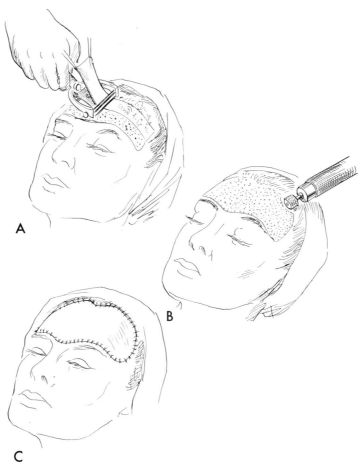

A

B

C

Another excellent adaptation of the use of dermabrasion is in the surgical preparation of the recipient bed for the overgrafting technique, which is of particular importance in resurfacing burn scars so that an optimal cosmetic result can be achieved. Dermabrasion and overgrafting also constitute an effective technique for the treatment of decorative tattoos.

A scarred area, such as the forehead, is denuded of epithelium by use of a dermatome or by dermabrasion, or both (A and B). A split-thickness skin graft is applied to the abraded dermal bed (C). A complete "take" of the graft is practically assured because of the rich blood supply entering the undersurface of the dermis from the subdermal plexus. The cosmetic results of such unit grafts are superior to those of full-thickness excisions, because the integrity of the deep dermis is maintained and contraction is therefore minimal.

(From Rees, T. D., and Casson, P. R.: Plast. Reconstr. Surg. *38*:522, 1966. Reproduced with permission.)

230

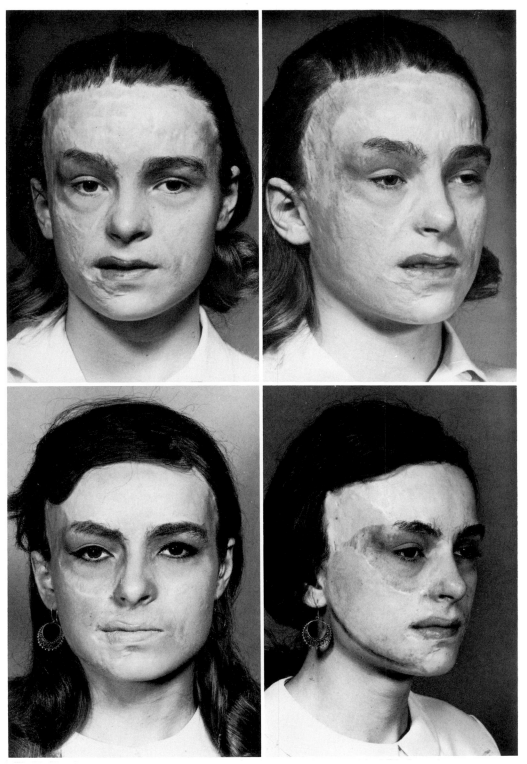

Results of overgrafting of the forehead and cheek in a young patient with extensive burn scarring. Note the improved texture of the overgrafted areas in the postoperative views. The application of camouflaging makeup is facilitated.

(From Rees, T. D., and Casson, P. R.: Plast. Reconstr. Surg. *38*:522, 1966. Reproduced with permission.)

Chapter 8

SILICONE INJECTION THERAPY

Thomas D. Rees, M.D.

Rumors concerning an injectable mixture which was being used in the Orient and Europe as a fat substitute for filling soft tissue contour depressions and especially for breast augmentation began to be widely circulated in the mid 1950's. At first it was almost impossible to get any scientific data about this material—its identification, its tissue reactivity, the technique of use or its range of clinical application. As surgeons everywhere became more and more interested, however, the main ingredient of these injectable mixtures was eventually identified as dimethylpolysiloxane fluid. The first report of the subdermal reaction of this silicone compound had been published by Rowe, Spencer and Bass in 1948. Its use for soft tissue augmentation was first suggested in the medical literature by Wegener (1957) and by Franklyn (1958a and b).

Surgeons have long sought the "ideal" alloplastic material for implantation, one which would fulfill a lengthy list of criteria. Such an "ideal" material would be:

1. Chemically and physically inert
2. Locally nonreactive
3. Nonantigenetic
4. Noncarcinogenic
5. Nontoxic and systemically nonreactive
6. Unchangeable with time, heat or pressure
7. Nonsupportive of bacterial growth
8. Easy to sterilize and prepare
9. Inexpensive

Materials for replacement of either hard or soft tissues in the human body that fulfill all these requirements will probably never be found. At present, living tissue is certainly best, when available without paying too high a price. However, as an alternative, dimethylpolysiloxane fluid does seem to meet many of the listed criteria.

In the search for the "ideal" material, various substances have been used as bone or cartilage substitutes, and a few have been tried as soft tissue replacements. These substances include ivory, homologous or heterologous bone and cartilage, various metals and, in recent years, plastic resins, polymers and other alloplasts. Many of these compounds have enjoyed a certain success in reconstructive plastic surgery, yet none have fulfilled all the criteria. Acrylics, polyethylenes, Teflon, Dacron and silicones, as well as silver, Mersilene, stainless steel and tantalum have been notably successful as tissue substitutes. In recent years the man-made plastics have been studied carefully. Of these, Teflon, Dacron, the acrylics and the silicone polymers have been most widely accepted for medical application.

Certain high viscosity liquids of animal and vegetable origin, such as paraffin and lanolin, were used as soft-tissue substitutes for a short time. However, as the sequelae and complications of their use became widely known, they were abandoned by most surgeons. The paraffin story is well known. The initial enthusiastic report by Gersuny (1900) was soon followed by reports of granuloma formation. Paraffin therefore enjoyed but a short life as an injectable soft tissue substitute in most clinics. Nevertheless, it is still used by some who are either not knowledgeable about the granuloma problem or who do not believe it is important. Boo-Chai (1965) recently reported on the continued use of paraffin compounds in the Orient. He also described granulomalike lesions resulting from paraffin injections, but advised that many of these benign lesions are self-limiting and often undergo resolution. As far as we are aware, no reports of carcinogenesis are available. Liquid lanolin has also been used for filling small contour defects. It causes localized inflammation that results in localized fibrosis providing soft tissue bulk. However, like paraffin, it is apt to result in granuloma formation.

Much has been written about the use and misuse of silicone fluid and its various mixtures in the past 10 years. Laboratory and clinical evaluation of the compound is still in the process of long-term study, and much work needs to be completed before the final facts are available. Research findings to date will be reviewed in this chapter.

Silicone (dimethylpolysiloxane) fluid seems to have suitable clinical applications, some of which cannot be equaled today by other methods or techniques. The treatment of hemifacial atrophy is a good example. Soft tissue augmentation by silicone fluid injections has, however, been met with mixed response by the medical profession. Some physicians have been intrigued by the possible advantages of its use for the treatment of severe contour deformities of congenital etiology such as the branchial arch syndrome, absence of the pectoralis major muscle, pectus excavatum and soft tissue loss from trauma or idiopathic deformities such as lipodystrophy and facial atrophy. Others have been understandably "bearish" on the subject because of past unhappy experience with other injectables such as paraffin. These men are concerned that premature availability of such a compound could result in untoward sequelae and widespread misuse.

The possible consequences of releasing silicone fluid for unrestricted use are worrisome indeed. The ease with which it can be used could place this material in the hands of some who may be untrained in its applications and unaware of the intricacies and complex problems involved. Silicone fluid injections should rightly be viewed only as an ancillary technique available to complement tried and tested surgical procedures and should be performed only by those thoroughly trained in all phases of plastic reconstruction.

In the United States a small number of investigators have been more or less officially engaged in the medical evaluation of this material until such time as its safety and efficacy can be established. Yet despite every effort that can be made by manufacturers and governments, liquid silicone injections are still being widely used with no restrictions for soft tissue augmentation in many other countries.

At this time the authors believe that silicone fluid does have a rightful place in the armamentarium of the plastic surgeon and that it is the current treatment of choice in certain deformities for which surgery is unsuccessful or sadly lacking in results. In our opinion sufficient research data are now available to delineate some of the parameters of use of silicone fluid. When used in the recommended volumes and dosage schedules, it is apparently a highly efficacious treatment modality for certain deformities. It is hoped that its use can soon be expanded to many more physicians to speed the collection of data.

Chemical and Physical Properties of Silicone

Silicone fluid is available for many industrial uses, and various techniques have been devised for "purifying" it for injection therapy. Silicone is a general term for the organopolysiloxanes, a class of polymers consisting of chains of basic units made up of silicon, oxygen and organic radicals of the formula CH_3-Si-O-CH_3. Its proper chemical name is dimethylpolysiloxane. This material is manufactured by the Dow-Corning Corporation and is available in many physical forms for medical purposes, including liquids, foams, resins, sponges and rubbers. The vulcanized (rubber) form of dimethylpolysiloxane is marketed as Silastic.

Silicone products, together with Teflon and Dacron, have revolutionized the attitude of most surgeons toward prosthetic implants. The inert nature of these materials and their nonantigenicity, high tissue tolerance, improved texture and malleability, along with the fact that local inflammatory response is minimal, has brought them into common medical use as prosthetic implants in a great variety of conditions too numerous to discuss here in depth. Their multiple uses in plastic surgery as chin, breast, nose, ear and other subcutaneous implants are well known. They have completely replaced the use of autogenous tissues or homologous (banked) materials in many common conditions in which the overlying tissue is healthy.

Silicone fluid has the distinct advantage over sponge or solid implants of being injectable in very small volumes. The fact that a surgical procedure is avoided is what has made this technique so attractive to the laity as well as to physicians not trained in surgery. Many of the complications and problems that have followed injections occurred because the compound was used by doctors without experience in the field of implantation. In fact, misuse of the material through inexperience was so great that it necessitated placing stringent restrictions on its use.

Silicone fluid, or mixtures of silicone fluid with various other substances such as vegetable oils, fatty acids and even snake venom, have probably been used for over two decades in Asia and Europe, and somewhat less in America. Many thousands of patients have been injected with such mixtures. However, the accumulation of meaningful follow-up data was woefully inadequate until recent years. Much of the early use of the injection technique was for mammary augmentation, a use now discarded in most clinics.

In the United States, silicone fluid is being investigated under "new drug" regulations of the government. Human research has been limited to a small number of treatment centers.

SILICONE FLUID AND SILASTIC

Some confusion exists about the different forms of injectable silicones that have been investigated. One type is known as RTV Silastic, an injectable liquid which, when injected with an added catalyst, vulcanizes in the tissues at room (or tissue) temperature; hence, the designation RTV (Room Temperature Vulcanizing). This vulcanizing fluid was investigated briefly, but for the most part has been abandoned for use in humans because the vulcanized rubber mass was hard and unyielding in the tissues.

Dimethylpolysiloxane *fluid*, on the other hand, remains permanently in a liquid state after subdermal injection, but becomes encapsulated within the tissues in a multicystic fibrous mass. It is this mass that displaces empty space and "fills up" contour losses. This is the "artificial fat."

This fluid was first designated as Dow-Corning 360 Medical Fluid. Its current designation is Medical Grade Fluid MDX 44011. It has been prepared in many viscosities, expressed in centistokes (the viscosity of water being 1 centistoke). The 350 centistoke fluid has been the most widely used in human research.

The higher viscosity preparations tend to remain in situ after injection, with the least loss of bulk, migration or absorption. Therefore, research is currently being conducted on such gel preparations, some of which can be vulcanized after injection by the addition of a catalyst. It is hoped that a material will be developed which will maintain the soft consistency of a gel after injection because it would remain fixed in place and yet reduce the already low tissue reactivity that has been demonstrated in the MDX 44011 fluid. Absorption of gel forms would also be unlikely.

Basic Research

In 1963 a series of experiments were undertaken at the Institute of Reconstructive Plastic Surgery, New York University, to investigate the local tissue effects and possible carcinogenic properties of dimethylpolysiloxane (silicone) fluid when injected into laboratory animals. These studies were under the direction of the author and Dr. Donald Ballantyne (Rees, Platt and Ballantyne, 1965). Early experimental work was done with the Dow-Corning 200 fluid. Later a purified form of the 200 fluid, known as 360 Medical Fluid, was used. Finally, the highly purified MDX 44011 became available. Most of the studies were performed with silicone fluid having a viscosity of 350 centistokes. However, the MDX 44011 fluid is now available in several standard viscosities for experimental use.

This preliminary study indicated that cutaneous injection of silicone fluid was well tolerated by tissues and did not induce tumor formation in the animals tested. Subsequent laboratory studies have been reported by us (Rees et al., 1967, 1968a and b, 1970) as well as by other investigators. From these data and from investigations now in progress, certain facts are emerging about the local and systemic responses to this liquid material in various species of animal.

More than 1000 animals (including mice, rats, guinea pigs, rabbits, dogs, monkeys and subhuman primates) have been used in silicone fluid studies. Most of the research was done on mice and rats. Monkeys, apes and baboons in smaller numbers have also been studied with perhaps more significant findings as related to humans. Therefore, current emphasis is on these primate studies.

The following summary of research findings is drawn mostly from a review by Rees, Ballantyne and Hawthorne (1970).

234

LOCAL TISSUE RESPONSE

The absence of measurable tissue response to the cutaneous injection of silicone fluid (viscosity of 350 centistokes) has been a constant observation in all animal species studied. Specific differences in the gross or microscopic appearances depend on the site, volume and procedure of injection. The injected material apparently diminishes in volume following single administration of large doses. This phenomenon of shrinkage also occurs when large volumes are injected into tissue planes where the fluid can disseminate, such as the suprapannicular, subpannicular, intramuscular, intraperitoneal or subcutaneous spaces.

Intradermal injections are difficult and impractical because the skin can accommodate only very small doses delivered through needles of very small caliber under considerable pressure. These physical limitations on intradermal injections do restrict the spreading or drift and also facilitate histologic evaluation of the local tissue response. Nonetheless, intradermal injection studies were soon abandoned because of technical difficulties and their impracticality in humans.

The gross appearance of subcutaneous injection sites shows multiple cysts resembling a honeycomb. There are infinite varieties in size of these compartments. The multiloculated cystic area eventually becomes localized by a pale, white, glistening capsule, the thickness of which varies with the number of injections and the total volume deposited.

Microscopically the early local response to single or multiple injections is a mild inflammatory one, characterized by a round-cell infiltration. This inflammatory phase usually subsides within six months. When massive doses are given, a fine membranous capsule forms around the injected material and divides it into delicate thin-walled spherical or ellipsoid spaces; the lining of these cysts consists of flattened endotheliumlike cells of connective tissue. Moderate fibrosis persists around the cysts six months after injections. Occasional giant cells are seen. Interestingly, the histologic appearance has been notable for the absence of significant chronic inflammatory response.

Varying degrees of a mild chronic inflammatory reaction are observed. In the interstices between the cyst walls, the collagen content of the dermal fibrous tissue appears increased and there is some disruption of dermal and subdermal architecture, along with a moderate number of histiocytes, a few lymphocytes and an occasional giant cell. Evidence of phagocytosis can be assumed from the presence of some large round cells with nuclei flattened aginst the cell walls, giving them an appearance similar to fat cells.

The presence of silicone fluid in the vacuoles, or cysts, and the swollen phagocytes can only be presumed, not proved. Inasmuch as this material does not stain with conventional stains, its presence could be demonstrated only by spectral analysis, a procedure extremely difficult to apply to the contents of microscopic cysts.

REACTION OF ADIPOSE TISSUE

When large doses of silicone fluid are given subcutaneously, adipose tissue seems transformed into cysts of varying sizes and shapes at the local injection sites. The fat cells surrounding the cysts appear shrunken and show varying degrees of atrophy, with small intracellular vacuoles present. Their nuclei are prominent and thin, and a "ground glass" appearance is sometimes seen.

When massive subcutaneous or intraperitoneal doses of silicone fluid are given, irregular foci of atrophy of omental and mesenteric fat are observed. These adipose tissue changes in animals suggest the possibility of a specific lipodystrophylike effect in their fatty cells, but the nature of any apparent affinity of silicone fluid for fat was not clarified. Other avenues of investigation, therefore, seem indicated, such as the possible effect of silicone fluid on cholesterol metabolism and its role in cardiovascular disease.

VISCERAL AND SYSTEMIC DISTRIBUTION

Silicone fluid has been shown to be phagocytized in rodents. It is also likely absorbed by other mechanisms. Following intraperitoneal injections or massive subcutaneous doses, vacuoles can be identified throughout the reticuloendothelial system—the regional lymph nodes, liver, spleen, kidneys, adrenals and elsewhere. These vacuoles are assumed to be silicone fluid until proved otherwise.

Accumulations of such vacuoles can be found in the corticomedullary junction of the adrenals of mice approximately 14 weeks after intraperitoneal injections. This area is very rich in reticuloendothelial cells and is a common site of drug accumulation.

Systemic distribution and depositing of sili-

235

cone fluid seems governed by the following variables: (1) the route of administration, (2) the amount given, and (3) the time interval after injection.

HEMATOLOGICAL EFFECTS

Andrews (1966) made a small incision at the injection site in a patient and collected blood samples from exuded bloody fluid, presumably mixed with silicone. He observed clear cytoplasmic vacuoles in several neutrophils and mononuclear cells. He believed these leukocytes could phagocytize silicone fluid.

We recently found similar vacuoles, presumably silicone, in leukocytes taken from the peripheral blood of mice and baboons after subcutaneous and intraperitoneal injections (Hawthorne et al., 1970). These transitory findings occurred several weeks after injection and persisted for a few weeks. Vacuoles were identified in leukocytes and a few monocytes. Vacuolization of some erythrocytes in the peripheral blood smears of rats has also been found. However, we were unable to duplicate this finding in other species.

These findings suggest that the injection of very large doses of silicone fluid may have some effect on the hematopoietic system. This effect bears further investigation. The hematocrit counts in a large number of rats remained within normal limits.

PERITONEAL AND PLEURAL ADHESIONS

The response of experimentally induced pleural and peritoneal adhesions in animals to the intrapleural and intraperitoneal administration of silicone fluid has been reported by several investigators (Cook and Butcher, 1964; Prachuabmoh and Eiseman, 1964, 1965; Malette and Eiseman, 1965; Furman and Denize, 1966; Perriard and Mirkovitch, 1966; Aboulafia and Polishuk, 1967; Frey et al., 1967; Brody and Frey, 1968). Work in our laboratory with rats demonstrated that the intensity and tensile strength of the adhesions are markedly diminished in animals receiving large amounts of silicone fluid. This suppression is considered a mechanical effect related to separation of injured serosal surfaces by the fluid volume.

ORTHOTOPIC SKIN GRAFTS

An evaluation of the effects of silicone fluid on the viability and revascularization of full-thickness suprapannicular skin autografts in rats was reported by Rees et al. (1968b).

Injections of 6 to 8 ml. of silicone fluid around and beneath fresh autografts do not adversely affect the vascularization or viability of these grafts in rats. No alteration in morphology of the grafted skin or in the blood vessels is indicated in histological sections. Other findings consist of multiple cystic spaces of varying sizes (presumably silicone) with disruption of the normal subdermal pattern and compression of the dermis. There are also minimal inflammatory reactions, similar to those previously described. No tumor or granuloma formation was seen in these studies.

According to Folkman and his associates (1964, 1966), silicone rubber sheets appear to possess certain unusual qualities related to metabolic processes. Gases (such as oxygen and carbon dioxide) as well as certain metabolites (particularly those of a fat-soluble nature) pass through silicone rubber sheets *in solution* — even though silicone sheeting is not considered to be a dialyzable membrane. It may be hypothesized that silicone fluid may possess similar qualities, which explains why the liquid is apparently innocuous to skin-graft survival.

Silicone fluid has been used advantageously in the treatment of burns (Gerow et al., 1963, 1964; Spira et al., 1967a and b). This use, coupled with the absence of adverse responses of skin grafts to silicone immersion and subsequent injections, prompted a limited investigation of the possible uses of silicone as a preservative medium for storing skin allografts at varying temperatures. Preliminary studies indicate that silicone does not significantly protect excised donor skin from freezing injury. Since silicone fluid has a high viscosity and repels water, this material cannot penetrate into skin tissue or cell membranes readily. Therefore, it does not prevent electrolyte imbalance (Lovelock, 1953), intracellular dehydration (Mazur, 1965) and mechanical damage from ice crystallization (Chambers and Hale, 1932; Luyet and Gehenio, 1940).

By contrast, when temperature is maintained at 12° C., the temporary storage of rat skin in silicone fluid is more favorable. The viability of skin segments under these conditions can be preserved for five days, but progressively declines during ensuing days. Successful autografts have been done following storage in liquid silicone at 4° C. for a maximum of four days.

Further work is needed to investigate the storage capabilities of silicone-treated skin at temperatures above freezing. Silicone fluid of differing viscosities should be investigated in this regard.

GRANULOMAS AND NEOPLASMS

The question of granulomalike response to the injection of silicone or silicone mixtures has been raised by several investigators. Sternberg and his associates (1964) reported two cases of "tumors" in apes following injection of silicone mixtures. They followed this by a second report (Winer et al., 1964) of three patients who received large volumes of silicone mixtures by injections into their breasts and subsequently developed benign tumors. They surmised the presence of silicone fluid in these tumors after examining routine histological sections. In two of their cases, polarized light illumination of the sections showed luminous crystals in giant cells and cellular infiltrates surrounding small cyst-like cavities.

All three patients were apparently injected not with pure medical grade silicone fluid, but with mixtures to which had been added various adulterants such as "1 per cent animal and vegetable fatty acids of unknown types."

Ben-Hur and Neuman (1963) reported development of "malignant epithelial tumors" in two out of 36 mice injected with 3 ml. of silicone fluid. However, their slides were reviewed by Grasso, Golberg and Fairweather (1964), who believed the growths to be adenomas of the mammary gland, a common tumor in mice.

Karfik and Smahel (1968) reported what they considered to be a subcutaneous silicone granuloma in a 29 year old Arab woman who had been injected for wrinkles between the brows. An excision of the area yielded histologic sections which demonstrated multiple cystic formations with cellular elements composed of lymphocytes and histiocytes, as well as multiple small "pseudocysts" lined by a fibrous capsule containing macrophages and giant cells. The exact chemical composition of the substance used was not known.

Since this time, reports of granulomatous lesions following injections of silicone fluid mixtures into the breasts have been made by Symmers (1968) and others. Symmers reported three such cases of breast lesions after injection of compounds presumably containing silicone fluid. According to his paper, it is not clear as to exactly what mixture was injected. The histological picture of the breast biopsies did, however, correspond to that described by previous authors and was highly suggestive of granuloma. In one of his patients, unusual histiocytes were identified in regional lymph nodes. It is known that after massive and rapid administration, silicone fluid can be found in the lymphatics (Ben-Hur et al., 1967). It is worthy of note that the amount of any material necessary to effect augmentation of the mammary glands constitutes a very high dosage. It is certainly not lmprobable that such high doses can instigate the formation of granulomas.

There is some confusion over the propriety of the term "siliconoma." Ben-Hur and Neuman (1965) coined this word on the basis of finding a collection of macrophages, presumably containing ingested silicone fluid, which were clumped together in one of a series of 60 mice. The word siliconoma would infer a tumor or neoplasm composed of silicone or silicone-containing cells. A collection of macrophages does not, however, constitute a tumor. "Oma" is a Greek suffix properly added only to words derived from Greek roots denoting a tumor or neoplasm. According to this definition, a siliconoma would be interpreted at least as a "proliferation of cells containing silicone." To the author's way of thinking, no one has yet convincingly shown that the injection of silicone fluid mixtures has produced a proliferating neoplasm. We do not, however, deny that intense local inflammatory reactions can be incited by the local injection of *adulterated* silicone fluid and, occasionally, it would not be unlikely to occur following the local misuse, by either technique or dosage, of medical grade silicone fluid.

TOXICITY

Examinations of several hundred experimental animals of different species have demonstrated no gross signs of toxicity, even when massive doses of silicone fluid were administered. All animals appeared to survive their normal life span without ill effect on their appetites or excretion, when compared to normal controls. However, injection of massive amounts did, sometimes, interfere with locomotion, as a matter of sheer weight (Ballantyne et al., 1965).

SUMMARY OF LABORATORY FINDINGS

So far, all studies indicate that injected silicone fluid with a viscosity of 350 centistokes apparently does not induce neoplasms in experimental animals. Local inflammatory response of a mild nature appears at injection sites, the severity of which seems to be proportional to the amount injected. Chronic lesions are represented by encapsulated silicone cysts and a low-grade reaction, characterized by some disruption of the dermis, some histiocytes and rare giant cells. Local fat cells, as well as some in

237

the omentum and mesentery, demonstrate varying degrees of atrophy.

Large doses of injected silicone result in some phagocytosis and absorption, with deposition throughout the reticuloendothelial system. These doses exceed any conceivable human use except possibly mammary augmentation.

Vacuoles which are presumably silicone fluid have been found in peripheral red blood cells and in peripheral leukocytes in mice and baboons following silicone administration. The significance of this finding is not yet clear.

Toxic manifestations have not been observed, even after administration of massive amounts of silicone fluid in mice, rats and subhuman primates.

The relevance of this experimental data to the possible applications of medical grade silicone fluid in man is not altogether clear. However, the total doses used in the animal experiments far exceed any conceivable dosage in man. The lack of toxic manifestations is encouraging for continued human investigation.

It is our belief that future research on silicone fluid and other alloplastic materials would be more relevant and valuable if carried out primarily in primates. Only limited information is obtained from animals of lower orders.

Clinical (Human) Use of Silicone Fluid

Dimethylpolysiloxane fluid has been used for many purposes in human tissue augmentation. Some of these uses have been questionable. Others have been efficacious, sometimes producing heretofore unbelievable results. Some of the clinical uses of silicone fluid injections will be discussed; however, the technique of injection will be described first, as the technique varies only in location and amount of silicone fluid used.

TECHNIQUE

Prior to injection, the skin of the area to be treated is thoroughly washed with pHisoHex or similar suitable skin soaps and painted with aqueous benzalkonium chloride (Zephiran). The silicone fluid should be of pure medical grade prepared in sterile ampules. A 1-ml. tuberculin syringe with a 20-, 22- or 27-gauge needle is best used for injection because the pressure gradient in such a long narrow syringe is sufficient to force the rather viscous fluid through the small bore needle with ease.

The most important aspect of the injection technique is to regulate the amount of silicone fluid given per injection. "Puddling" or "drifting" of injected fluid can occur if large volumes are delivered at each injection and the injectant is not sufficiently dispersed throughout the tissue planes. For small wrinkles 0.1 to 0.2 ml. at each injection site suffices, and for larger defects 2.0 ml. can be used in one area while constantly moving the needle. After each injection, a hand-held vibrating machine is applied to the area to ensure wide dispersement of the injected fluid so that localized cyst formation or accumulation does not occur. Such dispersement also prevents postinjection drifting. The injections should never be given intradermally, or permanent edema of the skin with an orange-peel effect will result.

Injections can be repeated at weekly intervals until the desired correction is achieved. It cannot be overemphasized that if a rather rigid scheduling of dosage intervals and amounts is not adhered to, untoward results can occur, such as "drifting," localized swelling and granulomalike lesions. A well intentioned attempt to increase the dose or shorten the interval between treatments to "help" the patient may well end in disappointment. The vibrating machine is especially important to disperse the fluid, and its use should be continued for several minutes after each injection.

In children, or patients with a low threshold for pain, local anesthesia can be used at the injection sites. However, it is best to inject only small volumes of anesthetic so as not to distort the soft tissue and thus interfere with judging the amount of silicone needed. Postinjection pain or discomfort is exceedingly rare. Edema and ecchymosis can occur, the latter if a vein is punctured. These persist for several days in some instances.

Loss of injected volume through absorption, spread along local tissue planes, or other mechanisms occurs to some degree, particularly early in the treatments. As the accumulated dosage builds up, volume loss diminishes. However, even after the final correction is achieved, "booster" shots may occasionally be required at intervals several months apart.

FACIAL ATROPHY

Facial atrophy can be mild or severe, unilateral or bilateral, and acute or progressive in behavior. Its causes are probably varied, and as little is known about its etiology today as was known 100 years ago. Various syndromes have been described, the most distinct of which are: (1) idiopathic facial hemiatrophy (first described by Romberg in 1846), (2) progressive atrophy associated with scleroderma, (3) congenital facial hemiatrophy (very rare), and (4) facial lipodystrophy with bilateral and symmetrical wasting of subcutaneous fat. The latter condition may also include atrophy of the trunk and upper extremities.

In addition, there are probably several other forms of facial atrophy which may be microforms of these more distinct entities or which may result from some form of idiopathic tissue insult such as trauma or inflammation. All forms of facial atrophy constitute a significant cosmetic deformity which, in the case of Romberg's disease (idiopathic hemifacial atrophy) in children, can be especially grotesque and tragic.

Many etiologic factors have been implicated throughout the years, yet none has been indicated as a common denominator in all cases. An analysis and review of 10,036 cases of facial atrophy in the world literature was made by Rogers (1963), and the interested reader is referred to his thorough and detailed presentation, in which he culled out 722 valid cases of Romberg's disease.

The author has had the opportunity of studying and treating over 30 patients with various forms of facial atrophy, mostly of a severe nature. A striking finding in the history and physical examination of these patients has been the absence of significant findings to corroborate any of the past theories of etiology such as trauma, infections, and so forth, and the absence of associated disorders such as grand mal seizures or other neurological disorders that have been reported to be frequently related.

It is difficult to separate the various clinical types of hemiatrophy into pure entities. Whether the problem is congenital or developmental in nature, or whether the individual case is associated with an inflammatory process such as scleroderma, is very difficult to establish. The exception to this is the bilateral atrophy of lipodystrophy, which usually presents a clear-cut clinical picture.

Hemifacial atrophy generally falls into two different clinical categories: the inflammatory and the noninflammatory types. The inflammatory type is often associated with sudden onset and cutaneous manifestations which are difficult, if not impossible, to distinguish from linear scleroderma. This naturally leads to considerable confusion surrounding the differentiation of these two entities. Hemiatrophy usually occurs with a rapid onset in childhood,

rarely occurs in early adulthood, and begins exceedingly rarely in middle age. We have seen only one such patient in whom the onset of hemiatrophy occurred after 40.

In the author's series, complete laboratory studies, including urinalysis, hematology and chemical studies, have yielded consistently normal results. Tissue biopsies have also been unrevealing. And, as noted before, there has been a striking absence of associated neurological disorders. Thus, our current scientific knowledge of this perplexing syndrome is as mystifying as it was when Romberg first described this condition over a century ago.

The treatment of facial atrophy, however, presents a more optimistic picture today than ever before. Previous methods of surgical treatment, including soft-tissue replacement by pedicle flaps or free grafts of dermis, dermis-fat or dermis-fat-fascia, as well as the augmentation of the skeletal framework with bone or cartilage onlay grafts or alloplastic implants, have been disappointing, usually ending in long-term failure. Dermis-fat grafts generally undergo absorption, as do bone or cartilage onlays, probably because of the pressure of the overlying atrophic integument and the absence of soft tissue padding. Facial bone x-rays and cephalograms have also shown that there is a hypoplasia of the facial bones in most cases of hemiatrophy.

The subcutaneous injection of dimethylpolysiloxane (silicone) fluid has, however, resulted in marked improvement in all patients treated by the author (Ashley et al., 1965; Ashley and Rees, 1965; Rees and Ashley, 1966, 1967). In many patients this improvement can only be described as remarkable; it even approaches normal appearance on long-term follow-up. The success of injection therapy has been limited primarily by the degree to which the soft tissues can be stretched by the injectant in the atrophic subcutaneous tissue and muscle layers. In severe atrophy, when the integument is literally stretched over bones (resembling parchment over skull), the results have been less satisfactory from the standpoint of firmness. In lesser degrees of atrophy, however, the postinjection results have approached normal in both consistency and contour. In all patients with lipodystrophy, excellent results in consistency and contour have been achieved, probably because the soft tissues are more supple than in hemiatrophy.

The technique of injection is essentially as described earlier in this chapter. The total amount of fluid needed usually varies between 10 and 40 ml.

Facial atrophy, either unilateral or bilateral,

constitutes one of the more positive indications for silicone fluid injections which have, in our opinion, become the treatment of choice. In very severe cases there is still a rare indication for pedicle flap reconstruction when the tightness of the skin does not permit significant distension because of almost total loss of elasticity.

Long-term follow-up observations continue on this perplexing clinical problem.

TRAUMATIC DEFECTS

Traumatic defects of facial contour can be improved by silicone fluid injections only to the extent to which the involved tissues are elastic or distensible. Tight, immature, adherent or rigid scars cannot be improved by injections. In such cases it is especially apparent that before silicone fluid injection can help to improve such deformities, basic principles of reconstructive plastic surgery must be taken into account; namely in these patients, the principle that scar tissue should be eliminated where possible and healthy soft tissue put in its place. This axiom is relative, of course, and must be modified to suit the individual problem. The pictures on page 246 are illustrative of the problem. The traumatic contour depression in this patient was markedly improved by silicone injections *after* the dense adherent cicatrix of the center of the scar was excised and more supple scar and soft tissue advanced over the defect. The principle illustrated by management of this patient can generally be applied in the treatment of traumatic defects.

A most interesting application of injection therapy is the elevation of depressed skin grafts, particularly of the forehead region. Defects of the face following burns, traumatic avulsion of soft tissue or cancer ablation are frequently covered by free skin grafts. These grafts do not replace the missing subcutaneous tissue, and a depression often results. Many months should be allowed for maturation of the grafts and cicatrix. When "softening" has occurred, injections beneath the graft can elevate it to almost normal skin levels. Obviously a suitable follow-up period after cancer excision must be allowed to elapse before injections commence so that recurrence is not masked.

Subgraft injections of the forehead region should be given in very small doses and should be well spaced out in time, since "drifting" is particularly apt to occur in this area because of the contiguity of the subaponeurotic tissue planes. An accumulation in the region of the nasion, brow or upper eyelid regions is particularly to be avoided.

NASAL DEFECTS

Depressed defects of the dorsum of the nose and minor degrees of postoperative asymmetry including sight external deviation, as well as certain aspects of the "butchered tip," can be successfully treated with silicone injections. Even saddle deformities from overly ambitious hump removal or resection of the dorsal septal border can be improved by injections when the defect is not too severe.

Silicone injections have proved most useful in "tidying up" these small postoperative defects. Drifting or migration is not a problem here, because the scar tissue resulting from the operation holds the injected fluid well in place.

Severe tip deformities following ill advised surgery are sometimes amenable to injection therapy, which yields a certain degree of improvement providing sufficient time has been allowed to permit softening and full maturation of the scar tissue. Indentations, clefts of the nasal tip and asymmetry also respond to injections. The illustration on page 260 demonstrates a severe deformity of the tip after surgery and the improvement which was gained from silicone fluid injections.

This technique seems to be excellently suited for the treatment of many postrhinoplasty defects for which secondary surgery might be hazardous and ineffective.

BRANCHIAL ARCH SYNDROME

In addition to the excellent results achieved in the treatment of hemifacial and bilateral facial atrophy, silicone injections have proved to be very helpful in augmenting the flattened hemifacial contour which is part of the first and second branchial arch syndrome.

This deformity is often accompanied by deformities of the ear and jaw. Correction of the mandibular asymmetry may require extensive procedures on the bone. Silicone augmentation of the soft tissue on the affected side over the hypoplastic mandible is helpful in restoring contour whether or not mandibular symmetry is improved by osteotomies, onlay grafting, and so forth.

CHIN AUGMENTATION

Silicone injections have a limited but useful role in chin augmentation. They are advisable, however, only for correction of minor degrees of microgenia.

CORRECTION OF SCARS

Contour improvement can sometimes be obtained by injecting very small volumes of silicone fluid beneath depressed, atrophic and thin scars, provided a rigid perimeter of scar tissue does not exist. Usually injections of 0.1 ml. to a maximum of 0.5 ml. are used for this purpose, depending on the surface area of the scar. The site should be thoroughly massaged with manual pressure or a vibrating machine. Good results have been achieved in the treatment of depressed scars resulting from certain inflammatory processes such as cutaneous leishmaniasis (Baghdad boil).

Acne, chickenpox and smallpox scars can sometimes be slightly improved by injections. However, deep acne scars of the "ice pick" type, with considerable scarring of the deep dermis and penetrating adhesion bands, are *not at all* improved by injections. When immature or thick scar tissue is present in the deep dermis or circumscribes depressed scars, silicone injections can even exaggerate the deformity. Because the nonelastic cicatrix does not yield, the surrounding healthy tissue receives much of the injection, thereby increasing in bulk and volume in all directions. Depressed and adherent scars therefore become further depressed because the surrounding tissue becomes elevated.

We have undercut these deep scars with cataract knives and filled in the resulting dead space with silicone fluid. However, these limited experiments have not proved particularly fruitful.

When subcutaneous atrophy is associated with acne scars of intermediate dermal depth, such as may be seen in microforms of facial atrophy, improvement can be obtained with a combination of deep dermabrasion and a series of silicone injections. (See page 251.) Sometimes further benefit is obtained by rhytidectomy in such patients, with wide undermining of the cheek skin.

WRINKLES

No one modality of therapy is entirely successful for the treatment of wrinkles (rhytides). Much depends on the configuration and contour of the wrinkle as well as the type of skin, i.e., whether it is dry, oily, thick or thin, and so forth. Often a combination of methods concomitantly or successively may be necessary.

Silicone fluid injection therapy is certainly useful as one of these techniques. The others include:

1. Chemabrasion (chemical peel)
2. Dermabrasion
3. Dermal electrodesiccation
4. Surgical undermining
5. Surgical excision

These techniques are variously discussed in appropriate chapters in this book. This discussion will focus only on the use or misuse of silicone fluid in this regard.

Deep furrows, such as vertical glabellar frown lines, nasolabial furrows and creases and the like are almost always improved (but not always eliminated) by injections of minute volumes of dimethylpolysiloxane fluid. A 1-ml. tuberculin syringe and a 27-gauge hypodermic needle are necessary to deliver these small 0.1- to 0.2-ml. volumes at strategic points subdermally beneath the wrinkle lines. In very deep frown lines as much as 0.5 ml. can be given at one dose. The material is injected evenly along the length of the crease. Repeated injections at weekly intervals or longer may be required.

Although creases and wrinkles are often improved and even eliminated, no guarantee of success can be made to the patient before treatment. There are a number of unpredictable factors which influence the result. Deep lines which are partly the result of dermomuscular connections, such as those produced by the insertion and action of the corrugator and procerus muscles on the vertical glabellar frown lines and by the lip levator group of muscles on the nasolabial fold, usually cannot be completely obliterated by any technique. When such lines are very deep, a combination of muscle section (page 174) followed by injections of silicone may yield the best results. Very small rhytides of the eyelids are not improved by injections. Furthermore, injections under the thin eyelid skin are definitely contraindicated. Unsightly discoloration, prominent bulging and persistent edema can result, all of which are difficult to correct.

Deep vertical lip wrinkles that persist after deep chemical peel or dermabrasion can often be further improved by silicone injections. However, they are rarely eliminated.

Marked rhytidosis of the face from prolonged actinic exposure or hereditary influence cannot be significantly improved by silicone injections alone unless relatively large dosage volumes are used which virtually "blow up" the skin of the face. Even then the skin cannot be made smooth, and a "basketball shape" of the face is the permanent price. This type of weather-beaten skin is best treated with chemexfoliation followed by injections of some of the

241

deeper lines remaining. Similarly, face lifting and blepharoplasty operations with wide undermining of the facial skin improve but do not eliminate fine wrinkles. Silicone injections can be helpful as an ancillary postoperative technique to help to "polish" the result.

MALAR EMINENCES

The high cheekbone effect so desirable to many patients can be simulated to some degree by silicone injections. Hypoplasia of the zygomatic arches or maxilla with recession of the infraorbital rim and anterior face of the maxilla can be considerably improved by injection therapy. Such augmentation is best done after rhytidectomy or blepharoplasty to add "finishing touches" to the operative result. However, if these surgical procedures are not indicated, soft tissue augmentation can be done as the definitive procedure.

Care must be taken to inject only beneath the skin of the cheeks and not to encroach on the thin eyelid tissues where permanent swelling may result.

Injections to build the malar prominence should begin at the most cephalic level of correction and proceed in a caudal direction very slowly and only after several injections of particularly small volumes. These measures compensate for any possible caudal "drift" of the injected material.

TRUNK AND EXTREMITY INJECTIONS

Since this book deals mostly with the correction of facial problems, a detailed discussion of other uses of silicone fluid in deformities of the trunk and extremities will be omitted. However, a brief description of some of these applications seems in order.

The injection technique of breast augmentation has been widely employed, particularly in the Orient, where an adulterated silicone mixture known as the "Sakurai formula" has been widely used (Kagan, 1963). This technique has not been legalized in the United States and was not included in the experimental protocol submitted to the federal government. Most investigators feel that this use of silicone fluid is not indicated as yet because of the likelihood of the formation of cysts or nodules which could interfere with cancer detection and because, once injected, the fluid is irretrievable. In addition, current methods of breast augmentation with prosthetic implants are quite acceptable.

Pectus excavatum, absence of the pectoralis major muscle, postpoliomyelitis leg atrophy and similar deformities have been treated with injections. Results have been encouraging, and wider investigations are currently in process.

REFERENCES

Aboulafia, Y., and Polishuk, W. Z.: Prevention of peritoneal adhesions by silicone solution. Arch. Surg. 94:384, 1967.

Agnew, W. F.: Biological evaluation of silicone rubber for surgical prosthesis. J. Surg. Res. 11:357, 1962.

Andrews, J. M.: Cellular behavior to injected silicone fluid: A preliminary report. Plast. Reconstr. Surg. 38:551, 1966.

Armaly, M. F.: Ocular tolerance to silicones. I. Replacement of aqueous and vitreous by silicone fluids. Arch. Ophthal. 68:390, 1962.

Ashley, F. L., Braley, S., and McNeil, E. G.: The current status of silicone injection therapy. Surg. Clin. N. Amer. 51:501, 1971.

Ashley, F. L., Braley, S., Rees, T. D., Goulian, D., and Ballantyne, D. L., Jr.: The present status of silicone fluid in soft tissue augmentation. Plast. Reconstr. Surg. 39:411, 1967.

Ashley, F. L., and Rees, T. D.: Facial hemiatrophy cases respond to DMPS injections. Surg. World 5:1, 1965.

Ashley, F. L., Rees, T. D., Ballantyne, D. L., Jr., Galloway, D., Machida, R., Grazer, F., McConnell, O. V., Edgington, M. T., and Kiskadden, W.: An injection technique for the treatment of facial hemiatrophy. Plast. Reconstr. Surg. 35:640, 1965.

Balkin, S. W.: Silicone injection for plantar keratoses. Preliminary report. J. Amer. Podiat. Ass. 56:1, 1966.

Ballantyne, D. L., Jr., Hawthorne, G. A., Ben-Hur, N., Seidman, I., and Rees, T. D.: The effects of silicone fluid on experimentally induced peritoneal adhesions. Unpublished findings, 1970.

Ballantyne, D. L., Jr., Hawthorne, G. A., Rees, T. D., and Siedman, I.: An experimental evaluation of skin graft preservation with silicone fluid. Unpublished findings, 1970.

Ballantyne, D. L., Jr., Rees, T. D., and Seidman, I.: Silicone fluids: Response to massive subcutaneous injection of dimethylpolysiloxane fluid in animals. Plast. Reconstr. Surg. 36:330, 1965.

Beckhuis, G. J.: Use of silicone-rubber in nasal reconstructive surgery. Arch. Otolaryng. 86:114, 1967.

Ben-Hur, N.: Breast augmentation by silicone. Letter to the Editor. World Med., Jan. 17, 1967.

Ben-Hur, N., Ballantyne, D. L., Jr., Rees, T. D., and Seidman, I.: Local and systemic effects of dimethylpolysiloxane fluid in mice. Plast. Reconstr. Surg. 39:423, 1967.

Ben-Hur, N., and Neuman, Z.: Malignant tumor formation following subcutaneous injection of silicone fluid in white mice. Israel Med. J. 22:15, 1963.

Ben-Hur, N., and Neuman, Z.: Siliconoma—another cutaneous reaction to silicone fluid. Plast. Reconstr. Surg. 36:629, 1965.

Berger, R. A.: Dermatologic experience with liquid silicones. New York J. Med. 66:2523, 1966.

Berman, W. E.: Use of silicones in rhinoplasty and chin implant. Presented before the American Academy of Ophthalmology and Otolaryngology, New York, October, 1963.

Blocksma, R., and Braley, S.: The silicones in plastic surgery. Plast. Reconstr. Surg. 35:366, 1965.

Boo-Chai, K.: Paraffinoma. Plast. Reconstr. Surg. 36:101, 1965.

Brody, G. L., and Frey, C. F.: Peritoneal response to silicone fluid. Arch. Surg. 6:237, 1968.

Brown, J. B., Fryer, M., and Ohlwiler, D. A.: Study and use of synthetic materials such as silicones and Teflon as subcutaneous prostheses. Plast. Reconstr. Surg. 26:263, 1960.

Chambers, R., and Hale, H. P.: The formation of ice in protoplasm. Proc. Roy. Soc. (Biol.) 110:336, 1932.

Cook, G. B., and Butcher, H. R., Jr.: The silicone serosal interface. I. Abatement of talc adhesion in dogs. Surgery 55:268, 1964.

Federov, S. N., et al.: Use of silicone liquid in the treatment of retinal detachment. Oftal. Zh. 20:527, 1965.

Folkman, J., and Long, D. M.: The use of silicone rubber as a carrier for prolonged drug therapy. J. Surg. Res. 4:139, 1964.

Folkman, J., Long, D. M., and Rosenbaum, R.: Silicone rubber: A new diffusion property useful for general anesthesia. Science 154:148, 1966.

Franklyn, R. A.: Chirurgische einpflanzung flüssiger Kuntstoffe. Zbl. Chir. 83:684, 1958a.

Franklyn, R. A.: Surgical implantation of liquid plastics. Cosmetic Surg. 1:7, 1958b.

Freeman, B. S., Bigelow, E. L., and Braley, S. A.: Experiments with injectable plastic. Use of silicone and Silastic rubber in animals and its clinical use in deformities of the head and neck. Amer. J. Surg. 112:534, 1966.

Freeman, B. S., Biggs, T., and Beall, A., Jr.: The use of injectable Silastic in treatment of deformities of the facial skeleton. Arch. Surg. 90:166, 1965.

Frey, C. F., Thorpe, C., and Brody, G.: Silicone fluid in the prevention of intestinal adhesions. Arch. Surg. 95:253, 1967.

Furman, S., and Denize, A.: Serous membrane regeneration: Use of interpleural liquid silicone. Surgery 60:733, 1966.

Gerow, F. J., Hardy, S. B., Spira, M., and Law, S. W.: Immersion treatment for burns. An experimental study. Surg. Forum 14:32, 1963.

Gerow, F. J., and Weeder, R. S.: Fluid silicone continuous immersion in the treatment of burns. Bull. Geisinger Med. Center 16:17, 1964.

Gersuny, R. R.: Ueber eine subcutane Prosthese. Z. Heilkunde 1:199, 1900.

Grasso, P., Golberg, L., and Fairweather, F. A.: Injection of silicones in mice. Lancet 2:96, 1964.

Hawthorne, G. A., Ballantyne, D. L., Jr., Rees, T. D., and Seidman, I.: Hematological effects of dimethylpolysiloxane fluid in rats. J. Reticuloendothel. Soc. 7:587, 1970.

Heuper, W. C.: Cancer induction by polyurethane and polysilicone plastics. J. Nat. Cancer Inst. 33:1005, 1964.

Kagan, N. D.: Sakurai injectable silicone formula. Arch. Otolaryng. 78:663, 1963.

Kalvin, N. H., Hamasaki, D. I., and Gass, J. D.: Experimental glaucoma in monkeys. II. Studies of intraocular vascularity during glaucoma. Arch. Ophthal. 76:94, 1966.

Karfik, V., and Smahel, J.: Subcutaneous silicone granuloma. Acta Chir. Plast. 10:328, 1968.

Levenson, D. S., Stocker, F. W., and Georgiade, N. G.: Intracorneal silicone fluid. Arch. Ophthal. 73:90, 1965.

Lovelock, J. E.: Haemolysis of human blood-cells by freezing and thawing. Biochim. Biophys. Acta 10:414, 1953.

Luyet, B. J., and Gehenio, P. M.: Life and death at low temperature. Biodynamica 3:33, 1940.

Malette, W. G., and Eiseman, B.: Silicone in the prevention of intestinal adhesions. Amer. Surg. 31:336, 1965.

Mazur, P.: Causes of injury in frozen and thawed cells. Fed. Proc. 24:175, 1965.

McGregor, R. R.: Toxicology of certain silicone fluids. Dow-Corning Bull. 2:15, 1960.

Miller, J., Hardy, S., and Spira, M.: Treatment of burns of the hand with silicone dressing and early motion. J. Bone Joint Surg. 47A:938, 1965.

Mullison, E. G.: Current status of silicones in plastic surgery. Arch. Otolaryng. 83:85, 1966.

Murray, J. E.: Factors for safety in use of silicone. Plast. Reconstr. Surg. 39:427, 1967.

Nosanchuk, J. S.: Injected dimethylpolysiloxane fluid: A study of the antibody and histologic response. Plast. Reconstr. Surg. 42:562, 1968.

Perriard, M., and Mirkovitch, V.: The effect of dimethylpolysiloxane on the prevention of abdominal adhesions in the rat. Helvet. Chir. Acta 33:536, 1966.

Prachuabmoh, K., and Eiseman, B.: Silicone fluids in prevention of pleural adhesions. J. Med. Ass. Thailand 47:1, 1964.

Prachuabmoh, K., and Eiseman, B.: Silicone fluid in prevention of intestinal adhesions. Amer. Surg. 31:336, 1965.

Rees, T. D., and Ashley, F. L.: Treatment of facial atrophy with liquid silicone. Amer. J. Surg. 111:531, 1966.

Rees, T. D., and Ashley, F. L.: A new treatment for facial hemiatrophy in children by injections of dimethylpolysiloxane fluid. J. Pediat. Surg. 2:347, 1967.

Rees, T. D., Ballantyne, D. L., Jr., and Hawthorne, G. A.: Silicone fluid research: A follow-up summary. Plast. Reconstr. Surg. 46:50, 1970.

Rees, T. D., Ballantyne, D. L., and Seidman, I.: Eyelid deformities caused by the injection of silicone fluid. Brit. J. Plast. Surg. 24:125, 1971.

Rees, T. D., Ballantyne, D. L., Jr., Hawthorne, G. A., and Nathan, A.: Effects of Silastic sheet implants under simultaneous skin autografts in rats. Plast. Reconstr. Surg. 42:339, 1968a.

Rees, T. D., Ballantyne, D. L., Jr., Hawthorne, G. A., and Seidman, I.: The effects of dimethylpolysiloxane fluid on rat skin autografts. Plast. Reconstr. Surg. 41:153, 1968b.

Rees, T. D., Ballantyne, D. L., Jr., Seidman, I., and Hawthorne, G. A.: Visceral response to subcutaneous and intraperitoneal injections of silicone in mice. Plast. Reconstr. Surg. 39:402, 1967.

Rees, T. D., Platt, J. M., and Ballantyne, D. L., Jr.: An investigation of cutaneous response to dimethylpolysiloxane (silicone liquid) in animals and humans—A preliminary report. Plast. Reconstr. Surg. 35:131, 1965.

Romberg, M. H.: Klinische Ergebrusse. Berlin, A. Forstner, 1846.

Rogers, B. O.: Progressive facial hemiatrophy: Romberg's disease, a review of 772 cases. Proceedings of the 3rd International Congress of Plastic Surgery, p. 68. Amsterdam, Excerpta Medica Foundation, 1963.

Rowan, R. L., and Howley, T. F.: Effects of dimethylpolysiloxane in the human bladder. New York J. Med. 63:1357, 1963.

Rowan, R. L., and Rowan, Y.: Method for coating bladder and urethral mucosal surface. U.S. Patent 3,239,414. Mar. 8, 1966.

Rowe, V. K., Spencer, H. C., and Bass, S. L.: Toxicological studies on certain commercial silicones and hydrolizable silane intermediates. J. Indust. Hyg. 30:332, 1948.

Rowe, V. K., Spencer, H. C., and Bass, S. L.: Toxicologic studies on certain commercial silicones. II. Two year dietary feeding of "DC Antifoam A" to rats. Arch. Indust. Hyg. 1:539, 1950.

Speirs, A., and Blocksma, R.: New implantable silicone rubbers. Plast. Reconstr. Surg. 31:166, 1962.

Sperber, P. A.: Chemexfoliation and silicone infiltration in the treatment of aging skin and dermal defects. J. Amer. Geriat. Soc. 12:594, 1964.

Spira, M., Gerow, F. J., and Hardy, S. B.: Silicone immersion burn therapy. Transactions of the 2nd International Congress for Research in Burns, edited by Wallace. Baltimore, The Williams & Wilkins Company, 1967a.

Spira, M., Miller, J., Hardy, S. B., and Gerow, F. J.: Silicone bag treatment of burned hands. Plast. Reconstr. Surg. 39:357, 1967b.

Sternberg, T. H., Ashley, F. L., Winer, L., and Lehman, R.: Gewebereaktionen auf injizierte flüssige Siliciumverbindungen. Hautartz 15:281, 1964.

Symmers, W. St. C.: Silicone mastitis in "topless" waitresses and some other varieties of foreign body mastitis. Brit. Med. J. 3:19, 1968.

Truppman, S., and Snyder, G. B.: Absorption studies of subcutaneous injection of dimethylpolysiloxane in mice. Presented at the 35th Annual Meeting of the American Society of Plastic and Reconstructive Surgeons, Las Vegas, Oct. 5, 1966.

Weeder, R. S., Brooks, H. W., and Boyer, A. S.: Silicone immersion in the care of burns. Plast. Reconstr. Surg. 39:256, 1967.

Wegener, E. H.: The problem of correction of forehead wrinkles. Med. Kosmetik. 5:136, 1957.

Winer, L., Sternberg, T. H., Lehman, R., and Ashley, F. L.: Tissue reactions to injected silicone liquids. Arch. Derm. 90:588, 1964.

243

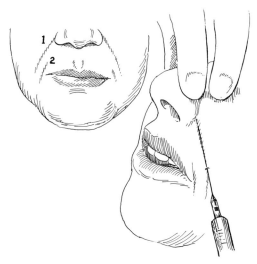

The technique for silicone injections to correct nasolabial furrows is shown in this drawing. A fine-gauge needle is passed along the length of the furrow at the immediate subdermal level. The injection is made as the needle is withdrawn. The procedure is best repeated two or three times. Not more than 0.5 ml. is injected each time. An alternate technique is to make multiple punctures with a 27- or 30-gauge needle along the nasolabial line, depositing 0.1 to 0.2 ml. at each site.

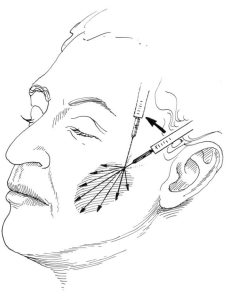

Injection treatment for buccal depressions or facial atrophy is best done by the "fanning" technique. Local anesthesia can be used at the needle puncture site. Injections are made radially, depositing small amounts of silicone as the needle is withdrawn.

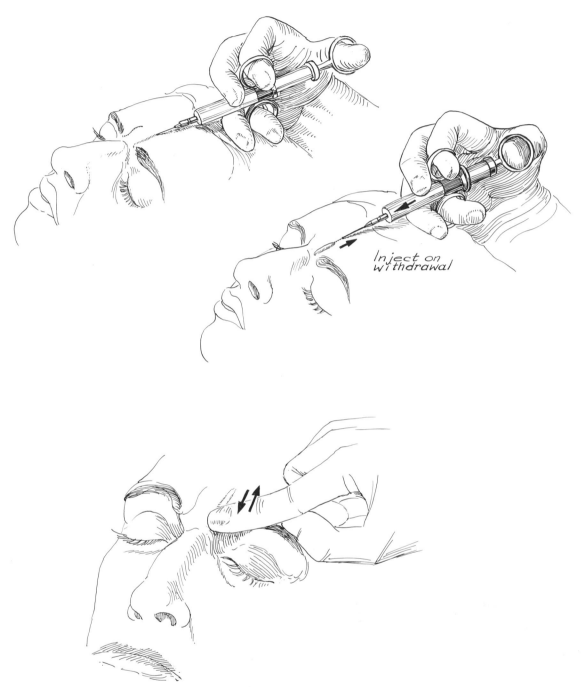

Inject on
withdrawal

Deep vertical glabellar frown lines are sometimes amenable to silicone injection therapy. A 27- or 30-gauge hypodermic needle is inserted subdermally along the length of the wrinkle, and silicone is injected as the needle is withdrawn. A tuberculin syringe develops sufficient pressure to inject the viscous fluid through such a fine needle. About 0.2 ml. suffices for each injection, and the injections may be repeated at weekly intervals for two to four doses. Immediately after the injection, the site should be massaged with the fingertip to distribute the injected fluid in the tissues. Overdosage will result in an unsightly elevation as well as "drifting" of the silicone into the loose areolar tissues at the root of the nose and the upper eyelids.

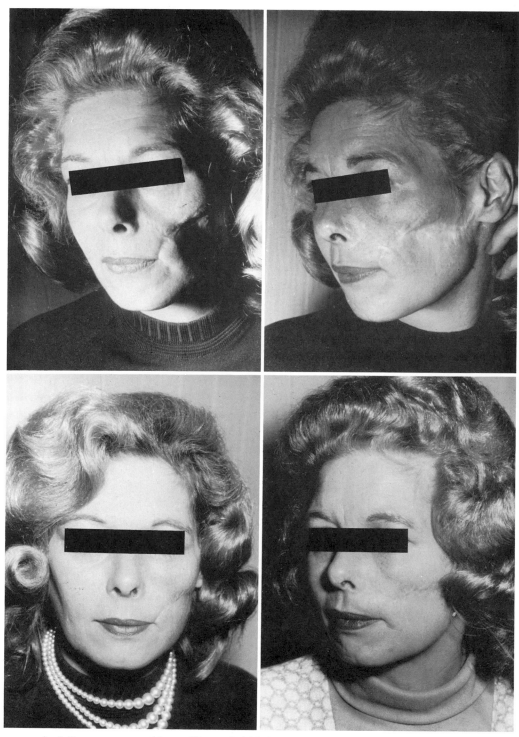

Certain traumatic defects are amenable to silicone fluid injection therapy. This young woman sustained a gunshot wound of the left cheek, with marked soft tissue loss, contour depression, and scar tissue formation. A large portion of the cicatrix was excised, followed by silicone injections to fill in the depression. A total dose of 45 ml. was given. Injection of silicone directly into scar tissue is rarely satisfactory because fibrous scar is inelastic. It is important to remove as much scar tissue as possible and to mobilize as much healthy soft tissue as possible before beginning silicone injection therapy.

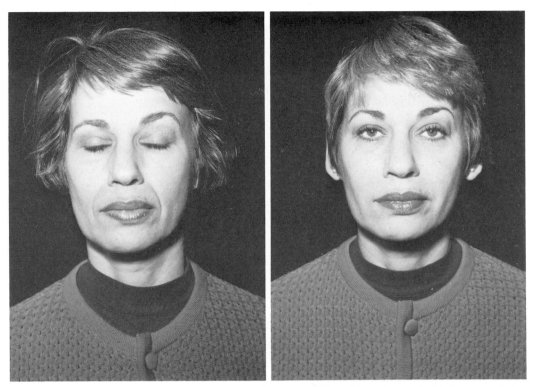

Nasolabial lines or furrows can sometimes be improved or even ablated by silicone fluid therapy. Animation accentuates all such lines. If they are more in the nature of furrows rather than etched wrinkles, and if the cheeks are not redundant so that the folds form over the nasolabial line, injections are more likely to succeed. The technique is shown on page 244. Caution must be exercised, and the dosage is delivered in small and multiple injections.

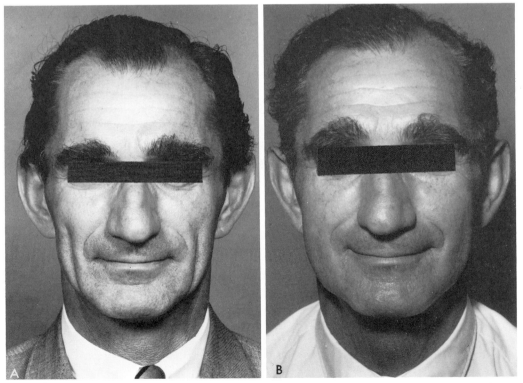

Deep furrows of the cheeks may be hereditary. They are similar to dimples. Some patients find them objectionable, and they can be eliminated by a series of silicone injections. This patient received a total of 16.1 ml. of injected fluid.

247

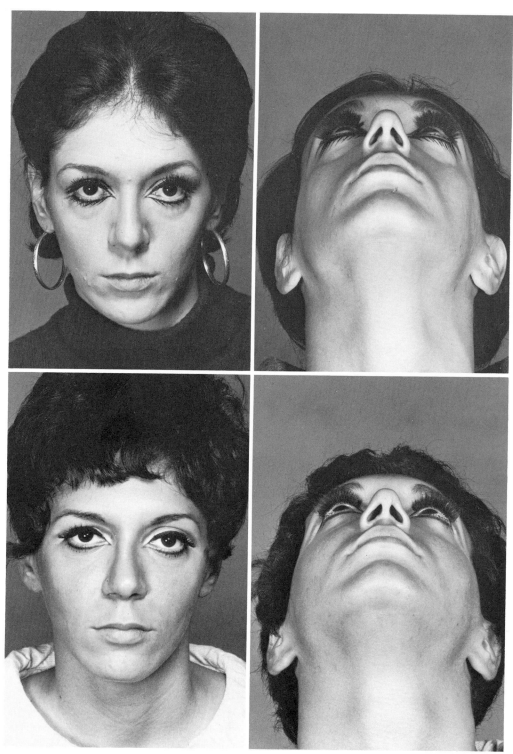

Prominent cheekbones are universally considered a mark of beauty. Hypoplasia of the maxilla may be traumatic or developmental in origin, and silicone injections can be most effective in adding substance to the soft tissues in this region. This young woman had a total of 15.85 ml. of silicone fluid injected bilaterally. She has been followed for five years and has maintained the correction without sequelae.

248

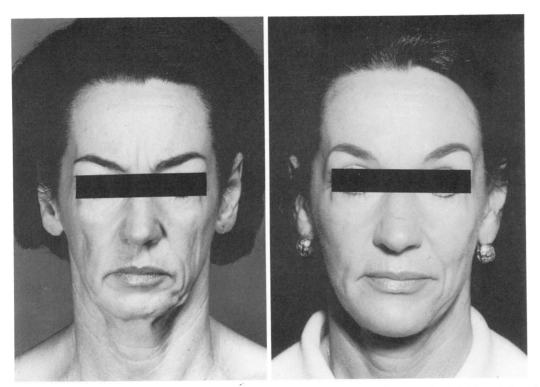

In patients with some degree of maxillary hypoplasia, silicone injections can be most helpful in adding the final cosmetic touch to a blepharoplasty and face lift operation. Injections should not be started until all swelling and ecchymosis have subsided following surgery.

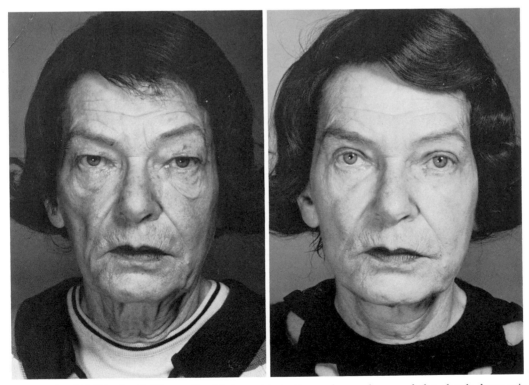

This patient received 7.35 ml. of silicone fluid injected into the malar regions and the cheek depressions in 10 injections, following blepharoplasty and rhytidectomy.

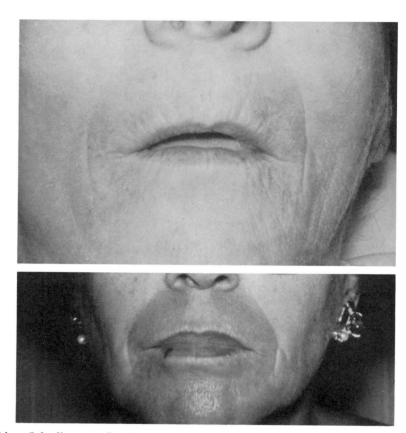

Deep vertical wrinkles of the lips are often improved by chemabrasion. Sometimes lines that remain after peeling are further improved by injections of minute doses of silicone fluid into each remaining line.

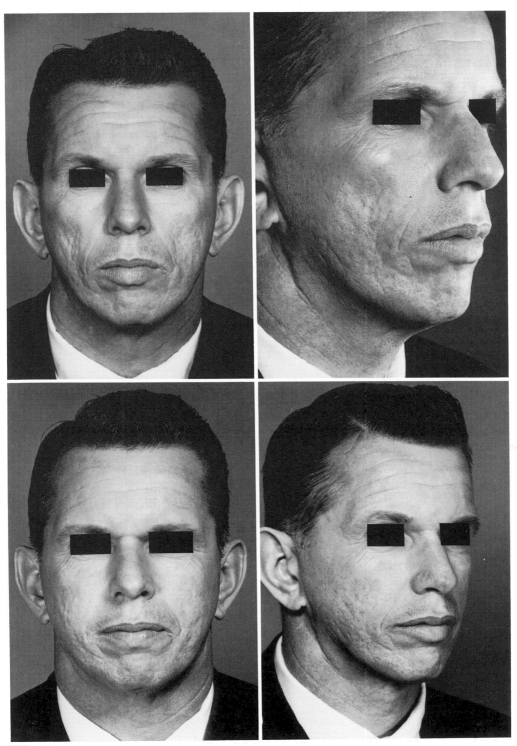

Mild subcutaneous atrophy of the cheeks in association with some scarring was improved with silicone injections. A total dose of 11 ml. was given. Contour filling improved the acne scarring, probably by stretching the skin. Attempts to improve deeper acne scarring by injecting silicone in the hope of elevating each individual pit have not been successful, and in fact the depressions can be accentuated because the surrounding healthy soft tissue becomes distended while the deep cicatrix of the base of the scar does not give.

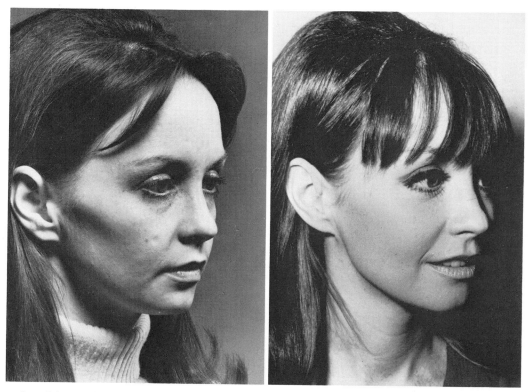

This attractive girl complained about the depressions visible on both sides of her face below the zygoma. An old inflammatory scar was also present on the right cheek. These facial depressions were accentuated by tangential light, a deterrent to her work as a photographers' model. The scar of the cheek was soft and atrophic. It was improved by dermabrasion followed by silicone injection therapy, and the facial depressions were eliminated entirely by injections of silicone fluid. The total dose was 9.9 ml.

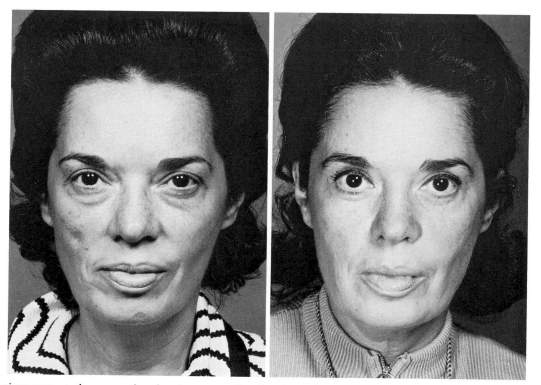

This patient reported progressive development of a dimple and atrophy of the right cheek, with no history of trauma or infectious disease. Wasting of the cheek had become noticeable in the past year. During pregnancy 10 years previously, the patient had taken large doses of cortisone and became "moon-faced"; the lesion first appeared after this effect of cortisone therapy subsided. The condition was corrected by the injection of 4.35 ml. of silicone fluid; a blepharoplasty was also done.

252

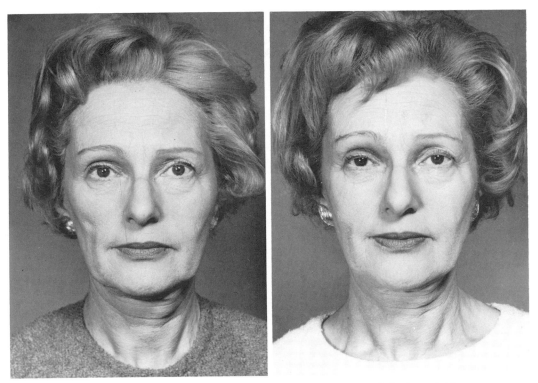

Progressive atrophy of the right cheek of unknown etiology, which developed during middle age, was successfully treated with 4.4 ml. of silicone fluid. Such atrophy affects the buccal fat pads and is a frequent occurrence as age progresses. Unilateral subcutaneous atrophy such as this is not rare and may represent a micro-form of hemifacial atrophy of a self-limited nature.

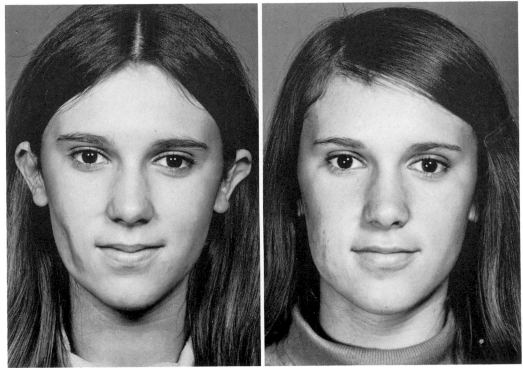

Depression deformity of the cheek was secondary to a resolved hemangioma of childhood which had been treated with irradiation. The deformity was highly distressing to the young patient. It was corrected with multiple silicone fluid injections; a total dose of 3.35 ml. was given.

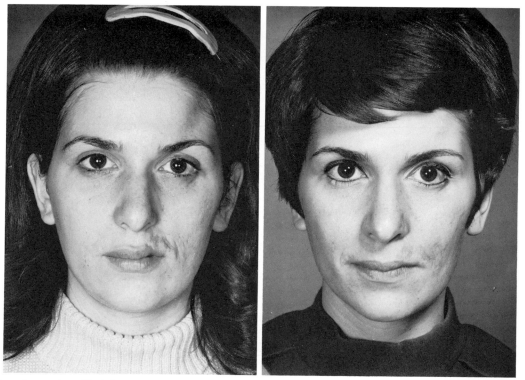

A case of moderate hemifacial atrophy in a young woman; note the coup de sabre mark on her forehead. The pigmentation spots and scarring of the upper lip and cheek suggest scleroderma as a possible cause. Correction was achieved with multiple injections of silicone fluid. It was not possible to obliterate the pigmented spots, but the soft, atrophic scarred area associated with them was considerably improved. The total dose of silicone was 11.55 ml.

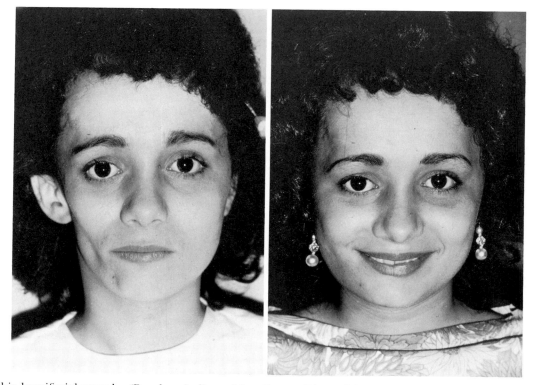

Idiopathic hemifacial atrophy (Romberg's disease) in a Puerto Rican girl was successfully corrected with silicone fluid injections. This patient has now been followed for nine years, and the correction has persisted without drifting, absorption, or loss of effect. Facial animation is normal, an advantage of silicone injections over implants or dermis-fat grafts. (From Rees, T. D., and Ashley, F.: Treatment of facial atrophy with liquid silicone. Amer. J. Surgery, *111*:531, 1966. Reproduced with permission.)

254

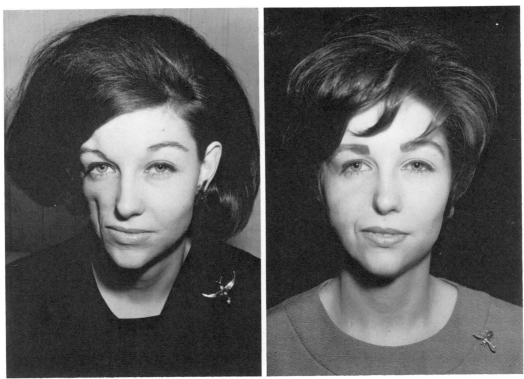

Severe hemifacial atrophy previously treated with alloplastic implants, which had to be removed because of their firmness and unnatural effect, was definitively corrected with 28.25 ml. of injected silicone fluid. The patient has been followed for four years without loss of the correction or untoward sequelae.

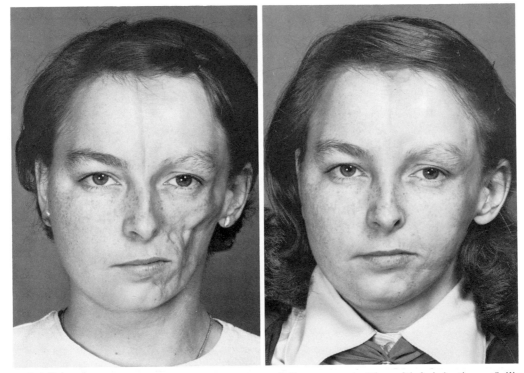

Severe hemifacial atrophy of the Romberg type was successfully corrected with multiple injections of silicone fluid to a total dose of 16.9 ml. Despite severe atrophy, the skin of this young woman was supple and stretchable, which facilitated the results. If the skin will not give, the results of injection therapy are limited, and supplemental iliac bone grafts may be required.

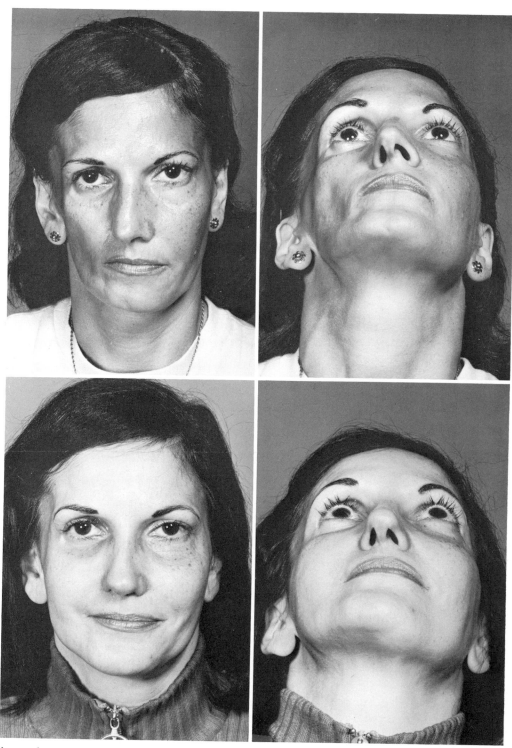

Hemifacial atrophy was treated with 28.45 ml. of silicone fluid. Note the marked deviation of the nose toward the atrophied side caused by hypoplasia of the maxilla and the nasal bones on that side—a common component of this condition. Rhinoplasty enhanced the result achieved by silicone injections.

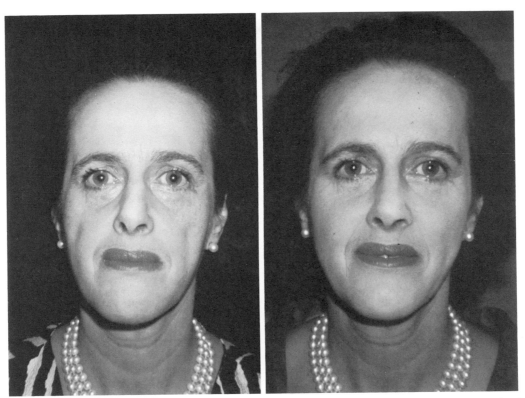

Bilateral contour depressions of the cheeks, probably of familial origin, were eliminated by the injection technique. The total dose in this patient was 6.35 ml.

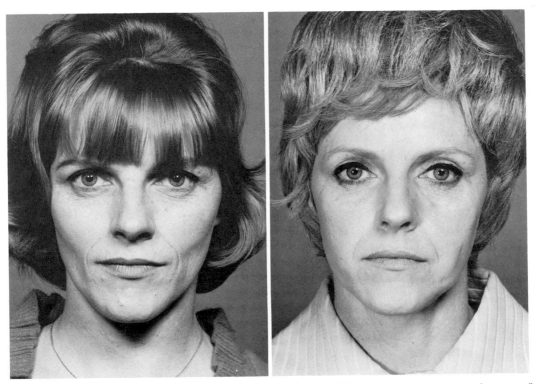

A patient had mild lipodystrophy of the face, a disorder that is probably much more common than was formerly believed—particularly in mild forms such as this. Correction was achieved with 11.9 ml. of silicone fluid.

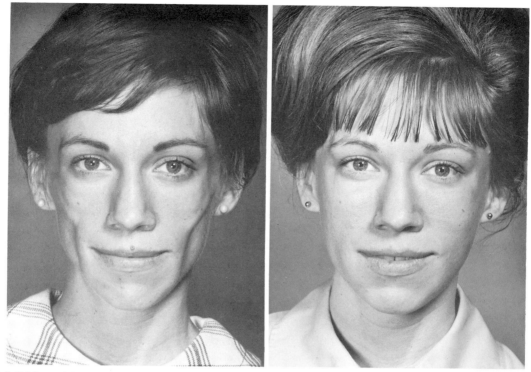

Typical full-blown bilateral facial atrophy caused by progressive lipodystrophy. The upper extremities and the trunk are also often affected. The results of silicone fluid injections approach perfection in such patients because the skin is not atrophic but elastic and distensible. The total dose in this patient was 38.35 ml.; a chin implant was also used.

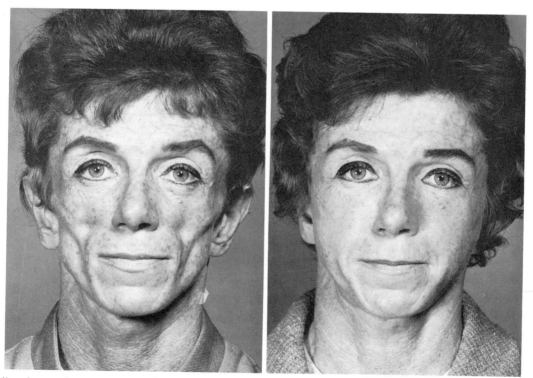

Marked lipodystrophy was corrected with silicone injections. A dose of 41.09 ml. was given in weekly treatments over several months.

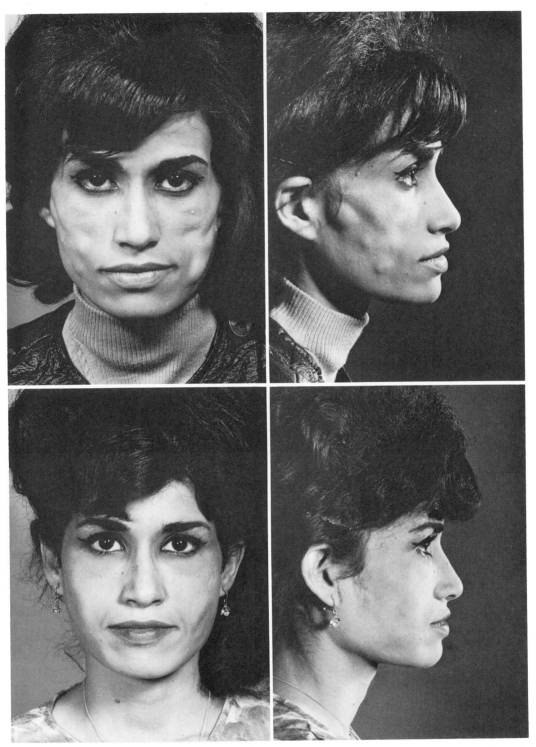

The pretreatment photographs of this patient show the long-term result of attempts to correct bilateral facial atrophy with multiple dermis-fat grafts. The fat has atrophied, and the dermis remnant has formed subcutaneous masses that are both palpable and visible. These graft remnants were excised through rhytidectomy incisions and subsequent correction was obtained with multiple silicone injections totaling 21 ml.

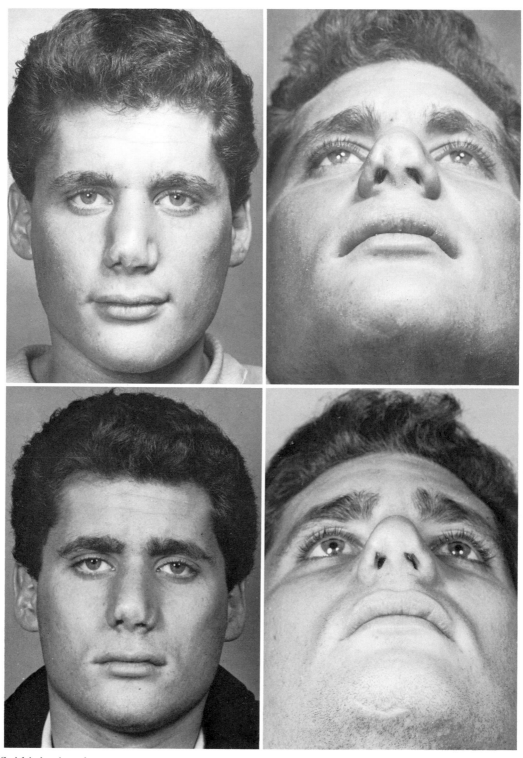

Silicone fluid injection therapy may play a decided role in the treatment of secondary nasal deformities when no other method, surgical or otherwise, offers much chance of success. This patient had marked scarring of the nasal tip with asymmetry, depressions, and scar contracture after rhinoplasty by an inexpert surgeon. Multiple injections of small doses of silicone fluid improved the symmetry after the nose was narrowed by lateral osteotomy and infracture. (From Rogers, B. O.: Secondary and Tertiary Rhinoplasty. Amsterdam, Excerpta Medica, 1969, pp. 1065–1071. Reproduced with permission.)

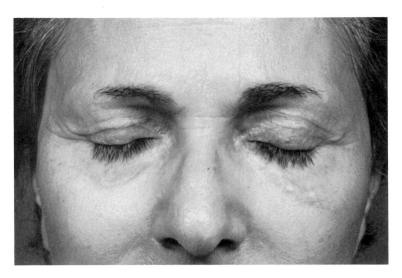

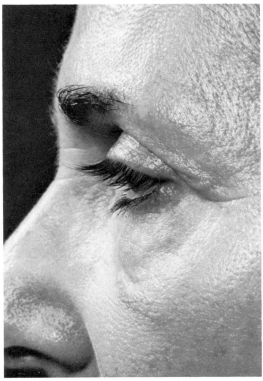

These photographs clearly show the unfortunate result of a common misuse of silicones—attempts to correct wrinkled eyelid skin. The skin of this region is much too thin to conceal the injected material, so that small subcutaneous masses of it are readily seen.

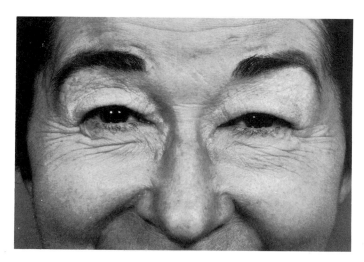

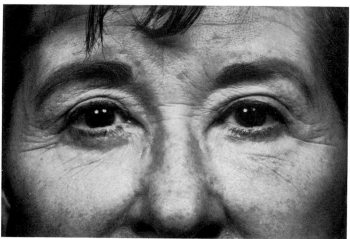

This patient had an undetermined amount of a silicone fluid mixture injected into her eyelids by a quack in an attempt to eliminate wrinkles. Marked palpebral bags resulted from this evident overdosage, as did chronic edema of the lids. A standard blepharoplasty improved the situation, but it was not possible to remove all of the injected material. (From Rees, T. D., and Ballantyne, D. L., Jr.: Brit. J. Plastic Surg., *24*:125, 1971. Reproduced with permission.)

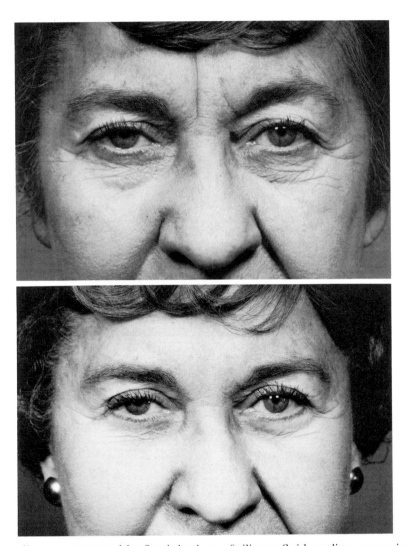

A deep frown line was corrected by five injections of silicone fluid totaling approximately 2 ml.

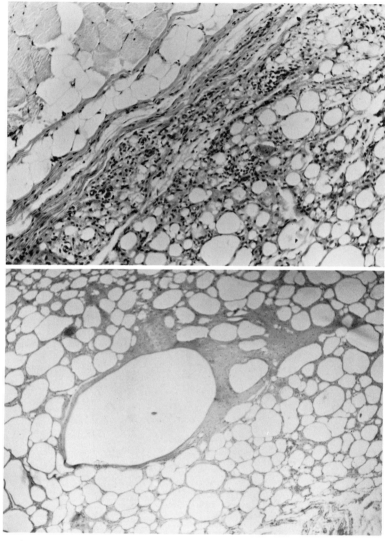

Photomicrographs showing the typical appearance of the subcutis following injections of dimethylpolysiloxane fluid of medical grade and without adulterants. Note the minimal evidence of inflammatory response. Multiple microcysts of different sizes are present and act as the contour-filling substance. Occasional giant cells are seen. The lining of each microcyst is composed of flattened epithelial cells resembling mesothelium. ($\times$ 3.5.)

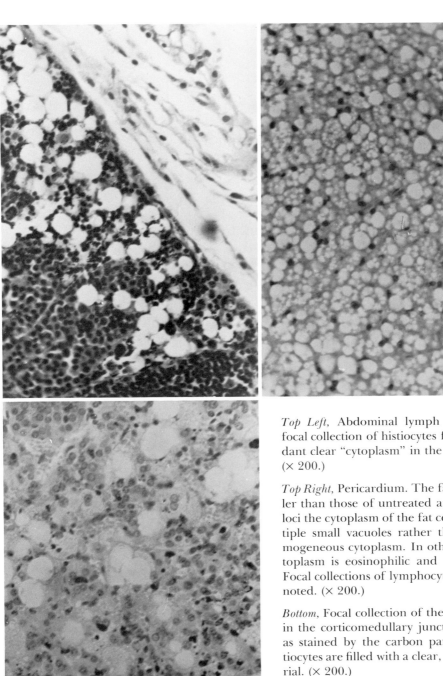

Top Left, Abdominal lymph node, showing focal collection of histiocytes filled with abundant clear "cytoplasm" in the marginal sinus. (× 200.)

Top Right, Pericardium. The fat cells are smaller than those of untreated animals. In some loci the cytoplasm of the fat cell contains multiple small vacuoles rather than a clear homogeneous cytoplasm. In other areas the cytoplasm is eosinophilic and finely granular. Focal collections of lymphocytes are regularly noted. (× 200.)

Bottom, Focal collection of the histiocytes seen in the corticomedullary junction of adrenals as stained by the carbon particles. The histiocytes are filled with a clear, unstained material. (× 200.)

(From Ben-Hur, H., Ballantyne, D. L., Jr., Rees, T. D., and Seidman, I.: Local and systemic effects of dimethylpolysiloxane fluid in mice. Plast. Reconstr. Surg., *39*:423, 1967. Reproduced with permission.)

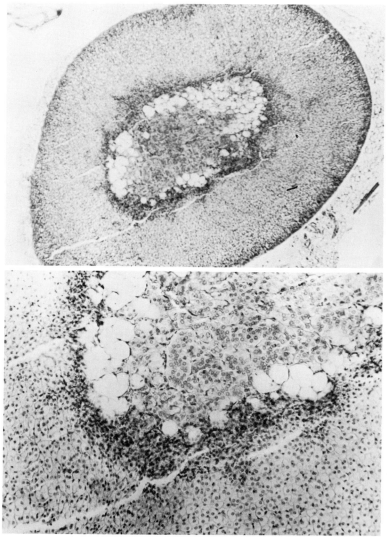

Adrenal gland. *Top*, Numerous histiocytes at the corticomedullary junction. *Bottom*, The clear cytoplasm presumably represents silicone fluid that has been phagocytosed. (× 10.)

(From Rees, T. D., Ballantyne, D. L., Seidman, I., and Hawthorne, G.: Visceral response to subcutaneous and intraperitoneal injections of silicone in mice. Plast. Reconstr. Surg. *39*:402, 1967. Reproduced with permission.)

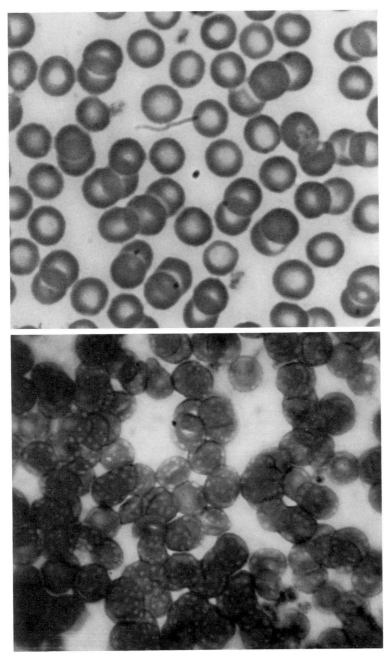

Top, Blood smear from a control rat; *Bottom,* blood smear from a rat injected with silicone fluid nine months previously. (× 970.) (From Hawthorne, G. A., Ballantyne, D. L., Rees, T. D., and Seidman, I.: Hematologic effects of dimethylpolysiloxane fluid in rats. J. Reticuloendothelial Society, 7:587, 1970, reproduced with permission.)

267

Chapter 9

RHINOPLASTY

Thomas D. Rees, M.D.,
and Donald Wood-Smith, M.D.

History

Over the centuries surgeons have been fascinated with the concepts of nasal reconstruction, and many methods have been devised for both replacement and modification of this all-important feature of the face. But it remained for Dieffenbach to record in 1845 the first attempts at reduction of the large nose. Many detailed accounts of the history of plastic surgery of the nose can be found in the standard texts of nasal surgery and in the original articles by Roe, Joseph, Weir and others reprinted in their original form in the Journal of Plastic and Reconstructive Surgery.

Plastic surgery of the nose was performed in India and Egypt between 2500 and 600 B.C. Denecke and Meyer (1967) cite the Egyptian hieroglyphics and ancient Indian writings in their review and quote the Edwin Smyth surgical papyrus hieroglyphic description of the first recorded use of pressure dressings applied to the nose. The use of a forehead flap for reconstruction of the nose following punitive amputation in India was described over 2000 years ago by Susruta Samhita in his work *Ayur-Veda*. It appears that these forehead flaps were unlined, the surgical work carried out by members of a caste of potters, the Comaas. The method of reconstruction described became known as the "Indian" method, although it was practiced during the same time period in both Egypt and the Middle East.

About 1450 A.D. knowledge of this technique reached the Branca family in Italy, and although they became practitioners of the "Indi-an" method of forehead flap reconstruction, a son, Antonio, began using a pedicle flap from the upper arm for nasal reconstruction. The method, usually credited to Gaspare Tagliacozzi and described in his work in 1597, became known as the Italian method. Tagliacozzi was persecuted for his efforts to repair the human form, the prevalent view of the church at the time being that deformities were the will of God and were best left alone. His teachings were lost for many years and rediscovered from time to time by other European surgeons, such as Cortesi of Messina and Graffon of Lucerne.

During this period nasal reconstruction began a two-century dormant period in Europe, while in India the ancient art, relatively unchanged, continued to flourish. A report appearing in the Madras Gazette in 1793 described the nasal reconstruction performed on an Indian bullock driver by Mahratta, a surgeon of Poona, using the forehead flap method. The report stimulated Joseph Carpue, an English physician, to use the same technique in 1814 to successfully reconstruct the nose of an English officer. The report of this successful case stimulated many of the great surgeons of Europe such as Dupuytren, Delpech, Syme, Beck, Zeis and Warren to modify and further develop methods of reconstruction of the nose as well as the lips and cheeks. Doubtless much thought had been given to possible operations for nasal reduction and modification of shape. However, it remained for the American surgeon Roe in 1897 and the German surgeon Joseph in 1898 to provide the first detailed accounts of reduction rhinoplasty without the benefit of external incisions. Indeed, Joseph's techniques have formed the basis for modern nasal surgery and are described in detail in *Nasenplastic und sonstige Gesichtsplastik nebst Mammaplastik* (1931).

It is virtually impossible to credit the many pioneers who have made meaningful contributions to the technique of rhinoplasty in the past 40 years. This surgery has caught the imagination of many surgeons the world over and has produced a voluminous literature, some of which is sound and constructive, and some of which is but interesting conjecture. Surgeons of various disciplines have become fascinated with rhinoplasty; most of the contributions to technique, however, have come from general plastic surgeons and rhinologists. The scope of this book does not permit a detailed chronology of the development of rhinoplasty, nor does it allow for proper credit to be given to each surgeon who has devoted his time and effort to this interesting subject.

Since cosmetic rhinoplasty is primarily a recent surgical development, much of the material is topical rather than historical. Rather than trying to summarize developments in the field since Joseph's time, the authors will attempt to credit, at appropriate places in the text, those surgeons who have made meaningful contributions. Unquestionably some will be overlooked, and to these we apologize in advance, but hope they will realize that it is not possible to cite every work on this subject. A most comprehensive reference work on nasal surgery is available in the book *Surgery of the Nose*, by Denecke and Meyer (1967).

Anatomy

THE SOFT TISSUES OF THE NOSE

The skin of the nose is tightly bound to the underlying alar cartilages but is quite loosely attached to the upper lateral cartilages and nasal bones. The skin of the nasal tip region carries an abundant supply of sebaceous glands which rapidly diminish in number as one proceeds superiorly over the lateral cartilages. It is important to note that the arterial and venous supply to the skin lies superficially in the soft tissues; hence, the need for maintaining the plane of dissection in nasal plastic surgery immediately adjacent to the underlying cartilage and nasal bones.

THE NASAL BONY FRAMEWORK

The bony framework of the nose is formed by the paired nasal bones projecting from the nasal process of the frontal bone superiorly and is supported laterally by the nasal processes of the maxilla in its lower portion and by the nasal process of the frontal bones superiorly.

The nasal bones are quadrangular in shape and thicker above than below; hence, the usual site for fracture of the nasal bones occurs at the junction between the thicker and thinner portions of the bone. They are supported in the midline by the osseous and cartilaginous septum and inferiorly over the upper portions of the upper lateral cartilages.

THE CARTILAGINOUS NOSE

The cartilaginous nose is a dynamic structure subject to constant motion and to the molding effects of the nasal musculature. The cartilaginous external nose lies anterior to the pyriform aperture, which is formed above by the inferior borders of the nasal bones and the nasal processes of the maxilla. Below this the thickened maxillary margins curve medially toward the anterior nasal spine of the maxilla.

The paired lateral cartilages are attached to the medial portion of the nasal process of the maxilla and to the inner aspect of the nasal bones above. In the midline they are attached to the expanded portion of the septal cartilage and are connected inferiorly to the alar cartilages by a dense matting of connective tissue between the upper edges of the alar cartilage which laterally overlaps the lower end of the lateral cartilage. The lateral margin of the upper lateral cartilage does not articulate directly with the pyriform aperture but is connected by fibroareolar connective tissue of varying density.

The overlapping relationship of the nasal bones to the upper lateral cartilages is established during embryologic development, the nasal bones developing from membrane on the surface of the cartilaginous nasal capsule which forms on the inner aspect of the nasal bone. The overlap of the lateral cartilage and nasal bone may be as much as 1 cm., with an intimate fusion between the perichondrium and periosteum in this region. This firm adherence is of significance in fractures of the nasal bones, since any motion imparted to the nasal bone fragment is immediately reflected by the firmly adherent lateral cartilage.

The cartilaginous portion of the nasal septum shares in this embryologic formation from the cartilaginous nasal capsule and extends for a similar distance below the nasal bones. The dorsal border of the nasal septum is expanded, and

269

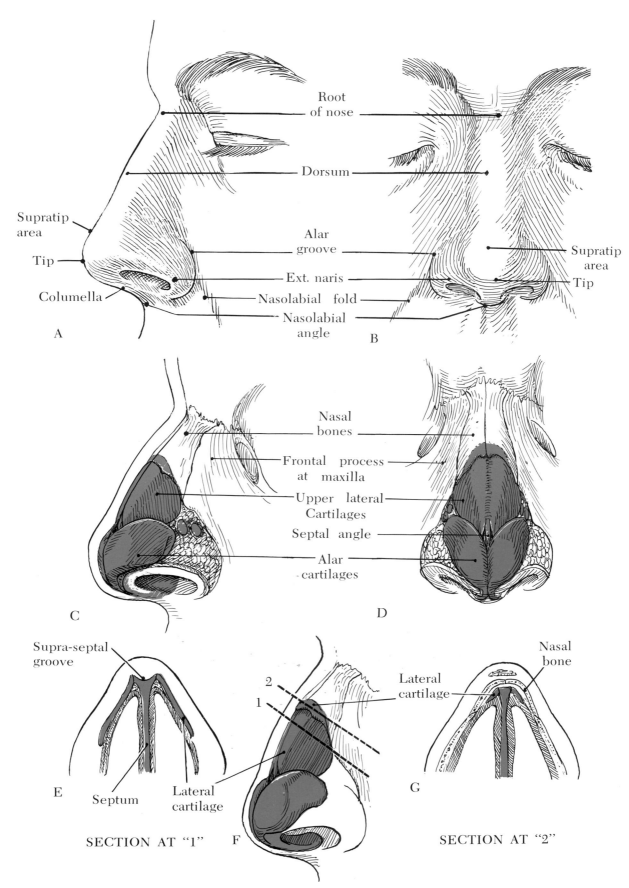

Root of nose

Dorsum

Supratip area

Tip

Columella

Alar groove

Ext. naris

Nasolabial fold

Nasolabial angle

Supratip area

Tip

A

B

Nasal bones

Frontal process at maxilla

Upper lateral Cartilages

Septal angle

Alar cartilages

C

D

Supra-septal groove

Septum

Lateral cartilage

E

SECTION AT "1"

2

1

Lateral cartilage

Nasal bone

F

G

SECTION AT "2"

The soft tissues of the nose.

270

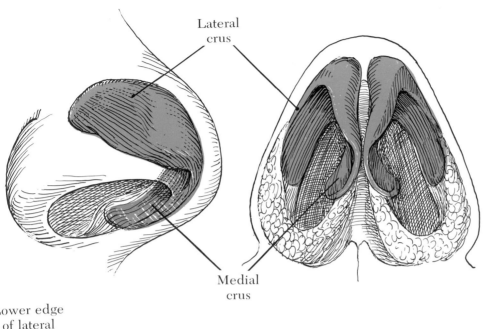

Lateral
crus

Medial
crus

Lower edge
of lateral
crus

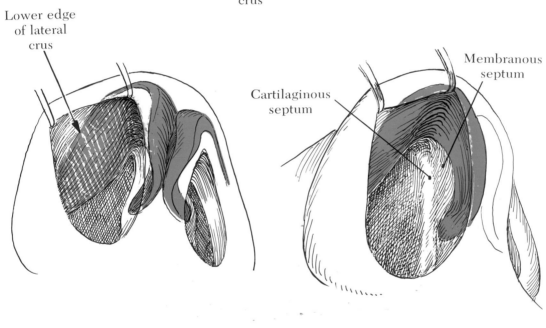

Cartilaginous
septum

Membranous
septum

Soft
triangle

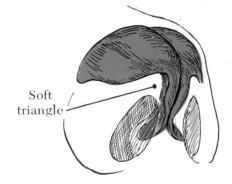

The cartilages of the nose.

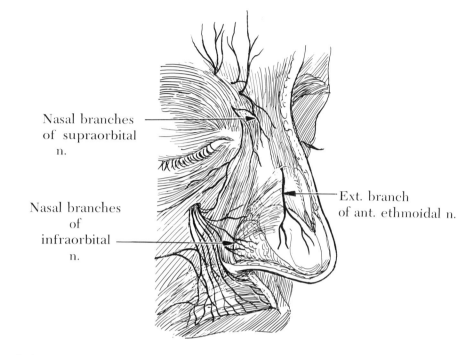

Nasal branches of supraorbital n.

Nasal branches of infraorbital n.

Ext. branch of ant. ethmoidal n.

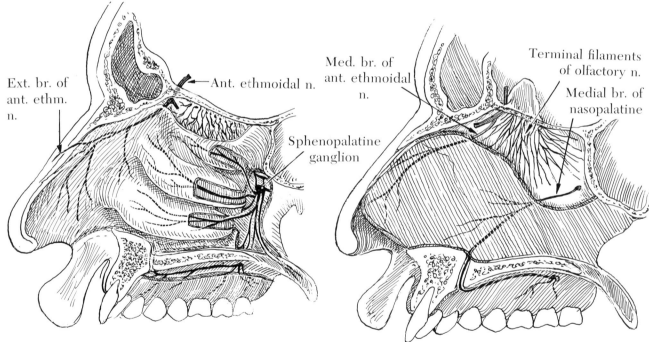

Ext. br. of ant. ethm. n.

Ant. ethmoidal n.

Sphenopalatine ganglion

Med. br. of ant. ethmoidal n.

Terminal filaments of olfactory n.

Medial br. of nasopalatine

The nerve supply to the nose.

the expansion becomes more marked as one proceeds superiorly; in some individuals the expanded area may be further accentuated by a midline groove which is readily palpable, but usually invisible on the surface. The junction between the upper lateral and septal cartilages is of an end-to-end type; the structures are intimately related near the nasal bones, but the appearance of cartilaginous continuity is not borne out by histologic examination, which always shows a separation between the ends. However, continuity of the perichondrium without passage into the false joint is frequently observed. The lower portions of the upper lateral cartilages are less intimately related and are bound by dense connective tissue. The connective tissue in this area permits motion of the upper lateral cartilages in an inward and outward fashion to enable expansion of the nasal cavity during heavy respiration.

THE SEPTAL CARTILAGE

The septal cartilage is a quadrangle-shaped structure protruding in front of the pyriform aperture below. The anterior superior angle of the septal cartilage forms the important nasal plastic landmark, the septal angle. This angle is located immediately above the alar cartilages in the superior tip area.

The septal cartilage is firmly bound to the vomer, the perichondrium of the cartilage passing imperceptibly into the periosteum of the vomer. The inferior portion of the septal cartilage extends over the smooth surface of the nasal spine and is quite mobile in this area; the considerable side-to-side motion is possible because of the flexibility of the cartilage and the weakness of the cartilaginous-osseous joint. Immediately anterior to the septal cartilage is the membranous septum formed by two mucocutaneous flaps packed with a layer of fibroareolar tissue. Anterior to these flaps lie the medial crura of the alar cartilage which form the cartilaginous support of the columella.

THE ALAR CARTILAGE

Paired C-shaped alar cartilages form the cartilaginous support for the tip of the nose. Each alar cartilage consists of the medial and lateral crus, which join medially to form the dome of the alar cartilage in their most anterior inferior point. The medial crura curve downward into the columella and diverge as they extend downward to the region of the columella base.

They are firmly attached to one another by means of fibroareolar tissue and they lie in intimate relationship to the skin of the columella.

The lateral crus of the alar cartilage forms slightly more than half the alar, the remaining portion being supported by the dense fibroareolar tissue of the nose. The nostril border is supported by a resilient, dense, collagenous tissue, fibers of which are arranged in a longitudinal fashion. At the junction of columella and alar "the soft triangle" of the nasal skin exists; this triangle-shaped area of skin bridges across from the columella to the nostril border and must not be incised in making a rim incision because distortion here is almost impossible to correct.

The lateral crura of the alar cartilages diverge in the supratip area, leaving a triangle-shaped defect between them, and into this area is inserted the previously noted septal angle. Relatively weak fibroareolar tissue connects the structures in this region, which is referred to as the weak triangle. The alar and lateral cartilages are connected by an aponeurotic tissue which maintains the attachment of alae to the septal angle and is referred to as the suspensory ligament of the tip of the nose.

The dome, the most prominent point of junction between the lateral and medial crura, is separated from the opposing alar dome by a varying amount of fibroareolar tissue; this degree of separation is more marked in the bifid nose and may present as a downward extension of the weak triangle.

THE COLUMELLA

The columella, which extends from the lip to the tip of the nose, is wider in the lip region; the width in this region is governed by the divergence of the medial crura of the alar cartilages. The lower ends of the alar cartilages embrace the lower margin of the septal cartilage as it articulates with the nasal spine. The shape of the columella is dependent upon the contour of the medial crura of the alar cartilages and is dynamically modified during breathing by the action of the nasalis muscles and the depressor septi nasi muscles.

THE VESTIBULE

The vestibule is limited posteriorly by the protrusion of the lower border of the upper lateral cartilage to form a fold, the internal nares. This fold extends laterally and inferiorly along the pyriform apterture, forming the posterior

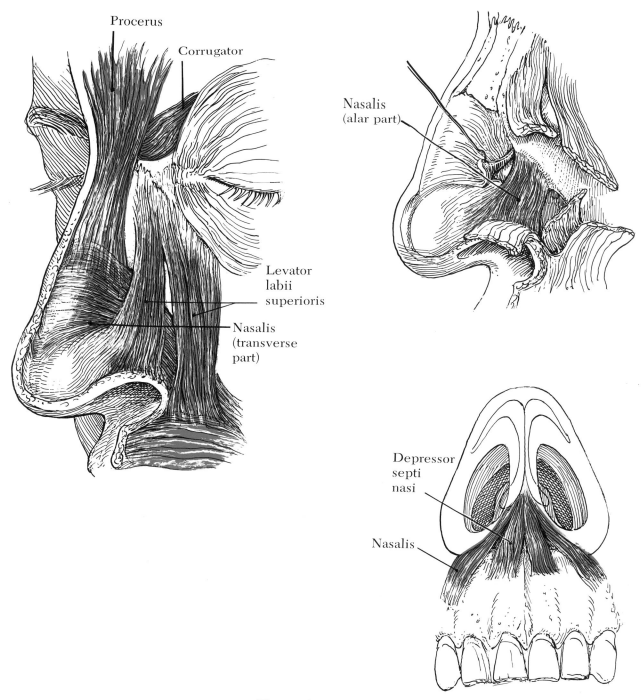

Procerus

Corrugator

Levator
labii
superioris

Nasalis
(transverse
part)

Nasalis
(alar part)

Depressor
septi
nasi

Nasalis

The nasal musculature.

274

extent of the vestibule. Motion of the upper lateral cartilage has a most important action on the control of the dimensions of the vestibule.

THE BONY NASAL SEPTUM

The bony septum is formed by the perpendicular plate of the ethmoid, the vomer, the nasal crest of the maxilla and the nasal crest of the palatine bone. Above, it articulates with the under aspect of nasal bones, and anteriorly, with the cartilaginous septum.

The septal cartilage lies in the vomerine plate groove, wherein it is loosely attached. The mobility of the cartilage in this region acts as a shock absorber and is instrumental in preventing frequent fracture of the septal framework.

Surgical Physiology of the Nose

BY AKIYOSHI KONNO, M.D.

FUNCTIONS OF THE NOSE

The nasal cavity, located at the entrance of the upper airway, functions to protect the lower respiratory passages by the warming, humidifying and filtering of the inspired air. Accessory functions are olfaction and action as a resonator for speech. Of all the portions of the respiratory tract the nasal cavity offers the greatest resistance to airflow, contributing some 47 to 54 per cent of the total airway resistance during quiet nasal breathing (Rohrer, 1915; Buttler, 1960; Speizer and Frank, 1964). This resistance is assumed by some investigators to be optimal in functioning as a servomechanism controlling the pulmonary ventilation (Forman, 1951; Williams, 1970). While the differing effects of nasal breathing upon pulmonator function have still to be completely investigated, the shape of the nose, both in its external and internal variations, is intimately related to its function. The most important function of all is to supply an adequate airflow to the lower airway, and it is to this single function that all other functions are subservient.

A deformity of the cartilaginous portion of the external nose of either congenital, traumatic or postoperative origin, especially when concentrated at the nostril and narial valve region, can result in marked airway obstruction. Congenital deformity of the bony portion of the external nose will result in a minimal airway disturbance, whereas the effect of trauma on the bony external nose and adjacent maxilla can cause disturbance of nasal breathing varying from minimal to maximal in degree.

In dealing with problems of nasal airway resistance, the entire nose, including both the area of deformity and the remainder of the nasal cavity, must be considered as a unit since nasal airway resistance is a summation of the resistance made at the various portions of the nasal cavity. The cross-section air space is not constant with the entire cavity and, indeed, the cavernous tissues of the turbinates may change the cross-sectional area of the nasal cavity in response to temperature or moisture changes in the atmosphere or to postural or emotional changes in the subject. However, even without apparent stimulation, the cavity changes its airway resistance periodically and reciprocally; this nasal cycle is seen in 60 to 70 per cent of normal people (Stokstead, 1952; Konno, 1969). This reciprocal change of airway resistance between the two nasal cavities can occur quickly, and may repeat itself every 30 minutes to three hours.

Postural change in the nasal airway resistance is brought about by change in position of the subject. In many patients it may be felt subjectively. However, since the changes occur reciprocally between the two nasal cavities, the total airway resistance will vary little in amount. While the air travels through the nasal cavity to the oropharynx it becomes humidified to a 75 per cent relative humidity and heated to 31 to 37° C. whether the inspired air, varying in temperature from minus 30° to 50° C., is dry or saturated. Approximately one third of this heat and moisture is recovered in expiration and transferred to the inspiratory air (Cole, 1953).

The efficiency of the nasal cavity as an air conditioner dictates that the surface area be of wide extent with a narrow width of airway, both factors contributing to a high resistance to air flow.

The turbinates and the anterior and posterior septal tubercles contribute to maintaining a fairly constant width of the nasal airway. The external nose, in particular the cartilaginous portion, contributes a certain degree of airway resistance and control to both the shape and the degree of turbulence of the nasal airflow.

AIRFLOW IN THE NASAL CAVITY

Diverse opinions have been voiced by Proetz (1953), Takahashi (1923) and Tonndorf (1939) on the pathway of nasal air through the normal nose. This is due entirely to the difference of the nasal model used in experiments and in particular to the comparative width of

275

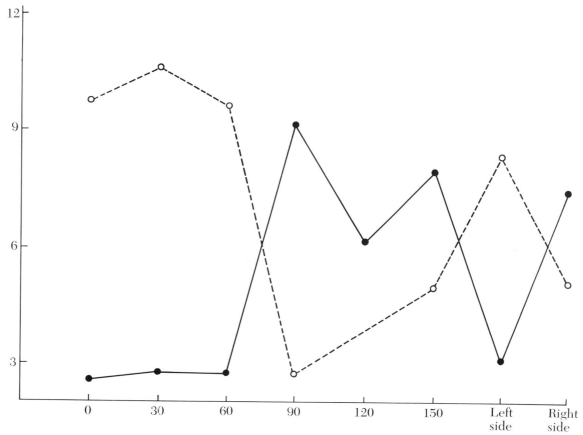

Resistance to airflow is not uniform in the two nasal cavities, and even without evident stimulation, there are periodic changes in resistance over time. If resistance in one cavity rises, the other falls reciprocally in 60 to 70 per cent of normal noses, as in the two subjects represented here. Resistance in the right nasal cavity is indicated by solid circles, and that in the left cavity by open circles. "Left side" and "right side" points are measurements taken after the subject had lain in the left (or right) lateral position for 10 minutes.

(*Illustration continued on opposite page.*)

the varying portions of the nasal cavity. Results of our measurements and observations of pattern and velocity of the airflow based on the nasal model obtained from a silicone cast of the human nasal cavity support the view of Tonndorf (1939). In the normal nasal cavity the main current of flow is through the middle portion of the cavity, making a parabolic curve (Cole, 1953).

This type of flow is due to the angle made by the nostril and the choanae and to the fact that the nasal airway adjacent to the olfactory tissues is much narrower compared to other portions of the cavity, making the airflow in this area smaller than elsewhere in the nose. However, as long as there is air space, the air flows throughout the cavity with a fairly high velocity. A portion of the air which flows into the nasopharynx passes through the choana on inspiration and impinges on the posterior wall of the nasopharynx, making various whirls. The whirl seen around the agger nasi, below the dorsum of the nose and anterior to the middle meatus, is

varied and is dependent upon the shape of the external nose, the nasolabial angle and the degree of development of the anterior nasal tubercle. This whirl is often seen in the apparently normal nose; even in the nose with a marked dorsal hump, the width of the airway in this area is kept constant and narrow as a result of the development of the anterior septal tubercle. In this instance no marked turbulence is noted in the airflow save for the regular whirl at the area of the agger nasi (Cottle, 1960).

In the instance of the long nose with a plunging tip and an acute nasolabial angle, the main air current will extend comparatively higher in the nasal cavity; conversely, in the nose with a larger labial angle or with a saddle deformity, the main air current level is lowered.

Following infracture and lowering of the nasal dorsum in rhinoplasty, the main air current is only slightly lower, and a change of flow pattern into the olfactory tissues is noted that, clinically, has little effect on olfactory sensibility.

It should be noted that the flow pattern is

276

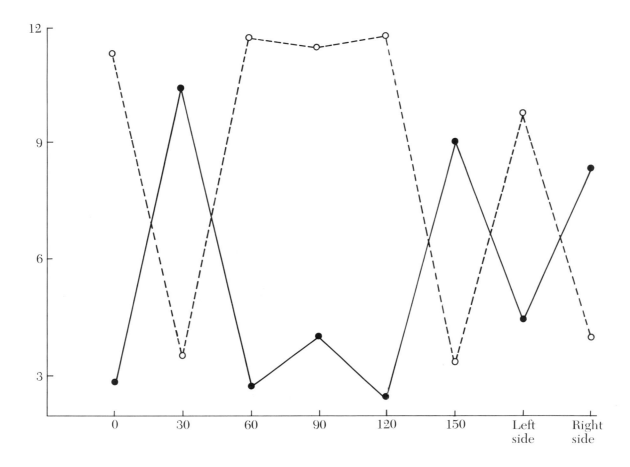

quite similar on both inspiration and expiration and that in the normal nose the air, having just passed through the external nares and the internal nasal valve area, has some degree of turbulence because of the sudden enlargement of the cross-sectional area. However, the flow in the nasal cavity proper is itself fairly stabilized (although not completely laminar flow in type) at a peak velocity of 12 liters per minute attained during quiet nasal breathing. This is because of the narrow width of the airway and the smooth contour of the concha; a moderate deformity in the shape of the external nose will have little effect on the character of airflow.

What will increase turbulence of the airflow is a deformity such as septal spur or scar contracture of the internal nasal valve area, but the most marked turbulence is seen in the nasal cavity of the patient with atrophic rhinitis when the normal narrow width of the cavity has been lost.

NASAL AIRWAY RESISTANCE AND THE SENSATION OF NASAL OBSTRUCTION

Pressure-flow relationships during quiet respiration have been measured by posterior rhinomanometry by Konno (1969). The accompanying illustration shows the variations ob-

served between the normal control, the patient with an atrophic rhinitis and the patient with hypertrophic rhinitis with a septal deformity. The pressure difference between the nasopharynx and nasal mask (P) at a determined flow velocity (V) indicates the nasal airway resistance.

Nasal resistance is found to correlate fairly well with various rhinoscopic findings, a fact well illustrated by gentle pressure on the lower portion of the upper lateral cartilages bilaterally, which will readily cause the sensation of nasal obstruction. This finding also holds true for deformity of the lateral crura of the alar cartilages.

The patient with a long, hanging nasal tip with long upper cartilages is apt to develop nasal obstruction and feel much less of a sense of obstruction when the tip of the nose is elevated to increase the lip columella angle.

When gas flows through a canal, laminar resistance increases in inverse proportion to the fourth power of its diameter (Poiseuli's law). This law can be applied to the nasal cavity, and when the effective diameter of the cross-section decreases by one half, the laminar resistance increases as much as 16 times. When the nasal cavity is wide, a decrease of the cross-sectional area will not affect airway resistance to any great extent, but in the narrow nasal cavity even a

277

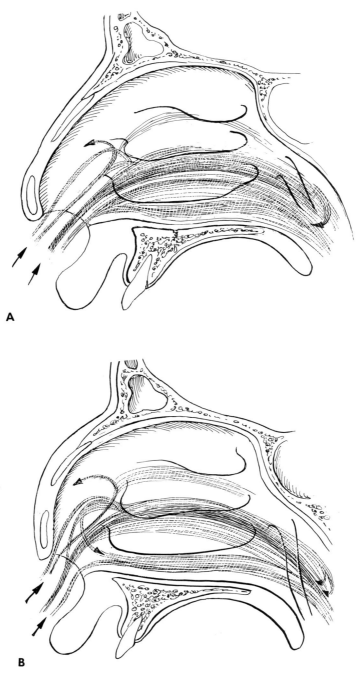

Pathways of airflow on inspiration in the normal nose (*A*) and in the long hanging nose with a dorsal hump (*B*).

278

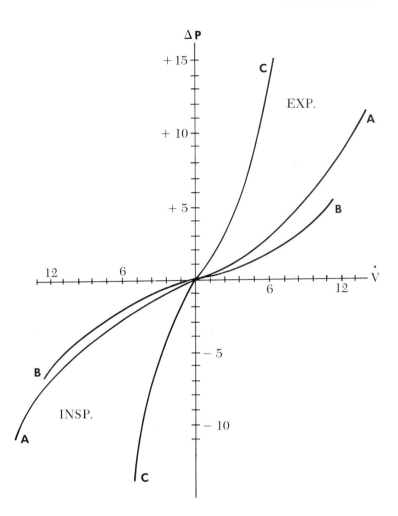

The pressure-flow relationship of the nasal air flow during inspiration and expiration in the normal nose *(A)*, the nose with atrophic rhinitis *(B)*, and the nose with hypertrophic rhinitis and a septal deformity *(C)*. ΔP is the pressure difference between the nasal mask used to measure the pressure and flow, and the mesopharynx (in mm. H_2O). $\dot{V}$ is the flow velocity (in liters per minute).

slight decrease of the cross-sectional area can cause a marked increase in the resistance to nasal breathing. However, the nasal cavity is not a canal with a constant effective diameter and, hence, the total nasal resistance is a summation of the resistances of the varying effective diameters of the cavity. A further fact to be taken into account is consideration of resistance in the turbulence formed by the irregular walls, which will also increase nasal breathing resistance.

Conversely, when the cross-sectional area of the cavum nasi gradually increases, the nasal airway resistance of the cavum nasi can decrease to the value of the resistance made by the nostrils and the internal nasal valve area. When the nasal cavity further widens, the turbulent resistance can increase slowly with a slight increase of the total nasal airway resistance, although in the actual nasal cavity, the turbulent resistance is always much smaller in comparison to the laminar resistance. When there is deformity in the nostril or the internal valve area causing an increase in nasal airway resistance, this cannot be relieved to any extent by operative procedures on the turbinates or septum.

Deviation of the septum which has devel-oped gradually is frequently accompanied by compensatory hypertrophy of the inferior turbinate and the septal tubercle on the concave side and hypertrophy on the convex side, which tends to maintain nasal airway resistance in the bilateral nasal cavities fairly equally. In doing a septoplasty or submucous resection the patency of the airway on the concave side of the cavity must be estimated before the effects of vasoconstrictors have occurred; infracture or submucous resection of the inferior turbinate should then be planned if indicated.

When the septal deviation is not accompanied by a compensatory change in the structures of the lateral wall of the nose on the convex side, this may cause a marked obstruction of the airway. A wide spur, particularly one extending into the area of the middle meatus near the concha, hypertrophy or edema of the posterior portion of the inferior turbinate, and synechia in this area can obstruct the airway to a marked degree because the area near the choana is also the narrowest portion of the nasal cavity proper.

The sensation of nasal obstruction is the subjective feeling caused by an increase of nasal

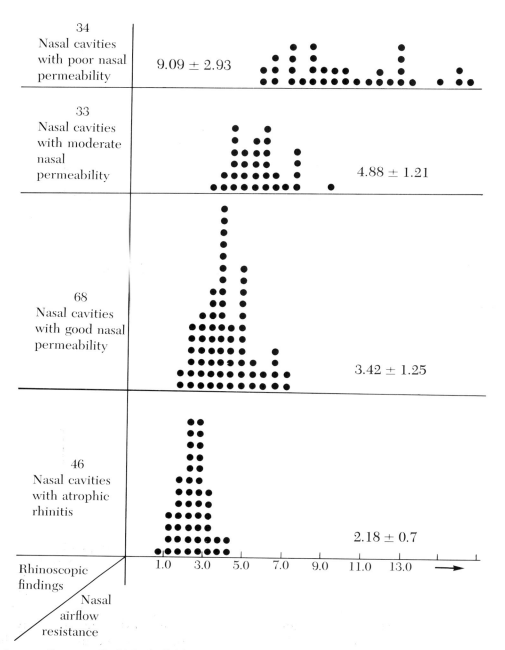

34
Nasal cavities with poor nasal permeability

9.09 ± 2.93

33
Nasal cavities with moderate nasal permeability

4.88 ± 1.21

68
Nasal cavities with good nasal permeability

3.42 ± 1.25

46
Nasal cavities with atrophic rhinitis

2.18 ± 0.7

Rhinoscopic findings

Nasal airflow resistance

1.0   3.0   5.0   7.0   9.0   11.0   13.0

Airflow resistance (in mm. H$_2$O) in individual nasal cavities with various rhinoscopic findings. Each dot represents a single nasal cavity.

airway resistance. The normal nasal cavity is so constructed as to have as narrow a width and as wide a surface area as possible. The surface is covered with mucous membrane with abundant cavernous tissue, secretory cells and glands, together with a loose submucous tissue which will easily accommodate to a vast amount of submucous edema. It is not abnormal that nasal airway resistance occasionally exceeds the threshold of sensation of nasal obstruction in a patient with only a minor deformity in the nasal cavity.

In most cases the sensation of nasal obstruction is consistent with nasal airway resistance as objectively measured, although there is wide individual difference in the value because of the differences of total volume, patterns of respiration and, thus, differences of peak intranasal pressures during the nasal breathing cycle. Most of all there is a difference of threshold and adaptation of sensation. An increase of nasal breathing airway resistance may be caused not only by organic changes in the external nose and the nasal cavity but can also be due to a reversible rapid change of the degree of filling the intranasal cavernous bodies. When the complaints of a patient do not correspond to subjective findings, the operator may have to repeat

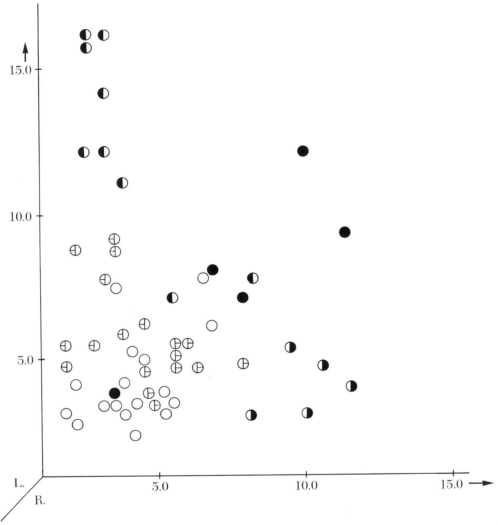

Relationship of nasal resistance to air flow (in mm. H$_2$O) and the subjective sensation of nasal obstruction. Each circle represents a single patient. Barred and filled semicircles indicate, respectively, sensations of slight and considerable nasal obstruction, which are seen to correlate reasonably well with objective measurements of resistance to air flow.

the rhinoscopic examinations with attention to the relationship of the complaints of obstruction to posture and periodicity at the time of examination. In some instances the sensation of nasal obstruction complained of is not caused by an increase of nasal airway resistance. This can be due either to other abnormal sensations of the nose or to factors of physiologic origin which cause the patient to pay constant attention to the nasal respiration.

The patient with atrophic rhinitis will frequently complain of nasal obstruction, which in most cases is caused by foreign body sensation or by a true increase of nasal resistance resulting from accumulation of crusts and secretions. In other instances this may be due to irritation or dryness of the nasal cavity and/or the nasopharynx or to changes of sensation to airflow caused by metaplasia of the mucous membranes

with degeneration of the glands and the cavernous body.

After removal of the crust in the nasal cavity the patient may still complain of a sensation of obstruction, although nasal breathing resistance is never higher than normal except in those rare patients who have scar contracture of the internal nasal valve area or saddle nose deformity involving the cartilaginous portion of the external nose.

RHINOMANOMETRY

As a qualitative method of measuring the nasal airway resistance, Glatzel's mirror is still used and, although lacking investigative sophistication, it serves for clinical purposes to determine whether the patient has nasal obstruction.

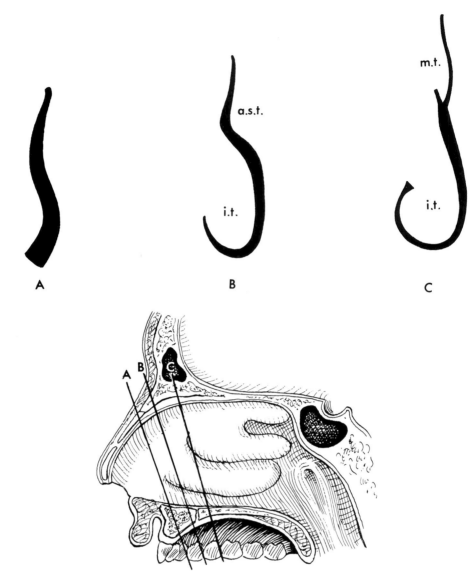

Top, Representations of cross sections of the nasal cavity taken at the planes indicated, drawn from a silicone cast of the nasal cavity of a living subject. *i.t.* is the inferior turbinate, *m.t.* the middle turbinate, and *a.s.t.* the anterior nasal tubercle. The septal wall accommodates its contour to that of the lateral nasal wall. *Bottom,* Longitudinal section identifies the turbinates on the lateral wall of the nose.

This method combined with a careful rhinoscopic examination and history of the patient's problems is frequently sufficient.

However, many quantative methods have been devised for the purpose of research examinations, all these methods being based for their design principle on Kayser's formula:

Resistance = pressure × time needed for passage of the flow, and constant volume.

Two major research methods exist in this instance and are grouped into those involving anterior rhinomanometry and posterior rhinomanometry.

In most methods natural respiratory air passed through the nose is used, but some techniques involve an artificial constant flow of air either through the pharynx to the nose or through the nasal mask to the pharynx, and the pressure in the nasal mask or in the mesopharynx at a certain volume in velocity represents the nasal airway resistance.

By these methods the resistance of the entire nasal cavity is measured under physiologic conditions, but it is difficult to measure airflow resistance of each nasal cavity separately.

The values shown in the illustrations were obtained by using posterior rhinomanometry with a nasal mask on which a pair of pneumotochometers is attached for measuring the velocity of nasal airflow through both nasal cavities and for measuring separately the velocity of nasal airflow through each nasal cavity.

Airflow through each nasal cavity is separated inside the nasal mask by the sponge septum which has been custom made to fit the contour of the nose of each subject. The illustration on this page expresses nasal airflow resistance as a pressure difference between the nasal mask and the mesopharynx when the flow velocity through one nasal cavity is 6 liters per minute.

THE CHANGE IN NASAL AIRWAY RESISTANCE AFTER RHINOPLASTY

Removal of the hump or infracture of the nasal bones may not affect the nasal airway resistance to a very great extent. The reason for this is readily appreciated in a cross-section of the area when one realizes that the area mainly affected by this procedure is restricted to the narrow supralateral portion of the cavity, or while the widely patent portion carrying the main airway flow is left undisturbed. Scar contracture or adhesion of the nasal valve area which is due to excessive removal of the upper lateral cartilage with mucous membrane can cause marked increase of the airway resistance.

Narrowing of the nostril, due either to alar base resection or to removal of the alar cartilage with or without the skin lining at the tip area, can cause, depending upon its degree, a marked increase of the nasal resistance.

On deep respiration nasal airway resistance is smaller on expiration and larger on inspiration. This is due to passive movement of the cartilaginous portion of the external nose by the intranasal negative and positive pressure. This is most marked when seen in the patients with congenital or postoperative collapse of the alar cartilage.

With collapse of the ala, marked increase of negative pressure is seen on inspiration together with visual evidence of apparent retraction of the ala. When the patient tries to breathe in more air, the greater the increase in the negative pressure in the nose.

When the patient has fragile alar cartilage preoperatively, any maneuver of the alar cartilage in doing tip plasty has to be most conservative.

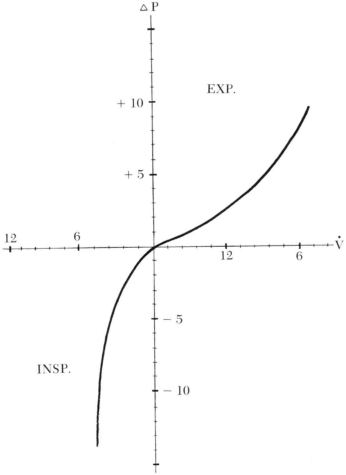

The relationship of pressure (ΔP, the difference between pressure at the mesopharynx and that in a nasal mask) to flow (V̇) in the nose of a patient with collapsed alae.

283

Preoperative Considerations

PATIENT SELECTION

The most common reason for rhinoplasty is a reduction in the size of part or all of the nose. However, as in the non-Caucasian (pages 473 to 483), it might be necessary to reduce the size of the tip while at the same time increasing the dorsal prominence by an implant. Overlying all these considerations are the standards of nasal beauty, which are surprisingly similar throughout the world, despite both ethnic and racial pride. The nasal form usually considered most attractive is the thin aquiline nose with a delicate "chiseled" tip. Many variations exist, of course; indeed, in some races the presence of a nasal hump is a sign of beauty. The profile most desired is that of a straight dorsum or one possessing varying degrees of retroussé, dependent on the ethnic criteria or area. The nostrils should be thin and delicate with a slight flare and, indeed, in nasal surgery of the non-Caucasian, excessive flaring of the alae is one of the common features for which correction is requested.

It is difficult to estimate the number of rhinoplasties performed adequately in the United States. A conservative estimate for New York City would be 5000 per year, and there is every indication that the frequency of rhinoplasty is increasing.

Unquestionably, nasal plastic surgery is the most technically difficult of all operations in plastic surgery. A part of this difficulty is the essentially blind nature of the procedure in which the success depends to a great extent on the tactile sense of the surgeon. This is further compounded by the difficulty in prediction of the final result; many factors combine to produce this result, such as the skill of the surgeon, anatomic variations in the skin and subcutaneous tissues and cartilages of the nose, healing idiosyncrasy of the patient, and complications. It is especially difficult to teach rhinoplasty to the student because of the above noted difficulties and the requirement for three-dimensional appreciation of the surgical results, not to mention the need for an artistic appreciation on the student's part. Although any surgeon can be taught the techniques of nasal plastic surgery, very few really become masters in the art; however, a great many are capable of producing an acceptable nasal plastic result.

One of the most difficult aspects of teaching rhinoplasty is to impart the limitations of each technique and the variable results that may occur due to the patient's physiognomy. Some of these limitations are predictable but others are not so clearly foreseen. One of the commonest causes of failure in rhinoplasty (the indifferent or disastrous result) is the pressing desire of the surgeon to accomplish a "perfect" job. Frequently such a result is completely outside the realms of possibility, and in such a case the failure is produced by the inability of both the surgeon and the patient to accept the fact that there will be some limitation in the final result. The experienced surgeon readily accepts these limitations and stops when a maximal practical correction has been achieved, whereas the inexperienced surgeon will resist these limits and court defeat and an unsatisfactory result. The overoperated nose is a tragedy because reoperation is rarely able to retrieve a satisfactory result; indeed, even minor improvement is frequently unattainable.

The routine (cookbook) patterned operation advocated by many surgeons is to be condemned; it is simply not possible to do a standard operative procedure on every patient and obtain satisfactory results. To attempt to correct each tip by the same technique shows a complete lack of understanding of the variations in size, shape and direction of the alar cartilages, as well as a failure to appreciate the influence of the subcutaneous tissue and overlying skin on the tip structure of each patient. The surgeon must appreciate these limitations and problems and command at least three or four basic surgical approaches in order to adequately treat the individual nasal plastic problem.

THE FIRST CONSULTATION

One of the most difficult and sensitive parts of the operation begins at the first consultation with the patient. At this time the surgeon must determine whether the patient is emotionally suited to the operation and to what degree the nose can be improved in contour. A poor decision at this time can result in the ultimate failure of the operation, even though a technically successful contour has been achieved. Of equal importance to the physical characteristics is the patient's concept of the outcome of the operation; this concept has to do with the self-image, so important in all of cosmetic surgery, the subject discussed in Chapter 3.

NASAL PLASTY

Although it is not possible to be absolutely accurate in predicting the result of rhinoplasty because of the many variables encountered, it is important for the surgeon to recognize certain anatomic problems which may pose difficulties during the surgery and will definitely limit the results to be obtained. The surgeon must learn to recognize just how these specific features will modify the outcome; many of these variations in anatomy have been discussed by numerous authors, but because of their importance bear repeated emphasis.

The factors which may influence the result of rhinoplasty are the thickness of the nasal bones, the presence or absence of the nasion and the thickness and position of the septum. If the nasal bones are thick, if the septum is shifted laterally at the level of the nasal bones or if the septum is excessively thick in this area, the possible degree of narrowing of the nose along its dorsum will be severely limited. A high deviation of the septum, unless corrected, will be reflected by an external deviation of the nasal framework after completion of the operation.

Deviations of the cartilaginous septum of the nose pose the most challenging and difficult problem. Despite all possible surgical maneuvers, the attainment of a completely straight dorsum may not be possible, and some curvature or external deviation of the nose may still be present after the operative procedure, or may become apparent only after a period of some weeks or months following completion of the surgery. Lowering of the nasal profile during rhinoplasty may expose a deviation of the cartilaginous septum present in the lower portion of the septum but not along its dorsal border. Trimming of redundant alar cartilages may also expose a crooked septum previously camouflaged by the lateral alar crura. The correction of deviated septum will be discussed further in the chapter, but it is important to study the septal conformation preoperatively in order to carefully plan the corrective procedure.

The mucous membrane should be shrunk with a topical vasoconstrictor during the preoperative examination so that all confines of the nasal cavity can be exposed. Patients with external nasal deformities, the result of septal deflections, should be advised that it may not be possible to obtain a completely straight nose at operation and that they must be willing to accept a possibility of a persistent small deviation. If a straight nose is obtained, little criticism can be directed at the surgeon, whereas if a small deviation persists, the patient has been adequately warned.

The tip frequently presents the most technically challenging part of the procedure. It requires considerable experience to be able to evaluate the tip preoperatively and to predict with any degree of accuracy the postoperative result. Some tips pose more difficult problems than others, and indeed some of these problems presented prove insurmountable; these patients should not, in most cases, be accepted for surgery. The most difficult tips to correct are those in patients with thick oily skin, usually associated with an abundance of sebaceous glands and a marked excess of subcutaneous fatty tissue. This kind of tip has an amorphous appearance (the underlying cartilage may or may not be hypertrophic) and cannot impress its shape on the external aspect of the nose because of the thickness of the overlying tissues. The thick skin frequently obliterates the normal supra-alar groove; in patients presenting with this sign, great care must be taken in examination of the nasal tip.

Correction of such a nose should be approached with caution since the results are apt to be indifferent or, if excessive surgery is done in an attempt to reduce the tip, the result will frequently be marred by added deformity and scarring. While a certain amount of improvement can be accomplished in such tips, it must be remembered that the memory of the patient and the patient's friends of the preoperative appearance can be very short and they may soon lose sight of what has been accomplished. Whether to accept a patient for surgery depends entirely on the surgeon's evaluation of the attitude of both patient and family, and it is frequently on the basis of the evaluation of this attitude that the patient is to be finally accepted or rejected for surgery.

It is well for the young surgeon, particularly when just starting practice in a community, to realize that he will be able to accomplish very little with conventional techniques operating upon such a tip and that if he becomes too aggressive with his surgery it will result in a disaster for all.

Occasionally despite the many obstacles in the path of obtaining acceptable surgical results in patients with some of these difficult anatomic problems, we find that the patients who seem to be helped the least are frequently most grateful and pleased. This problem certainly has to do with self-image. Conversely, we may find a patient who has obtained a superb technical result to be highly dissatisfied. Such patients usually have emotional problems that require, at the least, psychotherapy.

The decision of whether to operate depends on a meeting of the minds between surgeon and patient. If the patient is a minor, the family enters into the decision, and in this instance it is vital to keep in mind that it is the patient who is most important and that the wishes of parent or relative should be made a secondary consideration. Frequently more than one consultation may be necessary, and the surgeon must be convinced that the patient has a realistic concept of what can be accomplished and what is impossible.

The use of preoperative photographs is frequently helpful in discussing the proposed change with the patient; their use with careful retouching of a matt finished photograph can often show the patient's wishes to the surgeon, and at this time it will occasionally become very clear that the patient's concept of herself and what can be accomplished is grossly distorted. The surgeon must explore the depth and cause of this distortion and determine whether or not it can be channeled in a positive direction. The nuances of this type of situation are many, and clear guidelines do not exist. As the surgeon gains in experience he will make fewer and fewer mistakes in patient selection, but he will probably never reach the point where he is not in error in an occasional instance.

In our opinion the use of preoperative plaster casts and moulages on which the proposed nasal change is sculpted or carved is both misleading and inadvisable. Such three dimensional carvings are usually more fancy than fact, and frequently fail to convey the dynamic changes of the healing of the nasal tissues. The patient is apt to gain the impression from the plaster cast that the beautifully carved nose is exactly what to expect, and this expectation may turn quite sour if the exact result is not reproduced. It is well to remember that such casts provide excellent exhibits at legal proceedings.

In the younger rhinoplasty patient the handling of the family is frequently more difficult than handling the patient. Nevertheless, if the patient is a minor the family must be kept in the picture. A situation is not infrequently encountered in which the parents insist upon the operation while the minor patient does not wish the change to be made. Under such conditions it is both unwise and unethical to operate, since it is the primary job of the surgeon to help the patient and secondarily to aid the family. Our policy in such an impasse is to advise the patient that when, if ever, he or she desires to discuss nasal plastic surgery, a further consultation is available but that in the meantime no surgery will be performed.

Another difficult situation with the young patient is when the patient desires surgery but the mother or father or both are vehemently opposed to the procedure. This situation can be most troublesome because someone is certainly not going to be pleased with the results, and frequently a transfer of this dissatisfaction from the parent to the patient may occur. A similar situation may exist between husband and wife; emotional and psychological interplay may complicate proposed surgery and its results. Again it must be emphasized that when such problems are encountered, it is the surgeon's job to do his best for the patient. Thus, if consultation and careful appraisal of all relevant factors indicate the strong possibility of success and pleasing the patient, then we should proceed with the surgery.

Such situations are difficult to resolve and can often present a long and trying road for the surgeon, and yet when successful they are part of the pleasure of cosmetic surgery. Every surgeon must be prepared to assume certain risks which must be weighed against the chances of success; indeed, every cosmetic operation is a risk of sorts. However, the rewards for both patient and surgeon are such that the risk is well worth taking provided that the odds are not overwhelmingly weighted against success.

THE OLDER PATIENT

It has been emphasized in many studies that the older the patient seeking rhinoplasty the more the problems that are encountered from both the physical and psychological viewpoints. With increasing age, the self-image comes fixed, undesirable as it may be to the patient. Rhinoplasty often effects a profound change on self-image, a change which is much easier to assimilate at the age of 17 than at 40 or beyond. In the younger patient the mind soon erases the image of the old nose from the memory, whereas in the older patient who has lived with the same nose for many years this image may persist even after the nose is changed, creating a certain degree of mental confusion.

Extra caution must be exercised in evaluating the older patient for nasal plasty. The subtle signs of incipient psychosis should be watched for, and the perfectionist patient should usually be avoided since he has had many more years in which to practice this perfection and he will frequently be incapable of accepting any result. The foregoing is not to say that rhinoplasty cannot achieve highly satisfactory results in this age group. Indeed it can, but patient selection becomes all important, more so than in the eyelid or facial plastic surgery patient. The man who is approaching or is middle-aged must be carefully evaluated. The association between the nose and the genital organs does exist, and it can easily become confused in the emotionally ill or incipiently psychotic mind. Operations on such disturbed male patients have provided plastic surgery with some of its more tragic incidents.

It must not be inferred from this that every middle-aged man seeking cosmetic surgery should be rejected; there is a marked increase at present in the number of male patients in this age group who are interested in eyelid or facial corrective surgery. While one must be cautious with this group, one should be overly cautious with a rhinoplasty candidate. Rhinoplasty can be highly successful in certain older patients when circumstances are appropriate. A good rule to follow, nonetheless, is "when in doubt, get a psychiatric consultation."

HISTORY

Several facts in the general history of the patient can be especially pertinent to a rhinoplasty. A family history of bleeding tendency or a personal history of bruising or bleeding, particularly epistaxis, may indicate obscure blood dyscrasias. While females do not have true hemophilia, they may carry the potential for excessive or even dangerous postoperative hemorrhage by virtue of disorders of their blood coagulation mechanism. The usual bleeding and clotting time tests are generally of little or no value in these circumstances, and a complete hematologic evaluation of the patient's coagulation abilities is indicated if suspicion of a bleeding tendency exists.

A history of allergic disorders, particularly hay fever or vasomotor rhinitis, warns the surgeon that such patients may have an exacerbation of such difficulties in the postoperative period, often prolonged for several weeks or months. Vasomotor rhinitis can be distinguished by the intermittent nature of the nasal obstruction, often shifting from side to side, especially while the patient is in bed. Submucous resection is by no means always the answer to difficult breathing, and more observations on this problem will be made later in this chapter. The patient with a history or objective evidence of vasomotor rhinitis should be forewarned that the operation may accentuate his symptoms for a very long period of time. The surgery should be postponed if an active respiratory infection is present.

The routine use of prophylactic antibiotics before and after surgery is a frequently debated point, but in nasal surgery, where infections though rare are critical, it would seem wise to take advantage of every precaution; a thrombosed cavernous sinus with infection is a grave problem never to be forgotten. The authors employ antibiotics beginning 24 hours prior to operation; tetracycline 250 mg. four times a day is given and maintained for four days after surgery.

Premedication is discussed in Chapter 4. In rhinoplasty the premedication combination is most important, particularly if local anesthesia is to be used. A relaxed, sleepy and cooperative patient is apt to remember the experience, if indeed memory persists at all, without fear or discomfort, whereas the undermedicated or improperly medicated patient has only a disturbing and frightening memory to impart to friends.

The medication should be given sufficiently far in advance of the procedure so that the patient is well relaxed before transportation to the operating room. All too frequently patients placed on the schedule "to follow" are sent for with only a few minutes of time remaining for the floor nurses to administer the premedication. Such patients usually arrive in the operating room tense, worried and anxious because the medication has had insufficient time to take effect. Often it is not until the surgery is nearly completed that the medication finally works, so that during the most feared part of the procedure, in the period when sedation is most needed, the effects of the premedication are absent.

Local anesthesia is generally used, although general anesthesia can be employed in the extremely apprehensive or younger patient. Hypotensive anesthesia insures a dry field, but the technique requires the services of an anesthesiologist expert in its use.

For local anesthesia we prefer topical cocaine and epinephrine followed by infiltration with lidocaine (Xylocaine). The cocaine is applied with cotton packs wrung as dry as possible after soaking in a solution consisting of equal parts of 10 per cent cocaine and 1:1000 epinephrine. It takes a minimal amount of cocaine solution to achieve excellent topical anesthesia of the mucous membranes; because of the possibility of toxic reaction, it is important to keep the dosage as low as possible. Lidocaine and mepivacaine (Carbocaine) have proved to be excellent anesthetic agents in nasal plastic surgery. We use 2 per cent lidocaine with epinephrine added at the time of surgery to produce a 1:60,000 solution.

The Operating Room

POSITIONING THE PATIENT

Positioning of the patient for rhinoplasty is important. The hands should be lightly restrained; the table end is elevated so that the head is above the level of the heart. This simple maneuver is very important in diminishing bleeding during the procedure. The patient should be placed on the table so that the table break falls in the lower back region. This will enable the trunk and head to be raised to produce more postural hypotension if this should prove necessary. A foot plate should always be used to prevent sliding of the patient during surgery, and this should be adequately padded both for comfort and to prevent inadvertent grounding of the patient in this region should an electric cautery be used during the operation.

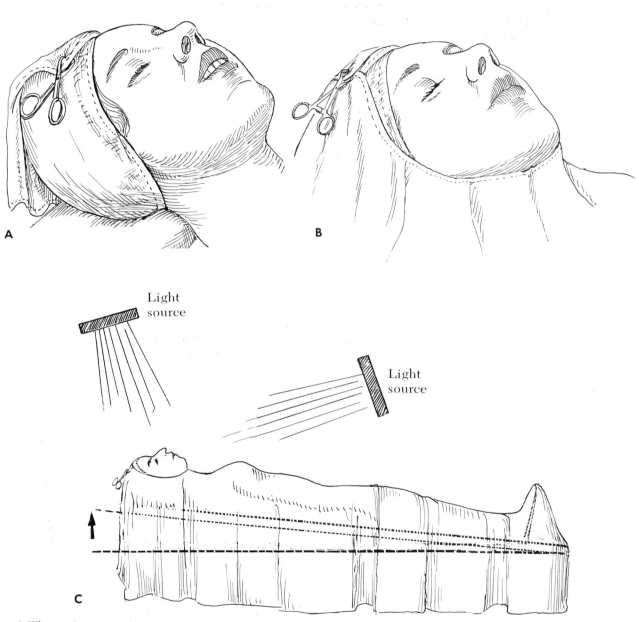

A, The optimum position of the patient on the operating table, with the head of the table elevated by about 10 degrees. The overhead lights are so arranged that one shines directly down onto the nasal dorsum and the other projects its beam into the external nares to illuminate the interior of the nose.

B, The patient's hair is draped back and held by a towel; it is important that the forehead be exposed in order that a true appreciation of the patient's full face can be attained during surgery.

C, A split drape is drawn about the patient's head (again note the importance of exposing the full face), leaving the mandibular borders exposed.

A good light source is mandatory. We prefer to have the whole face lighted directly from above, with a second light directed from below to illuminate the interior of the nose. When extensive septal work is done we prefer to use electric head lights rather than head mirrors and reflected light. However, this is a matter of individual preference with the surgeon. Fiberoptic "cold" lighting has been adapted for use for the dorsal nasal retractor of the Aufricht type, this instrument providing excellent illumination of the nasal interior.

The skin is prepared with pHisoHex and benzalkonium chloride (Zephiran) solution. The area will also have been washed with pHisoHex the night before surgery during the patient's preoperative preparation. Draping is done with the traditional towels and a split sheet, but it is important that the drapes not cover the entire face. Obscuring the forehead and chin will prevent the operator from appreciating the full nuances of facial contour. The nasal vestibule hair is trimmed and the external nares cleaned with cotton-tipped applicators soaked in Zephiran solution.

ANESTHESIA

Local anesthesia is generally used, although general anesthesia can be employed in extremely apprehensive patients. Hypotensive anesthesia insures a dry field, but this technique requires the services of an expert anesthesiologist well versed in its use. Hypotensive anesthesia for use in elective plastic surgery was pioneered and perfected in England, primarily at the Queen Victoria Hospital and Plastic Center, East Grinstead.

For local anesthesia, we prefer topical cocaine and infiltration with lidocaine. The cocaine is applied with cotton packs after diluting a 10 per cent solution with equal parts of 1:1000 epinephrine. It is important that the cotton packs be wrung as dry as possible. It takes very little cocaine solution to achieve excellent topical anesthesia of the mucous membranes, and it is important to keep the dosage as low as possible to minimize absorption. Toxic reactions are kept to a minimum in this way.

Lidocaine and carbocaine are excellent local anesthetic agents for nasal surgery because of their quick action and prolonged anesthesia. For nasal surgery we use 2 per cent lidocaine with epinephrine added so that a solution of 1:60,000 is obtained. Again, as with cocaine, it is important to keep the total dosage as low as possible. It is entirely possible to obtain excellent

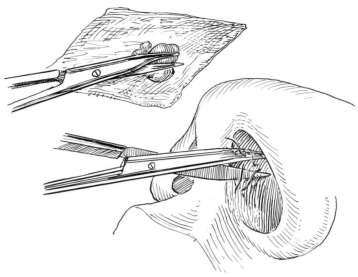

The nasal hairs are clipped after preparing the nares with Zephiran solution. The blades of a Stevens scissors are smeared with petrolatum so they will catch the severed hairs.

infiltration anesthesia with 6 ml. of this solution, 10 ml. at most.

The dorsum is infiltrated first, followed by field blocks just lateral to the pyriform aperture (p. 290). If the infraorbital foramina can be located without undue delay, intraforaminal blocks are done. The base of the nose is blocked by infiltration with 1 or 2 ml. near the nasal spine. It is helpful to wait at least 5 minutes for the anesthesia and the epinephrine to take effect before beginning surgery. Patience is rewarded by a much dryer field.

A recent innovation for apprehensive patients who are terrified of the injections required for local anesthesia is the administration of Brevital or an ultra-short-acting barbiturate during the few minutes necessary to give the injections.

When anesthesia is complete, the nose is packed with 1-inch gauze soaked in saline. This packing prevents blood and debris from draining into the posterior pharynx during the procedure.

The operator should learn to adjust the height of the table and the distance at which he operates so that he may work most comfortably. For most surgeons, with normal or corrected vision, the table is best located at elbow height.

THE OPERATION

The illustrations and their captions on pages 291 to 483 describe the basic procedures and their numerous variations. The text is resumed on page 484.

289

A, The full face is evaluated before the nose is injected. The nasal profile, the nasal tip contours, the columella-lip angle, and the relationship of the mental prominence are all examined with a sterile mirror. The use of such a reversed image often throws into prominence a minor defect that might otherwise be missed. This procedure is important throughout the operation.

B, Exerting gentle pressure with the thumb and forefinger, without displacing the nasal skin over the alar cartilages, brings the alar domes into prominence. At the point of skin blanching (the dome region), a single mark is made.

C and *D,* The usual points of prominence of the alar domes.

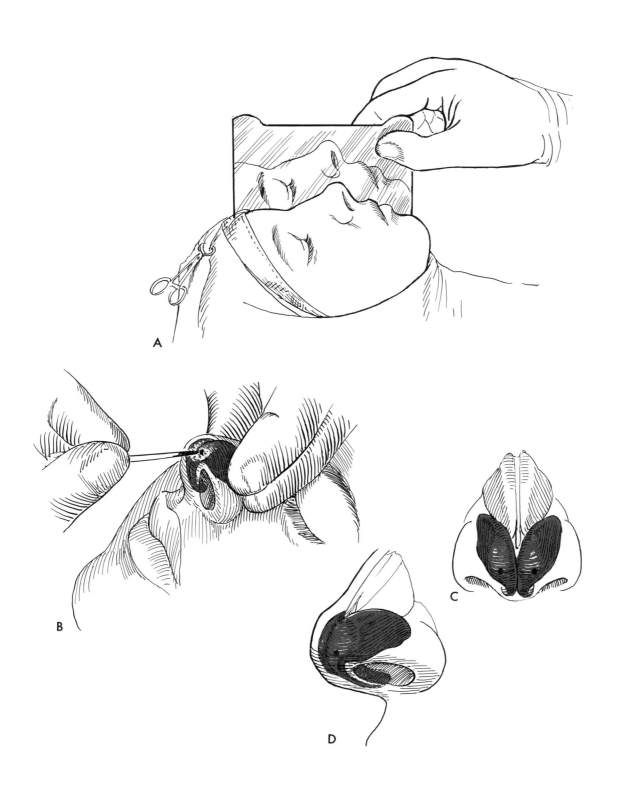

A

B

C

D

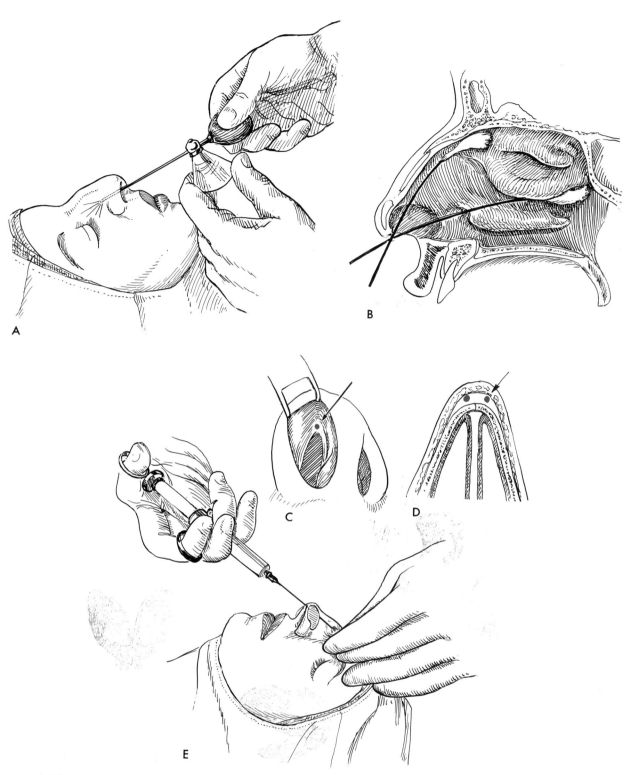

A, The nasal cavities are sprayed with a solution of equal parts of 10 per cent cocaine and 1:1000 epinephrine.

B, Pledgets of cotton on wire applicators carrying the same cocaine and epinephrine solution are placed first along the inner aspect of the nasal dorsum and the nasal bones to block the external nasal nerves. Similar applicators are placed beneath the middle turbinate posteriorly to block the sphenopalatine nerves.

C, The injection of the local anesthetic solution along the nasal dorsum.

D, The dorsal nasal skin is gently pinched between thumb and forefinger to elevate it from the underlying nasal pyramid.

E, The injection solution is deposited as close as possible to the nasal bones in order to raise the overlying soft tissues.

292

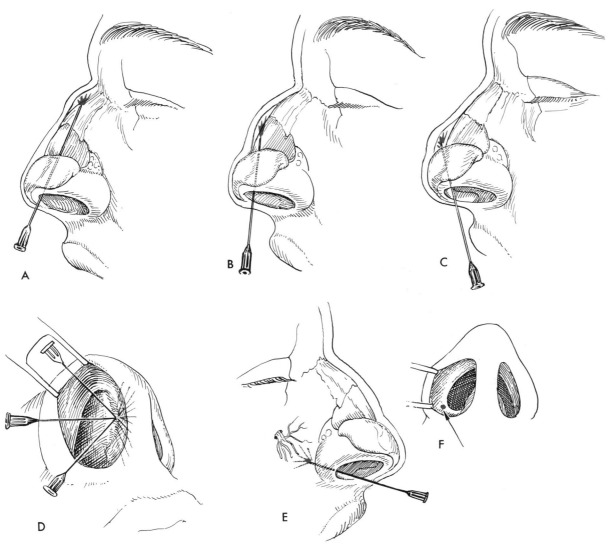

A, Local anesthetic solution is initially deposited at the nasal frontal angle, and as the needle is withdrawn, deposition of the solution is continued down to the point of withdrawal of the needle *(B).*

C, The weak triangle area is infiltrated with local anesthetic solution.

D, The needle is passed into the membranous septum and the base of the columella is first anesthetized to bring about a block anesthesia and diminish the patient's discomfort with the rest of the infiltration. Infiltration is continued up along the membranous septum to the interdome region.

E and *F,* The alar base is injected to block branches of the infraorbital nerve and the nasal branch of the anterior superior dental nerve.

Schematic steps in the nasal plastic operation. These steps may be carried out in any sequence deemed necessary by the operator. Each surgeon develops his own operative approach to rhinoplasty. The order of the procedure, whether the surgeon first removes the hump, trims the tip cartilages or does the submucous resection (if one is to be done), is not vital in the usual case. It is the authors' belief, as has been stated and emphasized in other chapters of this book, that each procedure should be adapted to suit the individual needs at hand. At times, it makes more sense to operate on the hump before the tip. At other times, conditions warrant a reversal of these steps.

A, Intercartilaginous incision and raising of the soft tissues from the upper lateral cartilages.

B, Raising the periosteum from the nasal bones.

C, Transfixion incision, which may be complete or incomplete.

D, Modification of the dorsal borders of the upper lateral cartilages.

E, Modification of the dorsal border of the nasal septum in its cartilaginous portion.

F, Resection of part of the lateral crura of the alar cartilages in the nasal tip plasty.

G, Modification of the osseous dorsal border.

H, Lateral osteotomy and in- or outfracturing procedure.

I, Shortening of the caudal border of the cartilaginous septum, with or without modification of the nasal spine.

J, Shortening of the caudal borders of the upper lateral cartilages.

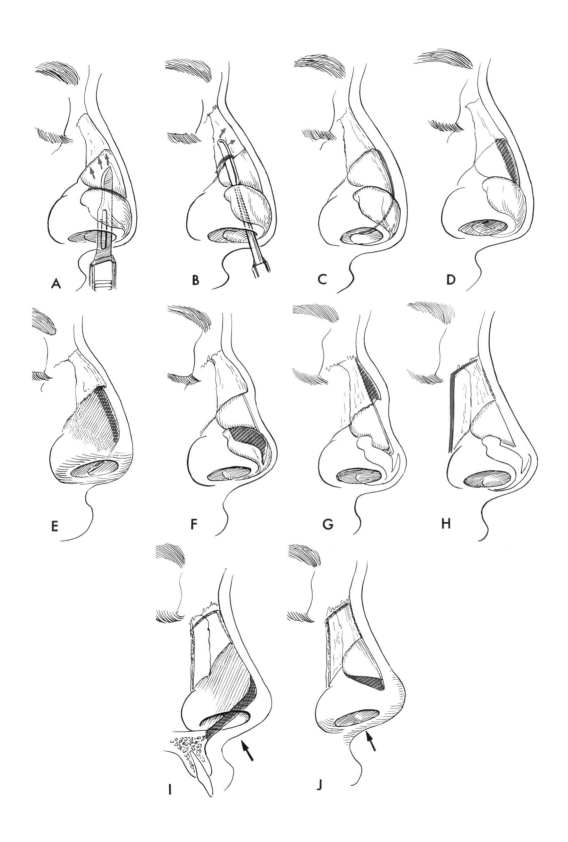

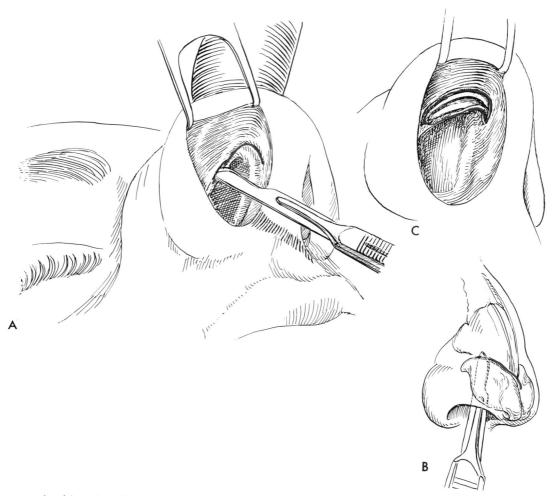

The first step in rhinoplasty is separation of the covering soft tissues from the underlying cartilaginous and bony framework.

A, Under direct vision, using a No. 15 blade, the first or intercartilaginous incision is made between the lower margin of the upper lateral cartilage and the upper border of the lateral crus of the alar cartilage. This is at the line of an internal narial fold, readily identified by retracting the nasal margin with a double-pronged retractor.

B, The relationship of the intercartilaginous incision to the upper lateral and the alar cartilages.

The intercartilaginous incision is carried along the dorsum of the septum, to and into the upper portion of the membranous septum. A similar incision is made on the other side.

C, Borders of the cartilages protruding through the wound.

A variation of this incision is preferred by Millard (1965) and by Pitanguy (1965), who utilize a transcartilaginous incision splitting the lateral crus as a primary procedure.

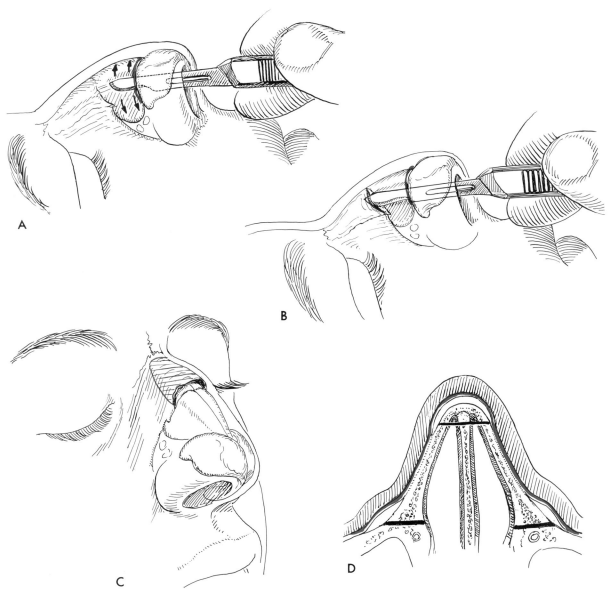

A, By gently sweeping the No. 15 blade over the external aspect of the upper lateral cartilage, the overlying soft tissues are elevated to almost the lateral extent of the cartilage. A Joseph double-edged knife may also be used for this maneuver.

Care is taken to dissect as close as possible to the perichondrium, in order to stay in the relatively bloodless deeper tissue plane and obviate possible damage to the skin of the nasal dorsum.

B, An incision is made along the lower border of the nasal bones through the periosteum to the underlying bone.

C, A usual line of osseous hump resection.

D, The sites of dorsal and lateral osteotomies, showing the raised periosteum. The periosteum is rarely raised intact and, in fact, is often lacerated.

297

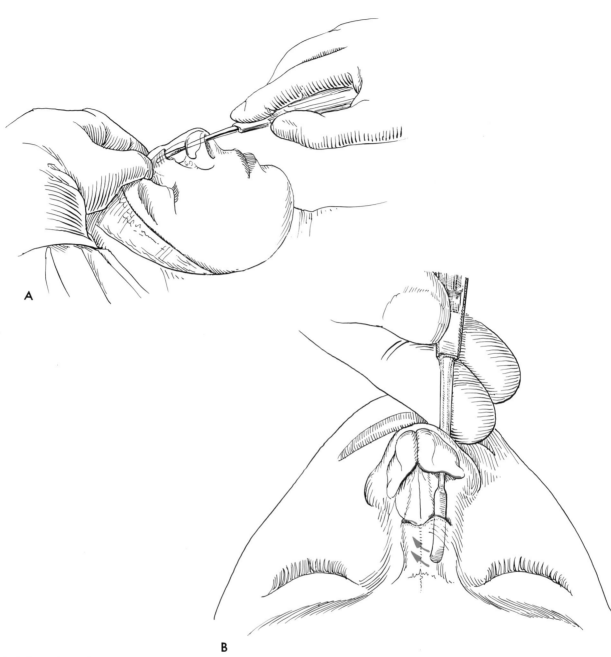

A, A Joseph periosteal elevator is introduced into the incision and the periosteum at the lower end of the nasal bone is raised. The elevator is passed directly upward to the nasofrontal angle.

B, The periosteal elevator is now swept medially over the nasal dorsum. It is important that the elevator be kept parallel to the midline of the nose during this maneuver so as not to unduly disrupt the periosteal envelope by perforating it with the tip of the elevator. The maneuver is then completed on the opposite side of the nose.

A frequently recommended maneuver is to raise the periosteum laterally and attempt to sweep both periosteum and soft tissues medially in the hope that they will be removed with the nasal hump. Whether such a maneuver is valuable is a moot point, particularly in the small hump excision, but where the hump is large, the procedure is worth attempting. We do not advocate the separate elevation of soft tissues and periosteum except in the extremely large nasal hump, and we rarely attempt this technique, believing that the extra trauma to the nasal skin caused by it is unnecessary and may promote the formation of excessive postoperative scar tissue.

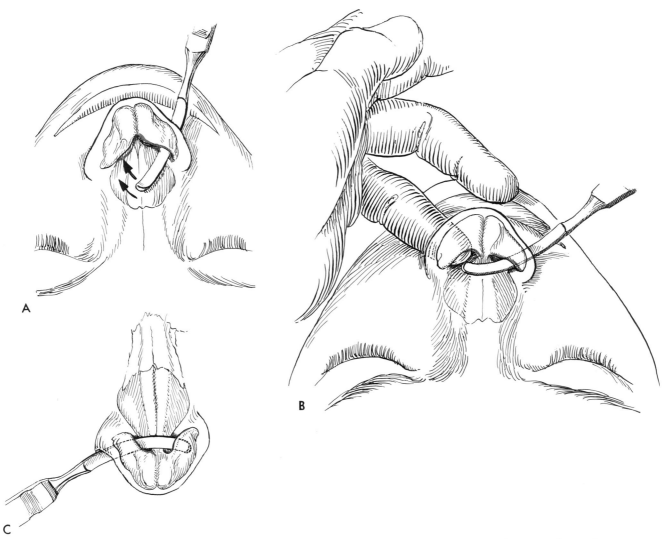

A, A Joseph button knife is introduced through the intercartilaginous incision and gently swept from the nasofrontal angle downward to sever any few remaining attachments of the nasal coverings to the deeper structures.

B, The operator's little finger inside the opposite nares guides the tip of the button knife out through the external nares.

C, The position of the button knife as it is about to turn posteriorly into the membranous septum. The knife should hug the dorsal and caudal borders of the cartilaginous septum.

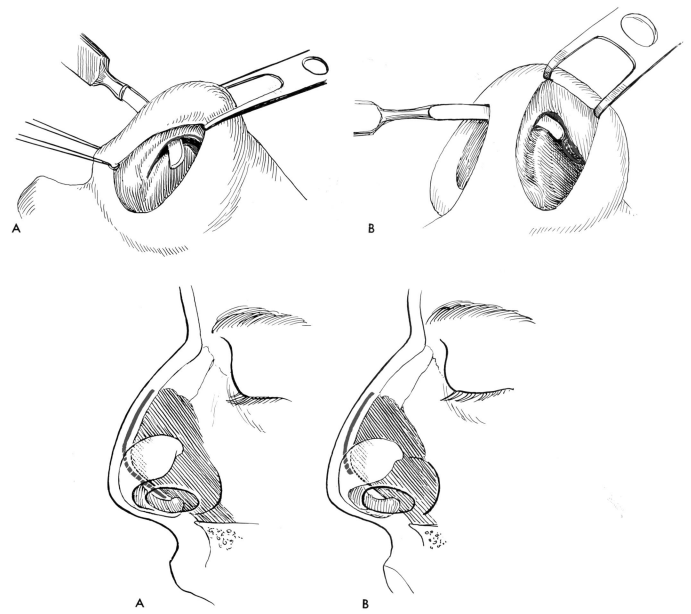

A, Under direct vision, staying as close as possible to the caudal border of the cartilaginous septum, pass the button knife posteriorly to incise the length of the membranous septum—the so-called transfixion incision.

B, In some instances, when no elevation of the nasal tip is desirable, the transfixion incision is stopped immediately after entering the membranous septum. This will result in no postoperative elevation of the nasal tip, but by just turning the corner into the membranous septum, the operator will greatly facilitate exposure of the nasal dorsum.

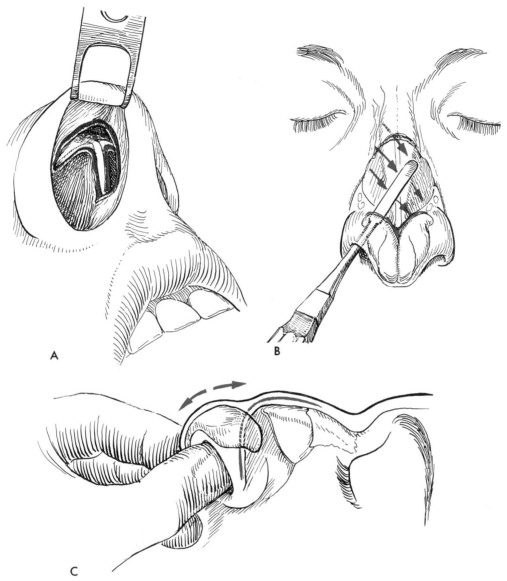

A, The membranous septum incised and the completed transfixion incision inspected.

B, A periosteal elevator is passed along the nasal dorsum to verify its freedom from attachment to underlying tissues and the completeness of the transfixion incision.

C, The nasal tip is dislocated from its normal position and the prominence of the dorsal border of the nasal septum and nasal bones is brought into view.

The question of whether to do a complete or an incomplete transfixion incision is frequently raised. In the majority of cases we make a complete transfixion incision, as this frees the soft tissues from the nasal skeleton and permits much more complete exposure of the nasal dorsum. However, we do not employ a complete transfixion incision in a patient with an obtuse lip-columella angle, since elevation of the nasal tip by even a few degrees may result in a most undesirable "pig snout" deformity in such a patient. A complete transfixion incision is of further benefit in mobilization of the tip so that the alar cartilages may be more easily manipulated during the operative procedure.

It has been argued that a complete transfixion incision should not be made because healing of the wound will result in straight-line contracture, pulling the tip inferiorly. In practice, however, this theoretical problem does not overcome the excellent mobility achieved by completing the incision, and it has not proved to be an undesirable feature.

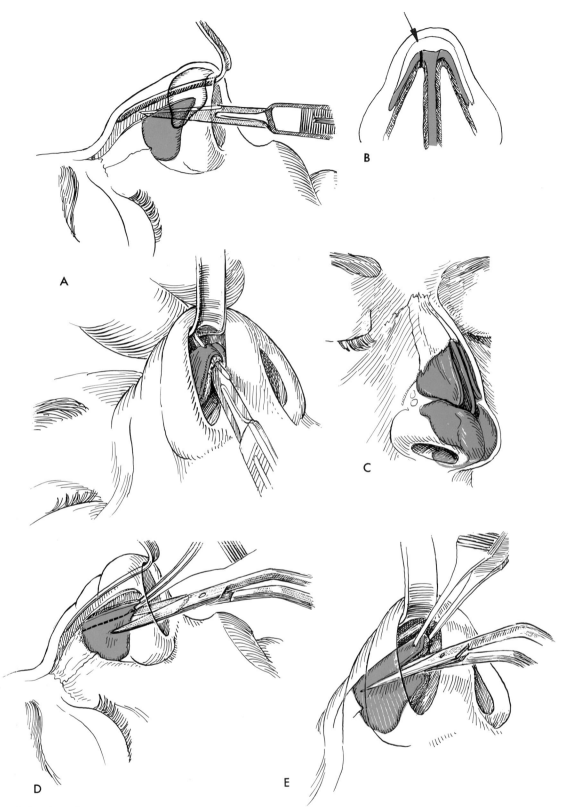

A, Protect the dorsal skin with an Aufricht retractor and pass a No. 11 blade from the upper lateral cartilage–nasal bone junction inferiorly to sever the attachment of the upper lateral cartilage to the cartilaginous septum.

B, It is important that the knife hug the nasal septum as closely as possible so that a shelf of upper lateral cartilage does not remain attached to the septum.

C, The detached upper lateral cartilages.

D, How much of the dorsal border of the upper lateral cartilage is to be removed is estimated and excised with a single closure of the scissors.

E, The cartilage is steadied by gentle inferior traction to produce a straight, single cut.

Once the upper lateral cartilage has been freed from the septum, the surgeon must determine the order of the rest of the operative procedure. Possible choices are hump removal, tip plasty, lateral osteotomies, or correction of septal deflection. Even in the hands of the expert operator, a change in the sequence may produce a significantly different result. Lipsett (1959) has emphasized that at times a smaller amount of dorsal hump can be removed if the septum has first been shortened—an important consideration in any patient with a minimal hump deformity and a drooping nasal tip.

If the caudal margin of the septum is prominent so that the tip is encroached upon or the columella displaced inferiorly or laterally, it is best trimmed at this time. The design of the excision of the caudal margin varies, depending on the deformity and on the extent of desired elevation of the nasal tip. To the novice it cannot be overemphasized that this excision must always be conservative. Always underestimate the cartilage to be excised and later, in the terminal stages of the operation, adjust the cartilage to the new nasal contour. The short, chopped-off nose or the retracted columella that may result from excessive resection of the caudal border of the nasal septum is at best difficult to repair and quite frequently impossible to improve upon.

When both the caudal border of the septum, at its point of junction with the nasal spine, and the nasal spine itself project into the columella-lip angle, the lip takes on the appearance of being foreshortened or tethered. This deformity may be further aggravated by the presence of a large dorsal hump. Resection of the caudal border of the septum together with the hump promotes relaxation and an apparent lengthening of the lip. If the nasal tip is to be significantly elevated, a triangular resection is done, with the base of the triangle at the septal angle. Where the lip is to be released with no or minimal elevation of the nasal tip, the triangular segment to be resected is reversed, the base lying at the nasal spine, which is resected at this time. By combining these resections, the operator may correct a variety of deformities in this region.

The decision whether to proceed with hump removal or tip remodeling from this point depends to a great extent on which of these two structures dominates the nasal deformity. On rare occasions it is necessary to modify only the nasal tip, without osteotomy or hump resection. This is not a common situation, and some modification of the bony structure is usually necessary. The surgeon should look most critically at the result of a tip modification before deciding that no changes are necessary in the nasal framework.

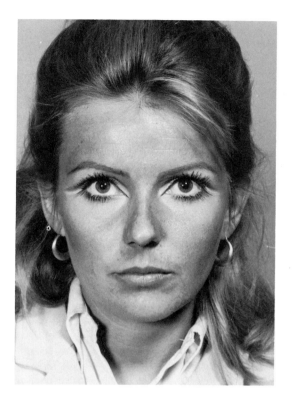
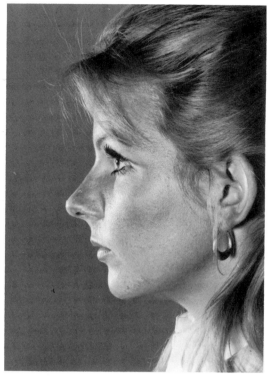
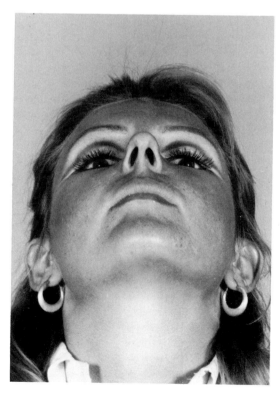

304

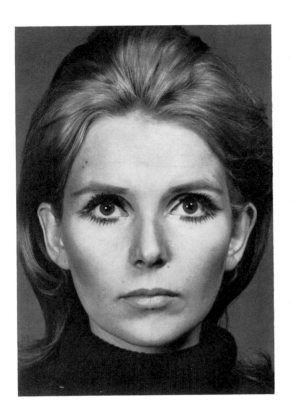

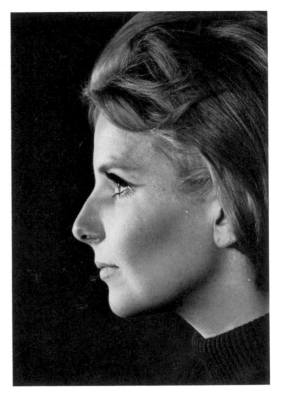

The effect of rhinoplasty when tip reduction is carried out without concomitant modification of the nasal profile. The postoperative views illustrate the small dorsal hump that became evident after tip reduction. The surgeon should always have permission to correct the entire nose, not just part of it.

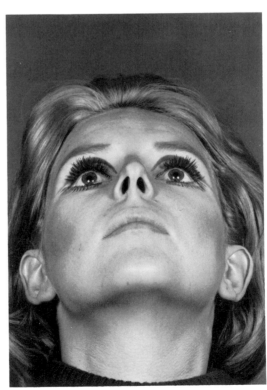

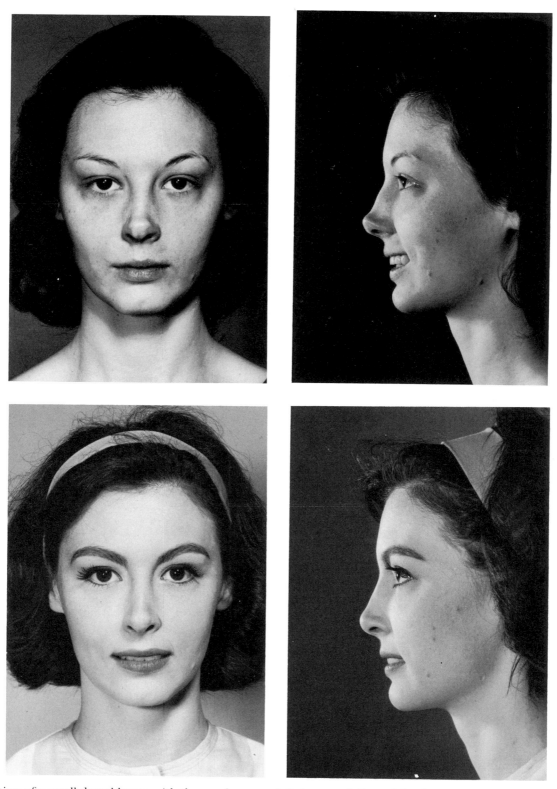

Resection of a small dorsal hump with the nasal rasp and slight remodeling of the tip were done for this patient. The postoperative photographs demonstrate the minimal amount of correction of the dorsum that was necessary.

If the bony and cartilaginous hump is of small to moderate proportions, we prefer to operate first on the nasal tip. On the other hand, larger humps are resected first, bone and cartilage being removed as a unit. A recent tendency has been to do the tip plasty first, as it seems easier to evaluate how much nasal hump to remove after this has been completed. In general, our hump removal is more conservative today than previously, as is true of all other steps in rhinoplasty.

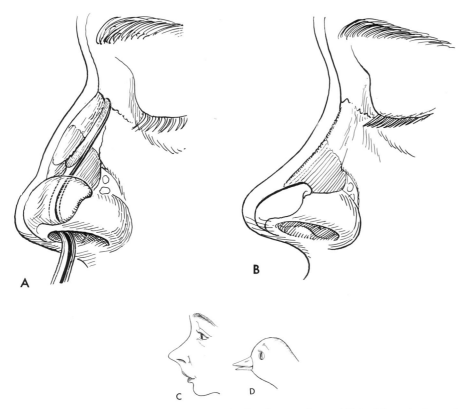

A, Resection of the osteocartilaginous hump in continuity by the nasal saw. With this technique the upper lateral cartilages are not detached from the nasal septum but are removed in continuity with the osseous hump.

B, Great care must be exercised in the use of the nasal saw, since it is easy for inexpert hands to remove too much of the nasal dorsum, as in this drawing.

C and *D*, Removal of excess nasal dorsum produces a so-called "birdlike" deformity.

Humps that are mostly cartilaginous and thus involve the lower third of the nose primarily are best removed after tip plasty and in a most conservative fashion. Conversely, humps that are mainly osseous and involve the upper portion of the nose can be removed before tip plasty, when it is much easier to judge how much dorsum to remove.

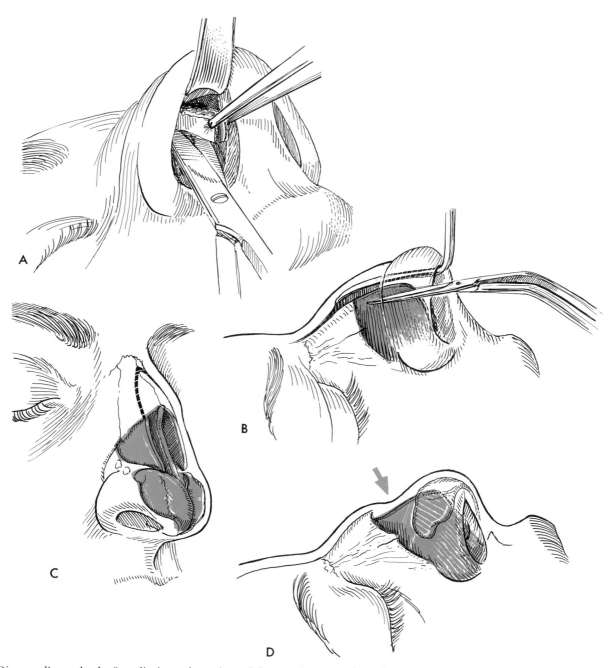

Diamond's method of preliminary lowering of the nasal septum in order to bring both the nasal tip and the osseous hump into prominence (Diamond, 1971).

A, The dorsal cartilaginous septum is lowered by the angled scissors to the estimated new profile line.

B, The dorsal borders of the upper lateral cartilages are resected to a slightly lower level than that of the septum.

C, The projected lines of the osteotomy, after cartilaginous resection.

D, The nasal tip and the osseous hump are brought into prominence; in many cases this facilitates the operator's judgments in planning tip cartilage resections and contouring.

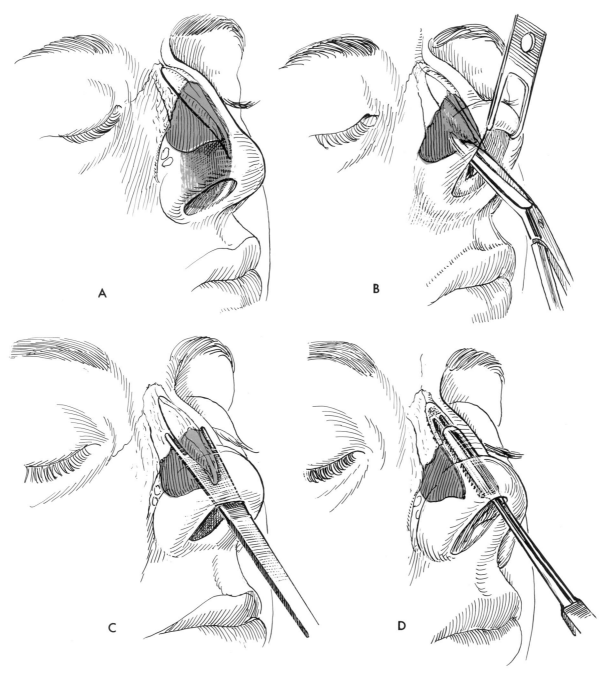

Removal of the osteocartilaginous dorsum in continuity with an osteotome.

A, The desired lines of osteotomy, transecting the upper lateral cartilages, osseous septum, cartilaginous septum, and nasal bones.

B, Cuts are made in the cartilaginous septum and upper lateral cartilages in the line of the desired nasal profile.

C, The osteotome is inserted along the lines of the cartilaginous cuts and gently tapped in to complete the new nasal profile.

D, Irregularities of the dorsum are eliminated by rasping, and the outer edges of the nasal bones are slightly rounded.

Correction of the dorsal profile with the Joseph nasal saw.

A and *A₁*, In a very large hump such as the one illustrated, a saw or an osteotome can be used for removal. The osteotome is particularly useful when the nasion is deep. The line represents a usual resection of the nasal dorsum.

B, The Joseph nasal saw is introduced with the blade lying flat on the underlying nasal structures. On reaching the site of the resection, the blade is turned so that a cut will be made in a plane across the face. The tip of the saw is intentionally brought through the apposing nasal bones, producing a small cut at their upper end.

C, The nasal saw is again introduced on the opposite side, the osteotomy felt for, and the saw cut begun at this point. This technique will result in a smooth dorsal resection. It is often more convenient not to detach the upper lateral cartilages until after the hump resection has been completed.

D, When the amount of correction is smaller, an osteotome is indicated to remove a minimal amount of bone. In this instance an inexperienced operator with a saw could easily remove too much and create a saddle deformity. A sharp osteotome of the McIndoe type with double guarded points to prevent skin puncture is inserted into a small cut in the dorsal cartilage of the septum. The small cut insures that the hump resection is begun at the desired point.

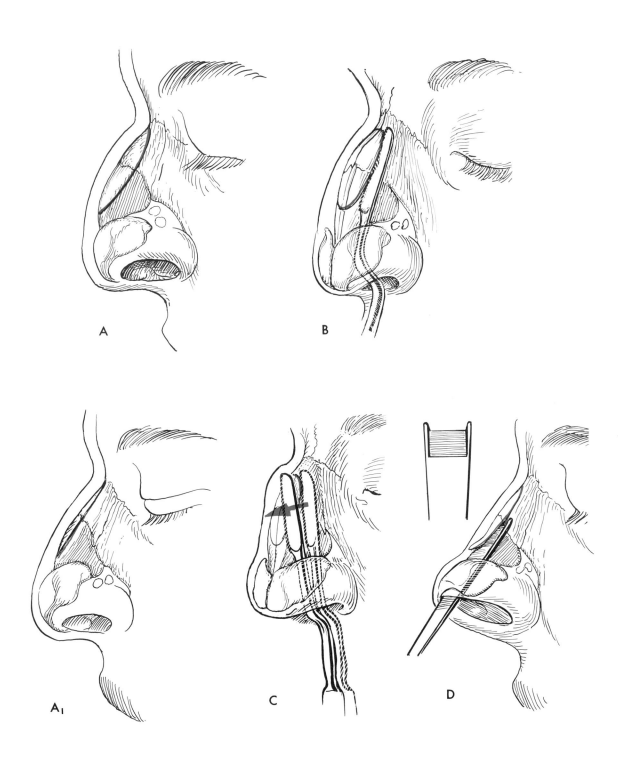

A

B

A₁

C

D

311

Removal of the osseous hump after reduction of the cartilaginous profile.

A, The Cottle osteotome, which has gently curved edges that make it more difficult to penetrate the overlying skin.

B, The Cinelli osteotome; two guarded prongs protect the skin.

C, The McIndoe-Cinelli chisel, whose rounded corners protect the overlying skin. The advantage of the osteotome over the chisel is that the direction of the cut can be changed without withdrawing it and reinserting it in a different direction.

D, The portion of the nasal hump to be resected.

E, The Cottle osteotome placed in contact with and along the line of the resected dorsal border of the septum.

F, The osteotome is gently tapped in to resect the osseous hump.

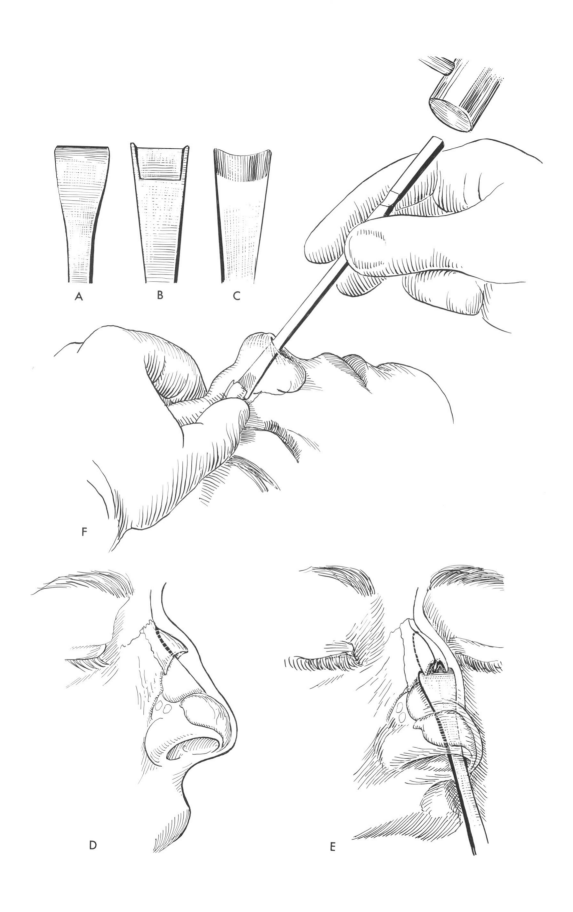

A   B   C

F

D   E

313

A, The remaining soft tissue attachments between the nasal hump and the septum, and the lining mucosa of the nose, are severed and the hump is removed. The attachments are completely divided in order to prevent inadvertent removal of excess nasal lining tissue.

B, The hump removed and the open nasal dorsum exposed.

C, A usual line of osteotomy, depicting the periosteum remaining in place after removal of the osteocartilaginous hump and the underlying mucosa. When removing very large humps it is desirable to include the overlying periosteum in order to facilitate shrinkage of the soft tissues to the new nasal framework.

D, Irregular bony surfaces are smoothed with a rasp; the sharp edges are rounded to simulate the normal convexity.

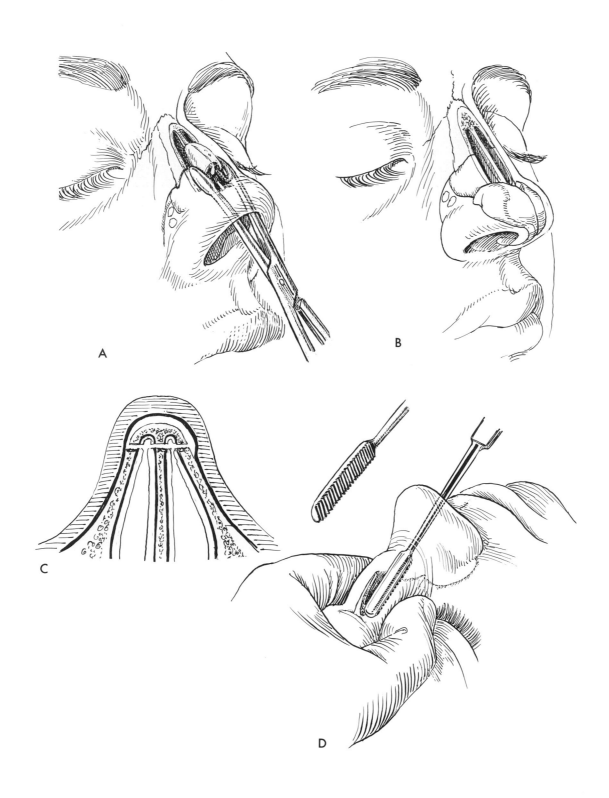

A

B

C

D

315

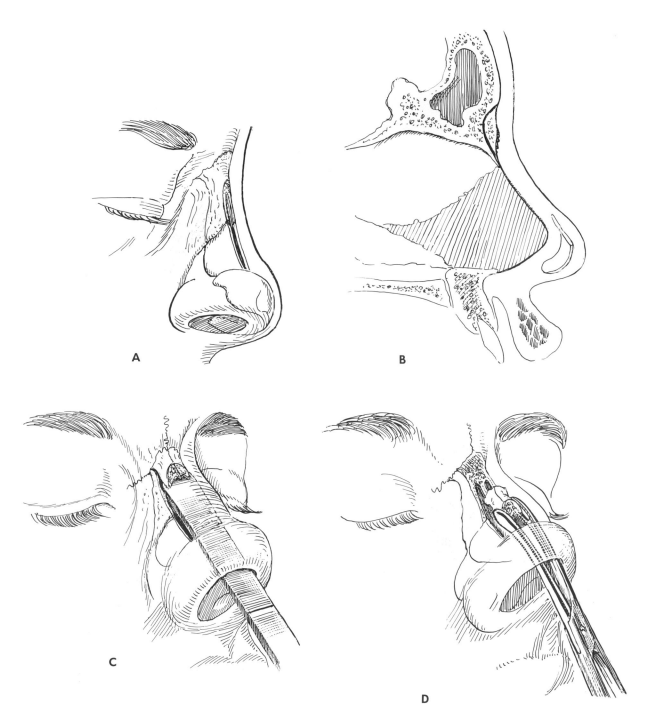

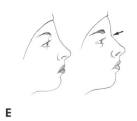

A, Excessive bone at the nasal-frontal angle after an otherwise adequate removal of nasal dorsum.

B, The area of nasal-frontal bone considered excessive, preventing the creation of a desirable new nasal profile.

C, A 10- or 12-mm. osteotome or chisel is passed along the new nasal dorsum and tapped into position. When adequate penetration of bone has been achieved, the instrument is levered slightly upward to produce a fracture at the upper end of the osteotomy.

D, The nasal bone is removed with the Converse forceps.

E, A common form of profile resulting from failure to remove nasal-frontal angle bone is shown in "before" and "after" states. It must be emphasized that in many patients there is a practical limit to the amount of deepening that can be realistically achieved in this region. An attempt to take out too much bone will frequently give rise to a webbing of soft tissue across the depression, obviating the correction.

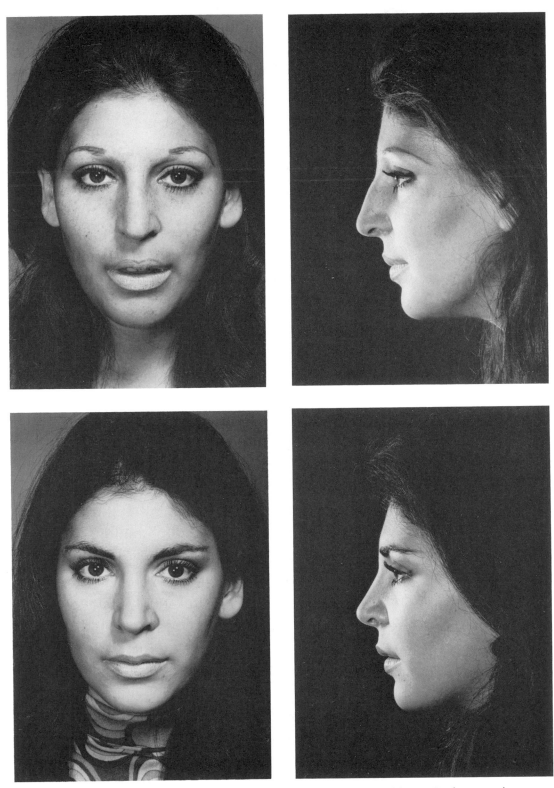

Deepening of the nasal-frontal angle by osteotome excision of a portion of bone. Such corrections are usually minimal.

The authors prefer a sharp osteotome to a saw for resection of the nasal hump. It is usually possible to be more accurate with an osteotome, in our opinion, but in the hands of an expert the saw can be a very precise instrument indeed. The osteotome is easier to control than the saw and can be angled quite exactly to fit the requirements of each operation; it is especially useful in deepening the nasofrontal angle. Use of the saw is particularly difficult in removing a small hump. The surgeon tends to turn the saw too far in order to gain purchase on the bone, and all too frequently excessive bone removal is the result.

A further advantage to the osteotome is that a cleaner cut is produced with less dust and less soft tissue debris in the wound. This debris can serve as a focus of infection. Of course, it is equally important for such debris to be removed following rasping to smooth the cuts of the osteotome.

Deepening the nasofrontal angle may be desirable after hump removal, but it is an extremely difficult feat because of the thickness of bone and shortage of skin in the region of the nasal root. Aufricht (1943) emphasized the importance of considering the nasofrontal angle in relation to the profile before completing the hump removal. He recommended that, if the radix nasi is tangential to the frontosubnasal line, the angle be left undisturbed. If it lies in front of that line, a deepening of the radix is desirable.

After removal of the nasal hump, it is usually necessary to adjust the dorsal borders of the septum and the upper lateral cartilages to the new nasal bone profile line. The cartilages are trimmed with sharp septal scissors; we find the Taylor dural scissors with serrated edges to be excellent for this purpose. Irregularities of the bony dorsum are rasped, and a further minor reduction of the height of the dorsum may be gained by this rasping. It is usually not desirable to reduce the hump directly by rasping unless it is quite small. However, once the operator has gained experience with the use of osteotomes, small humps are better managed by careful shaving with a very sharp McIndoe type of chisel controlled by manual pressure. By this means the bony dorsum can be decorticated, and only a minimum of tissue will be left to be removed by the rasp.

Removal of the nasal hump does not always result in an open bone defect extending superiorly to the nasofrontal angle. Frequently a web of bone of varying thickness remains at the apex of the dorsal aperture. This bony segment, if left in place, will cause difficulty during infracture and, indeed, may produce the "rocker" effect of Becker (1951) (see page 428). This bony webbing may be removed by the use of a curved, guarded osteotome (see page 452), or by the Converse nasal root forceps (see page 432).

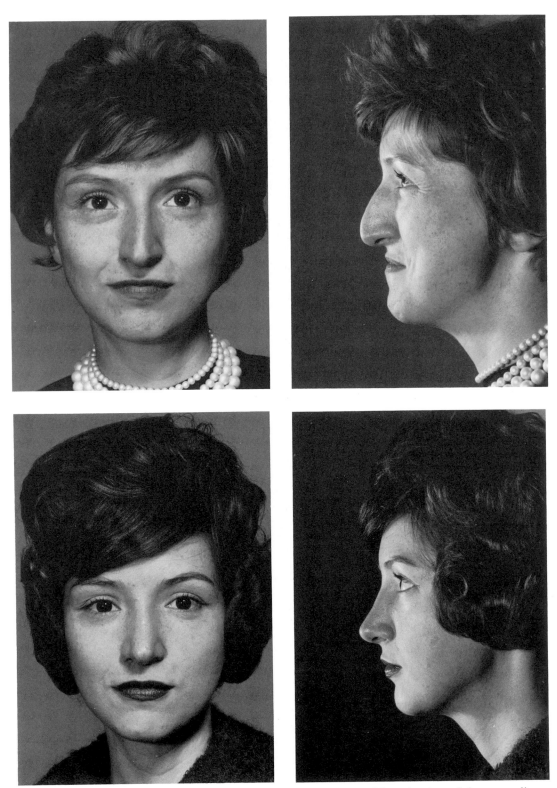

Resection of a large dorsal hump by the saw technique. Tip elevation and lengthening of the upper lip were carried out after correction of the hump. A saw can be used for such large humps with little danger of excessive resection of bone and cartilage. The entire redundant osteocartilaginous dorsum can be removed in one piece.

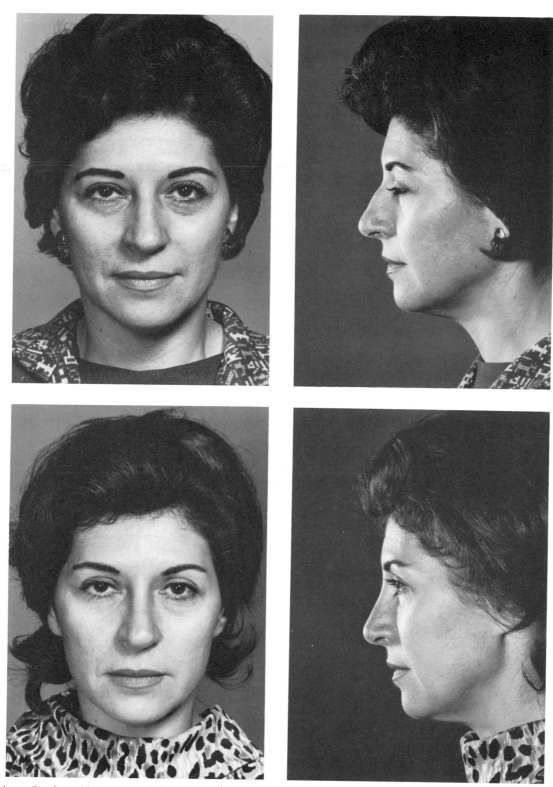

Resection of a dorsal hump consisting almost entirely of bone. Correction was achieved by osteotome resection, minimal shortening of the nose by removal of a triangle from the caudal margin of the septum, and conservative tip operation.

Minimal Rhinoplasty

The subtle or minimal rhinoplasty is an operation done to correct such minor problems as a very small hump, slight widening, or minimal deformity of the cartilages. Such minor irregularities can be quite distressing to some patients, whose complaints assume proportions which at first examination seem quite unrealistic.

Such patients should not be refused surgery until a thorough history, physical examination, and photographic study have been completed. Careful study of the photographs with these patients and inquiries about their aspirations will often make clear to the surgeon that the patient has a real problem and that there is a realistic approach to its solution.

Minimal surgery requires considerable care and experience, and even when the surgeon possesses these qualities, the results still may not be entirely satisfactory. Inasmuch as it is never possible to predict the final result of rhinoplasty, it is vital that patients be fully informed of this factor of uncertainty.

However, many minimal rhinoplasties produce gratifying results even though the physical change accomplished is small. A minor revision in the appearance of the nose can effect a great change in the patient's overall facial appearance—a point of particular importance to those who must work in the camera's critical eye.

Minimal rhinoplasties must be carefully planned to meet the requirements of each patient. Often a small readjustment or excision of alar cartilage is all that is required, or a minor dorsal modification may accomplish the desired correction. However, in most patients the entire rhinoplasty operation must be done, but with particular emphasis on removal of minimal amounts of tissue. It is in such patients that only those most expert in the use of a saw should attempt to resect a dorsal hump by this method, in our opinion, and it is here that we prefer to use only the sharpest of osteotomes and chisels to remove fine slivers of bone and cartilage. Our preference is the McIndoe hand-held chisel (page 313).

When removing such small pieces of bone or cartilage, the angle at which the chisel or osteotome is directed is of utmost importance. Chisels may not be redirected once the cut is started; they must be completely withdrawn and a new cut begun. The osteotome, however, may be shifted slightly by raising or lowering the handle, and until one becomes experienced it is the safer of the two instruments. If a mallet is used, only light taps should be delivered in order to guard against a sudden, unplanned dip of the sharp instrument into the nasal dorsum.

The use of a sharp rasp may also accomplish a sufficient dorsal correction, but it is our preference to reserve the rasp for final corrections after hump excision with a chisel. On occasion a lateral osteotomy with a 2- or 3-mm. osteotome and infracture may result in sufficient narrowing of the nose without disrupting the dorsum. When there is doubt about the wisdom of this procedure, the surgeon should resort to medial osteotomy without dorsal resection and follow this with lateral osteotomy.

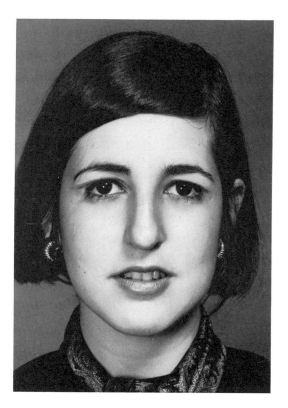
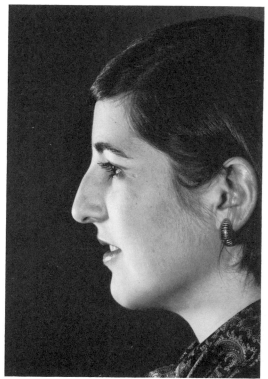
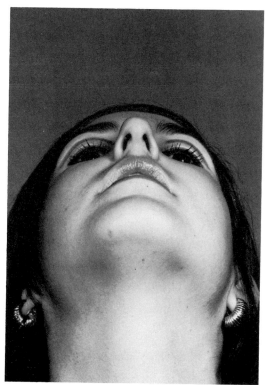

322

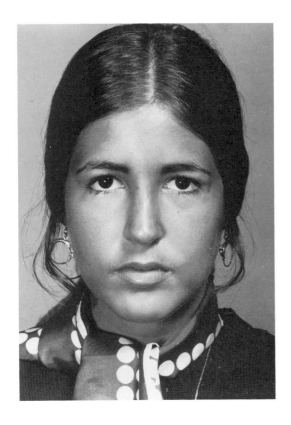

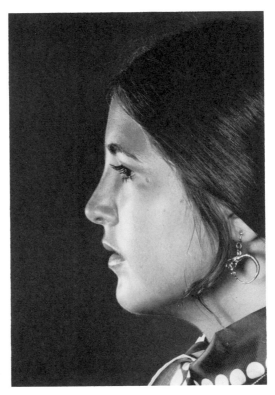

Minimal resection of the dorsal profile is required in a deformity of this type. The relatively large nose is balanced by the strong face. The postoperative views demonstrate the result of minimal tip elevation and only slight resection of nasal dorsum.

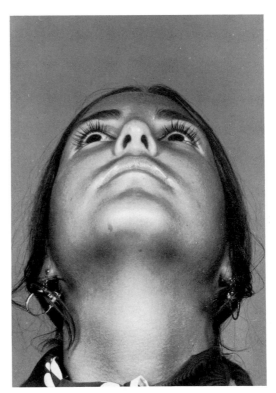

A tiny nasal hump was removed by rasping of the dorsum and this was followed by lateral osteotomies to achieve nasal narrowing and minimal lowering of the cartilaginous dorsum.

A conservative trim of the cephalic one third of the alar cartilages was also done, maintaining most of the cartilages intact. It is particularly important in post-teenage rhinoplasties to concentrate on these slight and subtle changes. Nothing is more disastrous than overoperation in the adult nose.

It has been said that successful nasal surgery is, for the most part, the surgery of "bits and pieces" — a little bit here and a little bit there. This is certainly a valid philosophy in a case such as the one shown on the opposite page. The aim is to modify the nose and not really change it much.

A small hump such as this can sometimes be rasped, although rasping is rarely sufficient for most bony humps. Actually small humps can be decorticated or shaved with a hand-held osteotome provided it is very sharp. A complete lateral osteotomy and adequate infracture probably contribute more to the result than any other single maneuver.

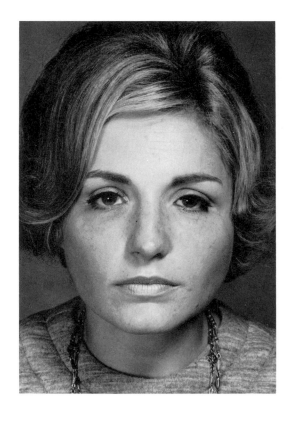
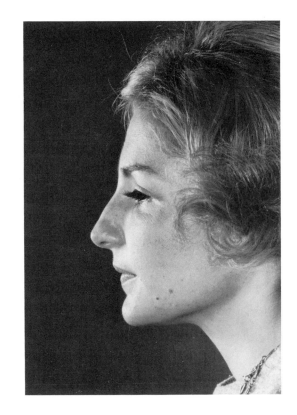
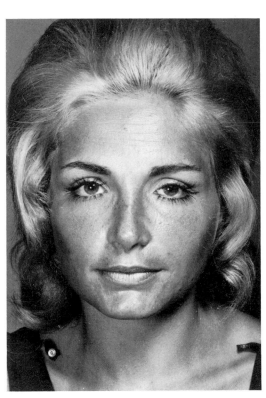
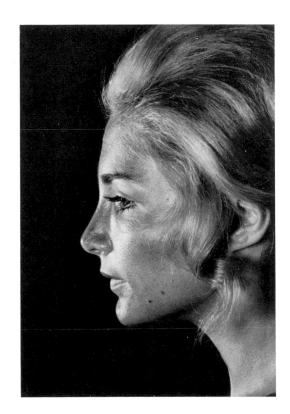

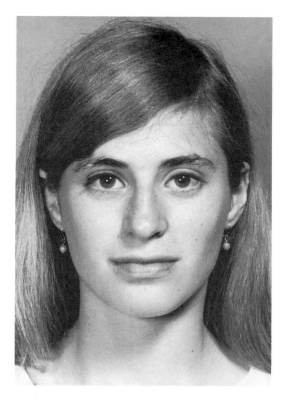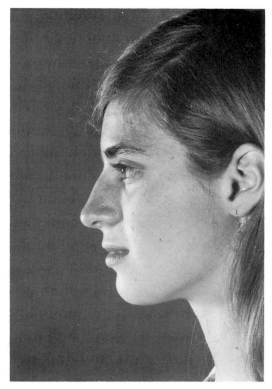

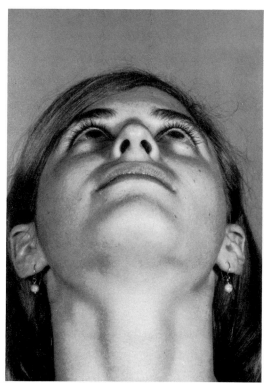

326

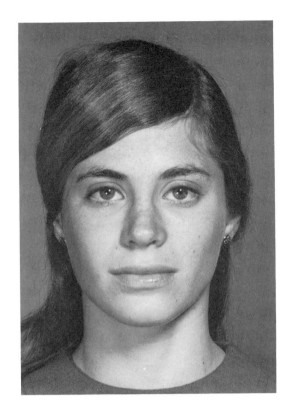

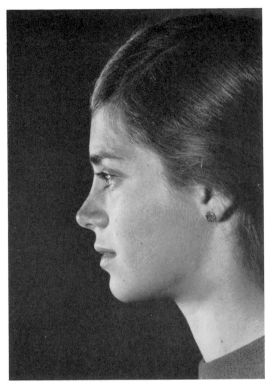

Removing a small extra amount of nasal hump can produce a pert upturned appearance. The slight overcorrection shown in these postoperative views, although producing a satisfactory result in this patient, would be disastrous in the patient adamantly opposed to any scooping of the nasal dorsum.

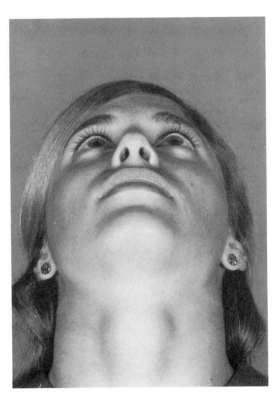

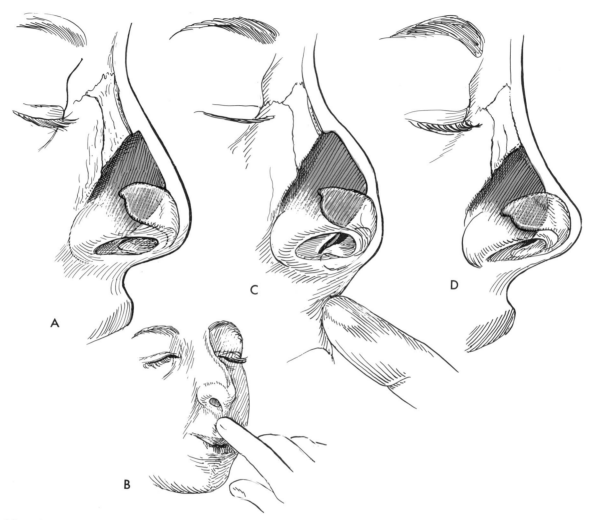

At this point in the operation, it is necessary to bring the cartilaginous septum into harmony with the new bony profile *(A)*. An estimate is made of the amount of excess cartilage by the Aufricht test, which is inferior traction of the upper lip by the surgeon's finger *(B)*. The dorsal border of the septum is brought into prominence *(C)*, and the nasal tip cartilages are dislocated from the septal angle.

In addition to looking for obvious dorsal irregularities, the surgeon can often detect invisible ones by gently passing his finger along the dorsum from the nasofrontal angle to the septal angle. Inspection is aided by using an Aufricht retractor, which enables one to determine whether the excess of dorsum is due to septum alone or involves the medial borders of the upper lateral cartilages. The recent addition of fiberoptic lighting to the Aufricht retractor has facilitated this procedure.

Excess septal and upper lateral cartilage is removed under direct vision until the new profile line is established *(D)*. Removal of this tissue should be conservative, for excision of too much tissue can be disastrous. We prefer to overcorrect in this region by about 0.5 mm., believing that we thereby obviate any tendency to later supratip prominence. Careful inspection of the dorsum at this point detects any remaining loose spicules of cartilage or bone and verifies the smoothness of the dorsal cuts.

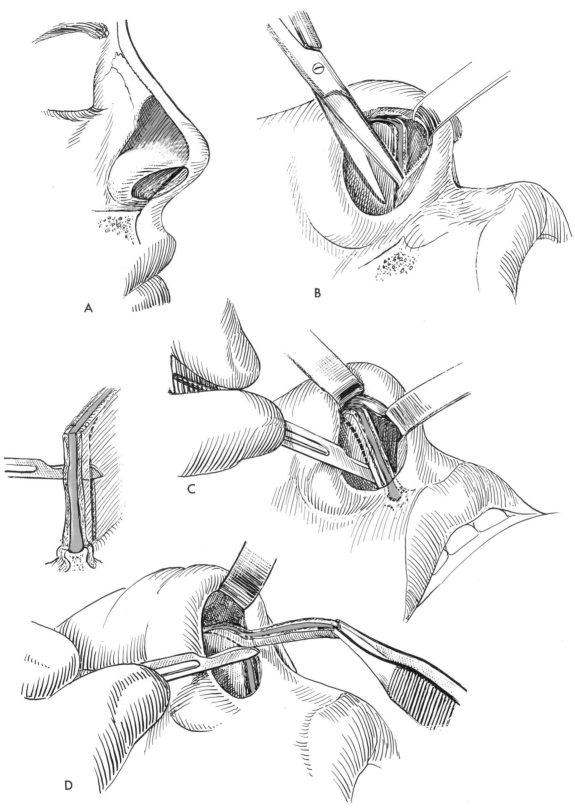

A, Short upper lip before the caudal border of the cartilaginous nasal septum is shortened. *B,* When necessary, the transfixion incision is deepened posteriorly with Stevens scissors to more adequately expose the caudal border of the septum. *C,* A segment of cartilage and mucosa is removed from the caudal border with a No. 15 blade. It is important that the line of resection preserve a natural curve in order to mimic the normal convexity of the columella. *D,* Removal of the segment is completed by curving the line of the incision into the dorsal border. The septal angle must be curved, not sharp.

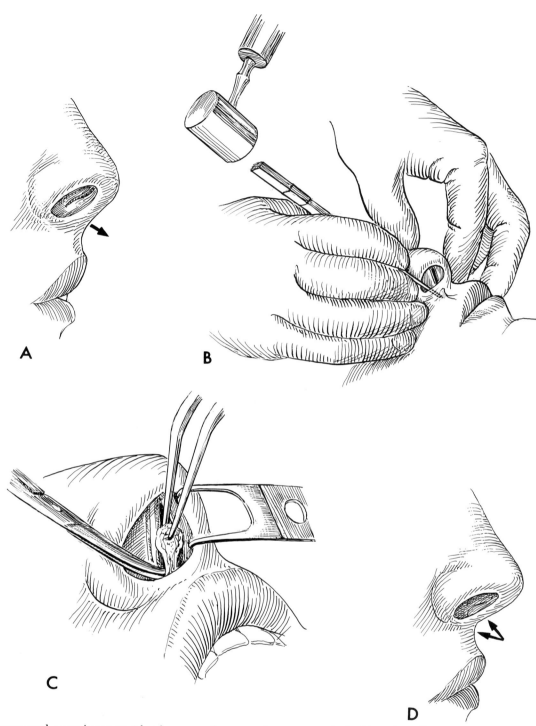

A, A large and prominent nasal spine sometimes produces an undesirable columella-lip angle and an apparent shortening of the upper lip. *B*, This nasal spine can be carefully resected with a 7- or 8-mm. osteotome. *C*, After osteotomy the bony segment is separated from the adherent soft tissue and removed. *D*, The new columella-lip angle.

Routine removal of the nasal spine has been advocated, but we do not believe in this practice. Removal of the bone may make it desirable to remove an additional strip from the caudal end of the septum, and this possibility should be considered in advance. Final adjustment of this region is best deferred until completion of the tip plasty.

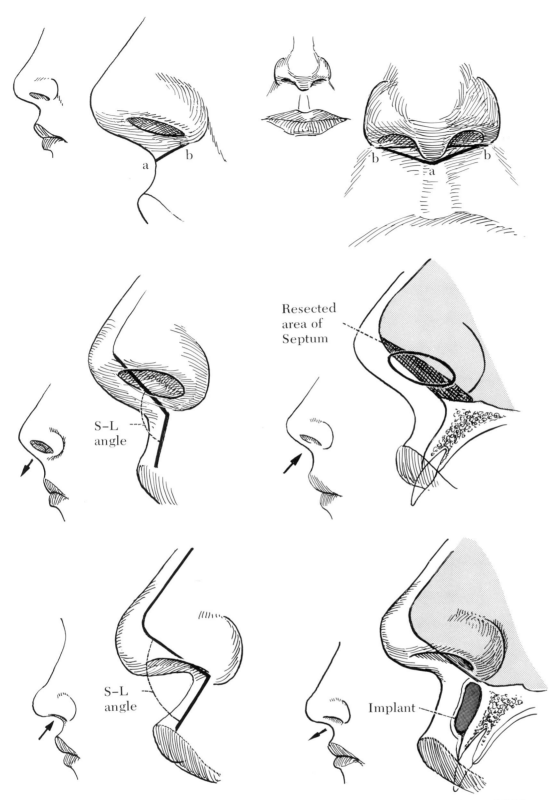

The columellar-alar angle (a–b) and the septolabial angle (S–L) are two important angles establishing symmetry of the nose in its overall relationship to the face. These angles are adjustable to a degree during rhinoplasty by excision of the caudal margin of the septum, the inferior margin of the medial crura, the nasal spine, and the alar bases. Great care must be exercised in the amount of resection of the nasal spine and the caudal margin of the septum in particular. Usually the amount of resection should be minimal to preserve naturalness of contour so that the columella is visible hanging below the alar margins and the septolabial angle remains obtuse. An acute septolabial angle either occurring naturally or as the result of excessive resection of the caudal septum and/or nasal spine is unsightly. An obtuse septolabial angle can sometimes be corrected by an implant of septal cartilage or other material in the region of the nasal spine during or after rhinoplasty (Aufricht).

331

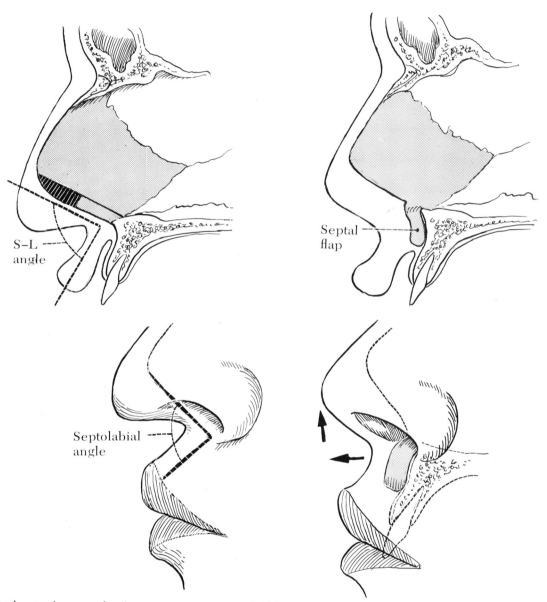

A method sometimes used to improve an acute septolabial angle is the rotation of a cartilage flap from the caudal margin of the septum as shown here.

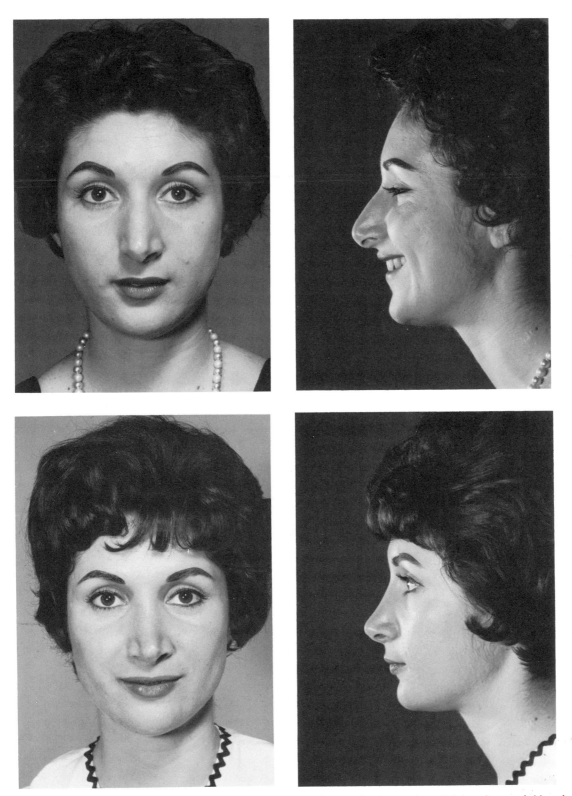

Lengthening of the upper lip was accomplished by removing the nasal spine and modifying the caudal border of the septum as well as trimming the inferior margins of the medial crura.

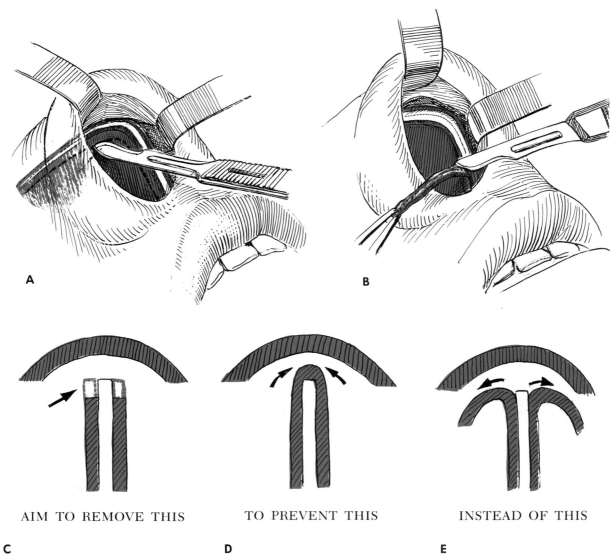

AIM TO REMOVE THIS   TO PREVENT THIS   INSTEAD OF THIS

C   D   E

Removal of a strip of mucosa from the septal cartilage protects against overgrowth of septal mucosa following surgery. This growth could result in either a mass of granulation tissue lying along the nasal dorsum, or in mucosa from each side meeting to form a passage across the dorsum. In either instance a sizable "poly" tip may result and mar an otherwise successful rhinoplasty.

A, A 2- to 3-mm. strip of mucosa is removed from the dorsal and caudal borders of the septal cartilage on either side.

B, Completion of mucosa removal along the caudal margin.

C, The suggested amount of tissue to be removed.

D, Where inadequate tissue is removed, failure of apposition of the overlying soft tissues and the dorsal border of the septum can occur. Septal mucosa may then enlarge, and the two sides may meet. This is not infrequently followed by the formation of granulation tissue and a supratip swelling which will require secondary surgery for correction.

E, The normal union of the septal mucosa to the mucosa underlying the upper lateral cartilages.

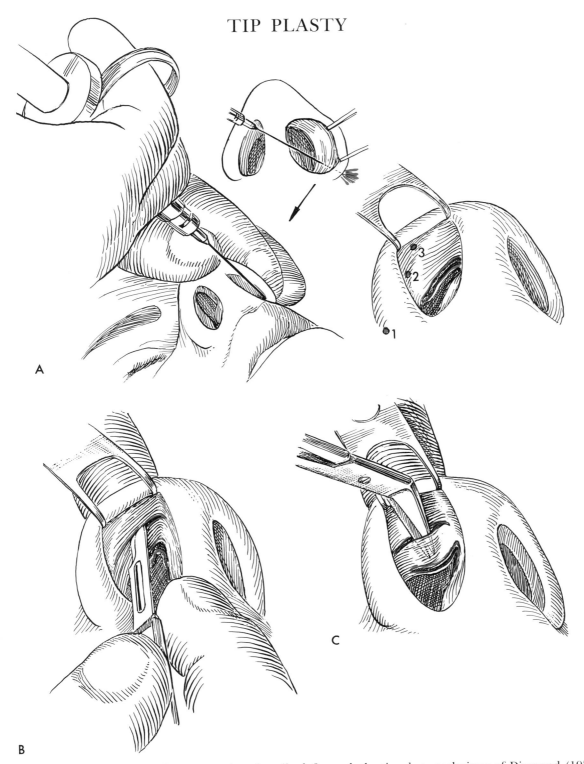

In patients with alar cartilages that are weak and easily deformed, the tip plasty technique of Diamond (1971) gives satisfactory results. It leaves a more substantial rim of cartilage than the other methods described, and this extra support softens the angularity that would otherwise tend to occur at the area of the new alar dome. The technique is excellent for routine use as well, provided the surgeon takes into account the need for weakening the cartilages of the alar dome region in the patient with normally strong cartilages.

A, Local anesthetic solution is infiltrated into the alar base to block branches of the infraorbital nerve and the anterior superior dental nerve.

B, After slight eversion of the nostril rim an incision is made through the lining skin approximately midway between rim and internal nares. The incision passes only through the lining skin.

C, The nasal tip scissors are used to lift the lining skin from the underlying lateral crus of the alar cartilage.

(Illustration continued on following page.)

335

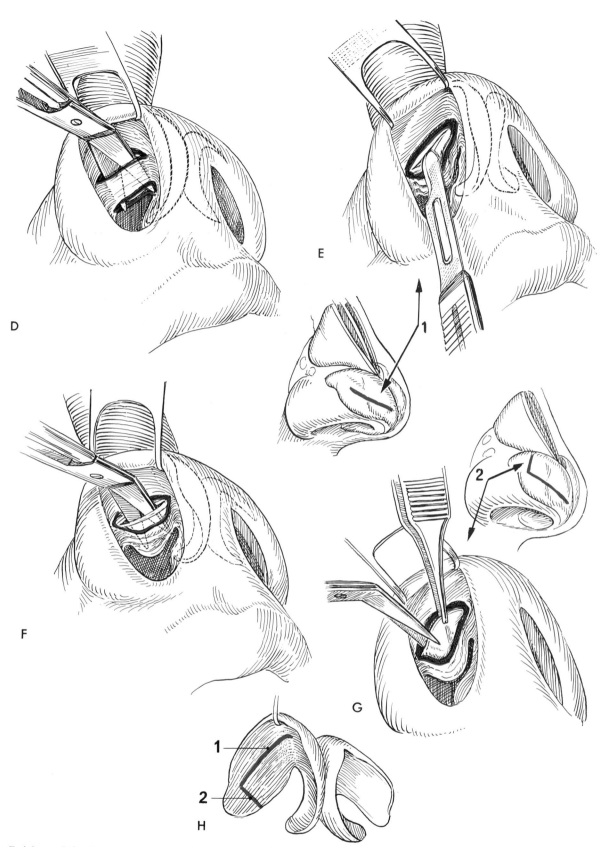

D, Raising of the lining skin is carefully completed by widely opening the nasal tip scissors.

E, The lateral crus of the alar cartilage is incised from the point of junction with the medial crus laterally in a line with the skin incision.

F, Nasal tip scissors are passed through the intercartilaginous incision, and soft tissues are raised from the external aspect of the alar cartilage.

G, The cartilage is pulled superiorly and transected laterally by a single cut with the tip scissors.

H, The alar cartilages from below.

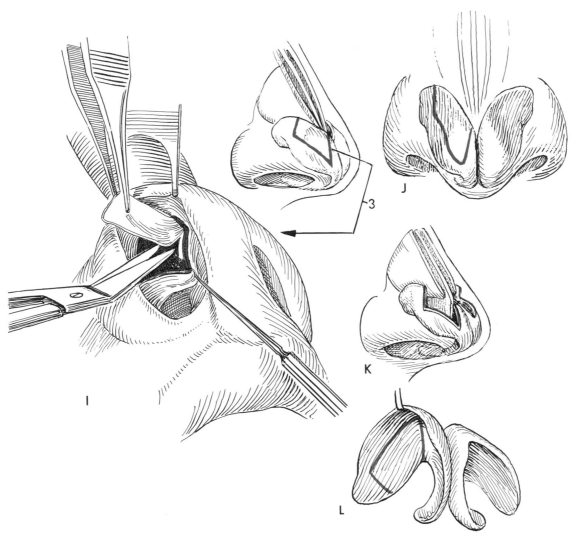

I, The alar cartilages are freed medially and the segment is finally removed by a cut directed anteroposteriorly, as shown in the accompanying diagram.

J, The usual area of cartilage to be resected.

K, The cartilage resected.

L, View of the alar cartilage that would be presented from below. The superolateral plate of the lateral crus is carefully maintained to prevent an unsightly groove at this point.

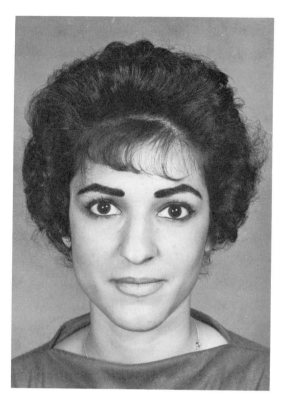
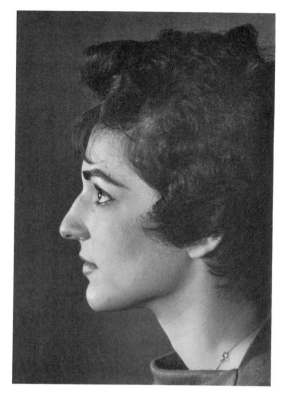
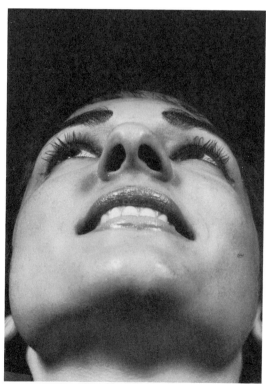

338

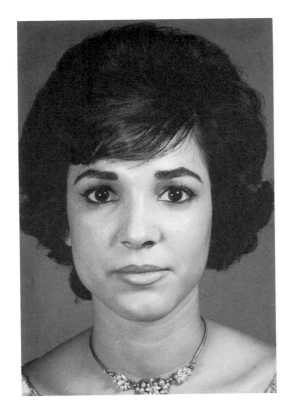

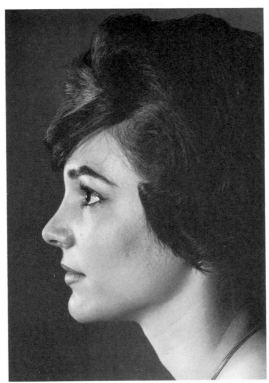

Correction of a nasal tip deformity by the Diamond technique.

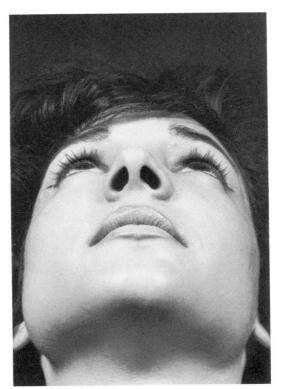

There is no one procedure that may be applied to all types of nasal tip deformities. The tip is the most difficult part of the nose to correct, and it requires ingenuity and flexibility in the approach of the surgeon.

We use three basic approaches to the tip cartilage. In order of frequency, these are (1) the transcartilaginous (intercartilaginous) approach, (2) the alar flap, and (3) the retrograde (eversion) technique. The transcartilaginous approach bisects the length of the lateral crus. Championed by Converse, this technique is indicated for the correction of most tips, being extended or adapted to suit the individual case. It is our technique of choice, except in patients with marked forward projection of the tip, very sharp angulation of the alar cartilages, bifid tips, and huge, "beefy" tips with excessive soft tissue or alar cartilage.

A, The nostril rim is everted after block anesthesia of the alar base is obtained. The vestibular lining may be elevated from the lateral crus by injection with local anesthetic, using a very fine needle. This infiltration aids the dissection by defining the subperichondral plane.

B, A hockey-stick-shaped incision begins medially at a point corresponding to the mark representing the alar dome on the external skin. The incision parallels the rim, extending from the apex of the dome laterally for a variable distance, usually about 1.5 cm. A slight medial or lateral shifting of the point where this incision is started will result in a corresponding diminution or increase in nasal tip width in this region.

C, Using the nasal tip scissors and spreading them widely, the nasal lining skin is raised from the underlying lateral crus of the alar cartilage.

D, Another incision of the same shape is made through the lateral crus. The incision leaves intact a margin of at least 3 mm. of alar cartilage, so that approximately two thirds or three fourths of the cephalic portion of the crus will be resected in the average patient.

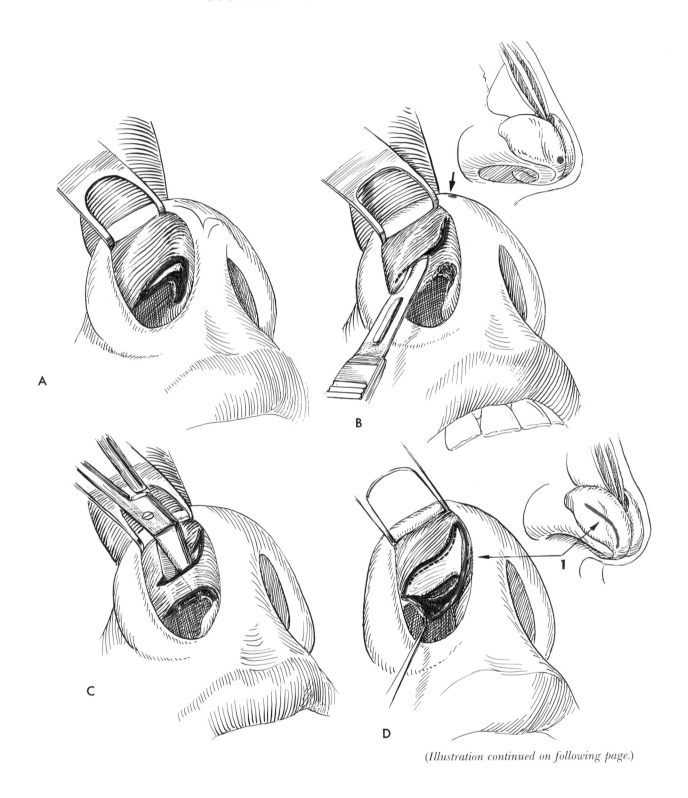

A

B

C

D

(Illustration continued on following page.)

E, The incision is made down to but not through the cartilage, and the lining is elevated subperichondrally with nasal tip scissors.

F, The cartilage is carefully incised and dissected free from the subcutaneous tissue. When traction is applied, the cartilage is transected laterally. Resection does not extend for the entire lateral width of the cartilage, for grooving of the overlying skin is apt to occur if this is done.

G, The redundant cartilage is raised medially with a forceps and resected to the dome, where it narrows markedly in width. The dome is not interfered with unless this is necessary for a contour change. The surgeon should endeavor to accomplish this third cut with a single movement so as to minimize the chance of leaving a small spicule of cartilage that may later become evident as healing progresses.

H, A few interrupted plain catgut sutures may be used to close the incision. They are not necessary, but they facilitate healing and flap apposition.

I, The cartilage resection from below.

J, The resection viewed from above.

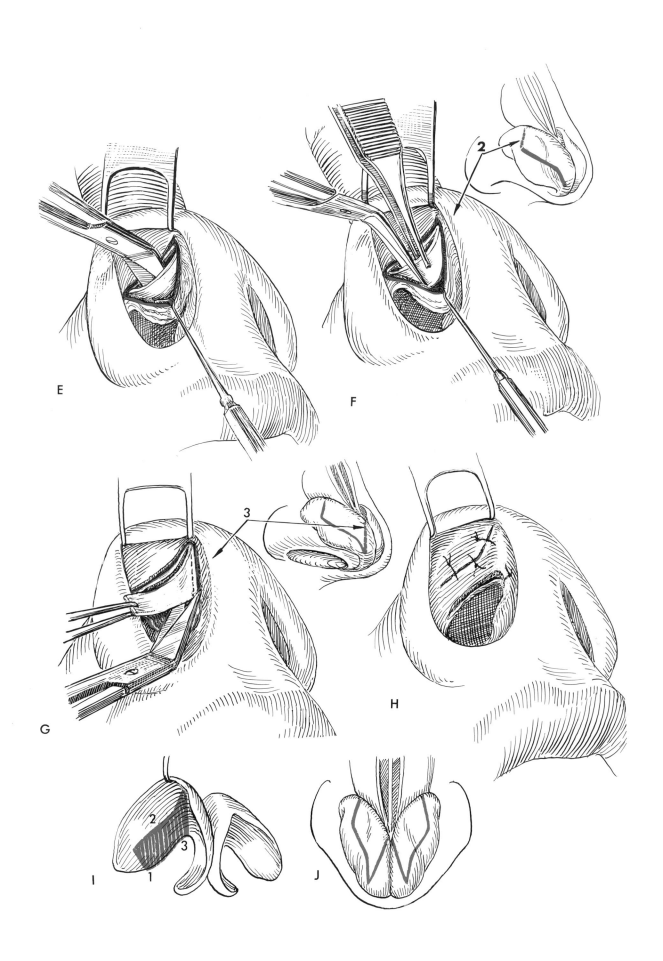

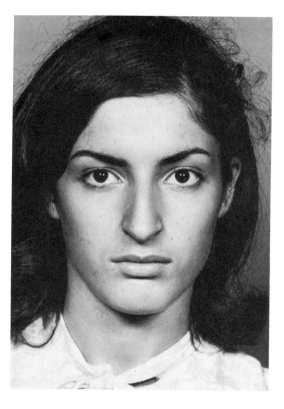
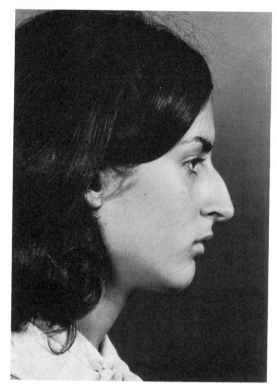
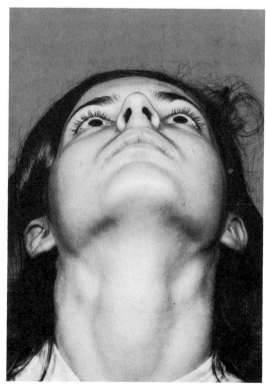

344

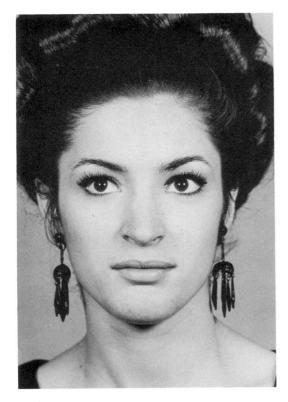
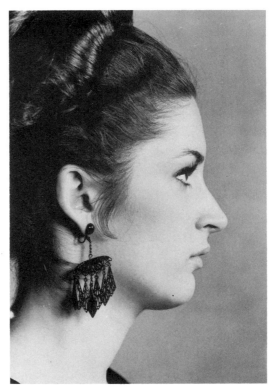

A patient with moderate drooping of the nasal tip and osteocartilaginous hump, which was corrected by the Converse intercartilaginous technique.

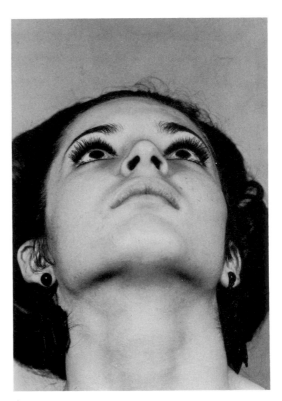

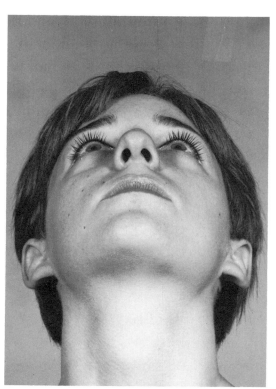
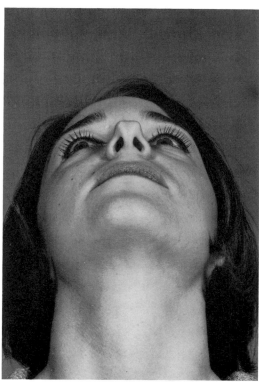

Development of a "boxed" tip after nasal tip plasty in which bifidity was not corrected and the alar "spring" was broken.

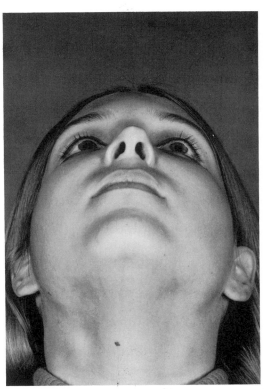 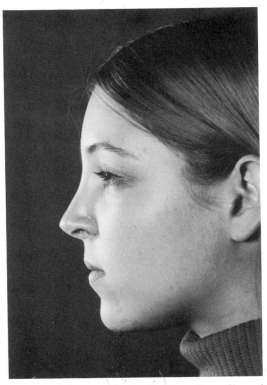

A complete breaking of the continuity of the alar cartilage may result in a small spicule of cartilage distorting the nasal tip skin, as in the postoperative view of this patient.

The rule in tip plasty is to be conservative, since there is nothing harder to repair than an overoperated nasal tip. If too much cartilage or lining has been sacrificed, little can be done to salvage the situation. Some surgeons have claimed that all the lateral crus can be resected without impairing the tip, either cosmetically or functionally. While this may be true in patients with thick, rigid skin and subcutaneous tissue, or in secondary operations where considerable scar tissue is present, it is not true in the average patient with more delicate tip cartilage and skin. Alar collapse can and does occur, and it is always preferable to leave a small margin of the cartilage to act as a spring. It is also better not to break this spring, though in fact this is often necessary, particularly at the domes. Dicing or morseling the cartilage so that it can be shaped or molded is a reasonable alternative.

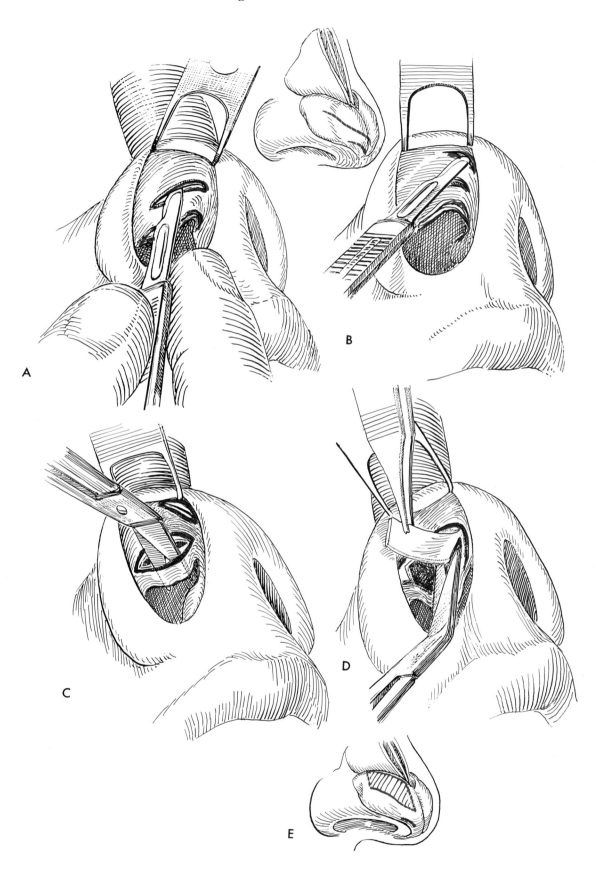

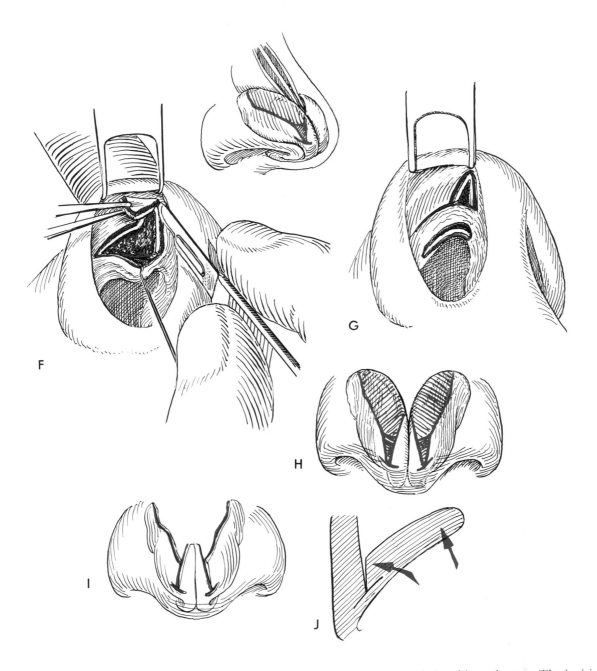

F

G

H

I

J

A, A transverse incision is made laterally from the point of junction of the medial and lateral crura. The incision may be made through both skin and underlying alar cartilage and is usually at the junction of the middle and lower thirds of that cartilage so as to straddle the region of the alar dome.

B, A similar but shorter transverse incision 1 to 2 mm. from the inferior border of the alar cartilage straddles the region of the alar dome.

C, With the nasal tip scissors, the lining nasal skin and overlying soft tissues are removed from both aspects of the lateral crus of the alar cartilage.

D, The segment to be removed is transected, both medially and laterally.

E, The area of cartilage excision.

F, A triangular segment of nasal lining skin and the underlying adherent alar cartilage is removed. The apex of this triangle lies at the alar dome.

G, The resection is completed.

H, The areas of cartilage to be resected.

I, Closure of the triangular defect by superior and medial rotation of the lateral crura of the alar cartilage.

J, A schematic diagram of the rotation: the intact narrow strip of cartilage at the alar border serves to soften the angle formed by this resection and produces a more rounded tip than does, for example, the hockey-stick resection procedure.

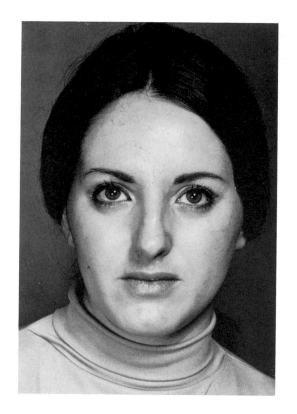 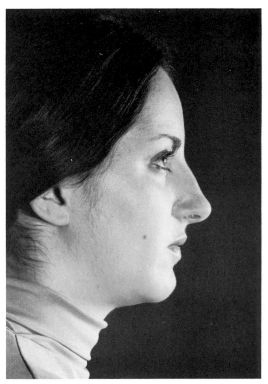

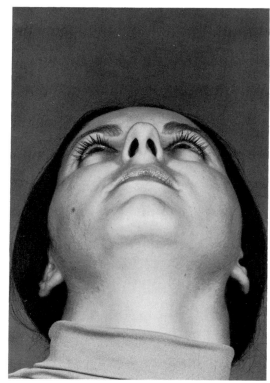

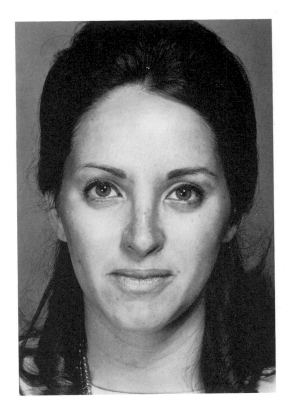

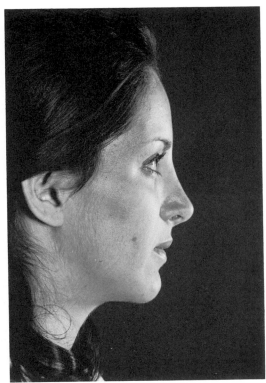

Correction of a nasal tip deformity by the modified Joseph technique.

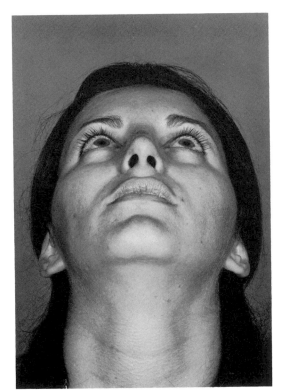

The entire dome of the alar cartilage, including most of the lateral crus, can be delivered as a bipedicle or laterally based unipedicle flap if the alar deformity is unusual and considerable dissection of the alar cartilages is expected. This technique requires a marginal rim incision that extends around the dome and continues medially into the columella, with care being taken to preserve the "soft triangle" of skin. The cartilage is left attached to the vestibular lining flap. Variations of this technique have been recommended for many years by Eitner (1932), Aufricht (1943, 1971), Goldman (1957), Dufourmentel (1959), Lipsett (1959), Fomon (1960), Safian (1970), and others.

We use the alar flap technique for those unusual conditions in which the transcartilaginous approach is unsatisfactory. It provides excellent exposure of the alar cartilages, permitting them to be carved, incised and resected according to need, while at the same time maintaining their blood supply and attachment to the soft lining skin. When this technique is used, the flap must be carefully repositioned and meticulously sutured. The tip can be molded without difficulty.

A, An incision through the entire vertical length of the alar cartilages is made along the line of junction between the medial and lateral crura.

B, The segment of skin and underlying alar cartilage is lifted laterally.

C, A triangular segment of both the nasal lining skin and the alar cartilage is removed from the region of the junction with the medial crus.

D, The triangular portion of the cartilage to be resected and the superior and inferior borders of the alar cartilage to be removed.

E, Resection of the superior and inferior segments, including attached nasal lining skin.

F, Cartilaginous section completed.

G, Closure is facilitated by the use of 4–0 plain catgut sutures.

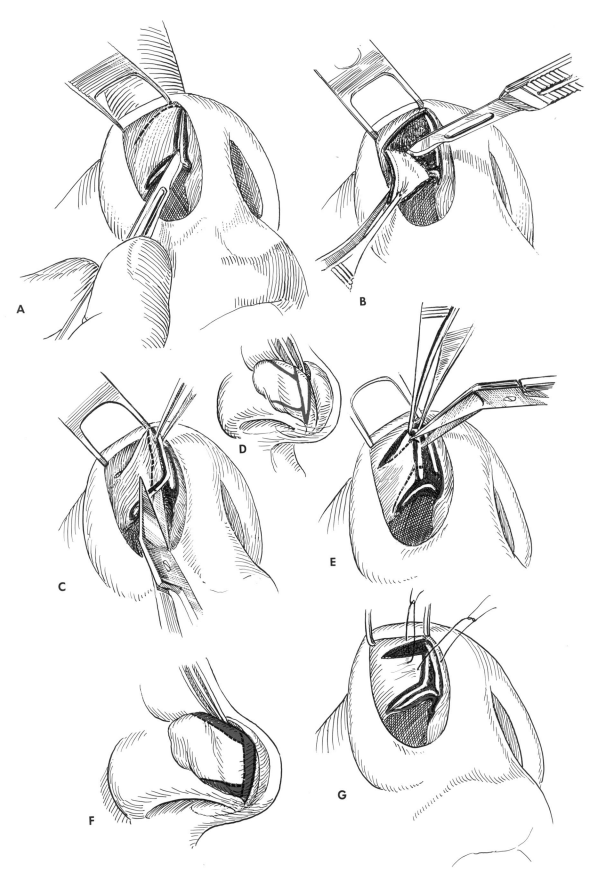

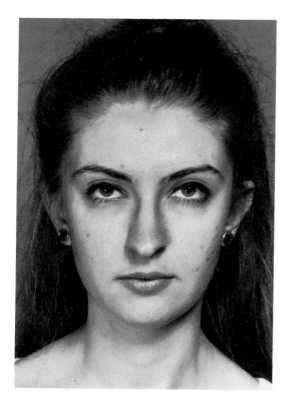
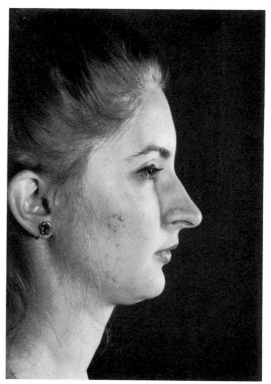
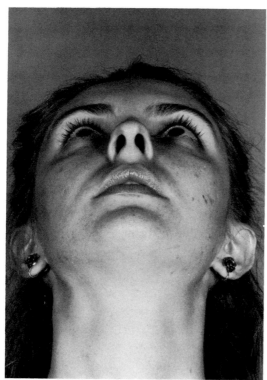

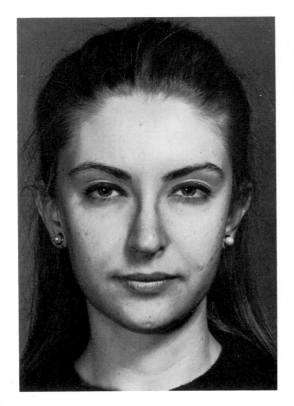

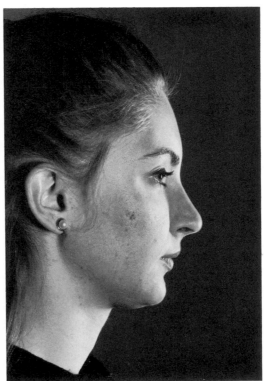

Correction of the nasal tip by the alar flap technique. The broad, flat alar cartilages plunging downward are best reduced and reshaped by this technique.

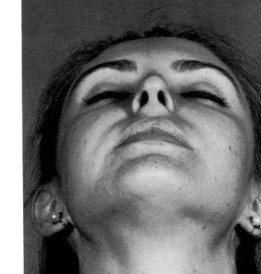

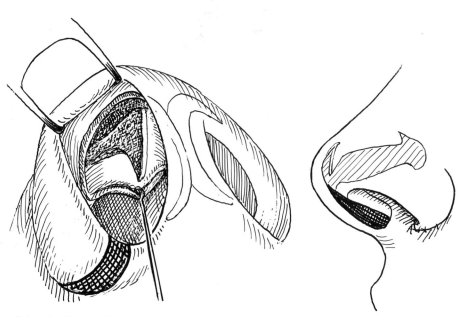

A modification of the alar flap and rim technique with preservation of the continuity of the alar rim, and alar base resection combined with a modification of the caudal border of the medial crura.

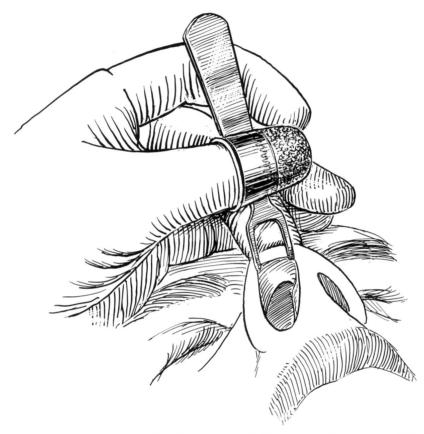

The thimble double-pronged retractor of Millard is a most useful instrument in surgery of the nasal tip. It facilitates accurate control of the alae during surgery and finger palpation of the external skin during cartilage excision.

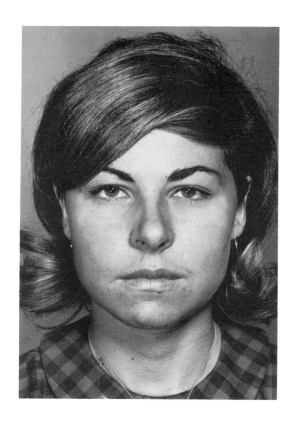
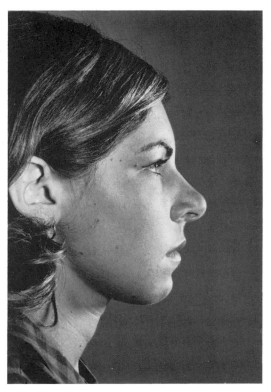
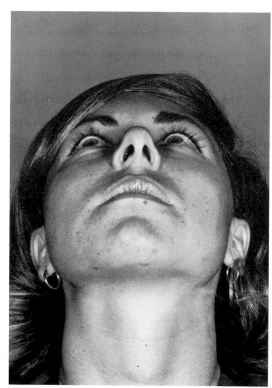

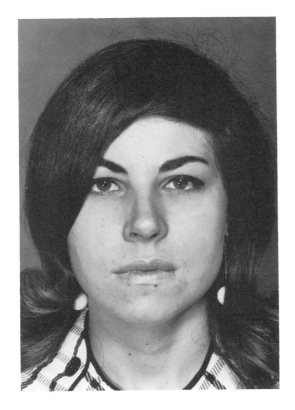

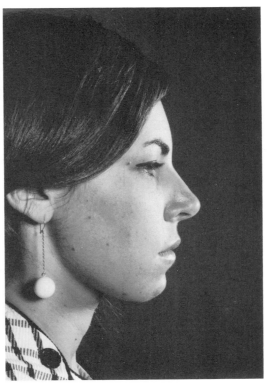

Correction of a tip deformity by the modified alar flap technique. Note the maintenance of the natural alar base following the resection.

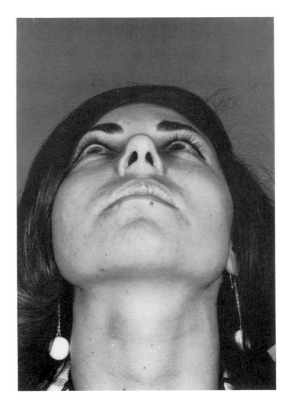

For the very bulky, thick-skinned nose, in which the surgeon wishes to sacrifice some lining skin as well as cartilage in an effort to reduce bulk, the eversion technique is useful. It is acceptable for most tips and, in fact, it differs very little from the transcartilaginous technique except that the dissection is retrograde. The method has been used extensively by Rode (1938), Brown and McDowell (1965), and others. The eversion technique of exposure facilitates the "hockey-stick" excision of alar cartilage under direct vision.

A, An incision is made anteroposteriorly along the junction between the medial and lateral crura. The incision extends from a point just inside the rim of the alar cartilage.

B, Both alar cartilage and nasal lining skin are lifted as a single unit by the nasal tip scissors.

C, The cartilage (only) is incised from its outer aspect with a No. 15 blade.

D, The area of cartilage to be resected is carefully raised, leaving the nasal lining skin intact.

E, The area of cartilage to be excised.

F, Closure of the triangular defect in the region of the alar dome by superior and medial rotation of the lateral crura.

G, The procedure completed. The vertical incision can be sutured.

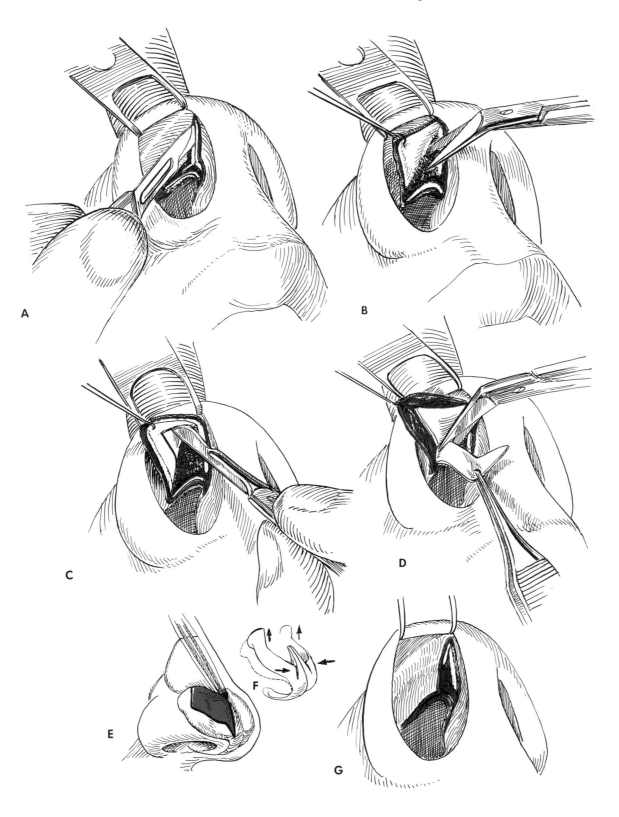

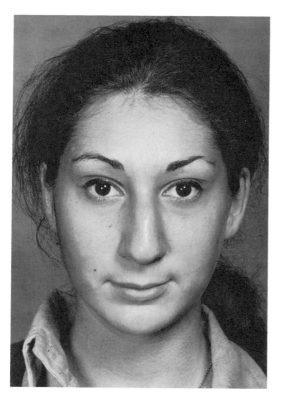
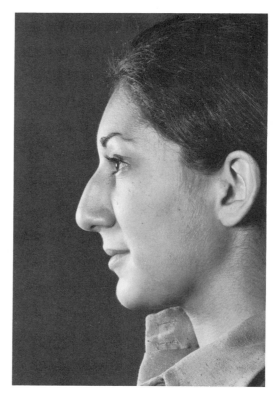
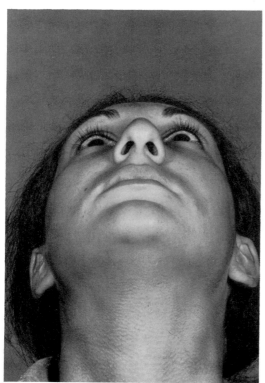

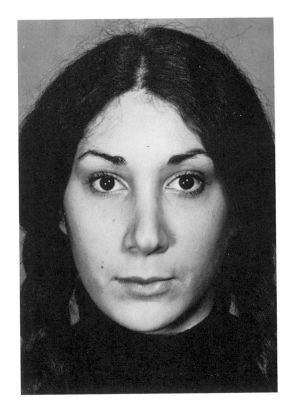

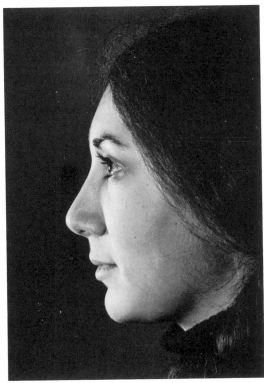

Correction of a thick nasal tip by the eversion technique. The postoperative result, while satisfactory, shows that limitations were imposed on the operator by the thick skin.

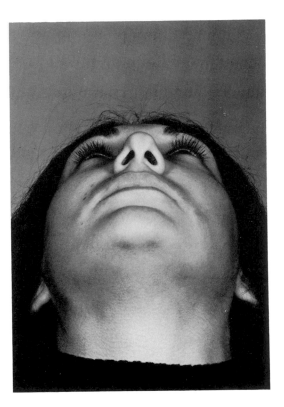

Exposure of the alar cartilages through a rim incision (Safian, 1970).

A, The inferior margin of the alar cartilage is carefully located and, with care taken to preserve the soft triangle, an incision is made immediately distal to it.

B, Nasal tip scissors are used to free both the medial and lateral crura of the alar cartilage, which are delivered into the external nares.

C, Supporting the area of junction between the medial and lateral crura, an incision is directed anteroposteriorly from the posterior border to a point about 2 to 3 mm. internal to the distal border of the alar cartilage.

D, A hockey-stick-shaped incision is completed laterally. The underlying nasal lining skin is protected from damage. The cartilage is then removed from the lining skin with nasal tip scissors.

It is essential that the incision be placed at the free margin of the lateral crus and the dome of the alar cartilage, and not at the nostril margin. Incision through the soft triangle will result in notching of this area, which is formed by soft tissue alone without any supporting cartilage. With care, the cartilage may be resected without damaging the vestibular skin. If it is necessary to cut completely through the dome, extreme care must be observed in the splinting lest the crura be displaced relative to one another, with a resulting twisting of the columella and asymmetry of the tip. Preservation of the lining intact will help considerably in preventing this deformity.

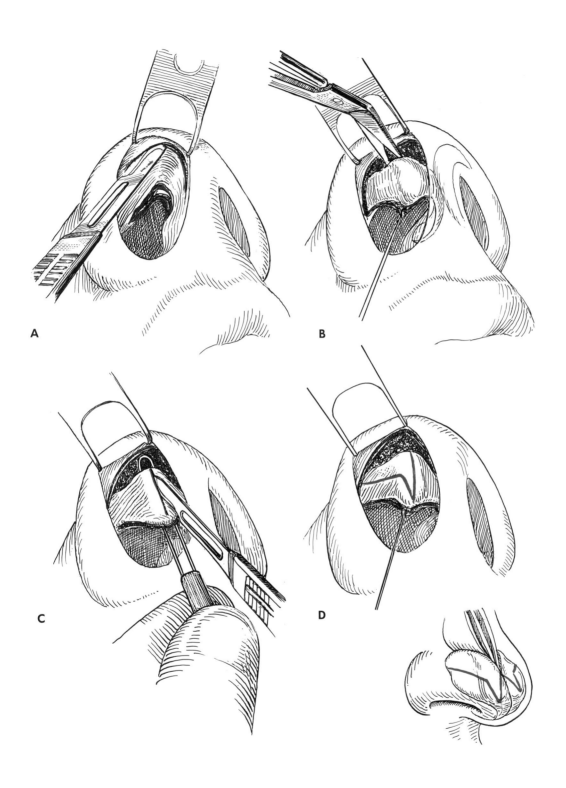

A

B

C

D

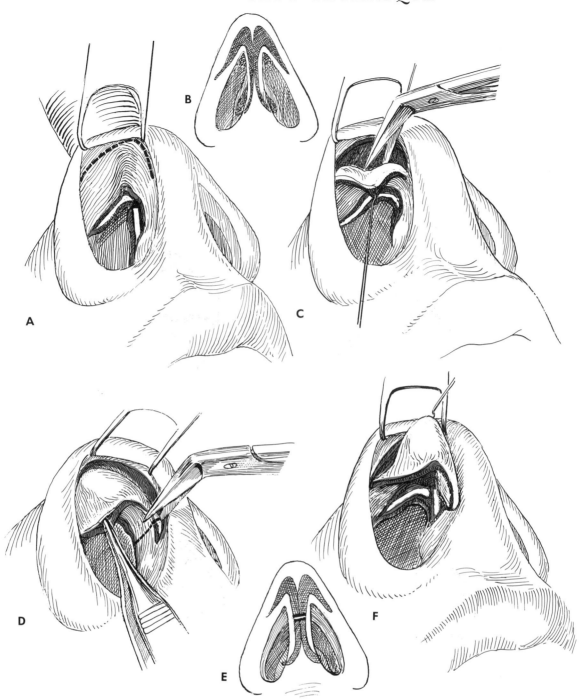

Though strictly speaking a variation of the alar flap method, the technique proposed by Lipsett (1959) is of sufficient importance to warrant separate consideration. Lipsett extends the marginal incision down along the anterior border of the medial crus to the point of junction of the middle and anterior thirds. At this point he incises through skin and medial crus back to join the transfixion incision; the cartilages are separated from each other and from the overlying skin, but remain attached to the vestibular lining skin and are prolapsed into the nostrils. The cartilages are then reshaped by a series of vertically directed incisions that spare the vestibular skin, and any excess of cartilage is removed from the medial crus. The new dome is remodeled with the now easily malleable cartilage.

A, A rim incision carefully preserves the soft triangle.

B, A phantom view of the cartilages from below.

C, The alar cartilages are freed from their attachment to the overlying nasal skin.

D, The alar cartilages and their attached nasal lining skin are pulled laterally, and the medial crus of the alar cartilage is transected at its approximate mid-point.

E, Transection of the medial crura.

F, The alar cartilage is prolapsed inferiorly.

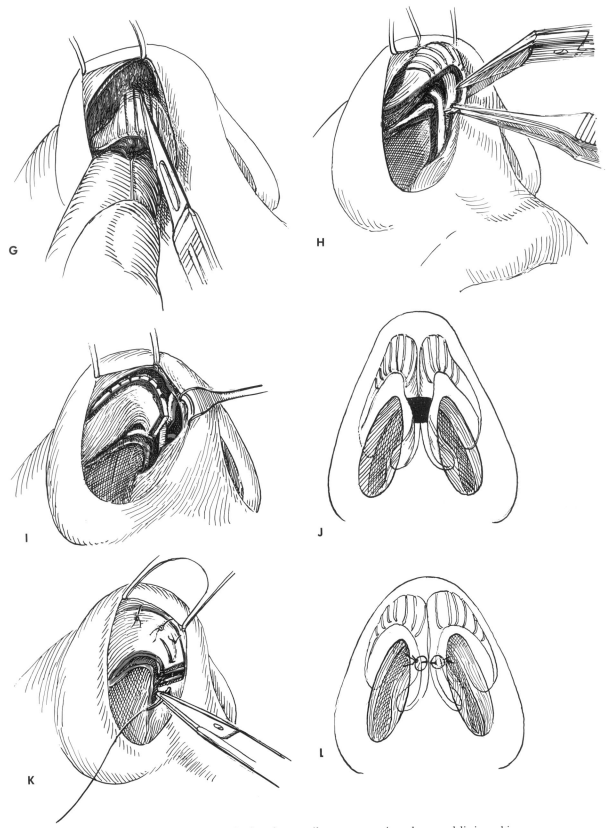

G, Anteroposterior cuts are made through the alar cartilage, preserving the nasal lining skin.

H, After the new nasal tip contour is formed, the excess length of medial crus is estimated and resected with its attached nasal lining skin.

I, The area of resection.

J, Phantom view of the nasal cartilages, showing the lines of incision and the area of resection.

K, Repair by 4-0 plain catgut sutures.

L, The completed procedure in phantom view.

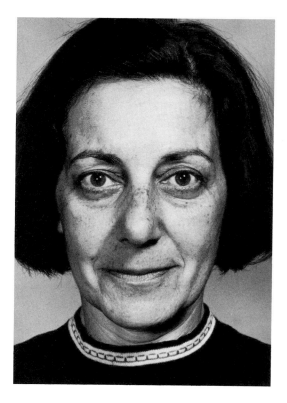
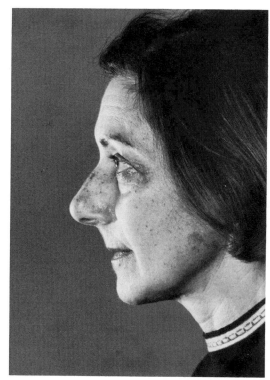
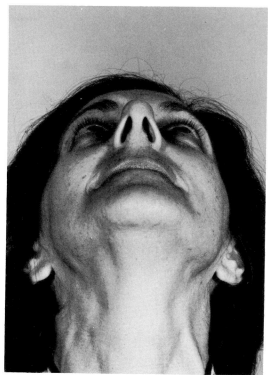

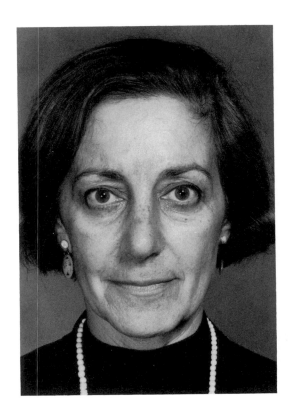

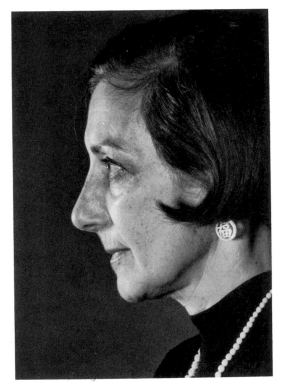

Repair of the nasal tip by the Lipsett procedure.

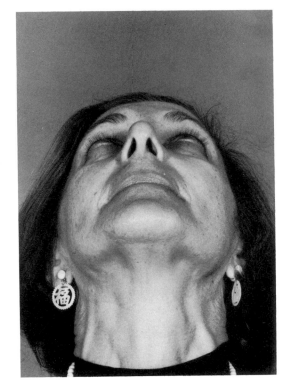

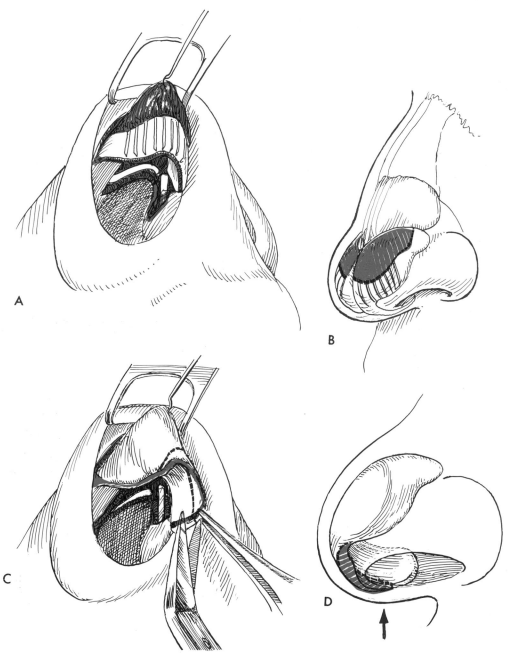

In complicated nasal tip deformities the Lipsett procedure shows great versatility in reshaping of the nasal cartilages.

A, The lines of incision and resection of the standard Lipsett procedure.

B, The Lipsett procedure combined with resection of a deformed, enlarged lateral crus.

C, The same procedure, this time combined with modification of the inferior border of the medial and lateral crus.

D, Elevation of the nasal tip achieved by this technique.

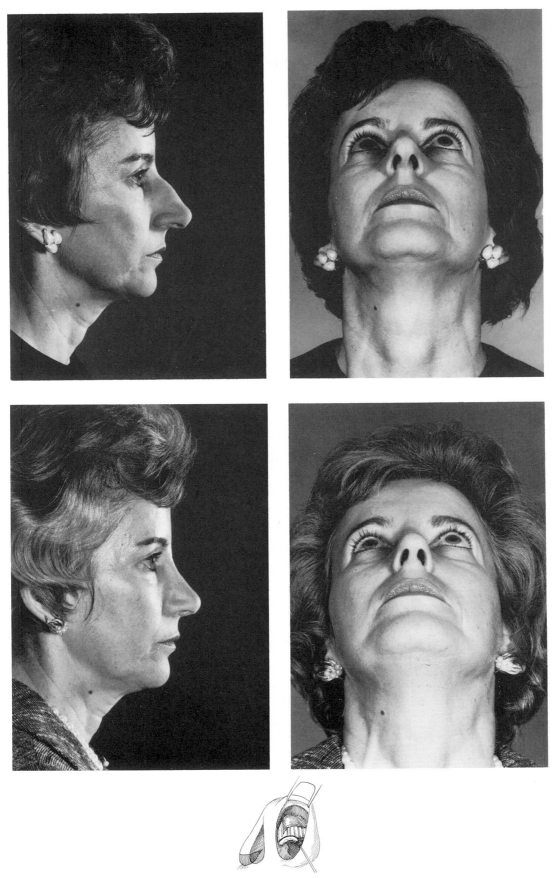

Correction of a complicated nasal tip deformity by a modified Lipsett technique. The drawing shows the technique employed: resection of the alar base, of the lateral crus of the alar cartilage, and of a portion of the rim in the dome region.

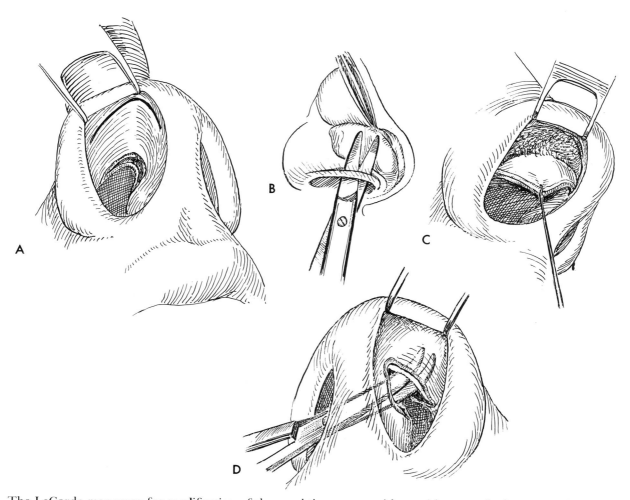

The LeGarde maneuver for modification of the nasal tip contour with or without cartilaginous resection.

A, A standard rim incision is made.

B, The nasal tip scissors are passed through the rim incision and the external aspect of the lateral crura of the alar cartilages to free these from their attachment to overlying skin.

C, The freed cartilages permit redraping of the skin.

D, Following a routine nasal tip plasty, the redraping is aided by freeing remaining alar cartilage remnants from the overlying skin.

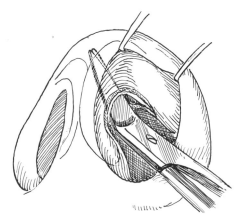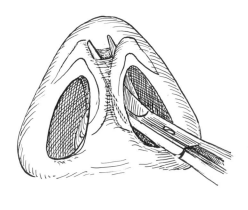

Moderate widening of the interdome proportion may be reduced by breaking up the fibro-areolar tissue in this region. Resulting scar contraction will pull the domes together. This technique is facilitated by resection of the supratip ligament (Pitanguy, 1965).

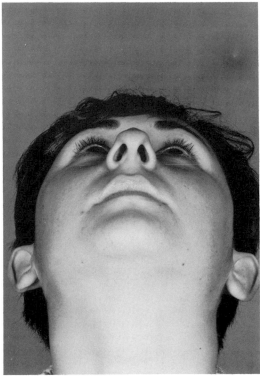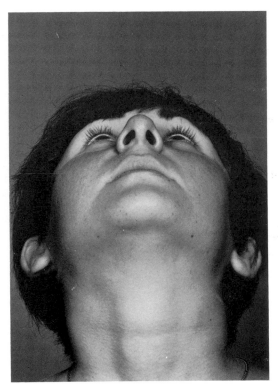

Moderate bifidity of the alar domes corrected by nasal tip plasty and breaking up of the interdome fibro-areolar tissues.

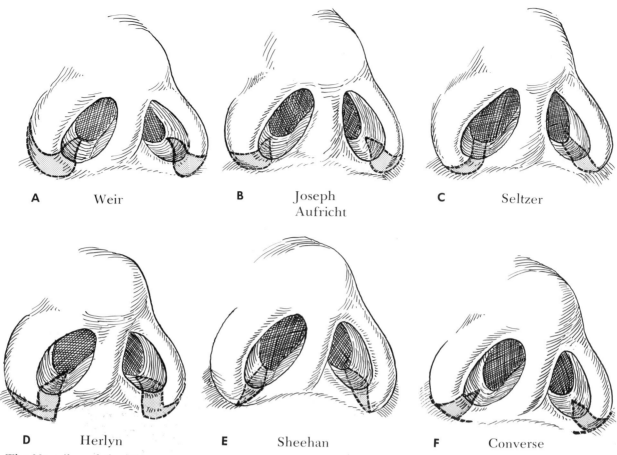

| **A** Weir | **B** Joseph Aufricht | **C** Seltzer |
| **D** Herlyn | **E** Sheehan | **F** Converse |

The Nostrils and the Alae

The shape of the nostrils is important to the final appearance of the nose. Certain surgical corrections can be undertaken at rhinoplasty which can measurably improve the result, but overly ambitious surgery of the nostril rims or alar bases can result in later deformities that are typical stigmata of the "operated nose." The surgeon should exercise care and discretion in his approach to these structures.

Flaring of the nostrils is a racial characteristic in blacks, Asians, and Indians, but it may also occur in whites. Furthermore, flaring may result from an operative procedure when it was not apparent before: lowering of the dorsum and setting back the tip relaxes the nostril margins and creates a slight flaring at the base. Millard (1965) claims that he excises a piece of the alar base in over 90 per cent of his patients for this reason, but this has not been our experience, and we average only 15 to 20 per cent.

Flaring can be improved or corrected by one of the several variations of alar base resections described classically by Weir (1892) and elaborated by Aufricht (1943) and others. It is best to maintain the scar in the natural vertical crease that is usually present in the floor of the nostril and extends slightly laterally. This is not always possible, and if significant reduction in the bulk of the alae or in the projection of the tip is required, the scar must sometimes extend laterally along the alar base. In this position it is apt to be more noticeable, as healing is not always perfect in this skin, laden as it is with sebaceous glands.

The different types of alar base resection shown in the drawings are used to achieve different goals:

A, Reduction in flare.

B, Reduction in both width and flare.

C, Reduction in width.

D, Reduction in width with a V-shaped staggering of the excision for a less pronounced scar.

E, Resection of a portion of the nasal floor to lessen flare.

F, Closure of the defect by advancement flaps of nasal floor and nasal cartilage; this has the disadvantage of creating more scars in this region.

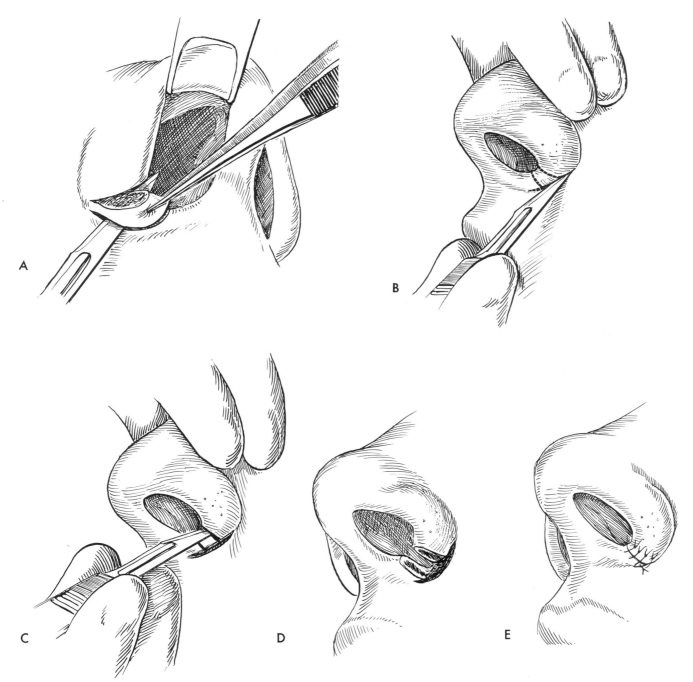

The classic alar base resection and a modified method.

A, Removal of an elliptical segment of the alar base gives the most natural result.

B, Removal of a square segment and closure by advancement of the nostril floor and the alar base.

C, Completion of the excision.

D, Freed medial and lateral flaps.

E, Closure by interrupted 5–0 nylon sutures. While it is possible to conceal the horizontal lines of the incision, these will always be more prominent than the lines of the classic elliptical resection.

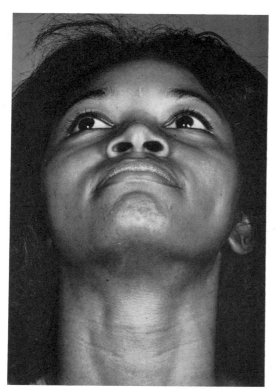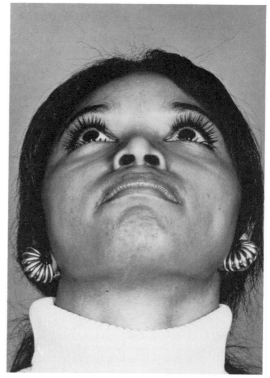

Alar base resection done as part of a nasal tip plasty produced this improvement in contour.

Reshaping a prominent nasal tip by resection at the alar base.

A and *B*, Resection of the alar base segment numbered 1 will almost always result in a somewhat unnatural appearance of the remaining alar base.

C and *D*, Excision of a triangular segment of the alar base and associated nostril floor, numbered 2, gives a moderate reduction in width.

E and *F*, A combination of these techniques can result in a significant reduction of projection and alar base width. But there will still be some degree of unnaturalness.

The novice surgeon must be cautioned that the use of alar base resection should be infrequent, for these are a major factor in the production of the "operated nose" look. Alar base resection ought to be a last resort, rather than a method of first choice.

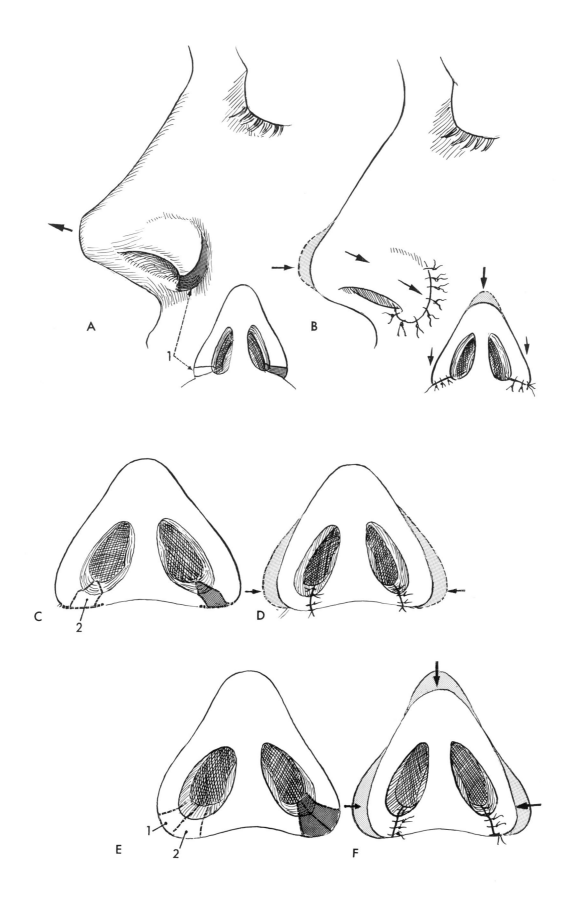

The alar base resection must be looked upon as an ancillary procedure. It is usually used in combination with other techniques to achieve a desired end-point and rarely as a single definitive procedure. Such a combination of techniques is required to reduce and remodel the prominent nasal tip shown on the opposite page. A simple alar base resection would reduce the forward projection of this tip, but would fall far short of the mark unless combined with other techniques. In this patient a combination of alar base resection with generous removal of the alae and a Lipsett approach to the tip, with foreshortening of the forward projection of the tip cartilages as well as lowering of the septal angle, resulted in a more pleasing profile. It must always be kept in mind during nasal reduction surgery that the nose must be considered as a three-dimensional whole. The surgeon should view individual techniques upon the nose only insofar as they affect the composite whole.

When in doubt as to whether or not an alar base resection should be done, it is generally wiser to postpone this procedure. A secondary re-evaluation of the results of the original surgery can often dictate the advisability of this simple maneuver, which can be carried out as an office procedure several weeks following primary rhinoplasty.

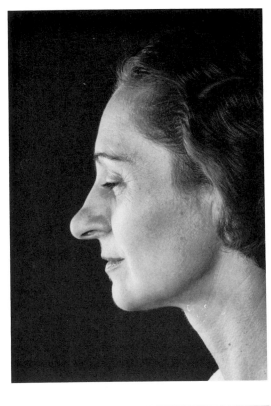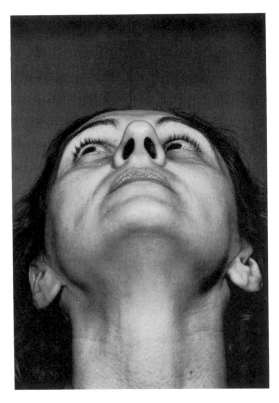
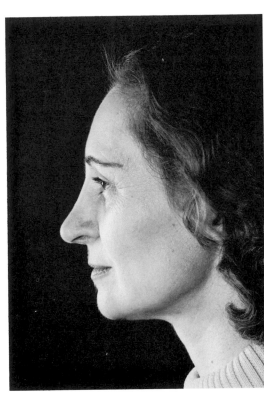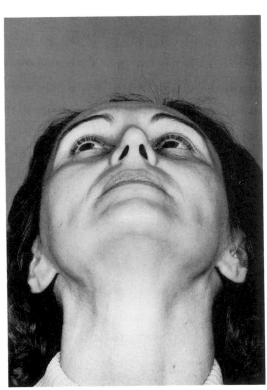

379

Thinning of the nostrils by the "piece of pie" excision technique can be combined with various designs of alar base resections advocated by Millard as shown here (*A*). The "hanging" nostril margin can be improved by the technique shown in *B*.

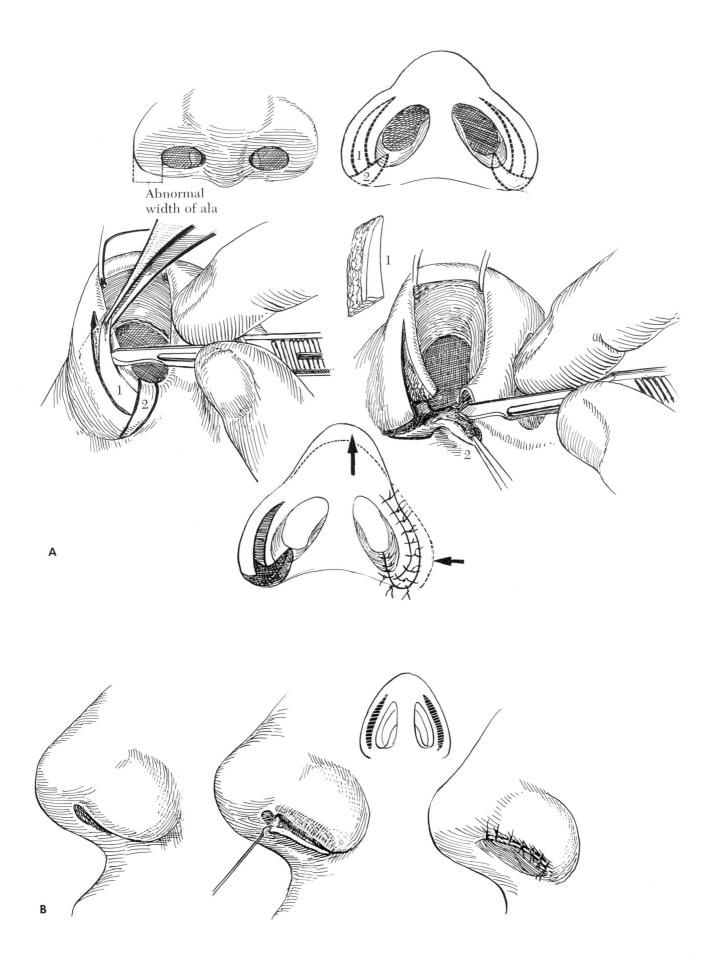

Abnormal
width of ala

A

B

381

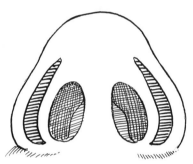

Correction of the nostril that is bulky and thick, often hanging like a curtain, sometimes to the level of the columella or below, is a difficult problem requiring resection of a wedge-shaped or "piece of pie" section of each nostril rim, sometimes in continuity with the alar base resection (Millard, 1960, 1965).

We use such thinning incisions only rarely, and only in those patients in whom no other approach is possible. Scars along the nostril rim heal quite well in most instances and are surprisingly inconspicuous, but the novice surgeon would be wise to proceed with care.

It is important to obtain the best possible scars from these external incisions about the nares, as they produce the only visible evidence of the surgery. Tension from suture lines is relieved with buried chromic catgut sutures. Skin sutures should be of fine 5–0 or 6–0 nylon and are removed on the third postoperative day.

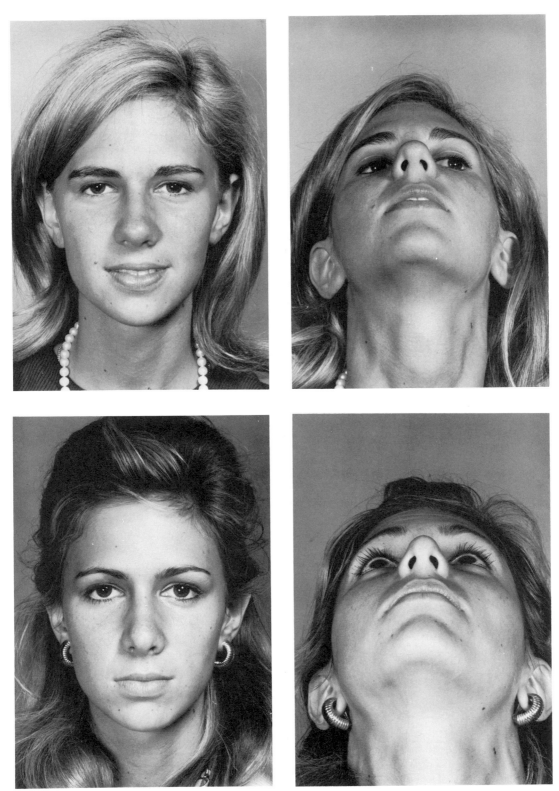

Thickened nostril rims in a patient with thick, oily skin and an ample pad of subcutaneous tissue. Some improvement was obtained by the eversion technique and with the nostril rim excision shown on page 380.

383

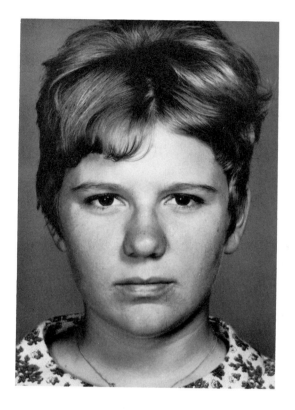 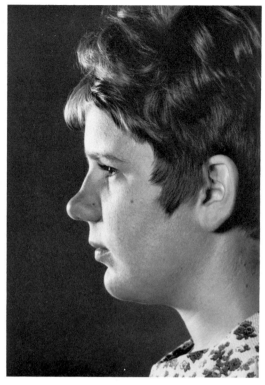

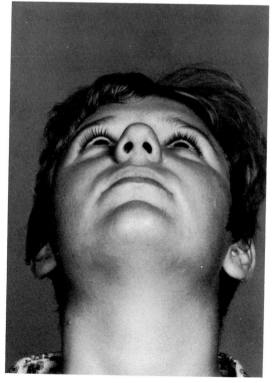

Correction of the thick or "beefy" tip is severely limited by the morphology of the problem, and both patient and surgeon must be prepared to accept limited improvement. If the patient and family do not seem to comprehend that only a *relative* improvement can result, surgery is best postponed or cancelled.

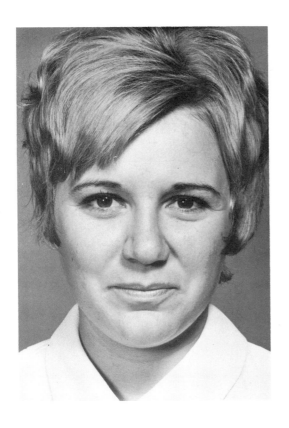 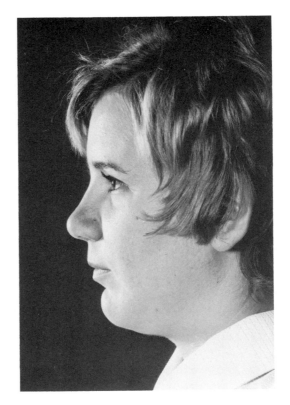

The principal limiting factor is the skin and subcutaneous tissue, which is usually quite unmanageable. Cartilage and bone can be reshaped, but not skin. Sometimes excessive subcutaneous fat can be resected, but the procedure is hazardous and can cause unsightly scar depressions and contour irregularities. Focal skin loss can occur. The alar eversion approach is often helpful, because as a rule some nasal lining can be spared, but excision of the lining must still be minimal.

In this patient, the tip was improved by complete removal of the lateral crura, including the alar domes.

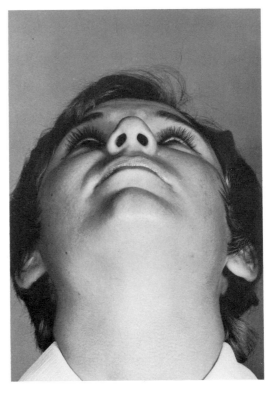

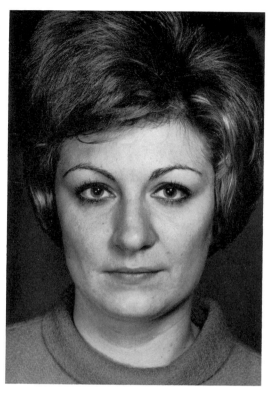 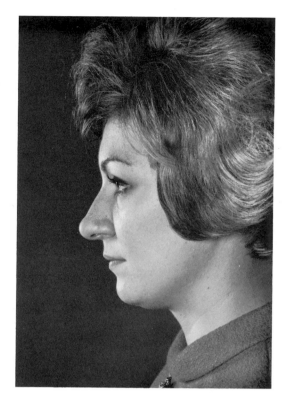

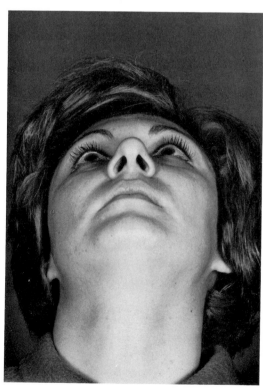

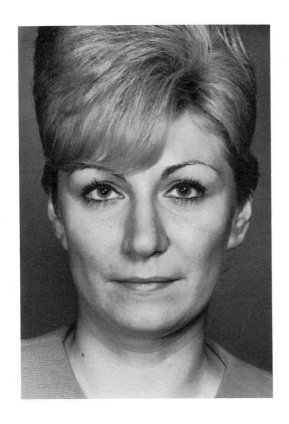

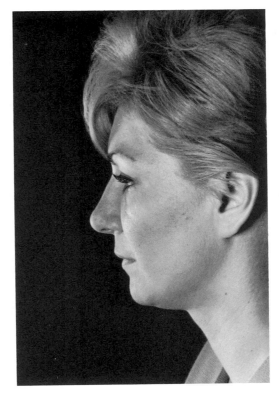

A nose that is slightly too wide and slightly too thick in the skin and subcutaneous tissues presents a real challenge to the surgeon. Careful excision of subcutaneous tissue beneath the dorsal skin and the nasal tip skin was the remedy applied in this case.

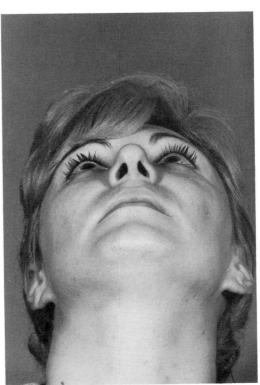

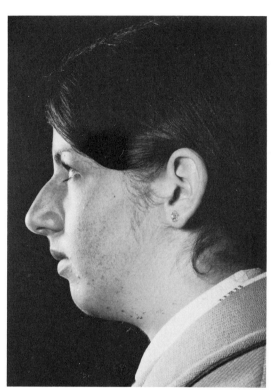 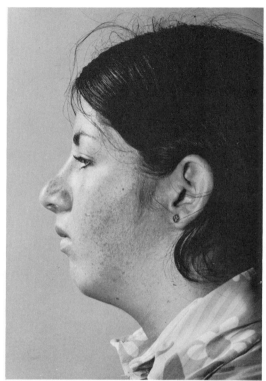

The result of an injudicious excision of subcutaneous tissues and damage to the overlying dermis. Note the depressed scar over the left alar dome area.

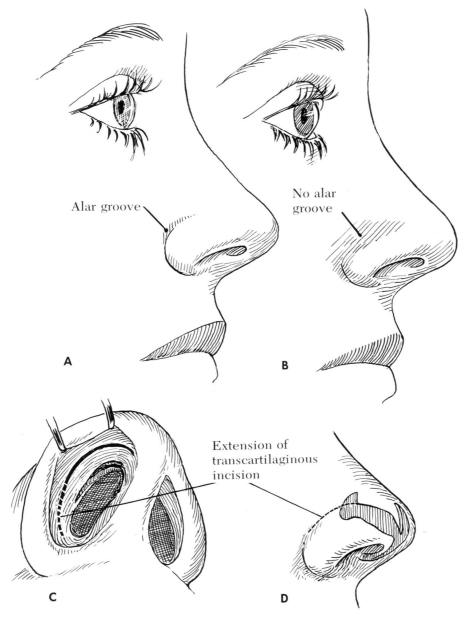

Alar groove

No alar groove

A

B

Extension of
transcartilaginous
incision

C

D

In a number of instances operations to improve thick nasal tips have produced satisfactory results, but without a supra-alar groove; to create one we have used the laterally directed vestibular incision of Diamond shown here. Some authors have advocated dermal scoring as a means of gaining further correction, but we do not believe that the attendant risks justify the small gain.

A, Prior to correction.

B, After correction.

C, Lateral extension of the transcartilaginous incision into the fibro-areolar tissues of the alar base.

D, The effect of this incision is to produce a bending of the rigid skin in this region and thus to imitate the natural supra-alar groove. Preservation of the supralateral plate of alar cartilage prevents unsightly extension of the groove, a common stigma of rhinoplasty.

389

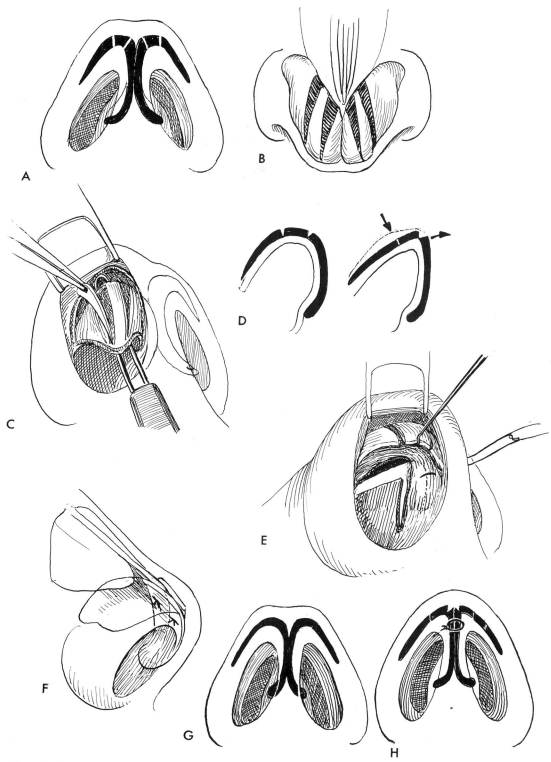

Modification of the squared and bifid tip.

A, Planned lines of incision through the lateral crura of the alar cartilages and the alar domes.

B, Excision of strips of alar cartilage to bring about an elevation of the rim and recession of the tip.

C, Strips of cartilage are removed, taking care to preserve the vestibular lining skin.

D, Medial motion of the medial crura brings about a flattening of the prominent alar dome region.

E, The two medial crura are sutured together by plain 4–0 catgut sutures.

F, Completed suturing of the medial crura, in this instance embracing the caudal border of the septum.

G and *H*, Preoperative and postoperative contours compared.

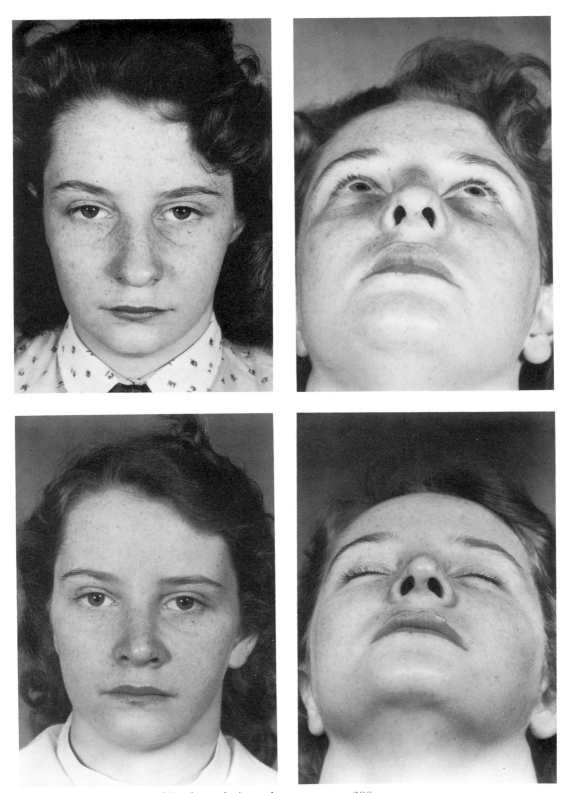

Bifidity of the nasal tip, corrected by the technique shown on page 390.

When bifidity is moderate to considerable, breaking up the soft tissues between the domes, as suggested on page 373, will not create enough fibrous scar tissue to correct the condition. Exposure of the dome and the lateral crura and remodeling of the area under direct vision will be required. The most important consideration is maintenance of continuity of the nasal lining skin. Final correction may be aided by the use of direct approximating sutures of 4–0 plain catgut. When bifidity is associated with asymmetry of the tip, the surgeon must make appropriate adjustments in the amount of tissue being removed on either side. This is a special problem in the case of the twisted nose (see page 397).

The most esthetically pleasing columella forms a graceful curve, with its convexity in a caudal direction. It should, in fact, hang slightly below the nostril rims when seen from the lateral aspect. The columella gains most of its shape from the medial crura of the alar cartilages, which are in close apposition at the dorsum and splay outward at the base, causing the columella to widen in this area. This width conveys a natural expression to the nose, and loss of it is an unfortunate stigma of nasal surgery. In the so-called "hanging" columella, the cartilages extend well below the nostril rims, the result of excessive curvature of the inferior margins of the medial crura.

A, The hanging columella.

B, An incision is made along the caudal border of the medial crura, just inside the vestibular margin and extending almost the full height of the columella.

C, Overlying vestibular lining skin is dissected from the superficial aspect of the crus.

D, The medial crura as separated centrally.

E, The crura prolapsed into the nostrils.

F, The columella is gently raised to its correct position and the excess segment of the medial crus is estimated.

G, The excess cartilage is removed, usually in a semilunar shape.

H, Appearance after correction and closure with interrupted 5–0 nylon sutures.

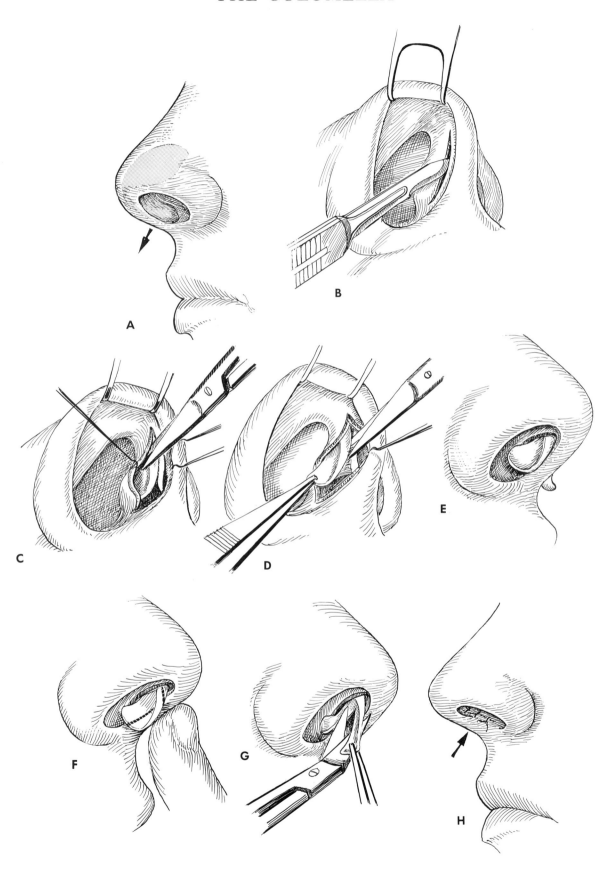

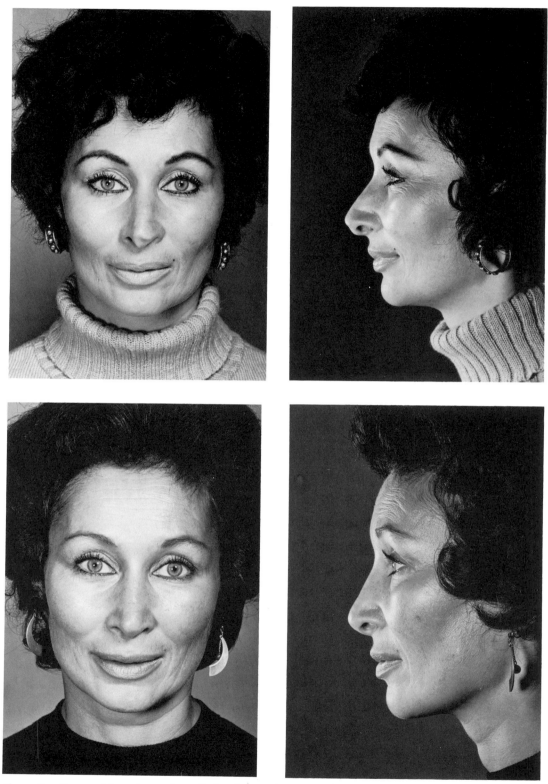

Correction of a distorted hanging columella by the method described on the preceding pages.

In addition to the cartilages themselves, it is often necessary to resect a corresponding strip of columellar skin. Marked curvature of the caudal margin of the septum can also contribute to a hanging columella and in some cases is the sole cause. The septum is easily corrected by resecting the convex portion.

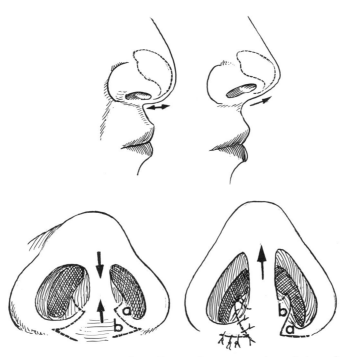

Another method of improving an acute labiocolumellar angle or retraction of the columella is the use of small interpolated flaps (*a, b*). The columella can also be lengthened by this technique.

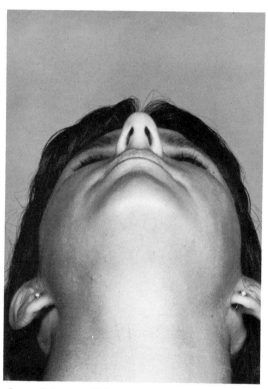 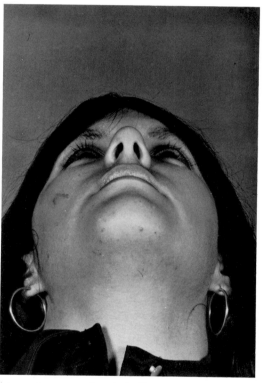

If the feet of the medial crura flare laterally to such an extent that resection is indicated to narrow the base of the columella, they can be delivered and resected through an incision similar to that described for trimming the caudal edge. Sometimes it is necessary to suture these structures when lengthening of the columella is desired. This maneuver can also increase the breathing space.

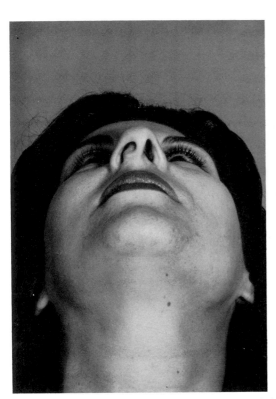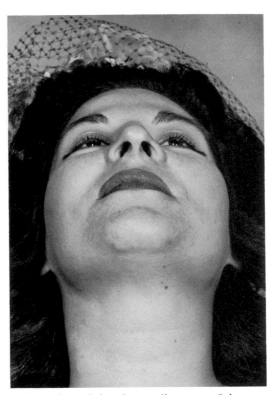

A twisted columella can result from a developmental deformity, either of the alar cartilages or of the septum, or both. Simultaneous correction of these two structures may be necessary. These photographs demonstrate correction of a twisted medial crus, a deviated caudal septal border, and an asymmetrical tip. Improvement required nasal plasty, anterior septal plasty, and correction of the tip asymmetry by bilateral columellar rim incisions, everting the alar cartilages and correcting their points of distortion.

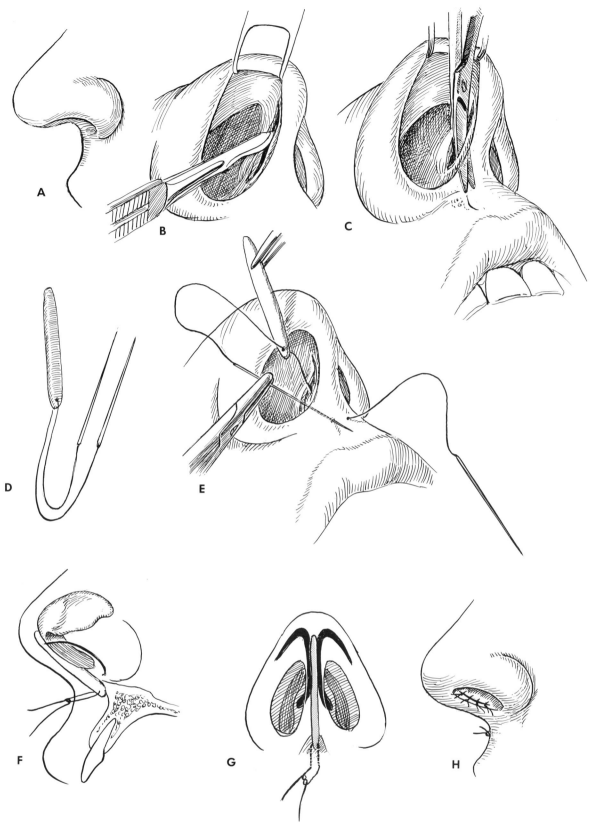

The retracted columella is often the result of old trauma, with destruction of the cartilaginous septum, or of section of the septum during radical septal surgery. Its correction is quite difficult. Cartilage, bone, or alloplastic struts can be inserted and may offer improvement, but generally the results are disappointing. In severe cases Millard (1969) has employed pedicle flaps from the side wall of the nose inserted into the septum, and good results are claimed. Dingman and Walter (1969) achieved impressive results with chondrocutaneous composite grafts transplanted to the lower septum.

A, The retracted columella.

B, An incision is made along the free margin of the medial crura.

(*Legend continued on opposite page.*)

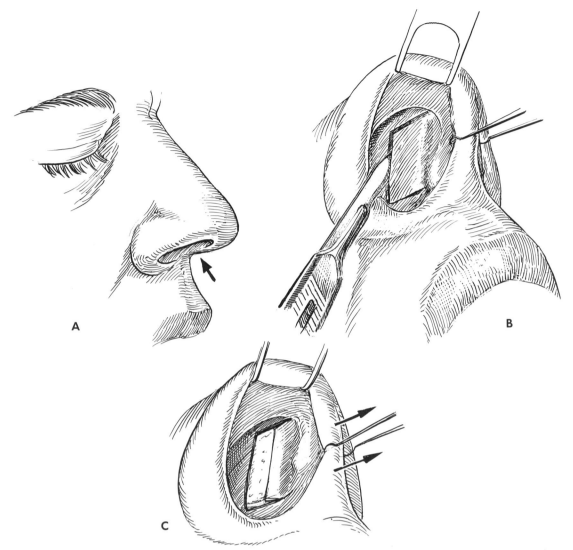

Retraction of the columella may also be alleviated by advancement of mucoperichondrial flaps from the caudal border of the septum, the result being to free the membranous septum to prolapse inferiorly. The correction that can be achieved in this way is limited.

A, The retracted columella.

B, Bilateral squared advancement flaps are raised, and the columella plus the remnant of membranous septum is drawn inferiorly.

C, The inferior correction achieved; it is maintained by the use of through and through sutures holding the advanced flaps in position, leaving the bare cartilage to re-epithelialize.

The classic Rethi (1948) external incisions across the columella, used for shortening the columellar length, are useful in extreme problems of the long tip.

(Continued from opposite page.)

C, The incision is deepened to the region of the nasal spine.

D, An appropriately shaped portion of cartilage has a double-armed suture threaded through either end.

E, Cartilage is placed in position in the previously formed pocket on the caudal aspect of the medial crura. Both double-armed needles are passed out through the lip skin, and the implant is thus stabilized.

F, The implant in position.

G, An inferior view of the position of the implant.

H, The defect is closed by interrupted 5–0 nylon sutures. Such a procedure is helpful, but it falls short of achieving complete correction.

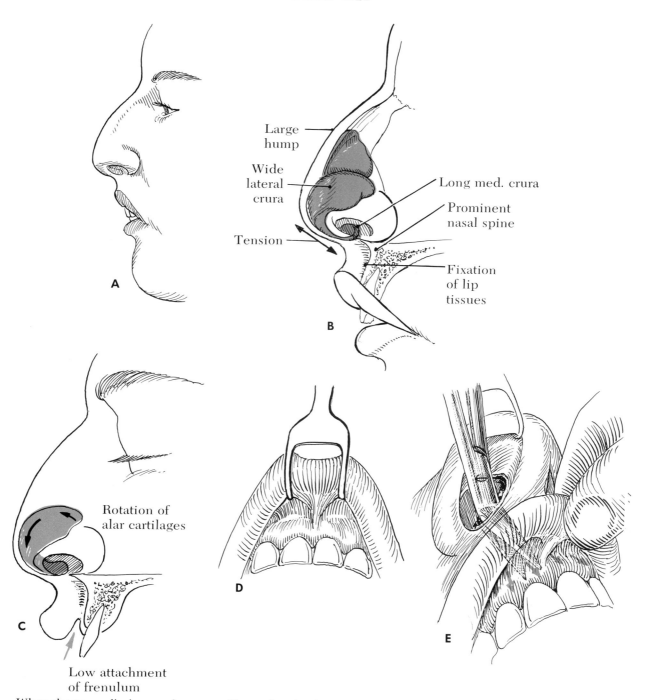

A, The "tethered" lip.

B and **C**, Anatomic characteristics of the deformity.

D, The strong, short upper lip frenulum.

E, Freeing of the frenulum and adjacent soft tissues by dissection through the lower end of the transfixion incision.

When the upper lip is very short, a malformation that is usually developmental in origin, extensive dissection of the gingiva from the upper jaw by subperiosteal dissection through the base of the transfixion incision at the columella is helpful to gain relaxation of the soft tissue.

A, The "tethered" lip.

B and *C*, Anatomic characteristics of the deformity.

D, The strong, short upper lip frenulum.

E, Freeing of the frenulum and adjacent soft tissues by dissection through the lower end of the transfixion incision.

400

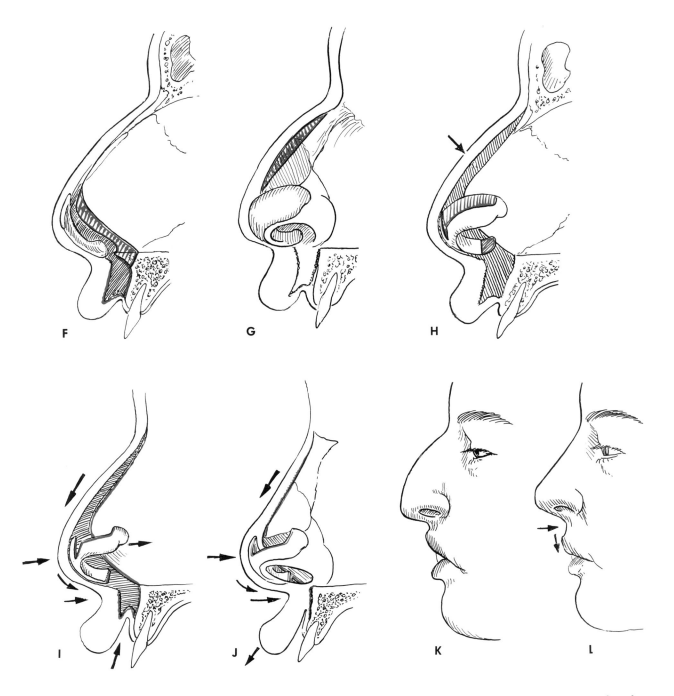

F, The lip is freed, the nasal spine is resected, and the caudal border of the cartilaginous septum is resected and shortened.

G, The nasal dorsum is corrected to a new profile line.

H, The tip is remodeled by resection of the outer portion of the lateral crus on each side. Further recession and correction of the flared, widened columella base is gained by resection of the bases of the medial crura.

I, The result of these resections, and the motion they impart.

J, The procedure will allow a drooping of the tip, recession of the columella base, and release of the transverse tightness of the upper lip, combined with some degree of lengthening at the expense of both the nasal skin and the adjacent lip skin.

K and L, Comparison of preoperative and postoperative profiles.

The relationship of the lip to the nose is important to facial contour. The posture of the lip depends on several factors, but primarily on the shape of the maxilla and of the upper dental arch and on the configuration of the nose. Rhinoplasty usually affects the lip to some degree, and sometimes the procedure must include some dissection of the lip's attachments to the maxilla.

The angle formed between the columella and the lip has been the subject of much discussion in the literature of nasal plastic surgery. The most pleasing angle is said to be 100 degrees, and numerous gadgets have been devised to measure the angle and to aid the surgeon in achieving the putative ideal—often easier said than done.

The lip-nose angle depends on the posture of the septum, the nasal spine, the columella, and the lip. The nasal spine is the most important element. Resection of this structure can result in retraction of the base of the columella and consequent overhanging or "plunging" of the tip. In many patients the nasal spine is poorly or not at all developed. The tip of the nose of such a patient often hangs down, and the nasolabial angle is acute. Aufricht (1969) recommends implantation of cartilage or alloplastic to simulate the normally developed nasal spine, and his results are impressive. However, we have resorted to this procedure on very few occasions because it produces a stiffness of the lip, of which the patient is quite conscious, and sometimes a loss of normal animation.

Excessive shortening of the nose, with removal of a large piece of the caudal margin of the septum, can relax the lip, sometimes to an extreme degree so that it hangs almost like a curtain over the upper teeth and appears overly long. The length of the lip, as well as the shape of the upper dental arch, should be thoroughly studied preoperatively in each patient. The surgeon should project in advance what the effect on the lip will be of the total operation. Often a judicious trimming of the lower nose and particularly the nasal spine is indicated in order to maintain a natural-looking upper lip.

If, on the other hand, a dropped or plunging tip is a part of the nasal deformity, which it is in a high percentage of patients, other adjustments in technique are required. In some instances the dropped tip can be improved only partially and not completely corrected without such excessive surgery that the secondary deformity would be more unattractive than the original. Such a result would certainly have all the stigmata of a "nose job."

Anatomical features contributing to the plunging tip are (1) the shape of the alar cartilages, (2) the relation of the septal angle to the alar cartilages, (3) the height of the nasal dorsum, (4) the shape of the caudal margins of the septum and the nasal spine, (5) the action of muscular attachments of the alae, (6) the length and shape of the maxilla and teeth, and (7) the shape of the upper lip.

Resection of the caudal septum and "overshortening" of the tip with fixation at a high angle by mattress transfixion sutures may be effective when a small correction is required, but can be disastrous when a plunging tip is a significant feature of the patient's deformity. Maintaining the tip in an elevated position may require shortening of the side wall of the nose, which involves resection of a large part of the caudal end of each upper lateral cartilage. The lateral alar wings can be elevated to fill the raw defect when they are fixed in their new position.

Generally speaking, the trimming of the caudal septum and nasal spine should be conservative. Ambitious removal of the spine or the base of the caudal septum can increase the plunging deformity by increasing the acuteness of the lip-columella angle. Overshortening of the nose is a common problem after incompetent surgery and is an almost irreparable defect. The caudal margin of the septum is used as a buttress to maintain the tip in its new position. The mucosa from each side is trimmed so that the denuded septal cartilage is inserted tongue-in-groove fashion between the medial alar crura, which are held apart by scissors; mattress sutures fix the tip in position. This technique has been criticized, but when used in the proper circumstances it has been successful in our hands. Further improvement can be obtained in some instances by a retrolabial implant of bone, septal cartilage, or alloplastic (Aufricht, 1969).

402

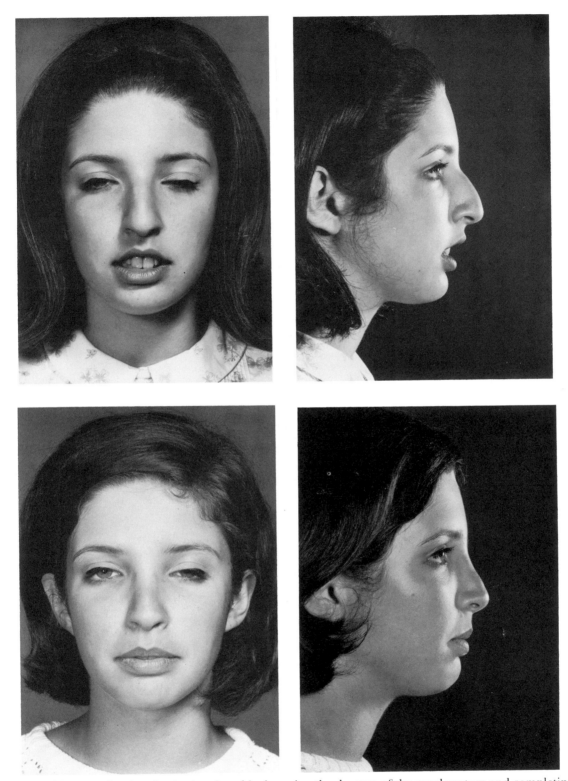

The tethered lip can often be pleasingly relaxed by lowering the dorsum of the nasal septum and completing the transfixion incision. In this patient, the upper lip and gingiva were freed from the anterior surface of the maxilla in the region of the nasal spine.

Correction of a plunging tip.

A, Dislocation of the tip structures of the septal angle.

B, After resection of part of the lateral crus; the arrow shows an excess of upper lateral cartilage which will require resection in order to suspend the tip.

C, Lateral view, showing the prolapsed nasal tip.

D, Correction of the dorsal and caudal borders of the septal cartilage.

E, The dropped tip replaced in position. The remnant of lateral crus overlaps the upper lateral cartilage.

F, The medial crura of the medial cartilage are sutured in a tongue-and-groove fashion to the caudal border of the septum.

G, The suture placed through the medial crura and caudal border.

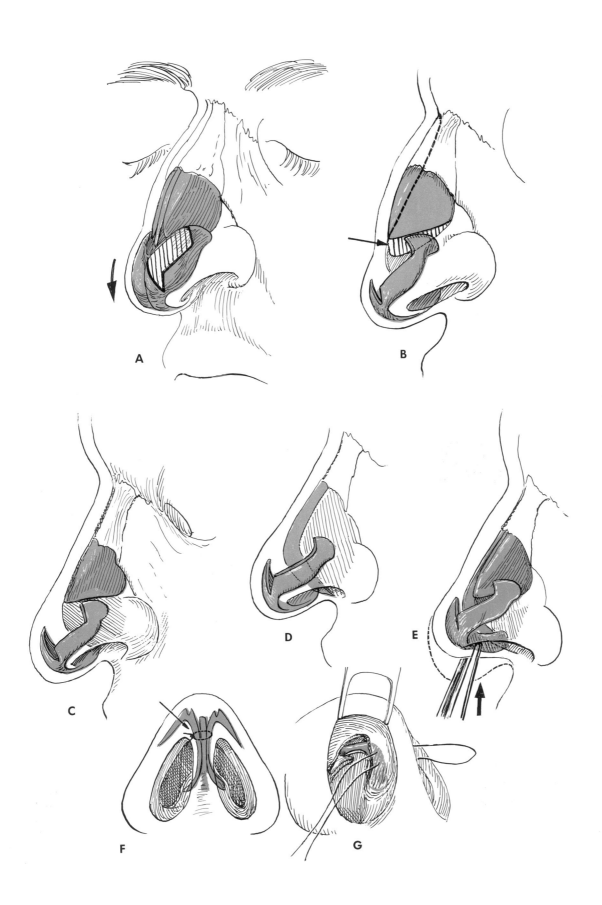

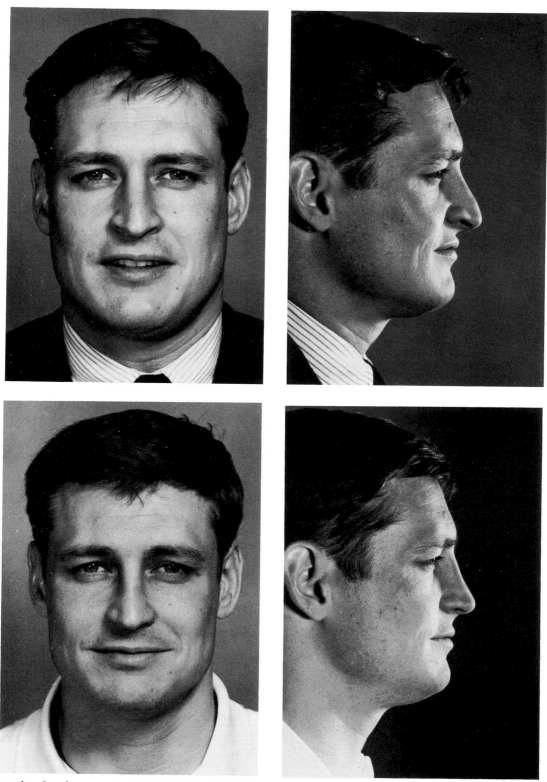

An example of a plunging tip that constituted the primary part of a patient's problem. The operative procedure combined alar cartilage revision, reduction of the nasal dorsum, and tongue-and-groove insertion of the caudal septal border between the medial crura. A small alar base resection completed the correction. The result was somewhat limited by the short columella.

Of obvious importance in these procedures is the method of suturing as well as splinting the tip, so that it will remain in the corrected position.

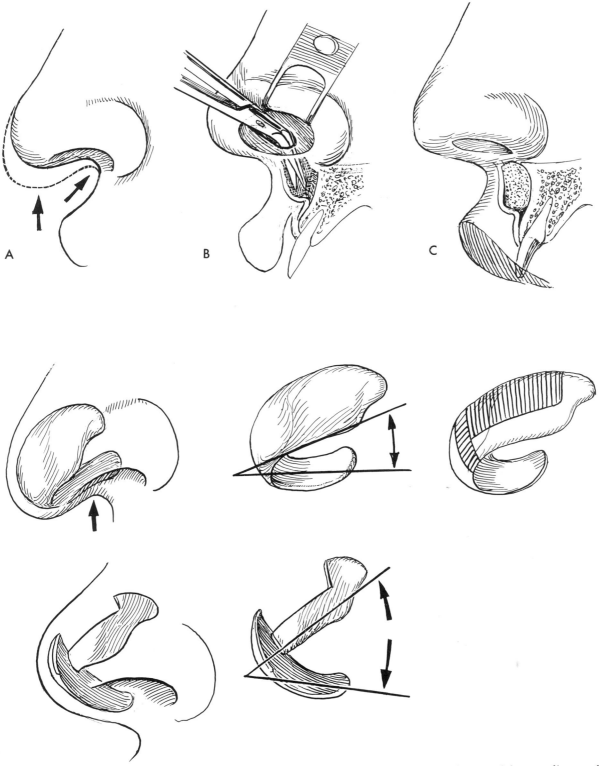

Correction of an acute nasolabial angle by an implant of bone, cartilage, or alloplastic material, according to the technique of Aufricht.

A, The prolapsed nasal tip.

B, Formation of a pocket in the region of the nasal spine.

C, The implant in place and correction achieved.

The lower series of drawings demonstrate the necessity of remodeling the nasal tip by breaking through the alae at the level of the domes in order to change the angle between the medial and lateral crura in some patients with plunging tips, which are the result of such an anatomical angulation of the alar cartilages.

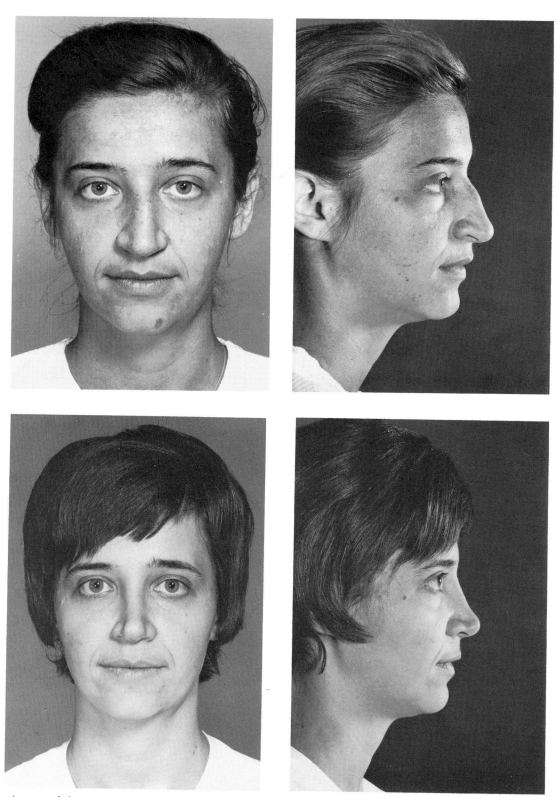

A plunging nasal tip was accompanied by a large bony hump and flaring of the alar cartilages in this patient. The improvement shown was achieved by a quite radical shortening of the upper lateral cartilages and superior shifting of the alar cartilages to fill in the defect. The medial crura were used to embrace the caudal border of the septum and hold it in position. It should be noted that excessive resection of the caudal margin of the septum in such a patient would be disastrous and would only increase the deformity.

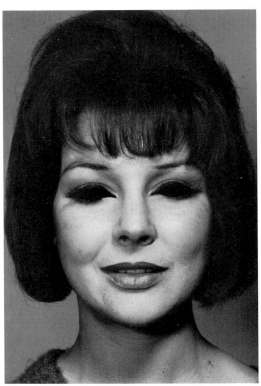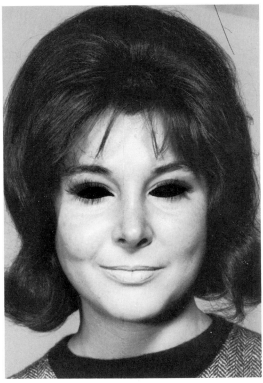

Narrowing or infracture of the bony pyramid may be all that is required in some patients, or it may be the focal point of the operation, tip plasty and other modifications being incidental. In such patients it is often not even necessary to remove any cartilage or bone from the dorsum of the nose. In spite of this fact, it is possible to perform a lateral osteotomy with small osteotomes introduced through pyriform incisions or transcutaneously through the cheek skin, cutting the bone along the nasomaxillary groove. Pressure on the side wall of the nose will then cause infracture and narrowing. It is particularly important that the lateral osteotomy extend superiorly to the level of the inner canthus or above.

This patient had an acceptable nasal profile preoperatively. Narrowing was accomplished by a simple lateral osteotomy and infracture.

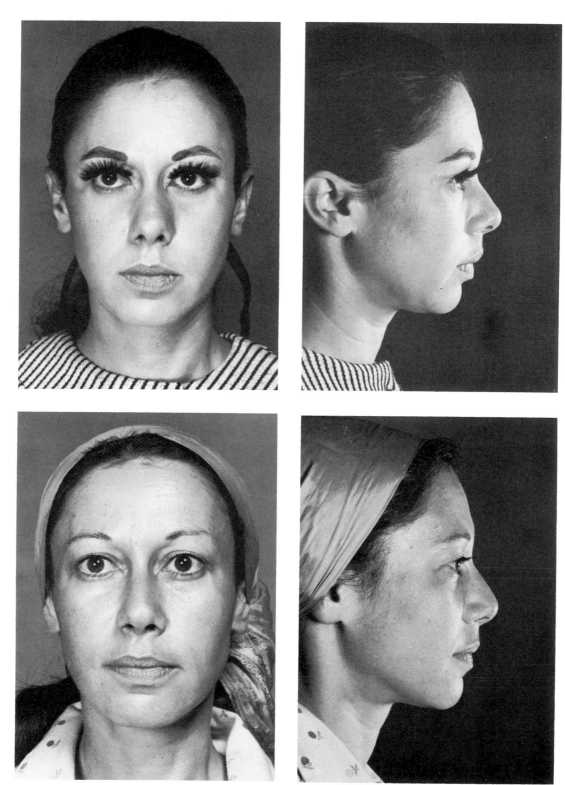

This patient's wide nose was due in part to the width of its bony base along the pyriform aperture and in part to increased thickness of the subcutaneous tissues. In such a case the upper lateral cartilages and the alar cartilages must be reduced in size to achieve narrowing of the nose. Great care must be exercised in trimming the upper lateral cartilage, a structure of importance in breathing through the nose. After separation of the soft tissue from the nasal skeleton, excessive subcutaneous tissue can be resected from the flap overlying the upper lateral and alar cartilages, with care being taken not to damage the dermis.

410

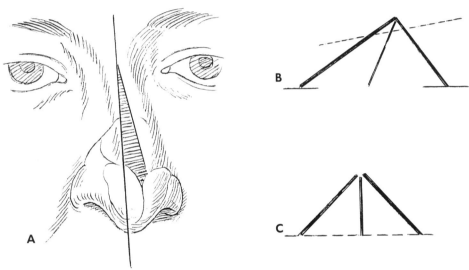

The externally deviated or twisted nose with unequal walls *(A)* can be likened to an off-center pyramid *(B)*. The nature and extent of the deviation dictates the steps required to straighten the nose. In high deviations, simple removal of the hump (lowering the profile) sometimes suffices. Asymmetrical removal of the hump *(C)*, allowing for the discrepancy between the nasal walls, is also most helpful.

411

Correction of the deviated or dislocated lower portion of the septum may require any of a variety of techniques, from the simplest procedure to complete resection of the septum followed by carving and subsequent insertion of the thinned and straightened fragment as a free graft. In correction of the long nose, as shown here, resection of the caudal border of the septum may remove the deviated portion. Caution must be exercised and the caudal border must not be overcorrected, for the retraction of the columella that will result will be difficult to repair.

A, Drooping of the nasal tip and retraction of the columella secondary to traumatic loss of the caudal border.

B, An incision is made parallel to the inferior border in the middle crura and deepened posteriorly to the nasal spine.

C, A cartilage implant of suitable size is placed in the incision, its anterior end in the interdome region. A double-armed suture passed through the lower end of the implant is brought through the upper lip skin to stabilize the implant during the early stages of healing.

D, The implant in position, with sutures passed through the skin.

E, Restoration of normal columella contour.

(After Converse, 1964.)

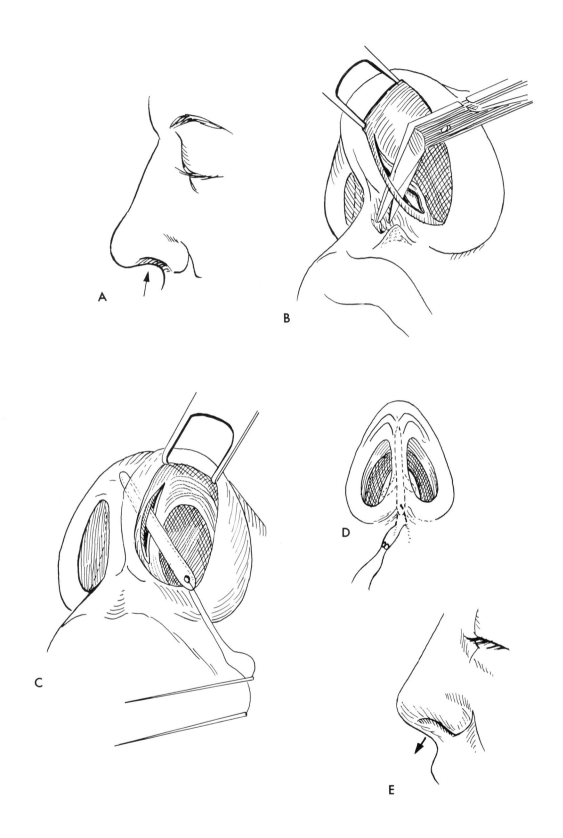

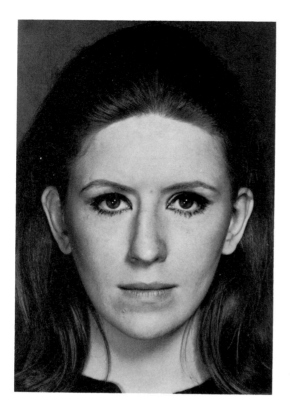
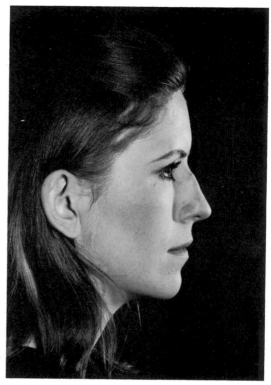
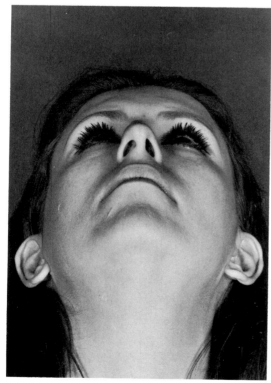

414

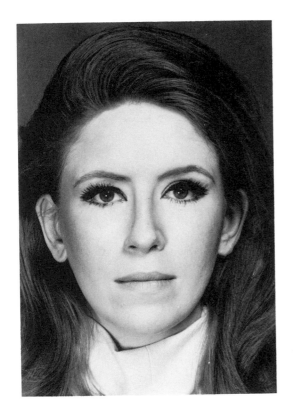

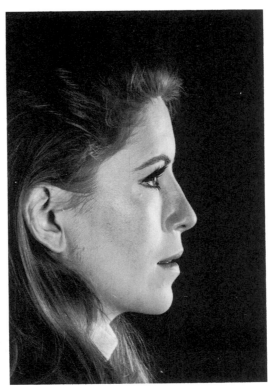

Post-traumatic deflection of the nasal bones with secondary deflection of the upper lateral cartilages, corrected by rhinoplasty that restored both bones and cartilages to their normal positions.

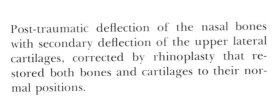

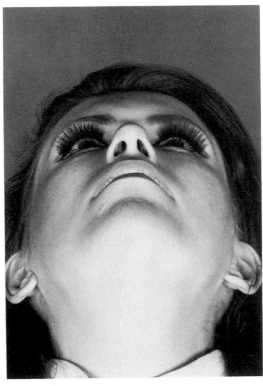

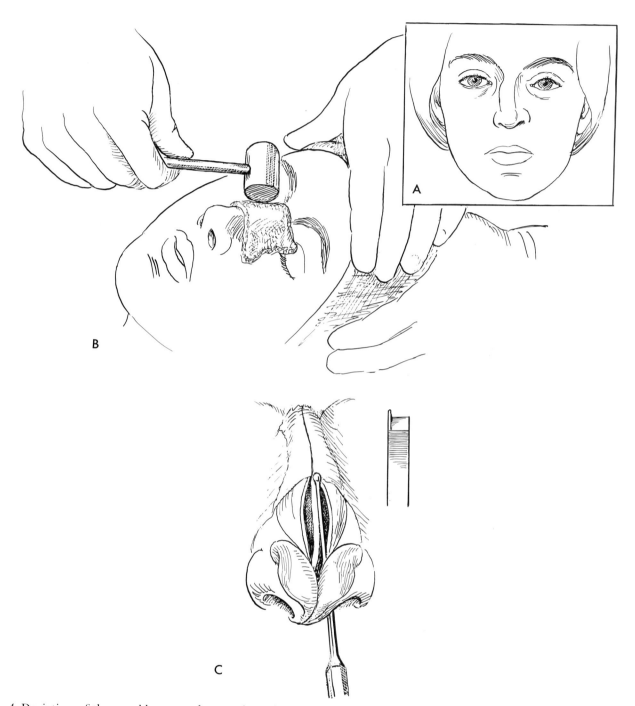

A, Deviation of the nasal bones and upper lateral cartilages of such a degree that repositioning the bones in the midline would not result in contour correction.

B, The Kazanjian maneuver: padding is applied over the nose and a sharp blow with a mallet comminutes the nasal bones. Care must be taken to protect the globe of the eye during this maneuver.

C, The guarded osteotome is passed along the nasal dorsum to separate the nasal bones and septum. The bones may then be straightened by manipulation and maintained in position by an external splint.

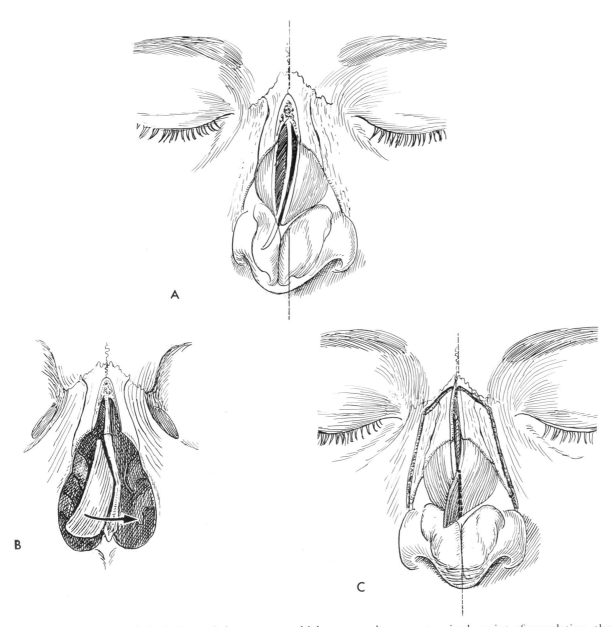

In simple developmental deviations of the septum, which commonly present a single point of angulation, the "swinging door" procedure will frequently suffice to correct the deviation. No resection of septal tissue is involved, and no risk of septal perforation exists.

A, Deviation of the cartilaginous septum, seen after correction of the dorsal profile.

B, A mucoperichondrial flap is raised from the side opposite the deviation through an L-shaped incision, with the lower arm of the "L" extending along the floor of the septum. No attempt is made to raise a flap on the deviated side. An incision is made along the point of maximal curvature and along the floor of the septum, allowing the septum to be bent into the midline and retained in this position without springing back.

C, Excess width of the upper lateral cartilage, which would tend to hold the septum in its deviated position, is removed.

(After Converse, 1964.)

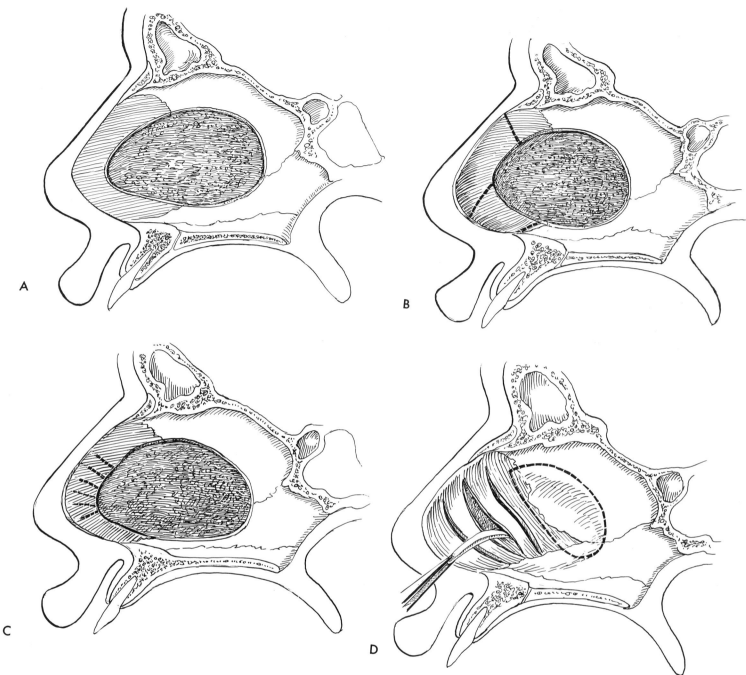

In the more complicated variety of septal deviation, especially where compound curves exist, it is necessary to perform a conservative submucous resection. No more tissue should be resected than is necessary to produce a straight septum, and in particular only a minimal portion of the perpendicular plate of the ethmoid is to be removed, since a considerable risk is run of dropping the dorsum in completing this procedure.

The submucous resection is preferably performed through an L-shaped incision, the horizontal arm passing along the floor of the septum. Mucoperichondrial flaps are raised on the side of the septal deflection, taking care to place the incision sufficiently posterior to the transfixion incision to allow a healthy band of mucoperichondrium to remain. If there is a complicated deflection in the region of the transfixion incision itself, so that direct surgery on the caudal portion of the septum is necessary, it will of course be mandatory to do the resection through the transfixion incision.

A, A submucous resection involving a somewhat more than conservative removal of bony septum. Note the remaining wide, strong dorsal and caudal borders of the cartilaginous septum.

B, Septal angle deflection can frequently be corrected by multiple vertical cuts which do not touch the dorsal or caudal borders of the septum. Overlapping cartilage must be resected.

418

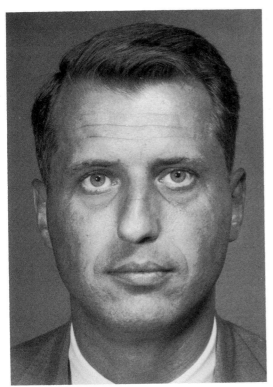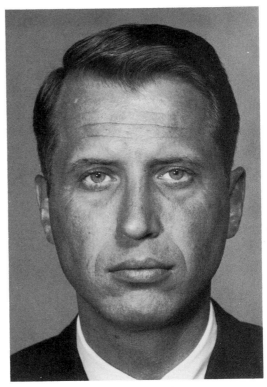

A deflection of the cartilaginous portion of the nose, including the tip, corrected by the "swinging door' procedure and nasal tip plasty.

C, On occasion the operator may be forced to allow one or two cuts to touch the dorsal or caudal borders. It is important that on one side the mucosa is not raised from the septal cartilage in this region, so that support of the cartilage is maintained and no break in the profile line results.

D, Multiple oblique cuts are sometimes made to straighten a badly deflected septum. Some of the most seriously deviated segments may be resected.

(After Converse, 1964.)

Approaching the septum through the transfixion incision.

A, The deviated nasal tip held in its deflected position by the septal angle.

B, The deflected dorsal border of the septum, with dislocation of the nasal tip into a central position.

C, Infiltration of the subperichondrial space by local anesthetic solution.

D, Mucoperichondrial flaps are raised with the anesthetic solution, a maneuver which will immeasurably aid the operator in dissection.

E, A transfixion incision is made along the lower border of the septum. It is frequently easier for the operator to begin the dissection by sharply removing the depressor muscles from the caudal border of the cartilaginous septum. After progressing superiorly for a distance of 4 or 5 mm., the operator will usually find a space appearing between the mucoperichondrium and the underlying cartilage.

F, Mucoperichondrial flaps are raised and the septal framework is exposed.

Submucous resection or septal plasty is best carried out after reduction of the hump, adjustment of the caudal septum and columella, and tip plasty, but before lateral osteotomy and infracture. Whenever possible, septal plasty (or readjustment of the position of the septum) is preferred over formal submucous resection (Killian).

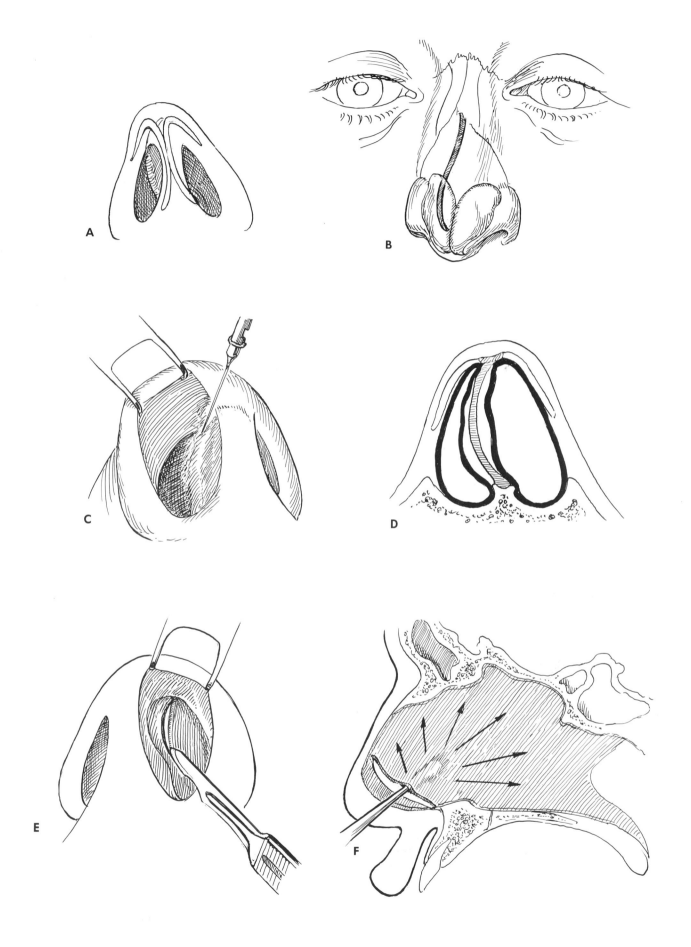

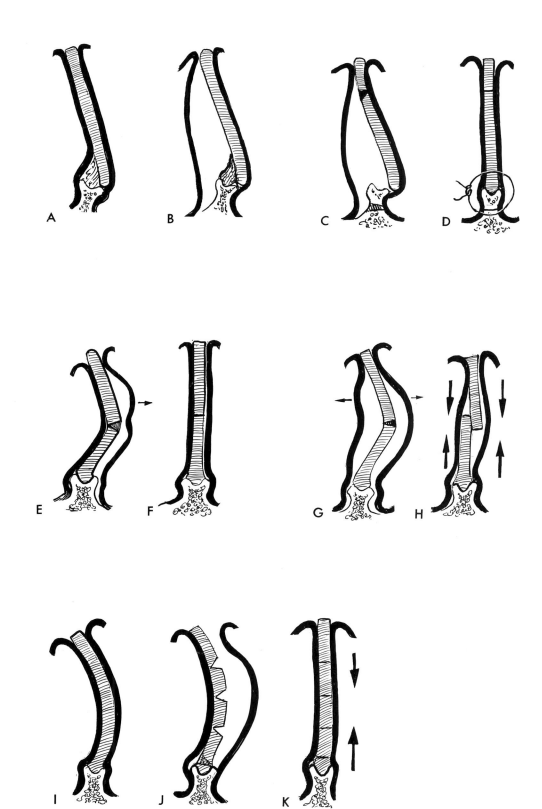

Surgical options available for straightening the deviated septum are illustrated; the choice depends upon the circumstances. Whenever possible it is wiser to strip only one mucoperichondrial flap in order to avoid postoperative bleeding, perforations, and unstable areas of septal mucosa which may be subject to ulceration.

A, Partial dislocation of the cartilaginous septum from the vomer groove.

B, Raising of the mucoperichondrial flaps.

C, Osteotomy of the deflected vomer and removal of a wedge section from the septal framework to allow it to swing to the midline.

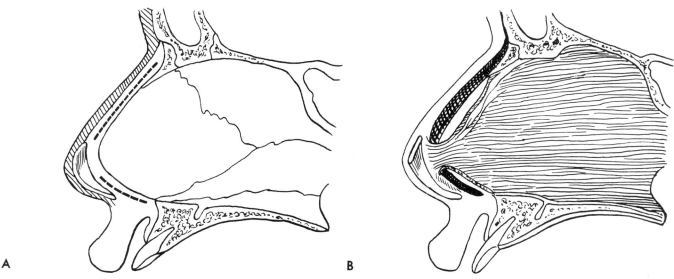

A

B

When marked serpentine curvature of the dorsal border of the septal cartilage cannot be corrected by conservative methods, it may be necessary to resect the entire twisted septal cartilage and replace it with a straightened portion of the cartilage to provide support for the nasal dorsum. This procedure is rarely indicated and should be resorted to only if the surgeon believes that all other techniques would fail. Many procedures have been described which aim at minimizing the risk of collapse following such extensive surgery, and principal among these is the interrupted transfixion incision, with the mucoperichondrial flaps of the septum acting as a sling for the nasal dorsum (Converse, 1959).

A, Interruption of the transfixion incision. *B*, The mucosa in the region of the interruption acting as a hammocklike support for the nasal dorsum.

The septal transplant may be fixed in any of a variety of ways to the lateral cartilage, and many ingenious techniques of suturing have been described, such as transcutaneous ligation or drawing of the transcutaneously placed sutures into the nasal cavity with a hook (Kazanjian and Converse, 1959).

D, Maintenance of the structures in the midline by catgut suture looped over the nasal spine.

E, Correction of a buckling septal cartilage by removal of a wedge.

F, Septum maintained in the midline.

G, Tension is frequently present when the perichondrium has been raised from both sides to return the septum to its uncorrected position. Overlapping of the fragments may result, with postoperative septal widening *(H)*. This will require correction by excision of the overlapping fragments.

I, Smooth, curved deflection of the septum.

J, Multiple wedges removed along the axis of the deflection, with raising of the mucoperichondrial flap only on the deflected side.

K, The septum held in its deflected position. Note the tension of the healing flap, which tends to hold the structure in its corrected position.

Allowances should be made for the normal healing contraction of the mucoperichondrial flaps (arrows). These forces of healing are often helpful in arriving at a straight septum during septal plasty.

423

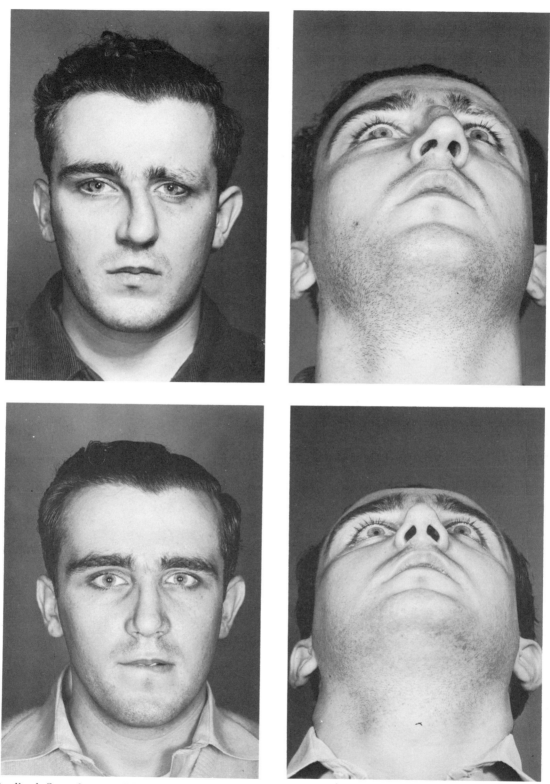

A badly deflected nose with a severely traumatized septum, corrected as shown on the preceding page.

424

LATERAL OSTEOTOMY

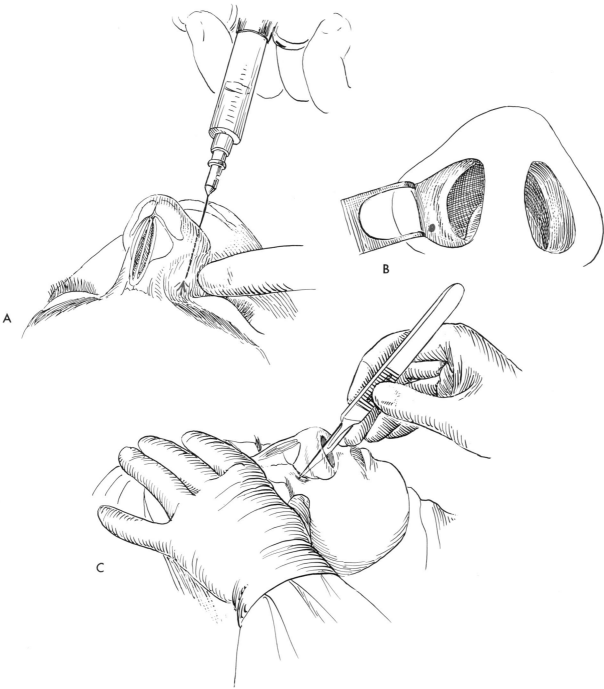

A, Through a point in the pyriform aperture shown at *B,* 2 to 3 ml. of anesthetic solution is injected along the line of osteotomy. The needle is directed to the immediate precanthal region; it is important that too much anterior inclination of the needle be avoided.

C, An incision is made in the pyriform aperture through the lining skin and soft tissues, to and through the periosteum overlying the maxilla. The pyriform aperture may be conveniently thrown into prominence by retraction laterally of the thumb on the adjacent cheek tissues, or with a nasal speculum.

(Illustration continued on following page.)

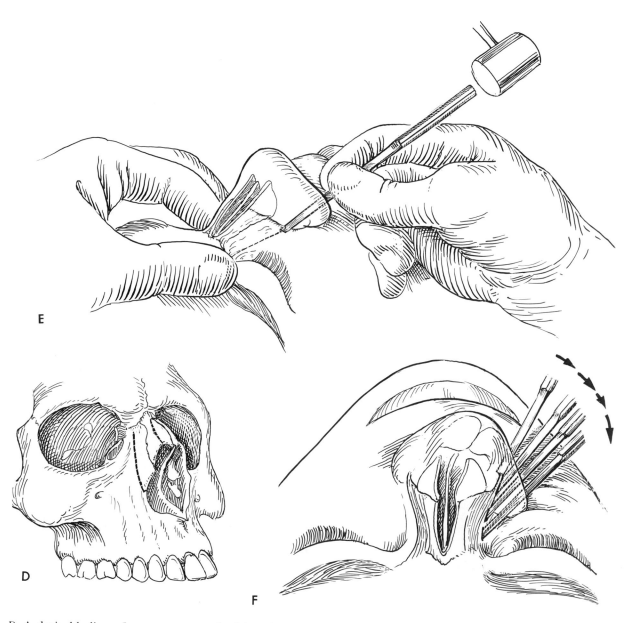

D, A desirable line of osteotomy, emphasizing that it lies on the nasal process of the maxilla rather than in the nasal bone proper.

E, The narrow osteotome (2 or 3 mm.) is inserted along the previously formed subperiosteal tract.

F, A series of osteotome perforations of the nasal process is made; usually four or five of these will suffice. As the osteotomy is continued upward, it is necessary to rotate the osteotome progressively laterally.

G, Infracture is accomplished by compression of the nasal dorsum between the thumb and forefinger. No "waggling" motion should be imparted, and the pressure is applied equally from both sides. Any twisting motion at this time creates a definite risk of fracture of the nasal septum.

Every precaution must be taken to insure that the bones are in the desired position at the end of the procedure; the surgeon should not hesitate to make as many cuts as necessary with the osteotome in order to obtain complete fractures. Comminuted fractures, or incomplete fractures with spicules of bone remaining attached to the frontal bones, may occur. Comminution, while worrisome to the novice, is not important provided the bones are in the proper position.

Up to this point it is not wise to separate the periosteum or soft tissue completely from the nasal bones. One of the main reasons is that if comminution does occur, the periosteum provides a sling or anchorage for the fragments.

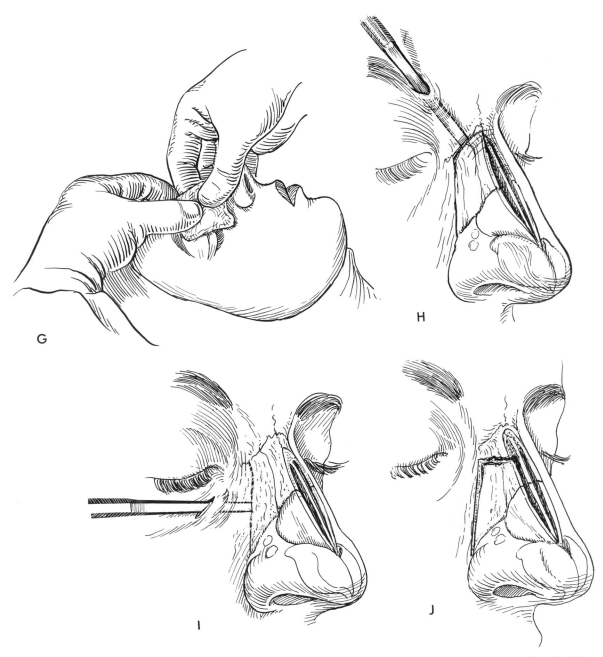

Greenstick fractures are acceptable if the bones are in their correct position. It cannot be overemphasized that if they are not, no amount of postoperative splinting, clamping, or other forms of pushing and pulling will put a bone into position. What the surgeon achieves at the operating table is the final result.

H, When infracture is difficult or impossible in the standard manner, it may be accomplished by passing a 2-mm. osteotome through a stab incision in the medial aspect of the eyebrow. The osteotome perforates the nasal bone in two or three places in the region of its junction with the nasal process of the frontal bone.

I, Lateral osteotomy may also be accomplished through a stab incision in the skin of the lower eyelid, but this technique will frequently give rise to considerable ecchymosis.

J, When excessive nasal root bone webbing is present, the superior osteotomy may be undesirably low. This will require removal of the nasal web tissue as shown on page 433.

Immediately following infracture, it is advisable to visually check and palpate the dorsum to make sure that no irregularities or projections of bone or cartilage exist. If they are present, they are rasped or resected. This last-minute nasal "toilet" is very important and can prevent much aggravation to patient and surgeon in months to come. It is disconcerting to both parties to have to schedule a second operation simply to rasp down a small spicule of bone or trim a small protrusion of upper lateral cartilage.

427

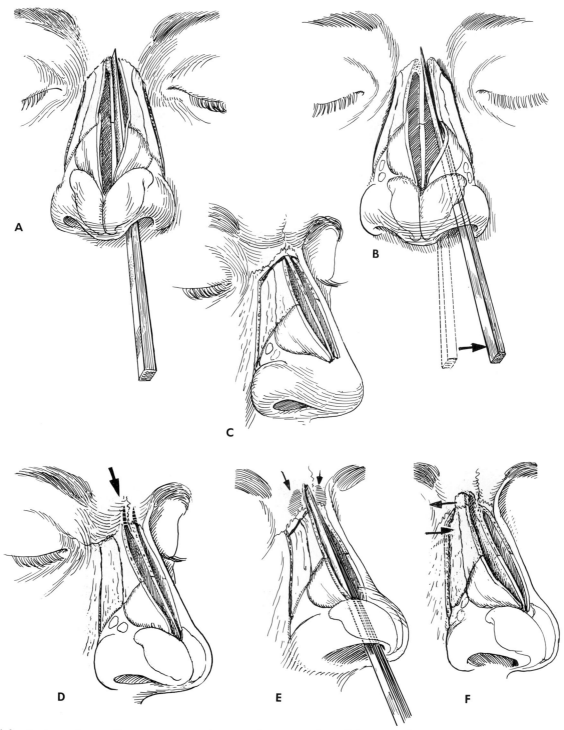

Medial osteotomy is usually not necessary in operative narrowing of the nose, but on occasion the bones do not fracture satisfactorily along the nasofrontal suture. In such cases they may be outfractured with an osteotome, or an osteotomy along the nasofrontal suture may be done with a 2-mm. osteotome.

A, An osteotome is gently guided along the bony septum and driven firmly into the nasal process of the frontal bone.

B, Pivoting on the nasal process, the osteotome is pressed laterally, with resultant outfracturing of the nasofrontal bone junction.

C, A satisfactory outfracture.

D, The usual limits of the osteotomy for outfracture.

E, Excessive passage of the osteotome into the nasal process of the frontal bone, resulting in a weakening of the bone laterally and its widening in this region.

F, The outfracture may be accompanied by a relative protrusion of an attached segment of the nasal process of the frontal bone (the "rocker effect of Becker"), which will require modification by rasping or comminution.

428

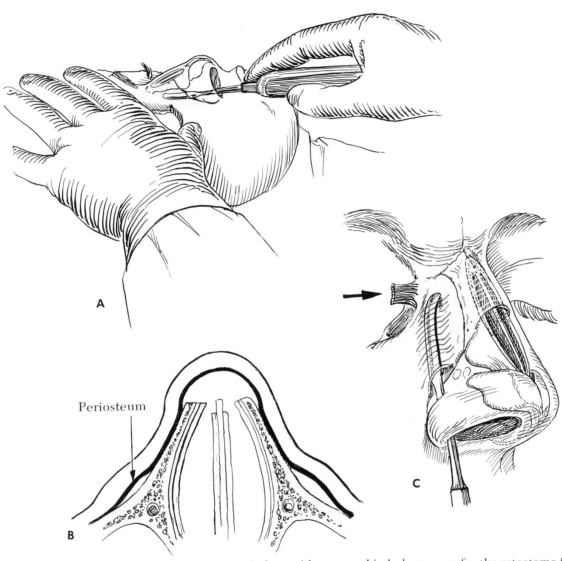

It is not important whether the lateral osteotomy is done with saws or chisels, but we prefer the osteotome for its ease of use and for the fact that it creates a less complete osteotomy, preserving periosteum as a sling. The osteotome also cuts without dust, is more easily controlled than a saw, and is much less fatiguing to use.

The saw technique illustrated on these pages requires that a tunnel of periosteum be raised first.

A, The periosteal elevator is placed through the incision and directed to the immediate precanthal region by a straight push. Excessive lifting of the periosteum in this region is to be avoided, as only a narrow tract is needed.

B, The line of elevation should be made to lie on the anterior aspect of the maxilla at the beginning of the nasal process. This is important to prevent the formation of a step in this region following osteotomy and infracture.

C, The elevator is pushed far upward to lie immediately in front of the anterior slip of the medial canthal ligament. The novice operator is frequently afraid of injuring this structure, but even in the most expert hands this has proved to be a difficult feat to accomplish.

429

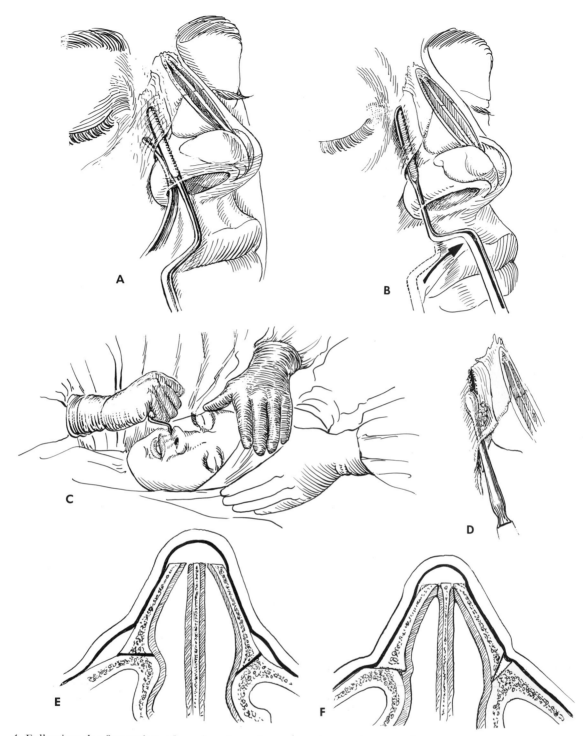

A, Following the formation of a subperiosteal passage, the nasal saw guide is inserted through the stab incision and the nasal saw is passed along the tunnel. This procedure is facilitated by keeping the saw teeth against the underlying nasal bone until the saw is in position.

B, The saw is turned so that it will pass directly across the face. The tip must be maintained in contact with the nasal bones to prevent entanglement with overlying soft tissues and the consequent production of ecchymosis. Correct use of the saw requires that a minimum of force be employed. Too much pressure jams the teeth and slows the cutting.

C, The patient's head is steadied between the two hands of the assistant during the entire sawing procedure. The operator's comfort and ease of working are aided by lowering the table and turning the patient's head to the side.

D, Bone dust and spicules are removed from the osteotomy site by a curette, frequently called a "nasal sweeper."

E, A correct osteotomy, passing straight across the face, contrasted to an incorrectly angled osteotomy.

F, Following infracture the natural shape is mimicked on the side of correct osteotomy.

430

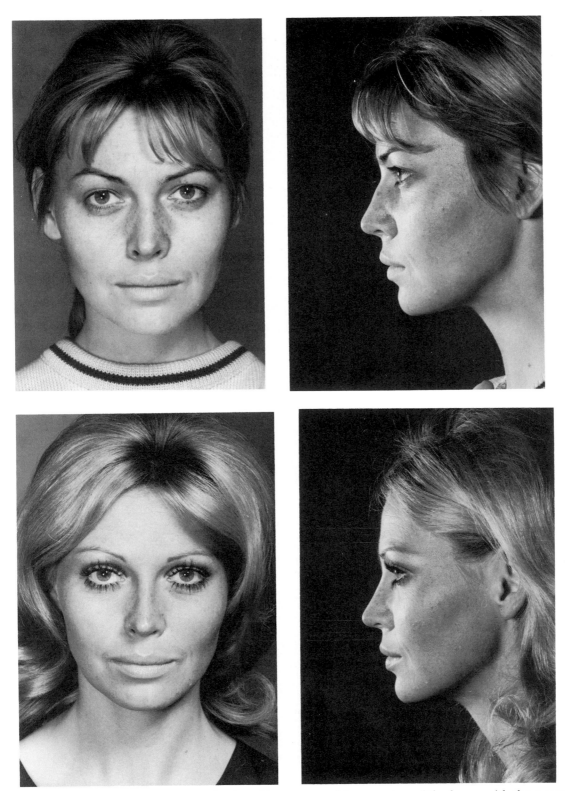

A patient with a broadened nose and a slight dorsal hump treated by resection of the hump with the osteotome and lateral osteotomies with infracture.

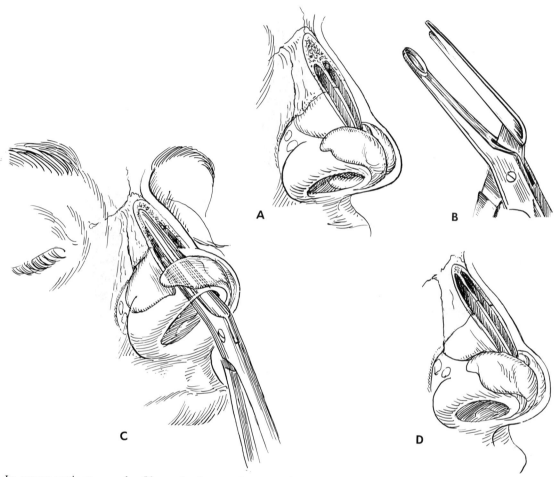

A

B

C

D

In many patients a web of bone in the nasal root region remains after the dorsum is modified. If this bone is left intact, it will prevent the complete narrowing of the nose in the upper third. The web may be removed with osteotomes or, as illustrated, with nasal root forceps.

A, A heavy nasal root web whose presence will impede the infracturing of the nasal bones and result in an excessively broad nasal septum with gaps between the nasal bones and the nasal septum.

B, The Converse (-Kazanjian) nasal root forceps, a heavy and specially designed style of rongeur, is available in broad and narrow shapes, the latter being more generally useful.

C, The nasal root forceps are inserted to the region of the web, which is encompassed by their tips. The forceps must be in good condition and they must be completely closed before removing nasal root bone. Failure to observe these two points will not infrequently result in total evulsion of the nasal bone, a calamity to be studiously avoided. Any resistance to removal of the forceps is to be regarded with suspicion, and the forceps should be reapplied and reclosed in such situations.

D, There is now no barrier to good infracture.

432

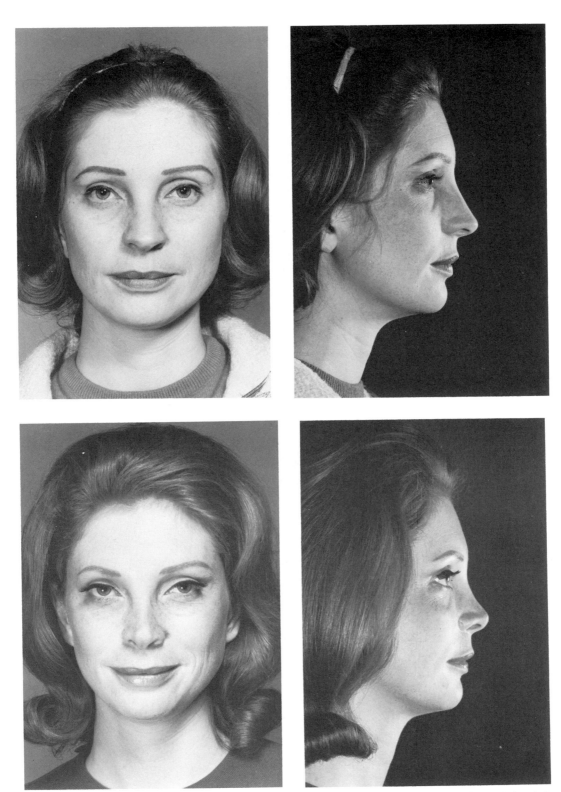

Excess width of the nose, particularly in the region of the nasofrontal angle, was corrected by minimal dorsal excision, removal of excess bone tissue in the region of the nasal root by Converse forceps, and lateral osteotomies.

433

THE SEPTUM

Whether a direct surgical approach to the septum is necessary in a rhinoplasty may be difficult to decide, as the septum is rarely straight throughout its length. There is almost no such thing as an undeviated septum. Correction should be undertaken only when a deviation causes a problem, for septal surgery always carries with it a risk of disturbance of the nasal dorsum, and such a risk is compounded when the surgery is done in connection with nasal plastic surgery.

The surgeon frequently sees patients with severe distortions of the septum with angulations in every conceivable plane and direction (for example, in fighters following repeated trauma to the nose), but with little or no difficulty in breathing. On the other hand, there are patients who complain of severe nasal obstruction with only mild degrees of septal deviation. There are obviously many factors to be considered in such a patient, and the surgeon must make every attempt to analyze them individually in order to assess the possible effect of nasal surgery.

The history of obstruction is important. Intermittent obstruction of the nasal passages, particularly when it tends to shift from side to side with the patient recumbent, indicates vasomotor rhinitis. A mild deviation of the septum, however, may contribute to the problem. In this situation the classic submucous resection at the time of rhinoplasty will rarely help. However, nasal obstruction from vasomotor rhinitis may be improved by rhinoplasty *without* submucous resection in the young patient, hinting that the phenomenon is very likely related to emotional stress which is being relieved by nasal plasty.

The typical allergic nose shows pale, swollen mucous membranes and hypertrophied turbinates. The patient experiences marked relief of symptoms when the membranes are shrunk with topical vasoconstrictors, and a history of their episodic usage (particularly in "allergy seasons") will often be given.

Because the airstream in the anterior part of the nose is apparently most important to the sensation of nasal respiration, respiration may be, or seem to be, obstructed if the septum is deviated in this region. Deviation of the septum at its point of junction with the upper lateral cartilages can also be disruptive. This triangle must be maintained high along the septal dorsum, and disturbance of the architecture here creates at least the sensation of nasal obstruction, if not obstruction itself. Severe deviation of the septum in its mid portion, with impingement on the lower and middle turbinates, can also cause respiratory interference of a type very difficult to correct without radical submucous resection and sometimes posterior turbinectomy.

Whenever possible, we prefer to avoid doing a submucous resection at the same time as nasal plasty. The caudal margin of the septum is modified in most operations, so that the surgery can technically qualify as an anterior submucous resection. The standard submucous resection, however, significantly lengthens the operative procedure and increases the morbidity, the likelihood of complications, and the possibility of postoperative epistaxis. Consequently this operation is best done after rhinoplasty, unless it is necessary to straighten a deviation of the septum.

Some surgeons, Aufricht prime among them, believe that a standard submucous resection is required in almost every patient in order to allow more room inside the nose for breathing. They believe that infracture and reduction of the nasal hump encroach on the available breathing space. Unless the cartilaginous septum is markedly thickened, however, the gain of 2 or 3 mm. from cartilage resection is really insignificant, and the internal nares are not appreciably altered by infracture in any event. Postponing radical septectomy until a later time, moreover, means that the surgeon is not limited in the amount of septal dorsum or inferior margin that can be removed at rhinoplasty.

It is actually impossible to separate the effects on the nasal physiology of submucous resection and rhinoplasty. Attempts to assign percentage values to the improvements achieved by the two procedures, as insurance companies do, are absurd in our opinion. Septal plasty, septal reconstruction and septal repositioning are preferred over formal submucous resection whenever they can be accomplished. It is rarely necessary to strip or to separate the mucoperichondrium from both sides of the septum—a step which can invite tears, perforations, and other complications. Much can be done to reposition the displaced or curved septum by elevating the mucoperichondrium from one side only and then making the appropriate cross cuts, which can be multiple and in all directions. Severely deviated portions or spurs can be shaved or partially removed where necessary, and the entire floor of the septum can be chiseled free and the septum moved. The advantage of maintaining the integrity of the septum instead of resecting large segments is obvious if one considers the anatomy of the nose. Techniques of septal reconstruction have been thoroughly examined by Converse (1950, 1964), Dingman (1956), Becker (1951), and Denecke and Meyer (1967).

The theory of Fry (1967) on the behavior of cartilage based upon its inherent system of response to stress may prove helpful in septal reconstruction. The observations stemmed from the work of Gibson and Davis (1958) on the biomechanics of cartilage. Fry has shown that multiple cross cuts (or "dicing") of cartilage disrupts the normal elastic forces on the side that is stripped of mucoperichondrium. Cartilages so cut will bend outward toward the cut side if the opposite side is left attached to undisturbed mucoperichondrium. Although this observation has not yet found widespread clinical support, we have found it useful in clinical trials. It bears a close relationship to the mechanical morseling process of weakening cartilage by crushing it or otherwise destroying the innate elastic forces of one side so that it can be made malleable enough to be molded into a desired shape.

We do not hesitate to do a conservative submucous resection, leaving a 1- to 2-cm. dorsal and caudal strut when it is obvious that this will correct a breathing difficulty at the time of rhinoplasty. Great care must be taken not to be lured into resection of the bony pillar, with the attendant risk of dorsal collapse.

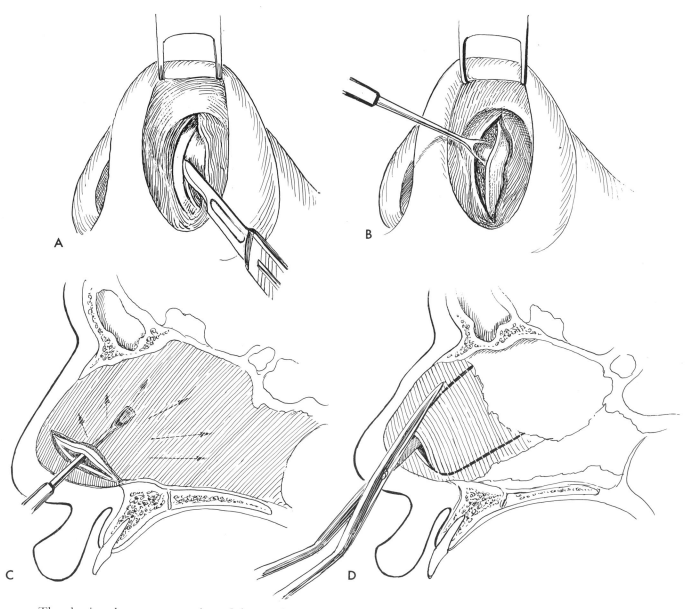

The classic submucous resection of the nasal septum.

A, An incision is made 5 to 10 mm. behind the corrected caudal border. Sharp dissection is required to separate the mucoperichondrium from the underlying cartilage, which is quite adherent in this region owing to the insertion of the depressor muscles.

B, Mucoperichondrial flaps are easily raised once the right plane is entered.

C, Similar flaps are raised on the apposing side after an incision is made through the cartilage. It is important to stagger this incision in relation to the first transmucosal incision so that the two do not overlie one another.

D, Resection of the deviated cartilage by the Knight nasal scissors.

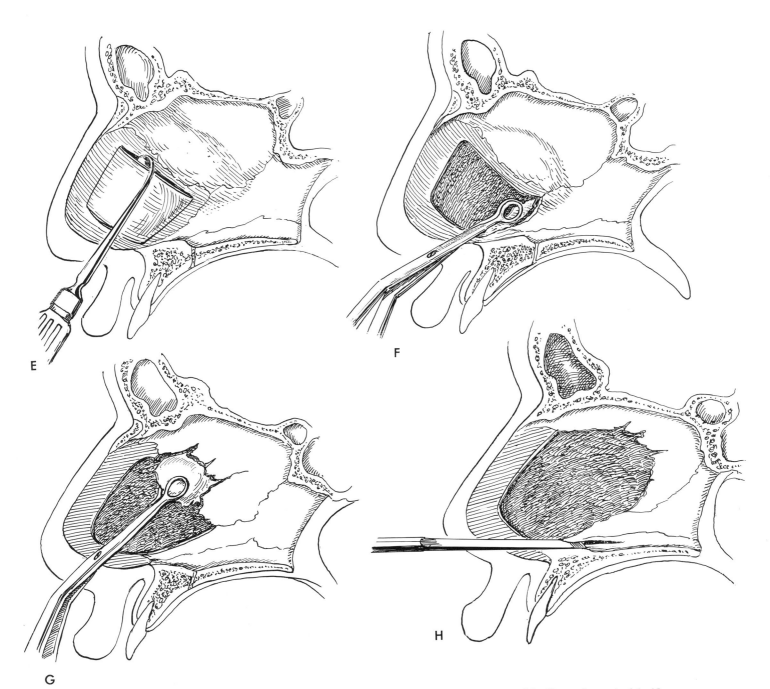

E, Resection of the deviated cartilaginous segment is completed by the Freer nasal knife or the swivel knife.

F, Deviated portions of bone and cartilage lying along the nasal floor are removed by Bruening forceps.

G, Where the submucous resection is more extensive than nasal plastic, the deviated bony septum is removed by Bruening forceps.

H, Further correction of the extensive osseous deformity may be achieved by passing an osteotome along the nasal floor.

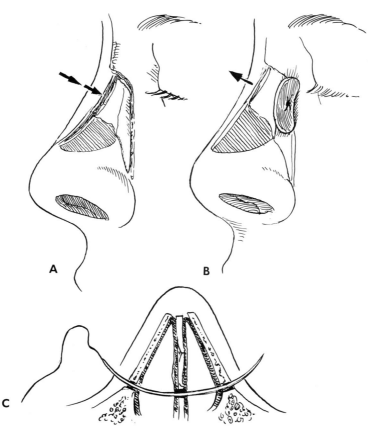

Radical resection of the septum, including the ethmoid plate and vomer, at the same time as a nasal plastic operation in which a large bony hump is removed, can result in a most distressing situation. Following lateral osteotomy with infracture, the bony and septal cartilage remnants can drop in their entirety into the pyriform aperture, just as is frequently seen in severe injuries of the middle face (A). This happens because the upper nose is literally hanging by a bony thread after radical septal surgery combined with hump removal.

This situation can be corrected only by bringing the nasal complex forward, as in a trauma case. The problem then is to maintain the complex in its new position. Suspension of the dropped structures on transnasal wires passed through lead plates (B) is the best answer. A curved needle is passed immediately anterior to the lateral osteotomies, and the nose is suspended from this in hammock fashion (C).

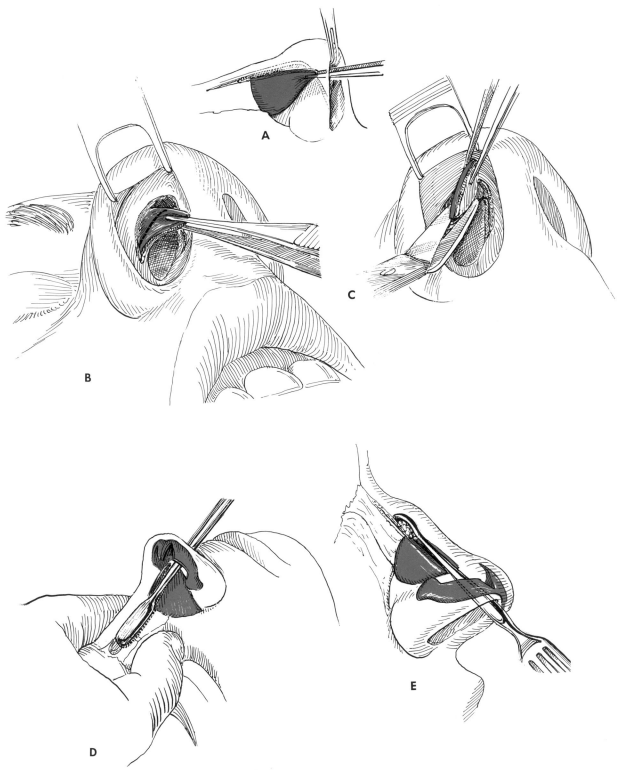

Finishing touches for the nasal plastic procedure.

A, Excess length of the upper lateral cartilages is estimated by visual inspection during gentle traction on their distal ends.

B, The excess amount of cartilage.

C, The excess is amputated conservatively.

D, Final smoothing of irregular nasal bones is completed when necessary with the rasp.

E, Bone and soft tissue debris is swept out by a small curette, and the entire region is carefully inspected with the aid of the Aufricht retractor to insure that all surfaces are smooth and that no small remnants of cartilage or bone remain. This measure is a most important step.

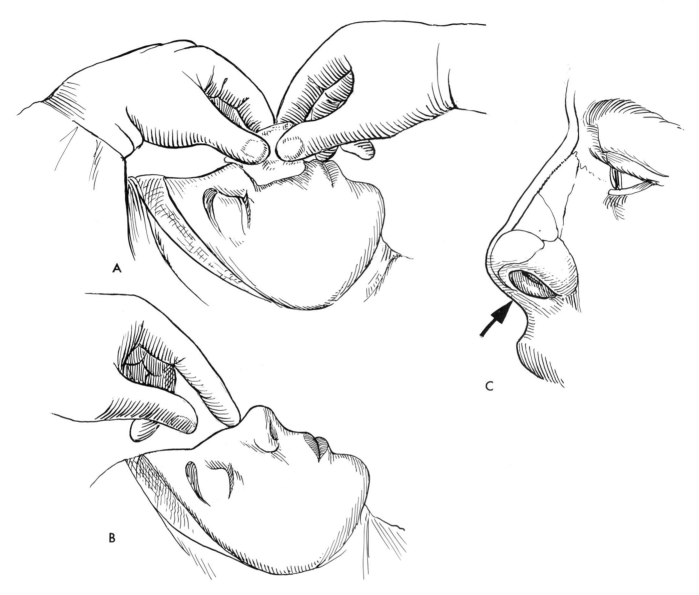

A, Operative edema of the nasal covering tissues is reduced by squeezing between the thumb and forefinger. The soft tissues are reapplied to the underlying nasal framework.

B, The finger is run along the new nasal dorsum and the soft tissues applied to it in order to determine the degree of correction achieved in the nasal tip and the dorsum. At this point it is important to palpate for any irregularities which will require secondary correction if left.

C, Pressure is carefully applied to reapproximate the margins of the membranous and cartilaginous septum, and the adequacy of the resection in this region is checked.

440

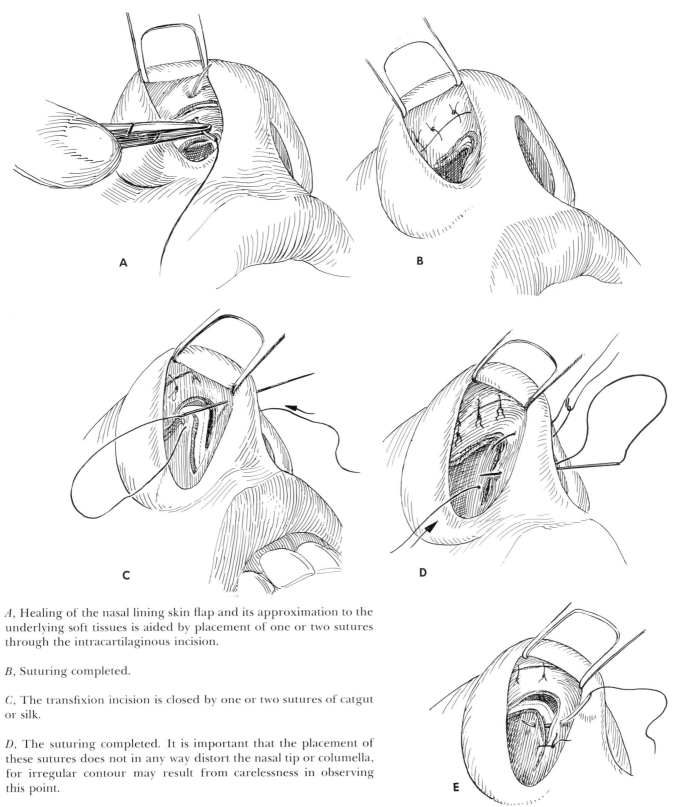

A, Healing of the nasal lining skin flap and its approximation to the underlying soft tissues is aided by placement of one or two sutures through the intracartilaginous incision.

B, Suturing completed.

C, The transfixion incision is closed by one or two sutures of catgut or silk.

D, The suturing completed. It is important that the placement of these sutures does not in any way distort the nasal tip or columella, for irregular contour may result from carelessness in observing this point.

E, Closure of the transfixion incision by reapproximation of lining skin to mucosa on either side of the incision. This method results in a minimum of tip distortion and is applicable when repositioning of the tip angle is not required.

A, Nasal packs of a single folded piece of Teflon-coated dressing placed in the nostril.

B, The packs in position, with a minimal amount protruding from the external nares.

C, Adhesive to support the soft tissues and to reduce dead space is applied to the exterior of the nose. The first tape to be applied is across the supratip region to appose the soft tissues to the dorsal portion of the septum.

D, The tip is supported by a sling of adhesive in the manner shown. This should be applied loosely about the tip and then tightened as shown in *E* to bring about accurate support of this area without skin wrinkling.

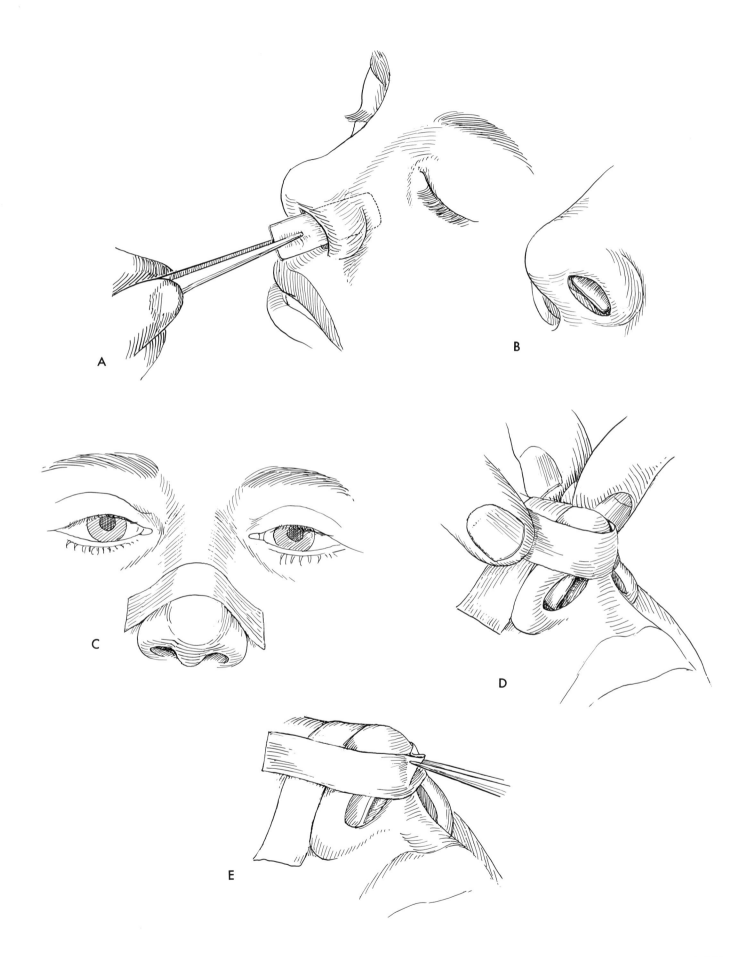

A, The adhesive support completed.

B, Seven or eight layers of plaster of Paris cut to the pattern shown.

C, In the patient with a deep nasofrontal angle, it is often necessary to cut into the precanthal area of the plaster splint to facilitate accurate approximation in this region. A piece of flannelette or Teflon-coated dressing is placed over the nose and the forehead in the manner shown to keep the plaster from adhering to the underlying adhesive tape.

D, The plaster of Paris is placed in tepid water to speed hardening, and the splint is molded into position.

E, The splint is held in place with additional adhesive strips. Prior to application of these strips, the skin should be protected with one of the many varieties of skin varnishes.

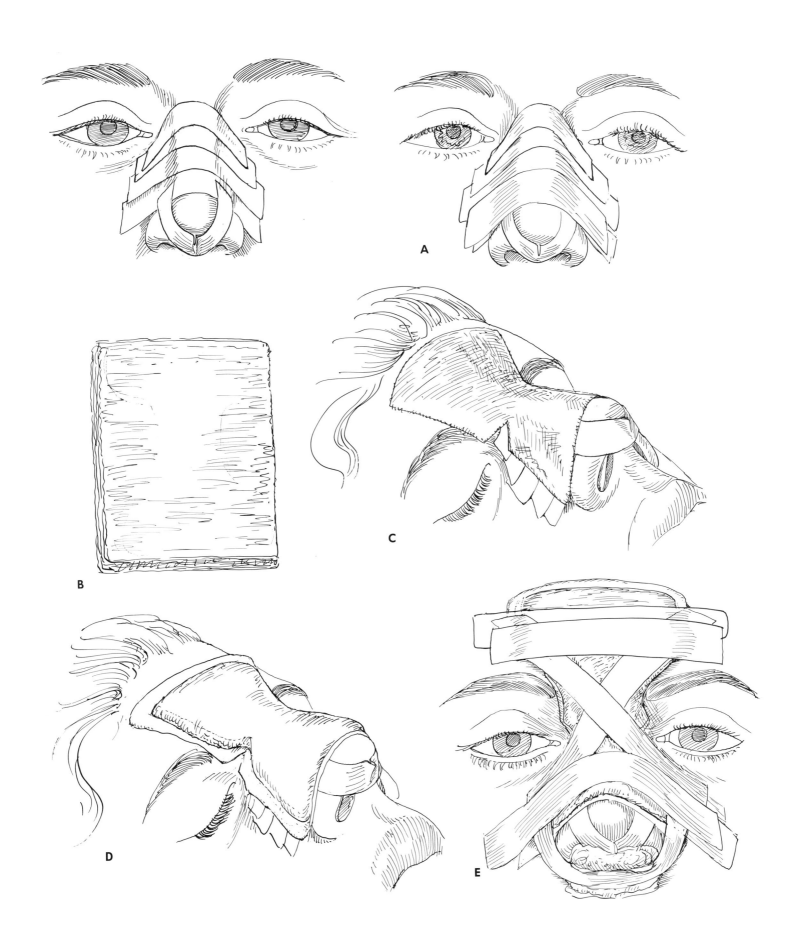

A

B

C

D

E

445

An alternate method of splinting the nose with dental compound.

A, A pattern is cut in Asche's soft metal to an approximate size, as shown.

B, A completed splint, showing the Asche's soft metal acting as a carrier for the dental compound.

C, The heat-softened (black) dental compound carried by the Asche's soft metal is placed over the nose and molded into position. Hardening is speeded by applying ice compresses. The soft metal carrier facilitates the handling of the dental compound and prevents transfer of excessive finger pressure to the nasal structure.

D, Transparent skin varnish is applied to the forehead and cheeks.

E, Adhesive applied to support the splint.

F, A 2 × 2 inch gauze is used to catch any nasal leakage.

446

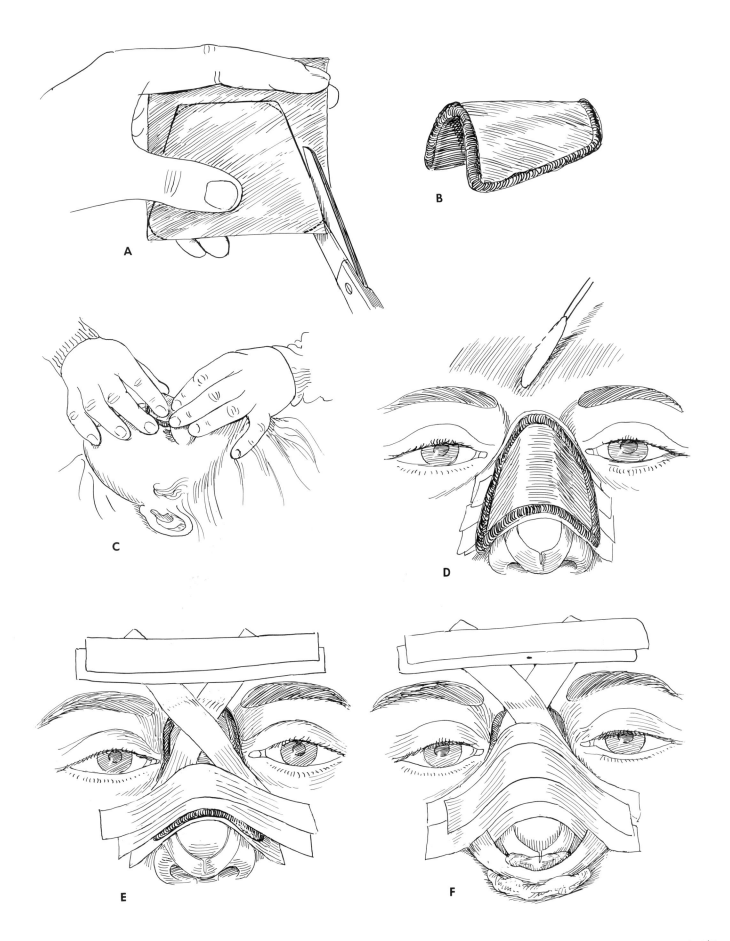

447

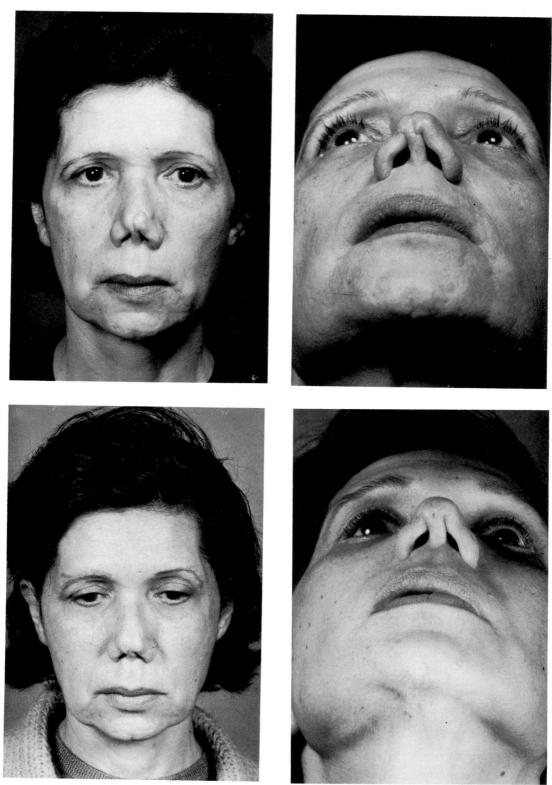

Severe nasal deformity following a number of inexpert operations on the nose. The postoperative views, taken after composite grafts from the concha were placed beneath the skin, illustrate the minimal success to be expected in such a difficult problem.

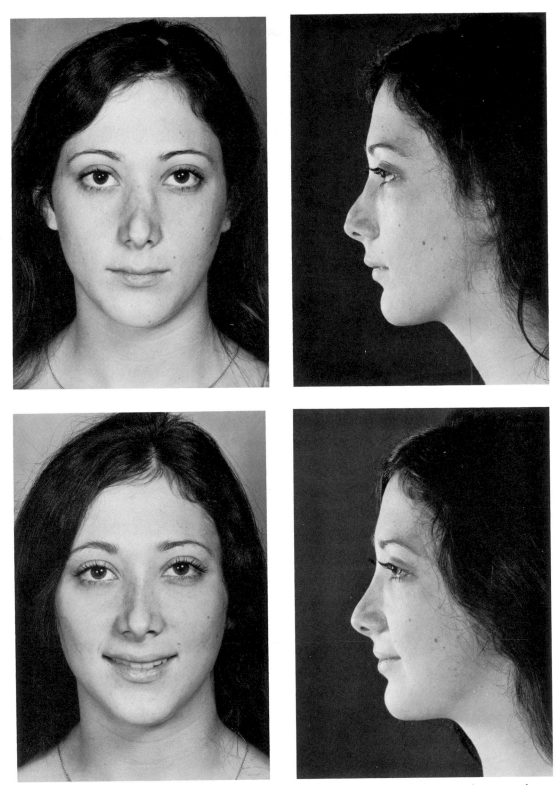

A favorable case for secondary repair. The first surgeon removed too much of the bony hump and practically none of the cartilaginous dorsum. He left only a minimal dorsal strut after completing a submucous resection. The secondary operation consisted of lateral osteotomy with infracture, trimming of the alar cartilage, and a careful lowering of the dorsal border of the septum. The slight dorsal hump was left, for it was feared that further lowering of the dorsum could result in sufficient weakening of the dorsal septum to bring about collapse of the nose.

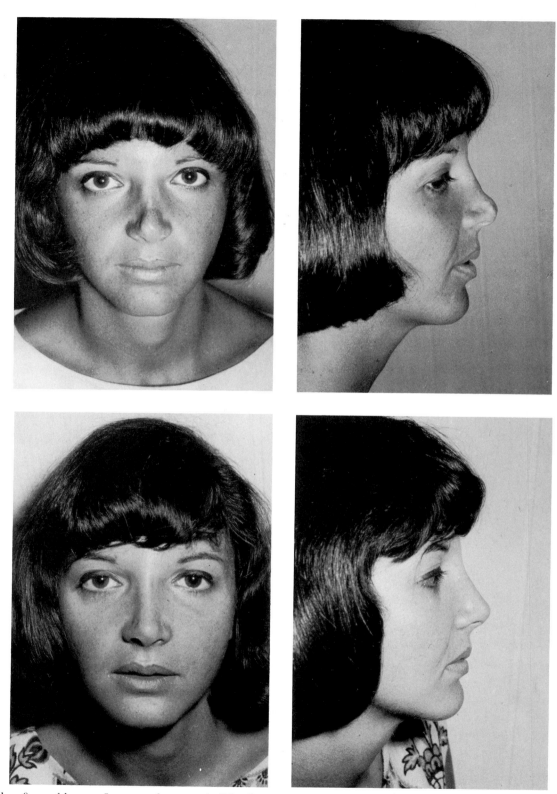

Another favorable case for secondary repair. The first surgeon apparently removed the hump unequally, so that a small dorsal bony hump remained, with a depression of the dorsal cartilaginous septal border. Additionally the alar cartilages were asymmetrically and insufficiently remodeled, and infracture was not done. The secondary procedure comprised lowering of the bony dorsum, nasal tip plasty, and lateral osteotomy with infracture.

(From Rees, T. D., Krupp, S., and Wood-Smith, D.: Plast. Reconstr. Surg. *46*:332, 1970. Reproduced with permission.)

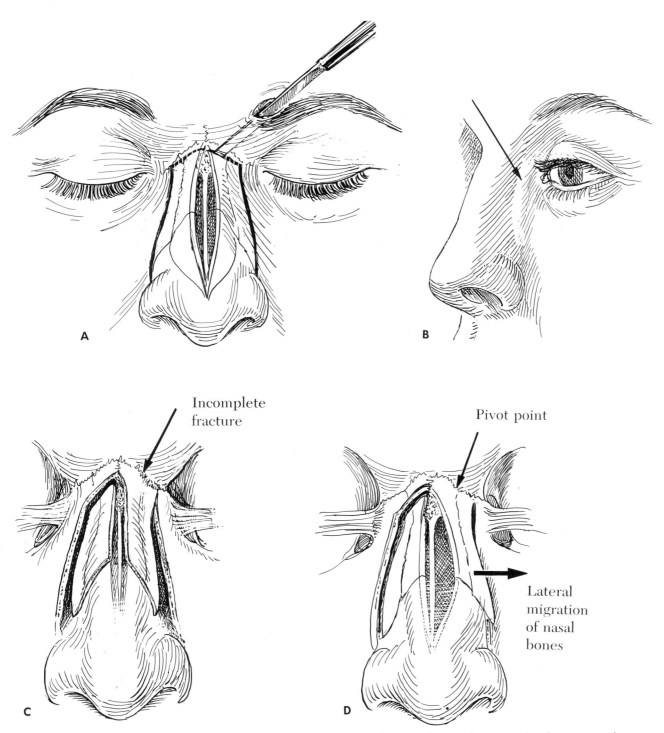

A

B

Incomplete
fracture

C

Pivot point

Lateral
migration
of nasal
bones

D

Lateral drifting of the nasal bones after rhinoplasty may result from an incomplete superior fracture at the root of the nose, or from a "greenstick" fracture. *A*, Direct superior osteotomy with a 2-mm. osteotome passed through the medial aspect of the eyebrow insures a complete fracture and prevents postoperative drifting. *B*, Lateral osteotomy should be low on the prefrontal process of the maxilla in order to prevent a "stair step" deformity. *C*, Postoperative widening of the bony vault may also result from incomplete fracture of the nasal bones or the nasal process of the frontal bone. This is particularly true if the bones are thick. *D*, Lateral migration may easily occur if a "greenstick" fracture is created, because the bone tends to pivot on the nasal process of the frontal bone.

451

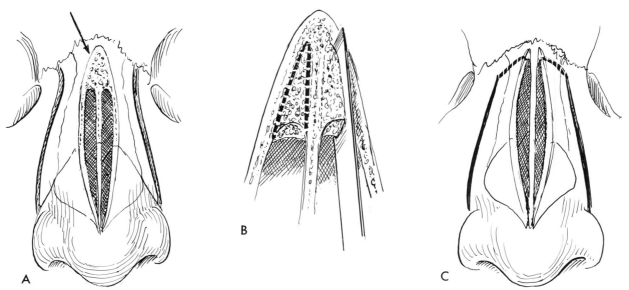

A, Sufficient narrowing of the bony nose requires complete fracture and, in addition, room for the fractured bones to move medially. *B*, Removal of a medial wedge of bone at the root of the nose may be necessary to achieve this medial movement. *C*, The complete lateral osteotomies and the clean superior fracture that are necessary for success.

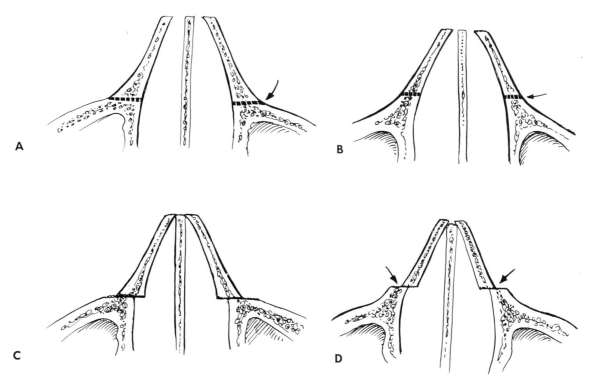

A common stigma of rhinoplasty is a visible ridge that can result from a lateral osteotomy at too high a level. The osteotomy must be made through the thick portion of the nasal process of the maxilla in order to prevent this "stair step" deformity. Osteotomy at this level by a surgeon inexpert in the use of a saw will be both tedious and difficult, and an osteotome will be easier to use.

A, The desirable lines of osteotomy. *B*, An osteotomy made too high on the bony vault. *C*, Ideal lines of osteotomy following infracture. *D*, Lines of osteotomy that will result in a typical "stair step" deformity.

(From Rees, T. D., Krupp, S., and Wood-Smith, D.: Plast. Reconstr. Surg. *46*:332, 1970. Reproduced with permission.)

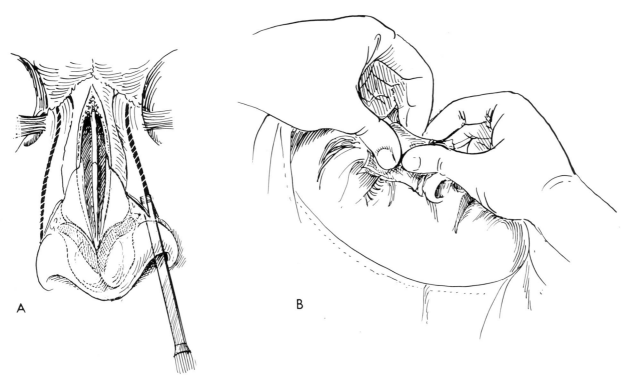

A

B

Narrowing of the nose after hump removal requires a complete lateral osteotomy to the level of the inner canthus. *A*, Lines of fracture of the lateral osteotomy. *B*, Complete infracturing by pressure concentrated on the upper halves of the nasal bones.

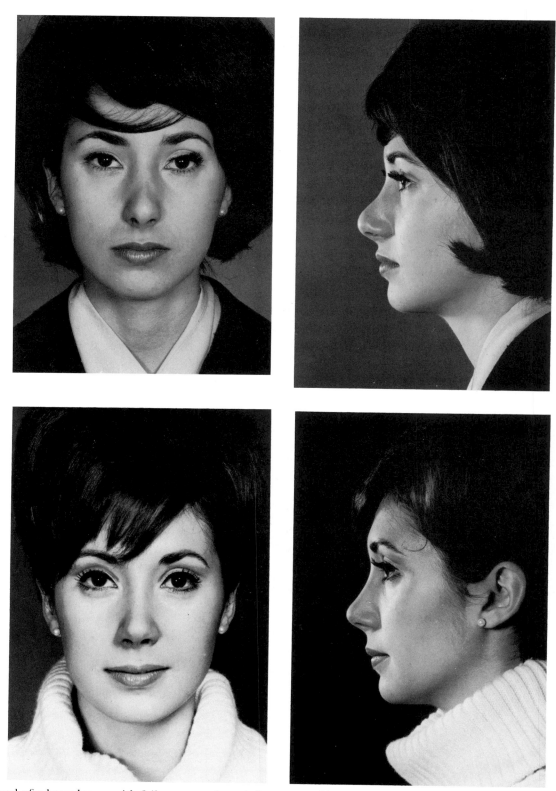

Removal of a bony hump with failure to perform infracture and lateral osteotomy; additionally there was insufficient lowering of the cartilaginous dorsal border of the septum. The secondary operation consisted of completion of lateral osteotomy, infracturing, and lowering of the dorsal border.

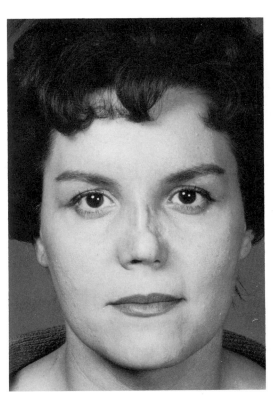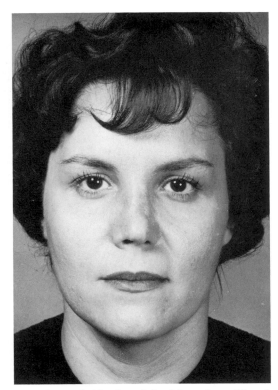

A series of inexpert surgical procedures resulted in scarring and actual skin slough in this patient. The situation was improved by full-thickness skin grafting and careful insertion of "matchstick" iliac bone grafts beneath the skin graft. (Courtesty of Dr. Ross Campbell.)

Supratip swelling, commonly called "polly tip" or "ram's tip," is perhaps the most common reason for a secondary nasal plastic operation. It is usually the result of scar tissue formation in the dorsal dead space secondary to granulation tissue *(A)*, inadequate reduction of the dorsal septal border *(B)*, or excessive resection of the alar domes *(C)*. The first two problems are usually correctable by a secondary procedure *(D* and *E)* and fixation of the soft tissues to the nasal framework. However, when too much alar cartilage has been removed, correction is almost impossible.

(From Rees, T. D., Krupp, S., and Wood-Smith, D.: Plast. Reconstr. Surg. *46*:332, 1970. Reproduced with permission.)

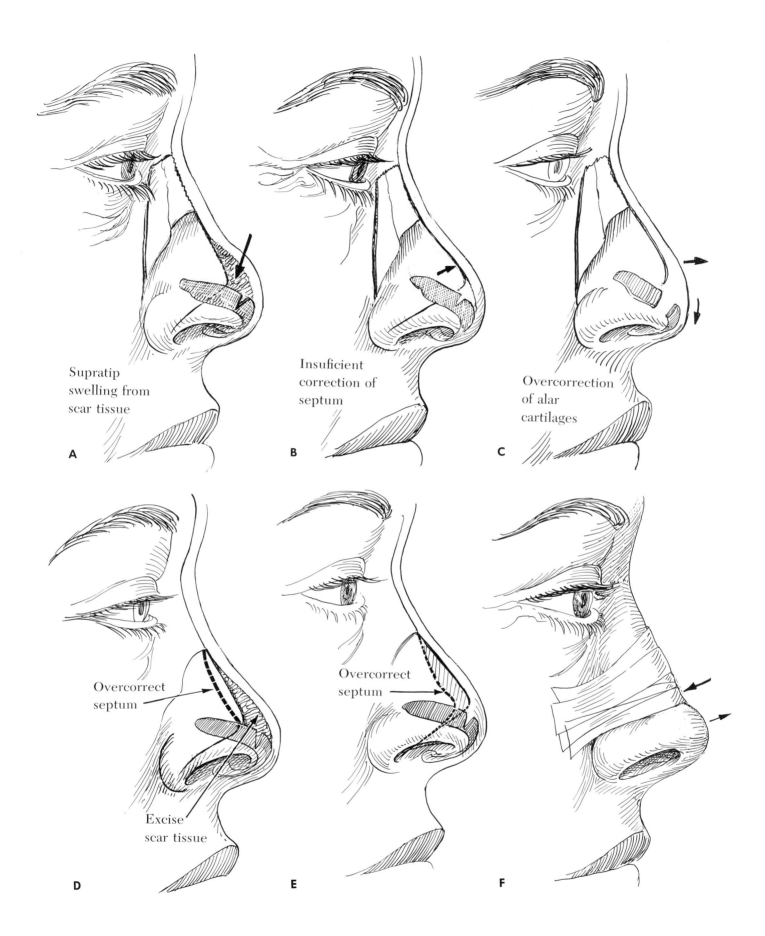

Supratip
swelling from
scar tissue

A

Insuficient
correction of
septum

B

Overcorrection
of alar
cartilages

C

Overcorrect
septum

Excise
scar tissue

D

Overcorrect
septum

E

F

457

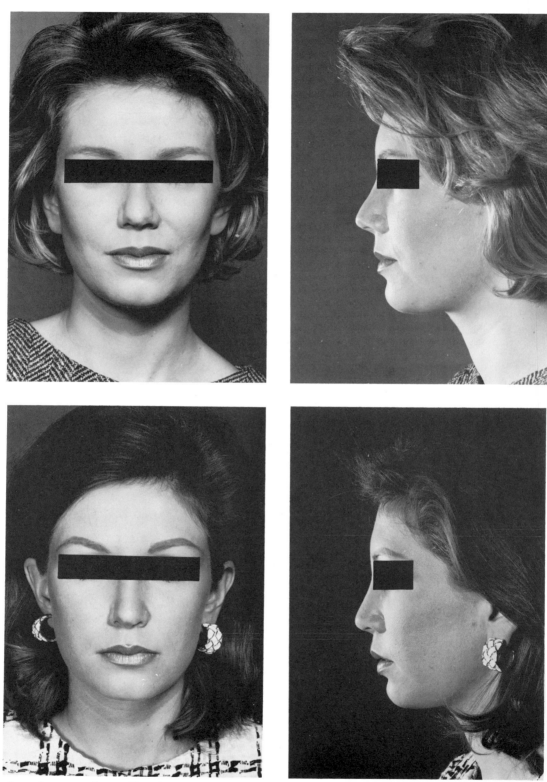

Correction of a supratip swelling by lowering of the dorsal border of the septum in the supratip region and removal of adjacent scar tissue with a secondary tip plasty. The two dimples on either side of the alar domes were filled with liquid silicone injected subdermally.

458

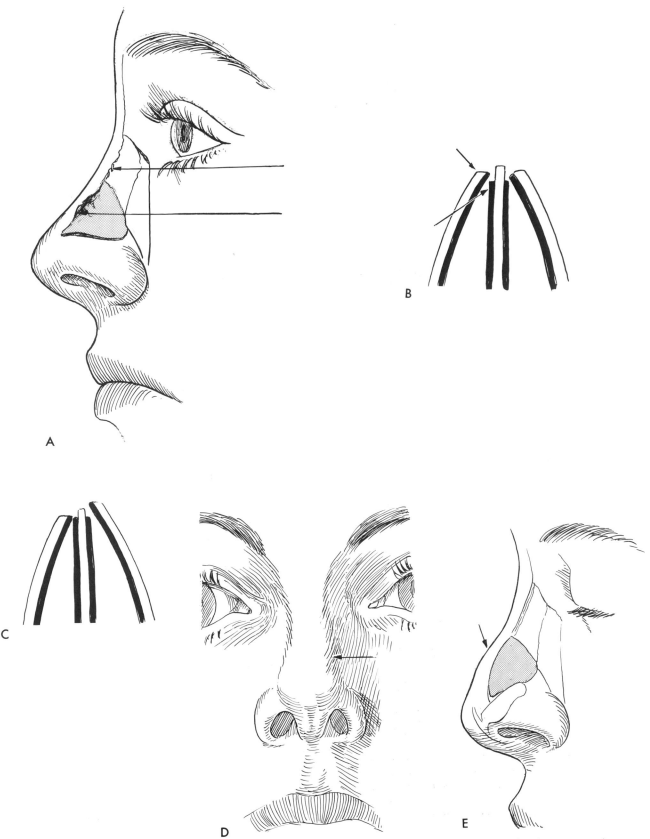

A, An irregular bony dorsum with excess protrusion of the upper lateral cartilages. No intervention is necessary in a patient whose irregularity is palpable but not visible. *B,* Ideal postoperative relations of cartilage and mucosa. *C,* An irregular upper lateral cartilage border. *D,* Fullness of the supratip area that may result from excessive upper lateral cartilage. *E,* In the thin-skinned patient, a supratip hump may be more noticeable.

459

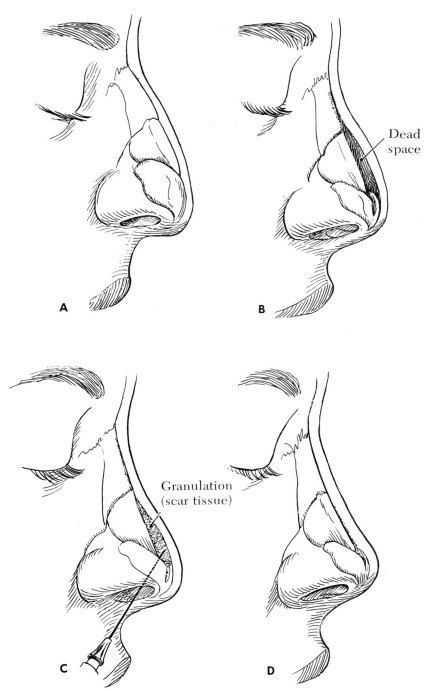

Intralesional injections of steroid compounds have proved helpful in hastening resolution of granulation tissue causing supratip swelling. *A,* The preoperative anatomy. *B,* Potential dead space between skin and cartilage created by the operation. Dressings help to eliminate this space. *C,* Granulation tissue in the dead space. Injection of triamcinolone directly into this tissue at weekly intervals for two or three weeks, usually in a dose of 5 mg. per injection, will help to eliminate this tissue. *D,* The result after dissolution of the granulation tissue.

460

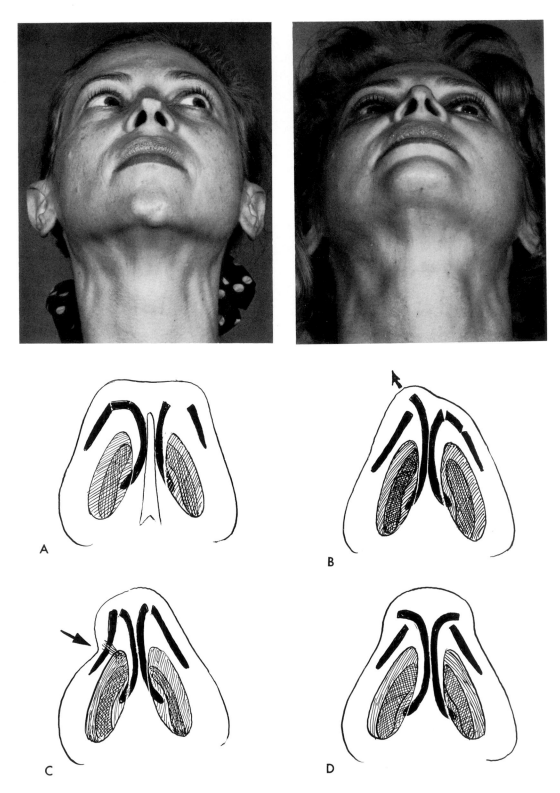

The asymmetric nasal tip and some of its common causes. *A*, Unequal excision of alar dome cartilage, with weakening of the dome support on the (patient's) left. *B*, Disruption of the continuity of the lateral crus of the alar cartilage, with projection of a portion of the cartilage expressing itself as a palpable skin irregularity. *C*, Damage to the skin overlying the lateral crus of the alar cartilage, resulting in dimpling. *D*, Breaking of the continuity of the lateral crura and failure to adequately resect their medial portions results in a so-called boxed tip.

461

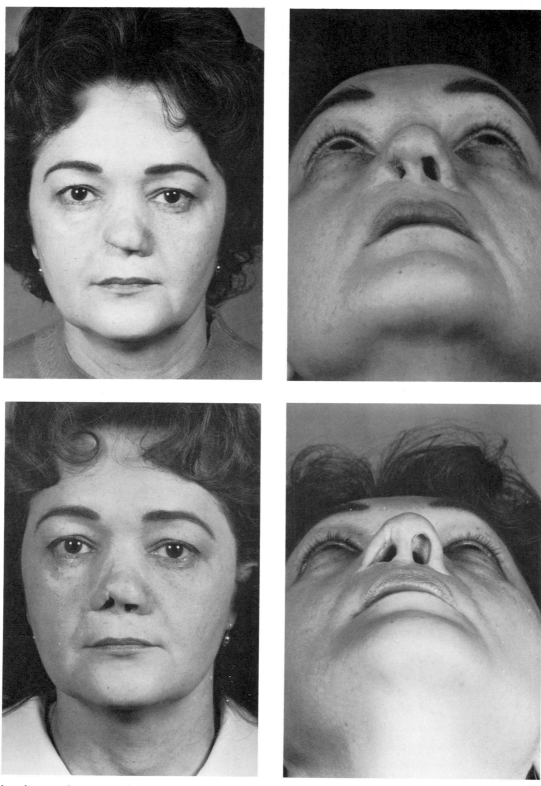

A mutilated nose, the result of many inexpert procedures done in rapid order. The right nostril was almost completely blocked, and loss of cartilage support on the left resulted in a flaplike action during inspiration. Postoperative views were taken after a chondrocutaneous composite graft to the right nostril; also illustrated is the use of a continuously worn acrylic shell prosthesis in the left nostril to prevent collapse.

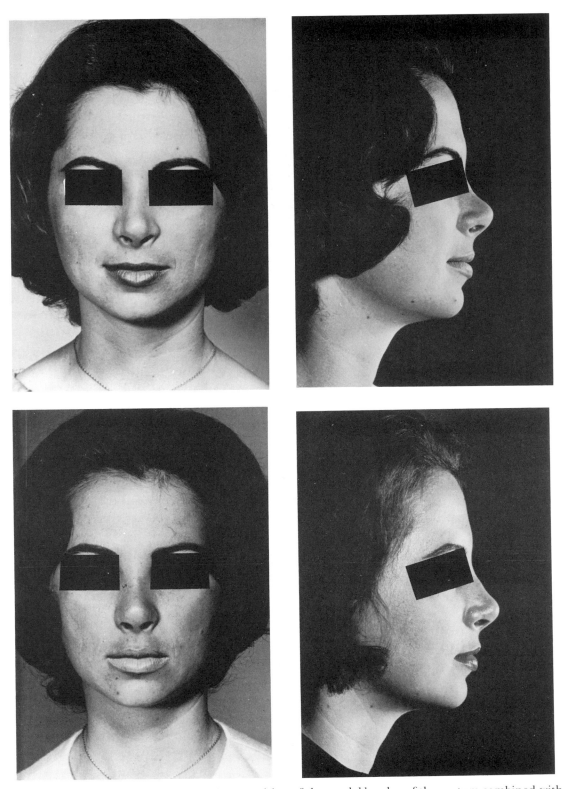

The preoperative views demonstrate the result of overexcision of the caudal border of the septum combined with total removal of the nasal spine—an overshortened nose. Separation of the soft tissues from the bony and cartilaginous skeleton of the nose, and their displacement caudally, achieved the lengthening shown in the postoperative photographs. Mattress sutures fix the soft tissues in their corrected position. The inferior displacement is further aided by lowering the septal angle. It must be emphasized that this is not the sort of result that can usually be achieved; frequently, there is little that can be done for these unfortunate patients.

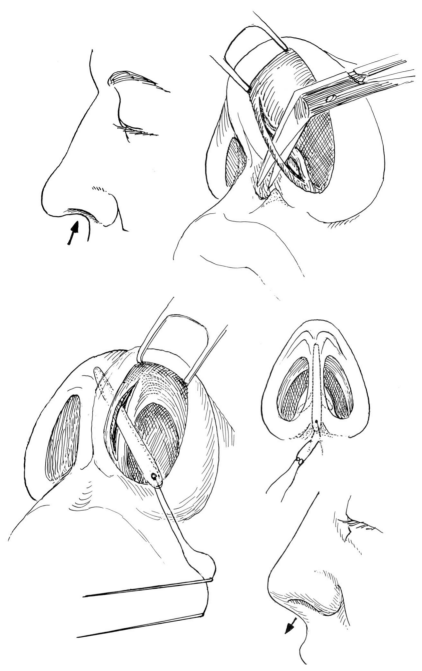

Retraction of the columella is a most distressing deformity following rhinoplasty or traumatic destruction of the nasal septum. It is *very difficult to correct.* When sufficient soft tissue is present—that is, when the membranous septum has not been destroyed—it is sometimes possible to improve the contour by an implant of bone or cartilage placed within the columella as a strut. The technique is illustrated here.

When extensive soft tissue and cartilage is missing, composite grafts to the region of the membranous septum from the ear, or flaps of nasal lining and alar cartilage from the side walls of the nose, can sometimes fill the gap, provided these structures too have not been mutilated or excised.

464

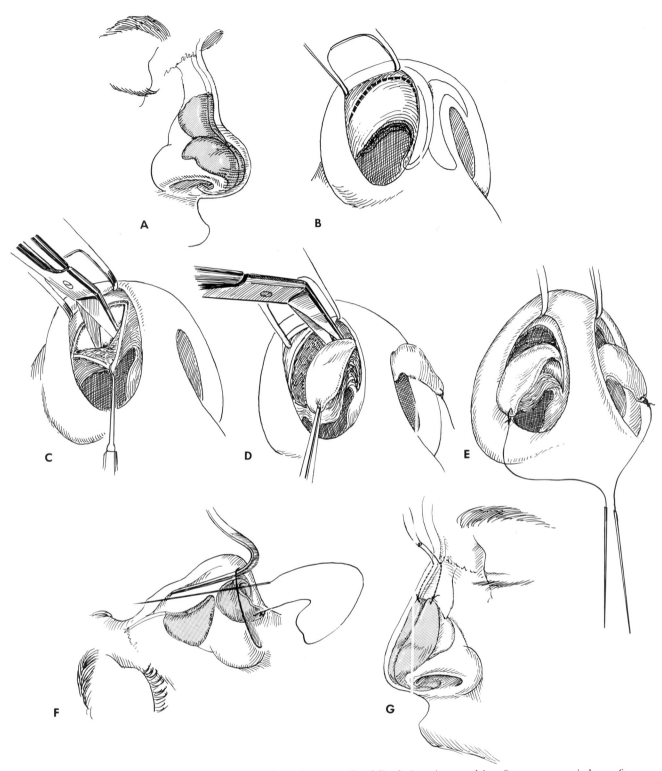

The "flying wing" technique for correction of minor degrees of saddle deformity resulting from traumatic loss of septum or from excessive resection of cartilaginous septum during surgery has been popularized in textbooks. The procedure has a place and is effective, provided sufficient lateral crus of the alar cartilage remains to provide bulk. The technique is illustrated here. We would emphasize that its use is to be limited to the most minor cases. Great care should be taken to adjust the cartilage flaps and suture them into position so that they are symmetrical.

The lateral crus is dissected free of lining and converted into a single pedicle flap (B to E). These flaps are then rotated into a pocket surgically created between the dorsal skin covering and the septal border, where they are fixed by sutures (F and G). The sutures can be fashioned as pull-out sutures passing through the dorsal skin.

Saddle defects are best repaired by implants. Prosthetic materials are rarely used because of the pressure of scar tissue and loss of pliability of the skin. Autogenous grafts, either septal or costal cartilage, or bone, are the materials of choice. Layered strips of septal cartilage rarely warp but are scanty in amount and difficult to shape, while costal cartilage tends to warp unless "eye round" cartilage is used (Gibson). Iliac bone is unquestionably the best material; it can be shaped exactly to suit, it is hardy, and it withstands contamination admirably. Some absorption and even spontaneous fracture can be found to occur on long-term follow-up, but those disadvantages are outweighed by the biological advantages of this excellent graft material.

The upper drawings illustrate the technique of placing a costal cartilage graft. *A*, Depression of the nasal dorsum.

B, Elevation of the soft tissues and periosteum via an intercartilaginous incision.

C, Cartilage from the costochondral junction carved to the appropriate shape for the particular patient.

D, The implant in position.

The remaining drawings demonstrate the insertion of a septal cartilage implant.

E, Depression of the cartilaginous dorsum.

F, Built-up dorsal cartilage implants held together with 4-0 plain catgut sutures.

G, The implant in place.

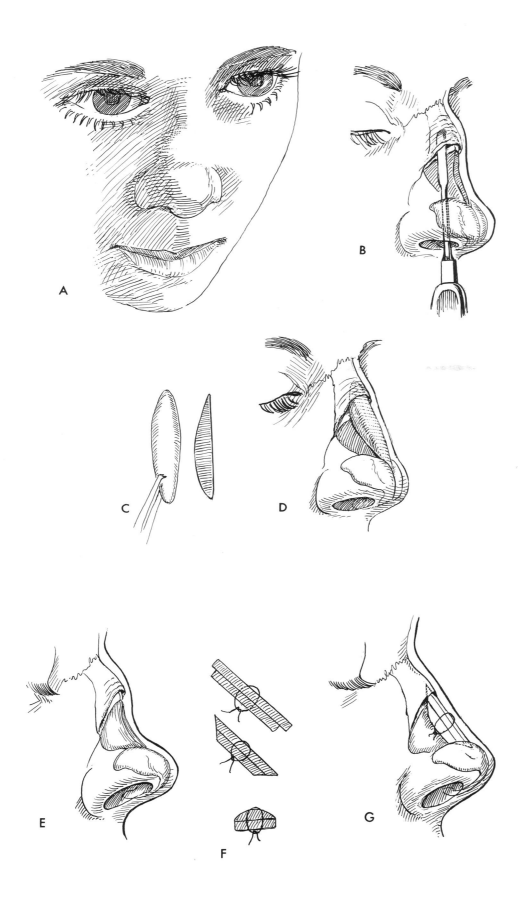

Bone grafting of the dorsum of the nose.

A, A saddle nose deformity.

B, The interdome region is exposed through a rim incision.

C, Soft tissues in the interdome region are divided.

D, After the soft tissues are raised from the dorsal aspect of the cartilaginous framework, a periosteal elevator is used to sweep the periosteum laterally from the nasal bones and to expose bare bone.

E, The shaped iliac bone implant; its shape varies considerably from patient to patient.

F, It may be necessary to remove a portion of the nasal bone in order to allow a sufficiently thick strut of iliac bone graft to be placed over the dorsum without overcorrecting the profile. The transnasal wires are placed in position by two small percutaneous punctures on either side of the nose.

G, The iliac bone graft in place and maintained in position by circumferential wire. Wiring is not essential to the success of the procedure and should be employed only when excess tension is believed present over the caudal aspect of the bone graft, which would make it difficult to maintain osseous contact above.

468

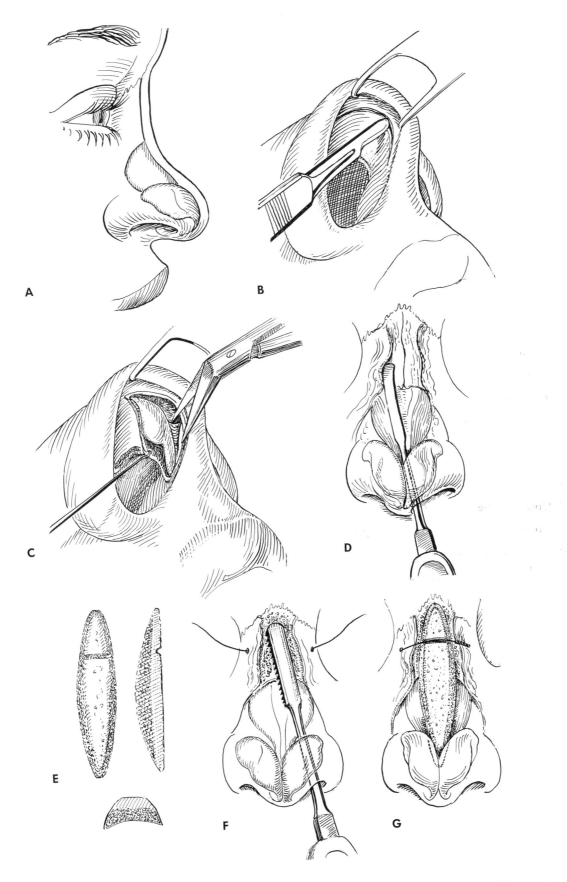

A

B

C

D

E

F

G

(*Illustration continued on following page.*)

469

H, Another view of the bone graft secured in place by circumferential wire.

I, Projection of the tip is maintained by 4–0 plain catgut sutures passed over the cantilevered tip of the nasal bone.

J, The nasal tip prior to correction.

K, The nasal tip after correction, showing how it is suspended from the bony strut.

L, The operative procedure completed, showing the tip projection achieved.

M, Periosteum undermined and raised.

N, The carved bony implant.

O, The implant held in position by the pressure of soft tissues over its upper end. It must be noted that such an implant will not stay in place where much tension exists on its lower end.

P, Undermining soft tissues in the columella to expose the nasal spine.

Q, An iliac bone graft with a nasal spine extension to support the tip.

R, The procedure completed and the support of the tip aided by the passage of a catgut suture between the alar domes.

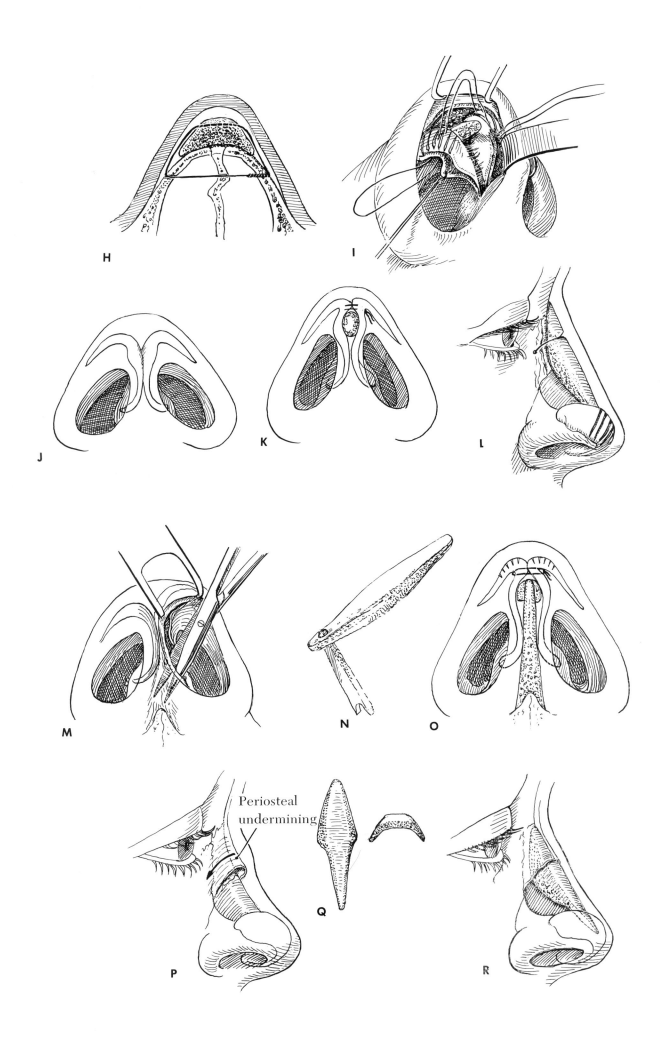

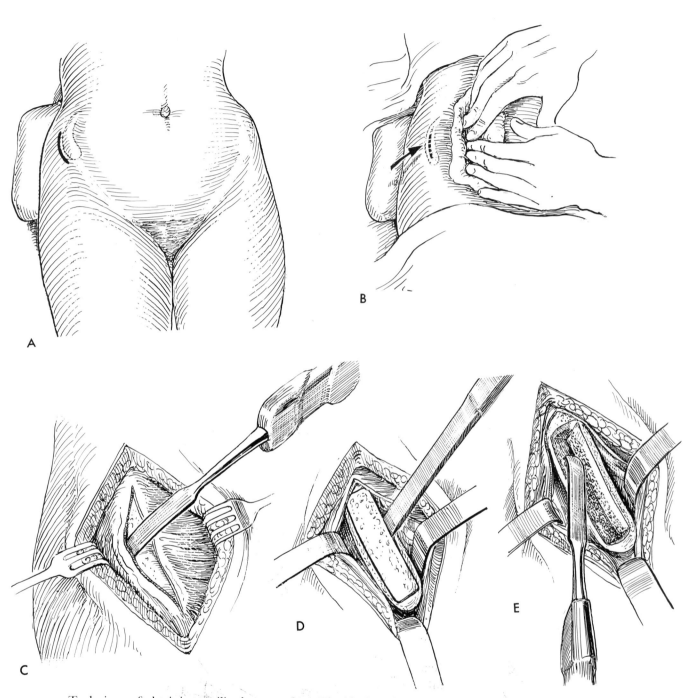

Technique of obtaining an iliac bone graft. *A*, The ideal site is shown; the patient is in the supine position and the incision is placed just below the iliac crest so that it will not be irritated by the pressure of belts or undergarments. *B*, The skin is displaced medially by pressure on the iliac fossa, and an incision is made through skin and subcutaneous tissues to the iliac crest. *C*, The periosteum is raised from the iliac crest. *D*, A suitably sized segment of bone, with the underlying cancellous bone, is removed. *E*, Hemostasis is aided by heavy pressure with the osteotome, which helps to bring about closure of the underlying cancellous bony spaces. The wound is closed in layers, with or without drainage, depending upon the degree of hemostasis obtained.

Rhinoplasty in the Non-Caucasian Nose

The desire for a more perfect nose is by no means limited to the Caucasian race. Increasing numbers of people of Asian, African and Indian extraction are undergoing rhinoplasty because of social, economic and personal pressures.

In Orientals augmentation rhinoplasty is a commonplace procedure, which Boo-Chai (1964) rates second in frequency among plastic procedures only to reconstruction of the superior palpebral fold. Like correction of the "slit eye," nasoplasty apparently answers a growing desire for Westernization of appearance, and many thousands of such operations have been done in Japan and the Orient.

The Oriental nose has many features in common with other types of non-Caucasian noses—flat bridge, flared alae, short columella; these are the nasal configurations for which cosmetic changes are most often sought. In his text on plastic surgery, Uchida (1958) described techniques for correction of the false saddle nose by various implants. Boo-Chai prefers medical grade silicone rubber as a carved implant to the dorsum because of extrusion of other substances, but has had little trouble with this material. Boo-Chai has emphasized the importance of remodeling the nasal tip to achieve consistently satisfying results. The favorite method of alar resculpturing consists of a standard Weir-type of wedge resection of the alar base and includes correction of the overhanging alae, as seen in profile, by excising a section along the rim of the alae similar to the technique of Millard (1959).

Reports of nasoplasty in Negroes are surprisingly uncommon, although there is every indication that increasing numbers of Negroes are seeking cosmetic surgery. With growing participation of Negroes in the advertising and entertainment fields, there is little doubt that the demand for rhinoplasty will continue to rise.

Rees (1969) and Falces et al. (1970) have reported several cases and discussed many of the problems attendant upon the procedure, including pertinent anatomic variations which are shared in general with other non-Caucasians.

The typical Negroid nose is flattened and broad and often shows some degree of "saddle" deformity. The tip tends to be flat and rounded, and there is an increase in the angle between the medial and lateral crura at the alar dome. The alae are often flared and the nostrils large.

There is frequently a low angle between the anterior and inferior border of the septum. This cartilaginous angle provides much of the tip projection of the nose. Whereas the projection of the septal angle must often be lowered in nasoplasty of Caucasians, in the Negro it is generally desirable for it to be increased. This is best done by inserting a graft or implant. The inferior septal margin of the Negro nose is usually somewhat concave or receded, much like the retracted columella that may result from radical submucous resection with removal of the lower edge of the cartilaginous septum. It is rarely necessary to shorten the nose or to resect any of the inferior margin of the septum during rhinoplasty in a Negro, but frequently necessary to graft the caudal border of the medial crura and the anterior aspect of the nasal spine.

The pyriform aperture is usually wide, with an increased distance between the nasal bones where they join the face. This may resemble the Caucasian nose after a direct blow to the dorsum has "splayed out" its bones. This increased distance between the facial attachments of the nasal bones gives the Negroid nose its wide frontal appearance.

There are many minor anatomical variations in the "typical" Negro nose; intermarriage with other groups has produced structural differences which require special consideration when performing nasal surgery. For example, Negroes from the West Indies or the northern regions of Africa often have dorsal hump deformities of the nose, probably because of Indian or Arabic genetic influences. Such patients require reduction of this hump as part of the overall correction.

473

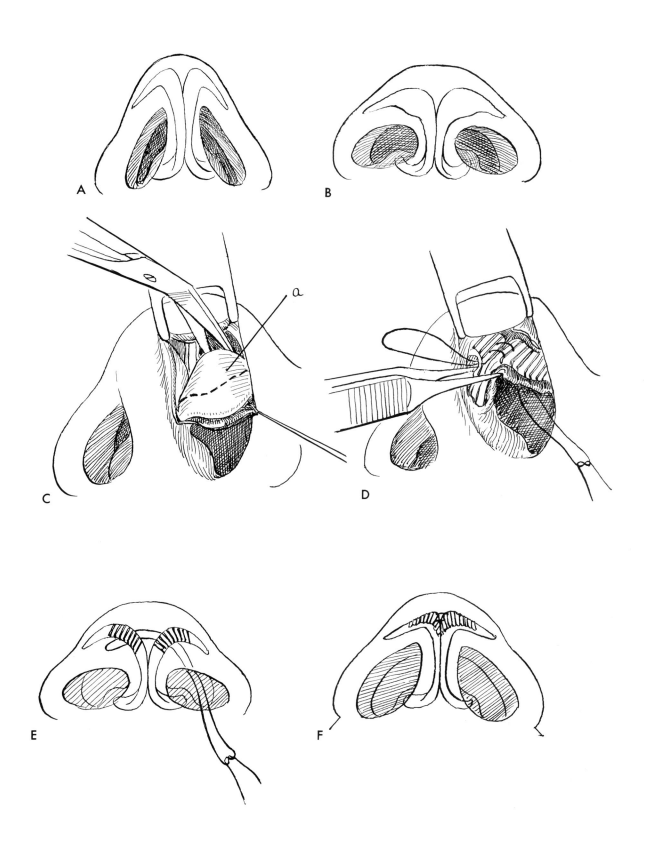

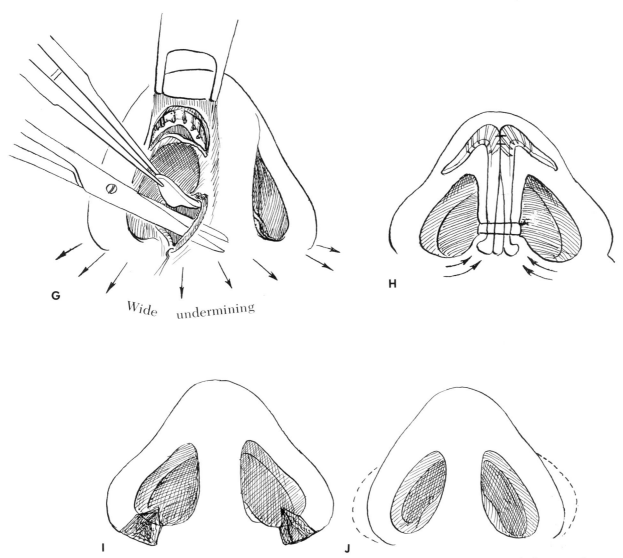

Rhinoplasty in the non-Caucasian nose requires a series of steps designed to alter those anatomic features that are different from those of the Caucasian. A prolonged and projecting tip with acute angulation of the alar crura and elliptical nares characterize the Caucasian nose *(A)*, while the non-Caucasian nose generally shows obtuse angulation of the alar domes, a short columella, flaring of the alae, and a low septal angle *(B)*.

The Lipsett maneuver used in reverse to achieve forward projection of the tip by suturing the scored alar cartilages has proved helpful. *C*, Exposure of the tip cartilages through a rim incision; "a" denotes the upper portion of the cartilage, which is to be removed (Safian, 1934). *D*, Weakening of the cartilage as in the Lipsett technique and "rolling in" of the lateral crura to form a new medial crus. *E*, A 4–0 plain catgut suture used to maintain the new medial crura in position. *F*, The medial crura in place (Rees, Guy, and Converse, 1966).

Another useful technique is to free the base of the columella and suture the feet of the medial crura together. *G*, Wide undermining of the base of the columella and adjacent lip, to allow for sweeping of these soft tissues into a new columella to increase tip projection. *H*, After removal of the soft tissues lying between the feet of the medial crura, a 4–0 plain catgut suture approximates the crura and gains further tip projection.

Finally, alar base resections can reduce flaring. *I*, In this instance the resection mainly involves the floor of the nostril. *J*, The alar base resection completed, achieving both reduction of flaring and increase of projection.

(From Rees, T. D.: Plast. Reconstr. Surg. *43*:13, 1969. Reproduced with permission.)

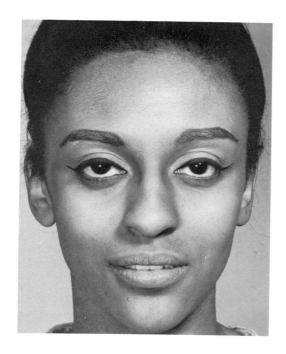

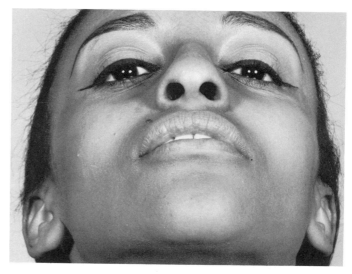

The non-Caucasian nose may have a slight hump deformity, resulting from a mixed heritage. Postoperative views show the results of hump removal, narrowing osteotomy, and tip plasty.

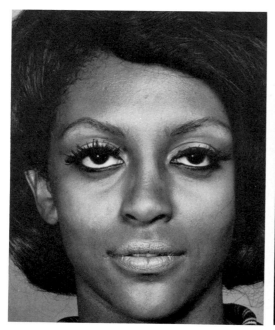

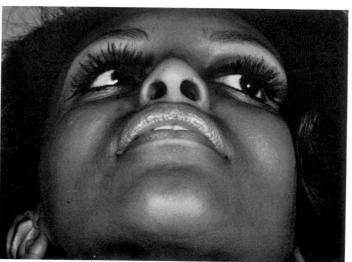

476

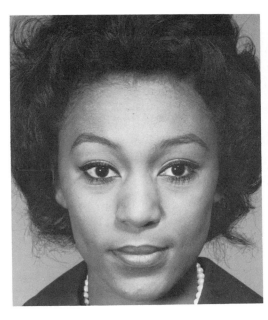

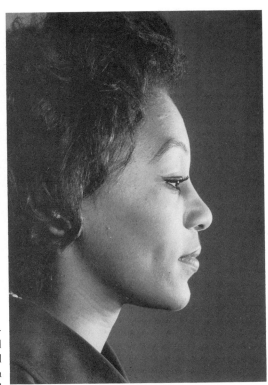

When the dorsal profile is not a major consideration but there is widening of the nasal pyramid, lateral osteotomy with infracture will not only narrow the nose but also result in a slight elevation of the nasal dorsum. This will often obviate the need for a dorsal implant. Osteotomy is done flush with the anterior surface of the maxilla to avoid "stair stepping" and is facilitated by the use of 3- or 4-mm. osteotomes.

(From Rees, T. D.: Plast. Reconstr. Surg. *43*:13, 1969. Reproduced with permission.)

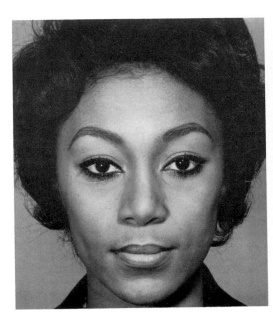

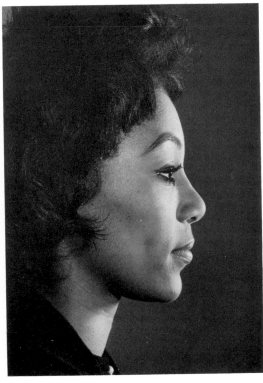

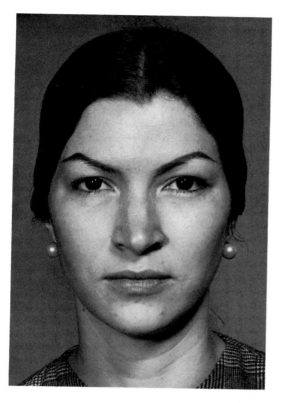

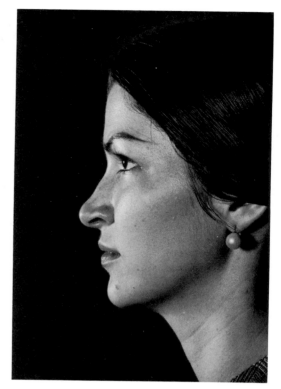

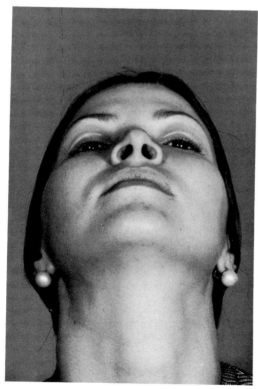

478

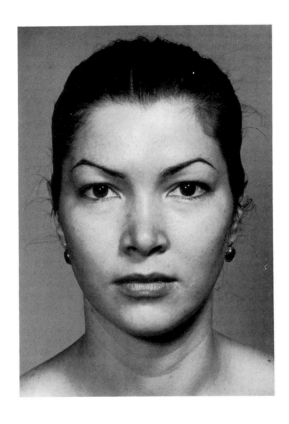

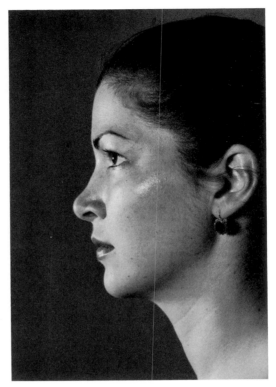

A patient of Indian extraction who exhibited a characteristic widening of the nasal base and flattening of the dorsum with a moderate degree of alar flare. The operative procedure consisted of lateral osteotomy, infracture, and a slight tip elevation. Flaring of the nostrils was diminished by alar base resection, and the supratip region was built up by inserting a small portion of septal cartilage under the dorsal skin.

In any patient with a significant degree of saddle deformity, a dorsal implant will be required. It may be inserted initially or secondarily. If the dissection has opened the nasal cavity into free communication with the submucous dissection, as is usual when the upper lateral cartilages are freed from the septum, a delay is advisable. This is especially true when alloplastic implants are being used for the correction.

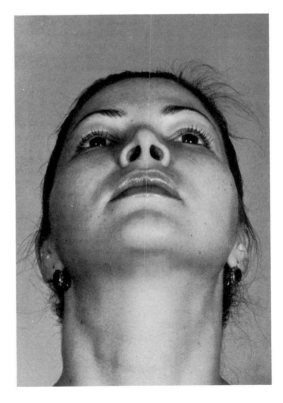

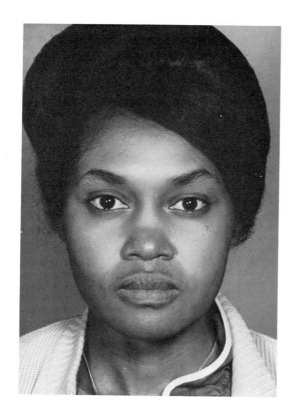

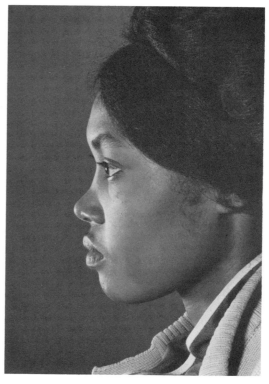

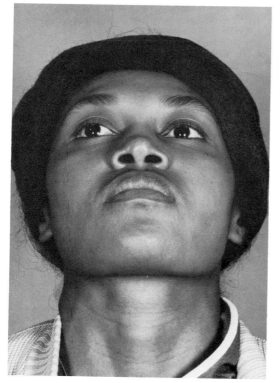

Correction of the supratip depression of a typical Negro nose. Correction in this patient was achieved in two stages: infracture with lateral osteotomy, followed after six weeks by insertion of a carved silicone dorsal implant.

Sometimes it is possible to infracture without disturbing the nasal lining, allowing dissection of a dorsal pocket for the graft with no connection to the airways except at the intercartilaginous incisions. In such instances the upper lateral cartilages are not freed from the septum, and the graft or implant is inserted through the intercartilaginous incision.

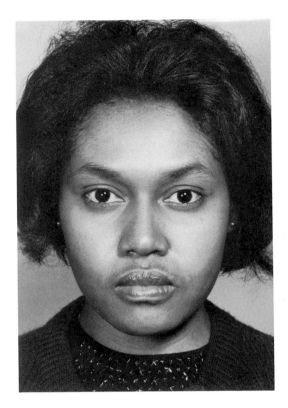

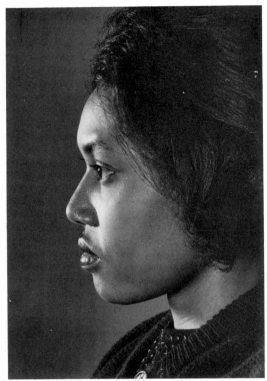

The choice between an autogenous bone graft and a prosthetic implant rests with the surgeon. The author prefers shaped silicone implants to correct natural saddle deformities in Negro or Asian noses, if the soft tissue is ample and unscarred. On the other hand, to repair a traumatized nose, where there is often considerable scarring, contraction, and even loss of tissue, cancellous iliac bone is preferred, as it is less likely to be extruded or to cause skin breakdown.

The graft or implant should extend well up into the nasofrontal angle and downward to the supratip area. It should be so shaped that it does not pivot on an underlying bony fulcrum. Iliac bone grafts can be secured to the nasal bones by wire, an option that is not available when alloplastic implants are used.

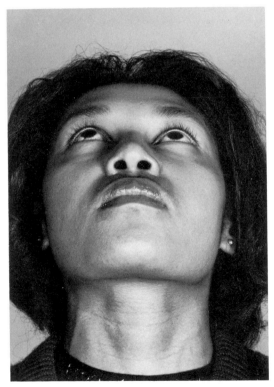

481

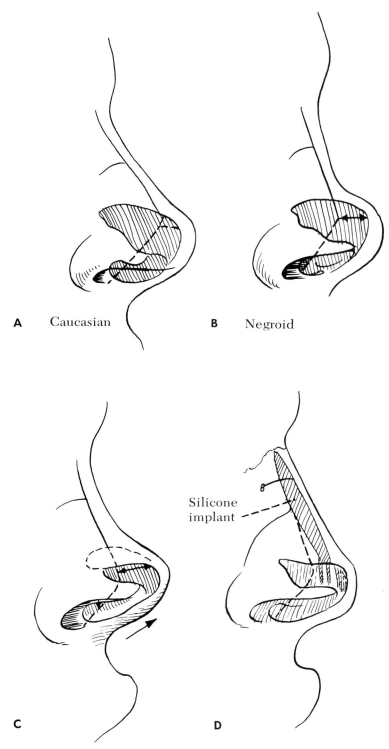

A B

A C D

A, Features of the Caucasian nose showing the sharp angle and good support achieved by the nostril rims from the lateral crura of the alar cartilages. *B,* The typical Negroid nose, illustrating a relative saddle deformity, the obtuse septal angle and poor support achieved by the tip. There is usually a relative smallness of the alar cartilages and poor support of the nostril rim.

The non-Caucasian nose may be corrected. *C,* Projection of the nasal tip achieved by "rolling" of the lateral crus into the medial crus and removal of the upper border of the lateral crura. *D,* A silicone implant is placed along the nasal dorsum to correct the relative saddle deformity made more apparent by the tip projection. It is usually not desirable to fix a silicone implant in position with circumferential wire.

482

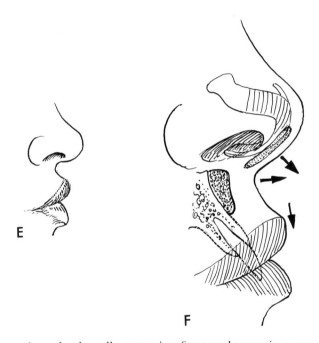

E, The acute lip columella angle and columella retraction frequently seen in a non-Caucasian nose.

F, Improvement by a columella implant and an implant in the region of the nasal spine. These implants may be of silicone, cartilage or bone.

THE FINAL STEPS IN THE OPERATION

After the transfixion incision is sutured, the final step in the procedure is removal of the redundant parts of the upper lateral cartilages. Mattress sutures of 4–0 silk or interrupted sutures of plain or chromic catgut can be used for suturing the transfixion incision.

It is usually necessary to overcorrect the tip slightly in an upward position, because the effects of gravity and scar relaxation will cause it to drop somewhat. Most patients prefer a nose that is slightly tilted rather than too long, and they often return to express disappointment as the tip relaxes from its immediate postoperative position. In patients with plunging tips, the tip must be markedly overcorrected and the caudal portion of the septum sutured between the medial crura in a tongue-and-groove fashion.

A separate incision in the mucoperichondrium to elevate a flap for submucous resection of the septum is sutured with fine catgut.

The suturing of the alar base incisions varies somewhat, depending on the design of the resection. A 4–0 chromic catgut suture with the knot tied inside the nose and incorporating a substantial portion of muscle and alar base is used to relieve tension from the skin sutures, which are removed on the third or fourth postoperative day at the latest. Interrupted nylon sutures of 5–0 or 6–0 size are used for the skin.

THE UPPER LATERAL CARTILAGES

The amount of upper lateral cartilage to be removed varies considerably from patient to patient and depends on how much of the lateral crus of the alar cartilages was removed and on the need to shorten the side walls to correct a plunging tip. It must be appreciated that the upper lateral cartilages are a vital part of the anatomy of breathing, and that the junction formed by the upper lateral cartilages with the septum is critical in nasal ventilation and should be maintained. Extra caution must be used when resection of the lateral wing of the alar cartilage has been generous and when some nasal lining skin has been resected in the eversion technique. Excess cartilage that projects after the tip is set at the desired angle and the transfixion incision is sutured is the only cartilage that is resected. It is not necessary to suture the upper laterals to the septum.

FINAL CHECKING OF THE NOSE

This is probably the most important single step in nasal plasty. The operator checks the nasal dorsum for spicules of bone or cartilage and for irregularities of contour. It may be necessary to smooth the nasal bones with a rasp, and care must be taken not to dislocate them. Finally, with a small curette the skin pockets are carefully swept for any bony, cartilaginous or soft tissue debris which may contribute to infection or contour deficiencies. This checking may be aided by gentle pressure to remove edema.

SUTURING

It is always better to suture an incision, and nasal incisions are no exception, particularly those in the vestibular skin used to deliver the alar cartilages. Such incisions, left unsutured, may be distorted by the tape supports or by the splint, with healing delayed across a gaping wound and scarring with distortion. Interrupted 5–0 catgut sutures are used in these incisions; one or two sutures suffice.

PACKINGS, DRESSINGS AND SPLINTS

Tight intranasal packs are not necessary except on the rare occasion when a wide submucous resection requiring bilateral elevation of mucoperichondrial flaps is done. The usual technique of accordion packing with strip gauze of a nonadherent type can then be used to approximate the flaps. A simple folded piece of Teflon-covered gauze is used to separate the incisions in the vestibule and the columella.

This minimum has proved to be all that is necessary. It is comfortable for the patient and suffices to separate raw surfaces. It also obviates outward pressure upon the nasal bones that can occur with tight intranasal packs. In our experience, there has been no increase in postoperative bleeding with this technique.

It is not necessary to apply external taping to all noses. It is difficult to assume that such taping does have a splinting effect on the underlying skeletal or cartilaginous structures. The exception to this statement may be when there has been ambitious remodeling of the alar cartilages, altering the "spring" effect. Under these circumstances, traditional tape strapping probably has a salutory effect as a fixation dressing to splint the cut ends of the cartilage in the desired position until fibrous union begins. Sterile paper tape has greatly reduced skin reactions.

A malleable splint is placed over the taping or on the skin to approximate the skin flaps to the bone and to help to prevent hematoma formation beneath the skin flaps. It is fallacious to assume that casts or splints will maintain inadequately fractured bones in place. Fractures must be complete, and the bones must be placed where desired *during* the operative procedure. A splint cannot do a job that the surgeon failed to accomplish.

Molded plaster of Paris applied directly to the skin is an excellent splint. It can also be applied over paper taping, when used; plaster rarely causes skin irritation. It can be accurately molded to apply to the skin over the nasal skeleton and conforms at crucial points such as the glabella and nasofrontal angle where small hematomas are apt to occur. It is difficult to apply too much pressure with plaster, so that focal skin necrosis is avoided. After the plaster has been molded and allowed to dry, it is affixed to the skin of the forehead and cheeks with 1-inch paper tape applied in such a way that some pressure is exerted on the splint to keep it firmly seated. Aeroplast, or a similar sticky substance, is helpful in achieving adherence of the tape to the cast. A dental compound splint may be used alternatively; it also provides satisfactory support.

Some surgeons remove the nasal splints soon after surgery, three or four days postoperatively. We prefer to leave all splints in place for seven to ten days because of the protection afforded the freshly operated nose. Edema is also controlled, and the patient has a sense of security knowing the new nose is being protected. Premature removal of the splint can accidentally elevate the skin flaps, so that accumulation of serum or blood can occur beneath. Healing is then prolonged.

All packs are removed on the second postoperative day, except when extensive septal reconstruction has been done in correcting the "crooked" nose. In such cases, the packing is left in place three or four days. It is not to be assumed, however, that this packing in any significant way prevents recurrence of the warping of the cartilage or the bending of the nose. Such recurrence of the distortion occurs throughout the healing period, including the prolonged period of scar contraction. It is inconceivable that packing for an extra day or two can influence the eventual outcome.

After extensive septal reconstruction, some surgeons employ the use of prolonged intranasal splinting with thin plates of polyethylene, silicone, Teflon or similar materials. These sheet splints are placed on either side of the reconstructed septum and sutured into position. They are left in place for several weeks (if the patient can tolerate their presence). Such splinting seems a reasonable technique. However, we have not employed it since we have not found it necessary. Surgical reconstruction of the twisted nose must at times, of course, be extensive, but postoperative splinting of parts cannot be accepted as a substitute for surgical correction.

Despite complete fracture lines, and what seemed entirely adequate infractures at the time of surgery, the nasal bones, one or both, sometimes seem to creep laterally soon after the splint is removed. This results in a widening of the upper nose, which can be unilateral or bilateral. When this lateral displacement of the bone occurs, it can sometimes be corrected by manual pressure applied by the surgeon at weekly or biweekly intervals. This is slightly painful but quite effective unless the bone is being held outward by a high septal deviation. Some surgeons prefer the use of a nose clamp, which Aufricht (1971) has attached to a pair of glasses. Nose clamps, if use is left to the discretion of the patient, can be dangerous by exerting too much pressure. It is our feeling that they are generally not very effective and are certainly no substitute for thorough fracture lines and proper infracture.

On the tenth postoperative day when all sutures and the splint are removed, patients are advised to gently cleanse the nose with one half strength peroxide solution and cotton-tipped applicators, after which the vestibule is coated with a fine layer of sterile petrolatum or baby oil.

The patient is instructed not to blow the nose until the second postoperative week. The use of nose drops is discouraged. Often the nose is stuffy, simulating a head cold, but this is caused by congestion and vasomotor changes in the mucous membranes as a result of surgical trauma. This problem usually clears within the first four weeks. If it persists, however, other causes should be sought, such as allergic rhinitis or mechanical obstruction aggravated by surgery.

In patients with severe pre-existing allergic rhinitis aggravated by surgery, a course of antihistamines is maintained throughout the healing period. In very severe problems the inferior turbinates are injected with a steroid solution. Postoperative nasal obstruction symptoms are common. When they persist for many months, however, the surgeon is apt to quickly blame a septal spur or an apparent minor deviation of the septum. He therefore suggests a submucous resection. This procedure may be very helpful if a true obstruction exists, but has been disappointing in many cases. Its worth has generally been overemphasized. It is not advisable to take the attitude, "when in doubt, do a submucous resection."

Many postoperative nasal obstruction problems are not structural but rather physiological in nature and can be treated with patience and medical care. Allergic problems often respond to only one or two of the many and varied antihistamines available. It may be necessary to try several different compounds before the effective one is discovered.

There is often a good deal of emotional overlay involved in nasal obstruction secondary to congestion of the mucous membranes. Such problems are highly challenging and sometimes obstinate to treat. The help of a psychiatrist can sometimes be obtained if the patient and family can be coaxed into accepting such help.

In cold climates where houses, especially the bedrooms, are heated artificially, the nasal mucous membranes often dry out during the night, causing small encrustations to form. These become separated, and often punctuate raw areas are produced which cause bleeding. Patients are advised to humidify their rooms. Placing a pan of water under the bed or a chair or on a radiator often helps. The use of a cold steam humidifier is most helpful.

Postoperative Care

PHYSICAL ACTIVITY

Moderation in physical activities is advised after surgery. This does not mean that the patient should be limited to a totally sedentary life for many weeks as some surgeons recommend. Most physical activities of a strenuous nature are limited for three weeks. Beyond this point, reasonable activities are begun. The exceptions, of course, are body contact sports such as soccer, volley ball, and so forth. These sports are limited for from four to six months.

The nose knits slowly at the fracture lines and can quite easily be disturbed during this period. However, sports activities which rarely cause injury to the nose, such as horseback riding, swimming (not diving) and tennis are permitted after the third week. The patients are advised that if the nose is injured, it can be reduced promptly (even more promptly than before rhinoplasty), so that they should not be overly concerned.

POSTOPERATIVE SWELLING AND ECCHYMOSIS

There is tremendous variation among individuals in the amount of time required after surgery for swelling, edema and ecchymosis to subside. Swelling of the tip is particularly stubborn in some patients and may take many months to resolve. For most patients it takes six to 12 months before all swelling has cleared and the final result can be seen. However, it is not rare for patients to have residual swelling for up to two years postoperatively. All patients should be advised of this eventuality prior to rhinoplasty, but gentle supportive handling by the surgeon through the long months following surgery may be necessary to bolster the patient's sagging patience. A good rule of thumb to use to determine whether the nose is still swollen and will therefore continue to improve is to ask the patient if he or she still notices a change in size with humid or rainy weather. If this is the case, then the surgeon can reasonably assure the patient that the swelling has not completely cleared.

Supratip swelling, causing a slight "ram's" tip or "polly" tip deformity is most exasperating. If this deformity is truly caused by swelling alone and not by the septum or upper lateral cartilages as discussed in the section on secondary rhinoplasty, it can be significantly and promptly improved by injections of small doses of steroids beneath the dorsal skin. This technique has proved highly effective in our hands and is often dramatic in reducing supratip swelling.

Ecchymosis usually subsides promptly within two to four weeks after surgery. However, there are some patients in whom dark circles remain beneath the eyes—presumedly blood breakdown products—for many months, even up to a year or more. The cause for this is unknown, but it usually occurs in patients of Mediterranean heritage, especially Italians. We are not aware of any patients in whom this condition has become permanent except in those with a family predisposition to darkly pigmented eyelid skin. A tendency to increased pigmentation of the lower eyelid skin should be looked for before surgery, as it is this type of patient who should be advised of the possibility of prolonged "black eyes." We are not aware of any effective treatment to hasten the absorption of the blood pigments.

COMPLICATIONS

Aside from the minor problems of prolonged edema and nasal congestion, the most common troublesome complication of rhinoplasty is hemorrhage or epistaxis. Bleeding can occur at any time from immediately after surgery to several weeks later. However, it is

486

most apt to occur during the first 48 hours or at 10 to 14 days postoperatively. The causes of bleeding can be many. Blood dyscrasias, particularly occult diseases (such as von Willebrand's disease), can, of course, cause troublesome and serious bleeding. As mentioned previously, if a history of bruising or a positive family history of bleeding is obtained, surgery should be postponed pending a complete hematologic work-up.

Bleeding which begins in the first 48 hours after surgery often occurs immediately after the vasoconstrictive effects of the epinephrine in the local anesthetic wear off. Such bleeding is usually from the incisions. It is particularly apt to occur from the raw edge of the septal mucosa along the dorsum and can be difficult to control because of this awkward location. When direct septal surgery, such as septal reconstruction or submucous resection, has been done, the likelihood of bleeding increases considerably.

When vigorous bleeding occurs at this early time after surgery, the intranasal packs should be removed and the nose gently repacked with epinephrine-soaked cotton pledgets. This maneuver must be done under excellent light, with a nasal speculum and all the instruments and packs needed to control the problem at hand. It is folly to attempt to pack a bleeding nose in a darkened hospital room without the proper equipment. Suction is an absolute necessity, as is an excellent light source. There is no substitute for a head light for this purpose.

Packing is removed, all clots are removed with suction and, using a speculum, every attempt is made to locate the exact site of bleeding. This same treatment is done whether the bleeding occurs immediately after surgery or several days later.

The second period when epistaxis is most common is from the tenth to the fourteenth postoperative day when the small protective eschars along the incisions separate.

In most instances, careful packing with epinephrine-soaked gauze controls the bleeding. It is then wise to insert a pack of Oxycel or similar material, which forms a natural clot and need not be removed.

If the hemorrhage is quite severe and the bleeding site cannot be located, the nose must be packed with a nonadherent or greased gauze packing extending as far posteriorly as possible and exerting pressure against the splint or cast. Posterior bleeding must be controlled with posterior nasopharyngeal packs as well as complete anterior packing of the nose. Every surgeon doing rhinoplasty should thoroughly familiarize himself with the technique of packing to control nasal hemorrhage. At some point in his career, if he operates on enough noses, he will be faced with very difficult epistaxis problems. This subject is well covered in most of the standard textbooks of rhinology, to which every reader of this book is most earnestly referred by the authors.

Infection following rhinoplasty is surprisingly rare and always has been, even before the advent of antibiotics. Operating on the nose from an internal approach transgresses one of the most potentially contaminated areas in the body. Fortunately most of the potentially invasive organisms of the nose are controllable by antibiotic therapy. Most surgeons utilize prophylactic antibiotics, a practice which seems to be effective. A most dreaded complication is septic cavernous sinus thrombosis, a rare entity today. If undiagnosed, this condition can lead to brain abscess and death. It must be treated vigorously with massive doses of wide spectrum antibiotics.

Localized abscess can occur at several sites on the nose. These include the transfixion incision in the columella, the tip (between the undermined domes of the alar cartilages), and the base of the prefrontal process of the maxilla along the lateral osteotomy. The lateral infection may begin as a periostitis and become a localized abscess. It is most apt to occur when the saw technique is used and sawdust or debris is left behind.

These localized abscesses are treated with incision and drainage as well as local heat application and wide spectrum antibiotics pending identification of the organism, whereupon the appropriate drug should be given in full doses. The offending organism is most often *Staphylococcus aureus*.

Periostitis along fracture lines in the bone can smolder and set up a low-grade infection that can last for weeks or months. It should therefore be treated vigorously when first recognized. The presenting symptoms are swelling and pain. Later, redness becomes evident.

Skin necrosis over the dorsum resulting from circulatory disturbances or excessive pressure from the dorsal splint can occur, but is very rare. It is our opinion that such a calamity is best treated much like frostbite, in a conservative "watch and wait" attitude. An eschar will form which eventually separates as healing progresses beneath. The final scar may require excision and even full-thickness skin grafting. If, of course, a full-thickness slough of dorsal skin is evident from the outset and there is danger that the bones will become exposed, the slough can immediately be excised and the defect covered with a small pedicle graft from the forehead.

The island flap or subcutaneous pedicle flap is most useful here.

Necrosis of the tip skin has also occurred. This probably results from excessive dissection of the tip and undue surgical trauma. It represents a surgical disaster, and little can be done, either at the time of the slough or subsequently, to save the day with a really acceptable result. Such patients become nasal cripples and often begin an odyssey from surgeon to surgeon to obtain help.

Minor skin complications include tape reactions, skin pustules, and the formation of telangiectases. Tape reactions have been minimized with the almost ubiquitous use of paper tape, but they still occur in highly sensitive individuals. (Allergic reactions are treated with topical steroid creams and systemic antihistamines.) Pustules are expressed as they occur, and a drying desquamating soap is prescribed. (A dermatology colleague can provide excellent advice in this regard.)

Patients with a diathesis toward capillary telangiectasis will sometimes develop these small spider lesions after rhinoplasty. They can be quite successfully treated by electrodesiccation, using an epilating needle which is passed under magnification into the lumen of the vessel. Several treatments may be required.

Secondary Rhinoplasty

Few statistics exist to suggest the frequency with which secondary rhinoplasty is necessary. Smith (1967) reported an incidence of 12 per cent in 221 patients, a figure that seems somewhat high. Each surgeon's personal incidence will decrease as his skill and experience increase. The experienced surgeon should not exceed a 5 per cent secondary operation rate.

Many surgeons are loath to undertake secondary surgery in patients other than their own, since such patients are often dissatisfied with the results of the second operation. Furthermore, if the deformity is severe, and particularly if scarring of the soft tissue exists, there may be little or nothing that can be accomplished by a secondary procedure.

The severely "butchered" nose is difficult to improve and presents a complex problem from both technical and psychological points of view. The novice would be wise to refer such cases elsewhere, and the experienced surgeon should give careful study and consideration to each case before he plans a surgical procedure. Of course, every surgeon is obliged to resolve problems arising in his own patients, if they are correctable.

Complications involving the skin of the nose such as hyperpigmentation, hypopigmentation, erythema, cyanosis, telangiectasia and scarring have been reported but are fortunately rare.

Secondary deformities following rhinoplasty are classified into those involving: (1) the bony framework; (2) the cartilaginous framework, including the tip; (3) the soft tissues; (4) the tip alone; (5) the nostrils, vestibulum and columella; and (6) any combination of the above.

THE BONY FRAMEWORK

The form of the upper portion of the nose is shaped by the nasal bones and bony septum and their junctures with the maxilla and frontal bones. A bony hump deformity is closely related to the remainder of the nasal framework and as such can be either a "real" or a "relative" hump. For example, Berson (1943), Goldman (1950), Converse et al. (1964), Calzolari (1965) and others have pointed out that a depressed vault in the lower cartilaginous part of the nose can simulate such a hump. Furthermore, the appearance of the hump also depends to a great extent on the length of the nose. Lipsett noted that a lesser amount of hump can be removed if the septum is shortened first. Therefore, it is often desirable to correct the cartilaginous nose before removing a hump, especially a small one. The nose with a recessed tip requires more extensive hump removal than the one with a projecting tip.

Insufficient resection of the hump during rhinoplasty may leave a secondary hump, requiring further removal, whereas removal of too much hump may result in a saddle deformity correctable only by a bone graft or prosthetic implant. Excessive hump removal most often occurs in those patients who had small humps to begin with. There is much less likelihood of this if the hump is removed with sharp osteotomes or rasps rather than saws.

Comminution of the nasal bones may result in palpable irregularities. If these are visible, they may be rasped or chiseled away. If they are not visible, no further intervention is indicated, and the patient should be reassured.

EXTERNAL DEVIATION

Asymmetry or external deviation of the bony framework, commonly due to deviation of

488

the bony septum, may have been caused by incomplete infracture or by failure to perform an adequate medial osteotomy on one side. Correction requires surgical comminution of the nasal bones or fracture of the ethmoid plate and nasal bones at the nasofrontal suture, and straightening of the septum. Percutaneous puncture with a 2-mm. osteotome is useful in accomplishing these fractures (page 451). Grignon (1963) claimed that extensive soft tissue uncovering of the lateral bony framework and improper lateral osteotomy may lead to healing of the mobilized bones without bony contact; this is rare in our experience, but a definite possibility.

POSTOPERATIVE WIDENING

Postoperative widening of the bony framework is usually the result of a high deviation of the septum which may have been unrecognized at the primary operation. This is difficult to correct; however, fracture with repositioning of the septum can sometimes solve this problem. Narrowing of the nasal bones, particularly at the nasofrontal angle, may have been prevented by incomplete osteotomy of the frontal process of the maxilla with a "greenstick" type of fracture. Marked thickness of the bone also may have prevented narrowing at the radix, and resection of a medial triangle or web of bone with osteotome or bone forceps may be necessary to allow room for medial displacement at infracture. These techniques have been reviewed by Levignac (1958) and Converse et al. (1964).

"STAIR-STEP" DEFORMITIES

Stair-step deformities have resulted from the lateral osteotomy having been placed too high on the prefrontal process. The lateral osteotomy should be located in the depths of the nasomaxillary groove and should pass through the nasofrontal process of the maxilla. "Stair-stepping" can be corrected by comminuting the prefrontal process with a 2- or 3-mm. osteotome or by rasping of the high bony ridge.

SADDLE NOSE

A saddle nose may have been caused by the fractured nasal bones dropping into the pyriform aperture. This most serious complication can often be avoided by making sure that the periosteum is never completely stripped from the nasal bones, using the soft tissues to support the fractured bones (Lewis, 1954; O'Connor and MacGregor, 1955). Correction of saddle-nose deformities is best done with autogenous bone or cartilage grafts, since alloplastic materials are frequently extruded after insertion into scarred soft tissue of the nasal dorsum.

Incomplete lateral osteotomy, incomplete fracture at the junction of the nasal and frontal bones, and incomplete infracture also present common postrhinoplasty problems. Refracture with comminution of the body complex helps to correct these problems.

THE CARTILAGINOUS FRAMEWORK

It is possible that an *external deviation of the nose* may have been apparent after rhinoplasty where none was visible before, with deviations of the dorsal border of the septal cartilage forming a C- or S-shaped curvature which is often very difficult to correct. Complete freeing of the septum along the vomer groove combined with multiple incisions in the deviated cartilage may be necessary for straightening. It is preferable to remove cartilage only when necessary to obtain an airway. Techniques to correct such deviations have been reviewed by Converse (1950, 1964), Becker (1951), Dingman (1956) and others.

Radical submucous resection with resection of the ethmoid plate and vomer as well as the quadrangular cartilage is ill advised during *any* rhinoplasty because of the danger of collapse of the nasal pyramid into the pyriform aperture. When radical resection appears indicated, it is best to plan it as a secondary procedure, since septalplasty and repositioning of the fragments usually sufficiently straightens the deviated nose without the risk of nasal pyramid collapse.

SUPRATIP SWELLING

If the dorsal septum was not sufficiently lowered, a *postoperative convexity of the supratip area may result*; this is the most common deformity requiring secondary rhinoplasty. It is referred to as a "parrot beak" or "polly tip." This can also result from: (1) insufficient removal of the dorsal borders of the upper lateral cartilages, (2) excessive resection of the alar cartilage domes, (3) insufficient trimming of the septal mucosa, (4) inherent thickness of the skin and subcutaneous tissue, and (5) a short columella. For example, if the septal mucoperichondrium was not trimmed lower than the dorsal border of the septum, it may have grown over the dorsum, uniting with the opposing mucosa and

489

becoming interposed between the covering skin and the septal cartilages. The supratip swelling may have been accentuated by the formation of granulation tissue in the dead space between the dorsal skin flap and the septal border; the granulation tissue results in scar tissue formation. The thicker the skin in the supratip area, the more obvious will be the deformity.

To avoid the "polly tip" in patients with thick skin, Wright (1967) advised shaping the nasal tip before reduction of the septal height and removal of the bony hump. Pitanguy (1965) believes the bulbous nose to contain fibrous ligaments between the dermis and the alar cartilages which need to be divided or resected in order to prevent postoperative supratip swelling. Rees (1971) has injected the supratip swelling with steroids with good results.

Correction of supratip elevation may be very difficult, involving lowering of the high septal dorsum, excision of scar tissue and resection of the upper lateral cartilages. Increasing the tip projection by rearrangement of the alar cartilages and lengthening the columella may be helpful. Implantation of alloplastic materials or autogenous grafts to increase tip projection is not advised as extrusion or resorption is the usual end result.

Excessive removal of the upper lateral cartilages may leave *oblique grooves on either side of the nasal dorsum* extending inferiorly from the lower border of the nasal bones. Such grooving is almost impossible to correct, although liquid silicone injection has been shown to be of some value in this problem.

Uneven trimming of the septum or upper lateral cartilages along their dorsal borders causes *palpable or visible irregularities* which will require secondary trimming when they are visible. In those patients in whom the irregularity is not visible but only palpable, a waiting course is advisable.

THE NASAL TIP

Common deformities of the tip following rhinoplasty are pinching, asymmetry, sharp points, the square or "boxed" tip, and pitting or depressions resulting from scar tissue. Asymmetry and pinching are frequently seen stigmata following nasal plastic surgery. These deformities are the result of injudicious carving of the alar cartilages along with, in the case of pinching, excision of excess vestibular lining. Many surgeons have been concerned with these problems, and their prevention and correction have been discussed by Cohen (1951), Lewis (1954), Grignon (1936), Hage (1964), Fomon and Bell (1967) and others.

Correction of irregularities of the alar cartilage remnants such as sharp points, asymmetry of the domes, or the "boxed" or square tip requires secondary trimming of the offending cartilage remnants.

BOXED TIP

The boxed tip may require total resection of the alar domes, a procedure safer in the secondary than the primary operation, since collapse or pinching is less likely to occur because of the added support given to the soft tissue by the cicatrix from the first operation. Patients with thick skin or excess subcutaneous tissue can afford loss of most or all of the lateral crura of the alar cartilage without nostril collapse. However, when the skin is very thin, resection of the alar cartilage must be conservative and accurate, with emphasis on shaping since support from the skin is weak.

When lining has been scarified, correction becomes much more difficult. Compensation for soft-tissue loss may possibly be accomplished by Z-plasty, but the use of local flaps, cartilage grafts, composite grafts or full-thickness grafts will be required both to cover the raw surfaces left by resection of the scar and to provide support. Unfortunately these procedures are often more attractive in articles or texts than practical in the living patient. Repair of the "crucified" tip is unquestionably the most difficult task in secondary rhinoplasty. When complete vestibular collapse is present, support can be provided only by a prosthetic insert which provides an airway at the critical junction of the nasal cartilages and septum.

"DROPPING" TIP

The dropping tip occurs if the upper lateral and alar cartilages have not been trimmed or sutured in suitable relationship to the shortened caudal margin of the septum. The tip also tends to plunge downward if excessive hump has been removed or if the nose has been shortened without tilting the tip. In the older patients their loss of skin contractibility may contribute to the dropped tip.

Correction of the plunging or dropped tip may require shortening the upper lateral cartilages or approximating them to the alar cartilages. Fixation of the medial crura of the alar cartilages to the caudal septal border by an "orthopedic suture" is frequently needed. If the alar cartilages are naturally shaped in such a way that they plunge downward at the domes, much like a spring or wishbone, it may be necessary to resect the domes and to reposition the medial and lateral crura in a new relationship.

Excessive shortening of the septum and/or the upper lateral and alar cartilages may have resulted in an elevated tip with undue nostril exposure. It is often found that the entire membranous septum has been resected in such patients and that correction of this problem is extremely difficult because too much tissue has been sacrificed. When the nasal spine is present or prominent, removal of this structure sometimes creates the illusion of lengthening the nose, although often at the expense of an unwanted lengthening of the upper lip. Undermining of all soft tissue and a complete transfixion sometimes allows a "stretching" downward of the degloved nose which can then be fixed by sutures in a lowered position to maintain the gained length. Severe cases associated with saddling may require bone grafts to the dorsum or composite grafts to the membranous septum to provide tissue to maintain length (Dingman and Walter, 1969). In some instances, if the septum has not been made too short, a septal flap can be used to elevate the base of the columella.

BIFID TIP

Bifidity of the tip requires suturing together of the alar domes or their remnants, a technique which is often more easily described than done. In many instances of bifidity we find that breaking up of the interdome fibro-areolar tissue will produce sufficient scar tissue contraction to correct the problem.

Many secondary deformities of the nasal tip cannot be corrected by surgery, which, in fact, can further damage the nose and compound the problem. The inexperienced surgeon is often tempted to take on these problem patients. Many patients with thickened, asymmetrical and scarred nasal tips, particularly in those instances where lining has been lost, should be advised against further surgery, or recommendations should be limited to provision of new lining and an acrylic prosthesis with a view only to functional improvement.

THE NOSTRILS, VESTIBULUM AND COLUMELLA

Cicatricial stenosis, synechiae or retraction of the nostrils has usually been the end result of secondary healing of raw surfaces left when lining was sacrificed (Wexler, 1952; Cohen, 1956).

The correction of such scarred defects is as difficult as the correction of the "crucified" tip. Rearrangement or replacement of missing soft tissue lining by Z-plasty, local flaps or skin grafts may be indicated, as are procedures designed to reproduce the cartilaginous support. Most such techniques utilize implants of cartilage or alloplastic materials, and end results are disappointing at best. From a practical standpoint we have found the provision of lining skin by full thickness retroauricular skin grafts and follow-up use of an acrylic obturator to provide the best and fastest answer to a usually unrewarding situation.

FLARING NOSTRILS

Flaring of the nostrils may be accentuated following rhinoplasty when the tip has been recessed and this may be remedied by alar base resection.

"HANGING" COLUMELLA

A hanging columella, a convexity or roundness of the caudal margin of the medial crura of the alar cartilages, may first become significant after nasal plasty. This can be corrected by marginal incisions in the columella and trimming of the rounded cartilage and, sometimes, the lining.

FLARING MEDIAL CRURA

Flaring of the feet of the medial crura in conjunction with abundance of soft tissue at the base of the columella can obstruct inspiration after rhinoplasty when the lateral crura has been resected. Correction can be achieved by resecting the soft tissue between the medial crura together with the feet of the medial crura.

RETRACTION OF COLUMELLA

Retraction of the columella may result from excessive removal of the inferior or caudal margin of the septum and sometimes from resection of the membranous septum and/or medial crura. Correction of this deformity is at best difficult and often impossible. When the retraction is minor, a septal cartilage implant is effective (Millard, 1965). Bone and alloplastic implants have proved to be disappointing. Replacement of soft tissue and cartilage by a composite graft in the region of the missing membranous septum (Dingman and Walter, 1969) or the so-called "banana split" operation of Millard (1969) follows sound reconstructive principles

491

and is often the only effective method of repairing the severely retracted columella, although results often leave much to be desired.

Aufricht (1969) has recommended cartilage implants in the region of the nasal spine to correct an acute angle. Such a technique is useful in improving retraction of the columella, the result of removal of the nasal spine. It is also a valuable means of correcting flatness of the upper lip resulting from overambitious surgery of both the nasal spine and inferior border of the septum.

NOSTRIL IRREGULARITIES

Irregularities or thickening of the nostrils which are accentuated after rhinoplasty can be improved by selective resection of the nostril rims by the methods of Pollet and Baudelot (1967) and Millard (1969). However, the scars are not infrequently unduly prominent, so this should be approached with caution.

Secondary deformities following cosmetic rhinoplasty are relatively frequent. Their incidence decreases, or should, proportionate to the experience of the surgeon.

REFERENCES

Aufricht, G.: Combined nasal plastic and chin plastic; Correction of microgenia by an osteocartilaginous transplant from a large hump nose. Amer. J. Surg. 25:292, 1934.

Aufricht, G.: A few hints and surgical details in rhinoplasty. Laryngoscope 53:317, 1943.

Aufricht, G.: Surgery of the radix and bony nose; Preliminary report of a new type of nasal clamp. Plast. Reconstr. Surg. 22:315, 1958.

Aufricht, G.: Rhinoplasty and the face. Plast. Reconstr. Surg. 43:219, 1969.

Aufricht, G.: Joseph's rhinoplasty with some modifications. Surg. Clin. N. Amer. 51:299, 1971.

Becker, O. J.: Problems of the septum in rhinoplastic surgery. Trans. Amer. Acad. Ophthal. Otolaryng. 55:244, 1951.

Berson, M. I.: Prevention of deformities in corrective rhinoplasty. Laryngoscope 53:276, 1943.

Boo-Chai, K.: Augmentation rhinoplasty in the Oriental. Plast. Reconstr. Surg. 34:81, 1964.

Brown, J. B., and McDowell, F.: Plastic Surgery of the Nose. Springfield, Ill., Charles C Thomas, 1965.

Buttler, J.: Work of breathing through the nose. Clin. Sci. 19:55, 1960.

Calzolari, L.: Rhinoplastica correttiva. Minerva Chir. 20:14, 1965.

Cinelli, J. A.: Correction of the combined elongated nose and recessed naso-labial angle. Plast. Reconstr. Surg. 21:139, 1958.

Cinelli, J. A.: Lengthening of the nose by a septal flap. Plast. Reconstr. Surg. 43:99, 1969.

Cohen, S.: Postrhinoplastic intranasal adhesions. Arch. Otolaryng. 54:683, 1951.

Cohen, S.: Complications following rhinoplasty. Plast. Reconstr. Surg. 18:213, 1956.

Cole, P.: Further observations on the conditioning of respiratory air. J. Laryng. 67:669, 1953.

Conroy, W. C.: Simple nasal tip setback. Plast. Reconstr. Surg. 33:564, 1964.

Converse, J. M.: Corrective surgery of nasal deviations. Arch. Otolaryng. 52:671, 1950.

Converse, J. M.: Maxillofacial deformities and maxillofacial prosthetics. J. Prosth. Dent. 13:511, 1963.

Converse, J. M., Wood-Smith, D., Wang, M. K. H., Macomber, B., and Guy, C. L.: Deformities of the nose. In Converse, J. M. (ed.): Plastic Reconstructive Surgery. Philadelphia, W. B. Saunders Company, 1964, pp. 869–948.

Cottle, M. H.: Concepts of nasal physiology as related to corrective nasal surgery. Arch. Otolaryng. 72:11, 1960.

Denecke, H. J., and Meyer, R.: Plastic Surgery of Head and Neck. New York, Springer Verlag, 1967.

Diamond, H.: Rhinoplasty techniques. Surg. Clin. N. Amer. 51:317, 1971.

Dieffenbach, J.: Die operative Chirurgie. Leipzig, 1845.

Dingman, R.: Corrections of nasal deformities due to defects of the septum. Plast. Reconstr. Surg. 18:291, 1956.

Dingman, R., and Walter, C.: Use of composite ear grafts in correction of the short nose. Plast. Reconstr. Surg. 43:117, 1969.

Dufourmentel, C., and Mouly, R.: Chirurgie Plastique. Paris, Flammarian et Cie, 1959.

Eitner, E.: Kosmetische Operationen. Berlin, Springer Verlag, 1932.

Falces, E., Wesser, D., and Gorney, M.: Cosmetic surgery of the non-Caucasian nose. Plast. Reconstr. Surg. 45:317, 1970.

Farina, R.: Plastica de navig; Tratamento do dorso esteo cartilaginosoe perfil nasal. Rev. Paul. Med. 64:23, 1964.

Fomon, S.: Cosmetic Surgery, Principles and Practice. Philadelphia, J. B. Lippincott Company, 1960.

Fomon, S., and Bell, J. W.: Rhinoplasty—A fine art. Arch. Otolaryng. 85:685, 1967.

Fomon, S., and Bell, J. W.: Rhinoplasty—New Concepts: Evaluation and Application. Springfield, Ill, Charles C Thomas, 1970.

Fomon, S., Bell, J. W., Lubart, J., Schattner, A., and Syracuse, V. R.: The nasal hump problem. Arch. Otolaryng. 79:164, 1964.

Fomon, S., Bell, J. W., Schattner, A., and Syracuse, V. R.: Postoperative elongation of the nose. Arch. Otolaryng. 64:456, 1956.

Fomon, S., Sayad, W. Y., Schattner, A., and Neivert, H.: Physiological principles in rhinoplasty. Arch. Otolaryng. 53:256, 1951.

Fred, G. B.: Postoperative dropping of the nasal tip after rhinoplasty. Arch. Otolaryng. 67:177, 1958.

Fry, H.: Nasal skeletal trauma and the interlocked stresses of the nasal septal cartilage. Brit. J. Plast. Surg. 20:146, 1967.

Gibson, T., and Davis, W. B.: The distortion of autogenous cartilage grafts: Its causes and prevention. Brit. J. Plast. Surg. 10:257, 1958.

Gnudi, M. T., and Webster, J. P.: The Life and Times of Gasparo Tagliacozzi, Surgeon of Bologna (1545–1599). New York, Reichner, 1950.

Goldman, I. B.: Rhinoplasty: Its surgical complications and how to avoid them. J. Int. Coll. Surg. 13:285, 1950.

Goldman, I. B.: The importance of the medial crura in nasal-tip reconstruction. Arch. Otolaryng. 65:143, 1957.

Goldman, I. B.: Rhinoplastic sequelae causing nasal obstruction. Arch Otolaryng. 83:151, 1966.

González-Ulloa, M.: Quantitative principles in cosmetic surgery of the face (profileplasty). Plast. Reconstr. Surg. 29:186, 1962.

Grignon, J. L.: Les eches des rhinoplasties. Ann. Otolaryng. (Paris) 80:51, 1963.

Hage, J.: Collapsed alae strengthened by conchal cartilage; The butterfly cartilage graft. Brit. J. Plast. Surg. 18:92, 1964.

Hilding, A.: Experimental surgery of the nose and sinuses. I. Changes in the morphology of epithelium following variations in ventilation. Arch. Otolaryng. 16:9, 1932.

Inoue, S., and Harashima, H.: Rhinomanometry. Otologia (Fukuoka) *24*:445, 1952.

Kazanjian, V. H., and Converse, J. M.: The Surgical Treatment of Facial Injuries. Baltimore, The Williams & Wilkins Co., 1972.

Konno, A.: Air flow and resistance in the naval cavity. Part 1. Observation on nasal airflow, using the model made from nasal and nasopharyngeal casts of the human body. Part 2. Bilateral rhinometry using a pneumotachometer. Its principles and clinical application. J. Otolaryng. Jap. *72*:36–48; 49–65, 1969.

Levignac, J.: Des petits et des gros ennuis dans la rhinoplastie. Ann. Otolaryng. (Paris) *75*:560, 1958.

Lewis, M. L.: Prevention and correction of cicatricial intranasal adhesions in rhinoplastic surgery. Arch. Otolaryng. *60*:215, 1954.

Lillie, J. C.: Methods in Medical Research. Vol. 2, edited by J. H. Comroe. Chicago, The Year Book Publishing Co., 1950.

Lipsett, E. M.: A new approach to surgery of the lower cartilaginous vault. Arch. Otolaryng. *70*:42, 1959.

Maliniac, J. W.: Prevention and treatment of sequelae in corrective rhinoplasty. Amer. J. Surg. *50*:84, 1940.

McIndoe, A., and McLaughlin, C. R.: Advances in plastic surgery. Practitioner *169*:427, 1952.

Millard, D. R.: External excisions in rhinoplasty. Brit. J. Plast. Surg. *12*:340, 1960.

Millard, D. R.: The triad of columella deformities. Plast. Reconstr. Surg. *31*:370, 1963.

Millard, D. R.: Adjuncts in augmentation mentoplasty and corrective rhinoplasty. Plast. Reconstr. Surg. *36*:48, 1965.

Millard, D. R.: Secondary corrective rhinoplasty. Plast. Reconstr. Surg. *44*:545, 1969.

O'Connor, G. B., and McGregor, M. W.: Secondary rhinoplasties: Their cause and prevention. Plast. Reconstr. Surg. *15*:404, 1955.

O'Connor, G. B., McGregor, M. W., Shapiro, L., and Tolleth, H.: The bulbous nose. Plast. Reconstr. Surg. *39*:278, 1967.

Ogura, J. H., Togawa, K., Dammkoehler, K., Nelson, J. R., and Kawasaki, M.: Nasal obstruction and the mechanics of breathing. Physiologic relationship and effects of nasal surgery. Arch. Otolaryng. *83*:135, 1966.

Ogura, J. H., Unno, T., and Nelson, J. R.: Nasal surgery. Physiological considerations of nasal obstruction. Arch Otolaryng. *88*:288, 1968.

Pitanguy, I.: Surgical importance of a cartilaginous ligament in bulbous noses. Plast. Reconstr. Surg. *26*:247, 1965.

Pollet, J., and Baudelot, S.: Séquelles de la chirurgie esthétique de la base du nez. Ann. Chir. Plast. (Paris) *12*:185, 1967.

Proetz, A. W.: Respiratory air currents and their clinical aspects. J. Laryng. *67*:1, 1953.

Rees, T. D.: Nasal plastic surgery in the Negro. Plast. Reconstr. Surg. *43*:13, 1969.

Rees, T. D., Guy, G. L., and Converse, J. M.: Repair of the cleft-lip nose; Addendum to the synchronous technique with full-thickness skin grafting of the nasal vestibule. Plast. Reconstr. Surg. *37*:47, 1966.

Rees, T. D., Krupp, S., and Wood-Smith, D.: Secondary rhinoplasty. Plast. Reconstr. Surg. *46*:322, 1970.

Rees, T. D.: An aid in the treatment of supratip swelling after rhinoplasty. Laryngoscope *81*:308, 1971.

Rethi, A.: Right and wrong in rhinoplastic operations. Plast. Reconstr. Surg. *3*:361, 1948.

Roe, J. O.: The deformity termed "pug nose" and its correction by a simple operation. Med. Rec. *31*:621, 1887.

Rode, B.: Zur Technik des Gipsverbandes in der Behandlung der Nasenbein-Frakturen und Deformitäten. Z. Hals. Nas. Ohrenheilk. *43*:294, 1938.

Rogers, B. O.: Secondary and tertiary rhinoplasty. Transactions of the 4th International Congress of Plastic and Reconstructive Surgery, pp. 1065–1071. Amsterdam, Excerpta Medica Foundation, 1969.

Rohrer, F.: Der Stromungsmiderstand in den menschlichen Ateurwegen und der Einfluss der unregelmässigen Verzweigung des Bronchialsystems auf den Atmungsveilauf in verschiedenen Lungenbeziken. Pfluger's Arch. J. Ges. Physiol. *162*:255, 1915.

Safian, J.: Corrective Rhinoplastic Surgery. New York, Paul B. Hoeber, Inc., 1935.

Safian, J.: Fact and fallacy in rhinoplastic surgery. Brit. J. Plast. Surg. *11*:45, 1958.

Safian, J.: The split-cartilage tip technique of rhinoplasty. Plast. Reconstr. Surg. *45*:217, 1970.

Seeley, R. D.: Reconstruction of the nasal tip: A new technique. Plast. Reconstr. Surg. *3*:594, 1948.

Seltzer, A. P.: Cautions in rhinoplastic surgery. Eye Ear Nose Throat Monthly *32*:35, 1953.

Seltzer, A. P.: The surgically induced saddle nose. Eye Ear Nose Throat Monthly *30*:250, 1951.

Silver, A. G.: Pitfalls in rhinoplasty. Eye Ear Nose Throat Monthly *31*:556, 1952.

Smith, T. W.: As clay in the potter's hand. Ohio Med. J. *63*:1055, 1967.

Speizer, F., and Frank, R.: A technique for measuring nasal and pulmonary flow resistance simultaneously. J. Appl. Physiol. *19*:176, 1964.

Steiss, C. F.: Errors in rhinoplasty and their prevention. Plast. Reconstr. Surg. *28*:276, 1961.

Stokstead, P.: The physiological cycle of the nose under normal and pathological conditions. Acta Otolaryng. *42*:175, 1952.

Takahashi, K.: Verläufige Mitteilungen über die Erfarochung. Z. Laryng. *11*:203, 1922.

Takemiya, S., Togawa, K., Unno, T., and Konno, A.: Bilateral rhinomanometry using pneumotachometer. Japan. J. Otol. (Tokyo) *66*:985, 1963.

Tonndorf, W.: Der Weg der Atemluft in der Menshclichen Nase. Arch. J. Orh-USW. H.K. *41*:146, 1939.

Uchida, J.: The Practice of Plastic Surgery. Tokyo, Kinbara, 1958, p. 62.

Weir, R. F.: On restoring sunken noses without scarring the face. New York Med. J. *56*:449, 1892.

Wexler, M.: Post-rhinoplastic complications. Eye Ear Nose Throat Monthly *31*:553, 1969.

Willemot, J.: Correction of old nasal deviations. Plast. Reconstr. Surg. *43*:430, 1969.

Williams, H. L.: Report of committee on standardization of definitions, terms, symbols in rhinometry of the American Academy of Ophthalmology and Otolaryngology. American Academy of Ophthalmology and Otolaryngology, 1970.

Wright, W. K.: Study on hump removal in rhinoplasty. Laryngoscope *77*:508, 1967.

Chapter 10

MENTOPLASTY, PROGNATHISM AND CHEILOPLASTY

THOMAS D. REES, M.D.,
SIDNEY L. HOROWITZ, D.D.S.,
AND RICHARD J. COBURN, D.M.D., M.D.

The Framework and Integument of the Face

The chin, the nose and the forehead are the three important balancing masses of the face. A well proportioned nose cannot reach its fullest esthetic impact without a chin that is in a proportionate and normal relationship. An understanding of the normal physical balance of these facial structures and of their position to each other are keys to diagnosis and to the selection of an appropriate operative technique. Many patients seeking rhinoplasty are not aware that a small chin is also contributing to their physical defect and that this also should be corrected in order to achieve the optimum operative result of a balanced face. The role of the chin has been emphasized as a balancing feature of the face by Converse (1950), Millard (1965), and González-Ulloa (1968) and others.

Deformities involving the chin are most apparent when normal maxillomandibular and dental relationships are disturbed. Thus, the relationship of the jaws to each other and the occlusion of the upper and lower teeth may contribute importantly to the total appearance of the face. Minor deviations, e.g., a slightly "weak chin" (microgenia), can often be corrected quite easily by insertion of a prosthetic implant. In contrast, major malrelationships of the jaw, such as marked recession (micrognathia, retrognathia) or asymmetry, may require corrective bone surgery to improve the skeletal framework. This may involve the upper or lower jaw, or both, in order to establish not only an esthetically acceptable result, but also to provide sound occlusion. Such severe deformities may be the result of hypoplasia, hypertrophy or malposition from developmental or traumatic causes.

Corrective jaw surgery, including the treatment of the small or recessive chin, falls into two main categories: those that can be corrected with camouflaging techniques (implant, onlays), and those requiring major surgery upon the jaws themselves, i.e., osteotomy or bone graft. Most patients present with deformities that fall into the first category. In this book only those procedures in which osteotomies on the mandible can be performed without interruption of the dentition, such as horizontal osteotomy (or ostectomy of the rim of the mandible), will be described, since they are of greatest interest to the esthetic surgeon. Description of the more complicated techniques can be found in works devoted to reconstructive jaw surgery.

Diagnosis and Treatment Planning

Facial harmony and balance involve complex relationships between the hard and soft tissues that are not easily evaluated either clinically or from photographs. Orthodontists, who have a special interest in the dental-skeletal-integumental balance of the lower face, have evolved the cephalometric roentgenogram as a diagnostic aid for this purpose.

The technique of cephalometric roentgenography was first described about 40 years ago and is now well standardized. The apparatus consists of two elements: an x-ray source and a head holder. The latter is used to fixate the patient's head by means of ear posts that enter the right and left external auditory meatus for a short distance. The source of radiation is similarly fixed so that the central beam is lined up with the ear posts. Enlargement and distortion are minimized for practical purposes by using a tube-midsagittal plane distance of 5 feet, which is now standard in cephalometric installations in this country.

The advantage of the cephalogram for the esthetic surgeon stems from the standardized technique, since the device makes it possible to obtain comparably oriented pre- and postoperative views of both the hard and soft facial tissues. The widespread use of standardized roentgenography by orthodontists led inevitably to the development of numerous schemes for analysis. Almost all of these are based on measurements of various angles and dimensions of the face and cranium. Although the diagnostic validity of such precise numbers may be questioned, the cephalogram does provide important information regarding the *relative* size and position of various facial structures. In this way, it assists the clinician in making judgments and in evaluating the changes that occur with treatment, whether surgical or orthodontic.

Accurate description of the human face has presented a challenge to artists, scientists and mathematicians for centuries. Attempts to establish basic mathematical or statistical rules for facial esthetics have all proved inadequate, which is simply a reflection of the variability between individuals that is the rule and not the exception. It is not surprising, therefore, that cephalometric research studies of persons with pleasing facial esthetics (motion-picture actresses and beauty queens, for example) confirm this observation. In these individuals, the dimensions and angular relations of the hard and soft tissues of the face, as measured on the cephalogram, fall within the ranges previously established as population norms but they show wide variability. It is apparent that even the most pleasing examples of facial harmony involve skeletal and integumental relationships that cannot be conveniently and simply reduced to average measurements that have any clinically useful meaning in diagnosis and treatment planning.

Soft Tissue Balance

The cephalometric x-ray is particularly helpful in visualizing relationships between the skeletal framework and three curves within the facial profile that are of the greatest significance esthetically.

Calvin Case, a physician turned orthodontist, described these facial curves in detail in his textbook published in 1921, and little needs to be added to his observations.

The lowest curve of the face shapes the character of the chin and should form (as Case said) a "graceful and concurve" arc from the chin to the border of the lower lip with the profile in repose. Below the nose, the curve of the upper lip should be slightly concave, "gracefully curving with a light deepening of the naso-labial lines where it joins the cheek." The uppermost curve in the facial profile, the frontonasal, is equally as important as this lower curve. It is important to recognize that the facial curves described by Case occur normally when the lips are closed with ease *in repose* and that the mandible is in "rest" position, i.e., with some distance between the upper and lower jaws so that the teeth are *not* in contact. Under normal conditions, therefore, the features are in unconscious repose when the lips are closed and the teeth are slightly apart. In a well balanced face the lips thus close without strain, and the curves of the face are neither abnormally deep nor straight.

The drapery of the facial musculature of the lower one third of the face also controls lip seal (lip competency). Rest position is established relatively early and involves not only the masticatory musculature, but the muscles of facial expression as well (Ballard, 1967). The orofacial pattern is characteristic of the individual, and under normal conditions it is instinctive for each individual to produce a lip seal of the soft tissues around the mouth in the rest position. If this does *not* occur, then adaptive postures are used and the muscles around the mouth are almost continually contracted and maintained in that position in order to accomplish lip seal. *Competent* lip posture implies adequate lip seal, with the lips able to contact one another without strain when the mandible is in rest position. *Incompetent* lip posture occurs when the lips are unable to form an adequate seal under similar unstrained conditions (see page 524). Most importantly, competent lip posture is functionally related to the soft tissue contour of the chin. Attempts to achieve adequate lip seal when there is lip incompetency often results in unsightly strain of the perioral musculature.

495

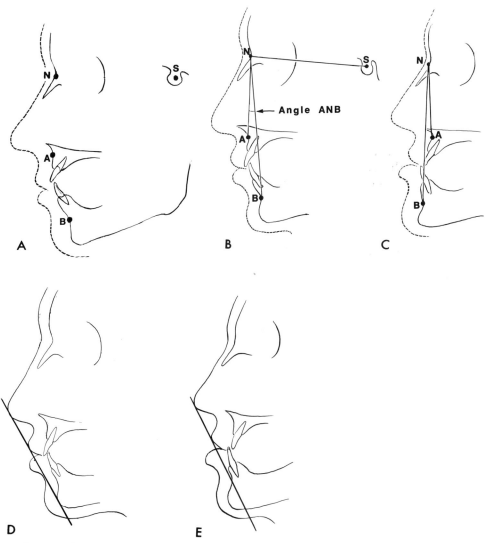

A, Reference points: S: Center of sella turcica; N: nasofrontal suture; A: most posterior point along junction of maxillary basal bone and alveolar process; B: most posterior point along junction of alveolar process and mandibular basal bone.

B, Reference planes: S-N: Plane through sella turcica and nasion; N-A: Plane through nasion and most posterior point along maxillary alveolus; N-B: plane through nasion and most posterior point along mandibular alveolus; Angle ANB: angle developed between planes N-A and N-B, normal range being 5 to −2 degrees.

C, Reverse, or minus, angle in prognathism of the mandible.

D, The esthetic line, a plane between the nasal tip and the upper lip, passes on or near pogonion, the most anterior bony chin point, when the lower and middle face are balanced.

E, The esthetic line falls behind pogonion in a prognathism.

Cephalometric Evaluation in Facial Surgery

Nonmetric techniques for using the cephalogram depend upon the evaluation of relationships between the underlying skeletal and dental structures and the integument that are judged subjectively. Despite the subjectivity involved, these methods have been helpful in (1) rapid evaluation of the initial discrepancy, and (2) stimulating profile changes that might result from surgical-orthodontic procedures. The cephalogram also makes it possible to evaluate the surgical result objectively by comparison of the pre- and postoperative films.

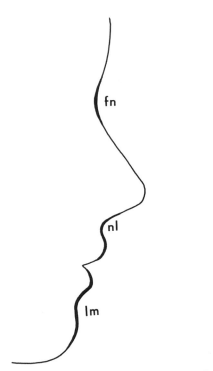

Curves of the face (after C. S. Case, see text): *fn* - frontonasal; *nl* - nasolabial; *lm* - labiomental.

CUT-OUT TECHNIQUE

This technique is particularly useful in evaluating nose-chin balance and in determining the site and extent of change required for improvement. When the maxillary anterior teeth are protrusive, for example, the chin may appear underdeveloped in consequence. Two possible treatment strategies for changing the profile must be considered in such cases; these are surgical-orthodontic set-back of the anterior maxillary dentoalveolar segment, or advancement of the chin point by implant or by horizontal osteotomy. In either instance, the anticipated result can be reasonably predicted by (1) moving the maxillary cut-out posteriorly, or (2) moving the mandibular cut-out anteriorly. The appearance of many such patients may also be improved by routine orthodontic therapy.

FACIAL PLANE

When the curves of the lower face are distorted in an attempt to obtain lip seal over a procumbent upper and lower dentition, the "facial plane" used by orthodontists is an excellent guide in planning treatment. In these conditions, "bimaxillary protrusion," the chin also appears to be underdeveloped because of the facial convexity.

The facial plane connects the points *nasion*—the most anterior point on the x-ray outline of the frontonasal suture—and *pogonion*—the most anterior point on the mental symphysis. In faces with acceptable dentofacial balance, this line usually intersects (or closely approximates) the outline of the lower central incisor crown.

The process of constructing this line is reversed in bimaxillary protrusion cases in order to obtain a guide to the amount of chin advancement required; that is, a line is drawn on the cephalogram tracing from *nasion through the lower incisor crown outline*. This line indicates the new position of the *pogonion* point that will provide an esthetically satisfactory lower face contour, and the result may be achieved either (1) by horizontal osteotomy with chin point advancement, or (2) in less severe cases, with an implant.

WEDGE REMOVAL

One type of bimaxillary protrusion occurs in extremely long faces. The mandible is characteristically deformed in such cases, showing an overdevelopment in height that results in distortion of the labiomental curve. The face must be shortened and the chin point advanced to gain profile improvement in these conditions. The facial plane line is again used to determine the new and more prominent position of pogonion, as just described. In addition, a wedge of bone is removed from beneath the tooth roots in order to reduce face height (pp. 504 and 505).

Prognathism

The scope of this book does not permit an exhaustive treatise on prognathism. Indeed, it was specifically not our purpose to discuss this complicated subject except as it pertains to most esthetic surgeons; nevertheless, most cases of true prognathism who do not have open bite or a strong potential for developing open bite after surgery, as attested by cephalogram, x-ray and dental casts, can be corrected by one or two current techniques which are quite simple and in wide use. These techniques are the "sagittal-split" operation and the vertical ramusection. The latter is particularly useful to the surgeon who does not operate on a large volume of prognathism patients, but is sometimes called upon to treat such patients. The collaboration of an orthodontist knowledgeable of the diagnostic

497

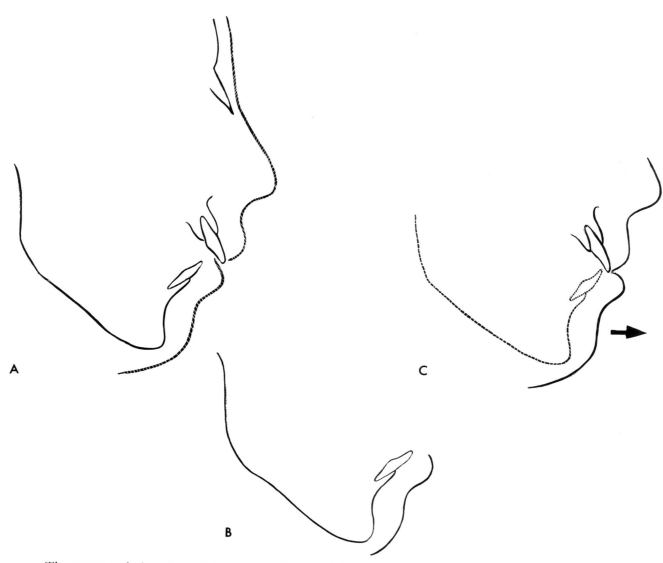

The cutout technique in cephalometric evaluation. *A*, The original cephalometric tracing of a patient with maxillary protrusion. *B*, Cutout tracing of the mandible. *C*, The cutout moved anteriorly into correct occlusal relationship, showing the hypothetical improvement in soft tissue contour to be expected as the result of chin point advancement. *D*, Cutout tracing of the maxilla. *E*, The cutout moved posteriorly into the correct occlusal relationship, again showing the hypothetical improvement that could be achieved by anterior maxillary dentoalveolar setback.

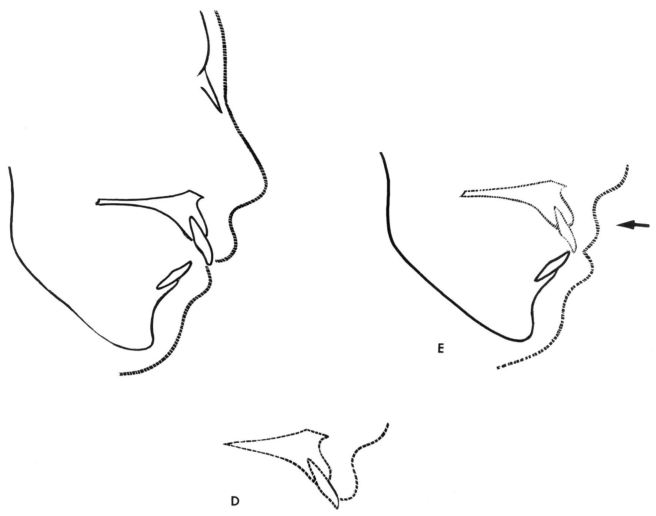

and surgical planning techniques of jaw surgery is mandatory to good results.

Mandibular prognathism, although seen less frequently than microgenia or maxillary protrusion, requires especially careful attention both in planning and in the surgical correction procedure. In order to fully understand this deformity it is necessary first to briefly describe some intermaxillary relationships as they are classified by orthodontists.

When the teeth make maximum occlusal contact under unstrained conditions, the interdigitation of teeth provides a guide to the *relative* positions of the maxillary and mandibular alveolar arches. Three broad classes of occlusion are categorized as follows: Class I, "normal" maxillomandibular relationship; Class II, the maxillary dentoalveolar arch *relatively* anterior to the mandibular arch; and Class III, the mandibular teeth and alveolar arch *relatively* anterior to the corresponding maxillary structures.

Mandibular prognathism may be defined by two criteria: (1) Class III malocclusion of the teeth; and (2) an unsightly appearance of the

lower one third of the face, with loss of the labiomental curve. It is, therefore, a dentofacial deformity, and while it is possible in many cases to correct the dental malocclusion by orthodontic treatment, esthetic improvement in facial contours usually requires a combined surgical-orthodontic approach.

Numerous other surgical procedures have been proposed for the correction of mandibular prognathism (Converse et al., 1964) and each has its champions. The interested reader is referred to the above reference.

CLINICAL ASSESSMENT OF PROGNATHISM

The surgeon confronted with the Hapsburg jaw problem must analyze the characteristics of the deformity and select an appropriate operative plan based on this assessment. Some considerations may be resolved in part by clinical inspection. Does the patient indeed suffer a forward overgrowth of the mandible, or is there an associated defect masquerading as a prog-

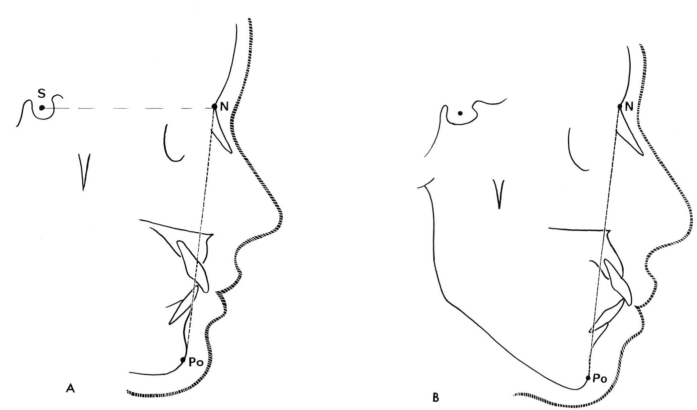

The facial plane. A line drawn on the cephalometric tracing connecting the points marked *N* ("nasion") and *Po* ("pogonion") usually intersects the crown outline of the lower incisors in a well balanced face (*A*). When the dentoalveolar area is procumbent relative to other facial structures (that is, when there is bimaxillary protrusion), the lower third of the face appears convex in profile and the facial plane falls posterior to the lower incisor crown outline (*B*).

nathism? Maxillary hypoplasia (or retrusion) often associated with trauma or cleft deformities must be identified to avoid a misdirected operative procedure. Careful clinical observation of the profile, coupled with study of the photographs, will aid in diagnosis and in establishing a treatment plan. Nevertheless, cephalometric and occlusal analyses are mandatory to confirm the diagnosis and to arrive at the correct modality of treatment. A prominent chin secondary to a posteriorly positioned or underdeveloped maxilla is referred to as a relative prognathism.

It is important to determine if the jaw prominence is associated with Class III malocclusion (a true prognathism) or if it is because of an overgrowth of the chin (macrogenia). Such cases are rare, but do occur. True prognathism connotes an anterior displacement of the mandible in relation to a normally positioned maxilla, with the lower teeth in mesio-occlusion to the uppers. The question is resolved by clinical examination of the teeth and alveolar arches and examination of the study models. A pseudoprognathism is a clinically meaningless term referring to those patients who can bring the

lower anterior teeth into end-on occlusion with the maxillary incisors.

When maxillary hypoplasia and macrogenia have been eliminated from the differential diagnosis, it must be determined whether the prognathism is surgically correctable. Mandibular growth should have ceased prior to operative intervention. Failure to await growth maturation invites the possibility of a relapse. A minimum age of 16 can be justified by the evidence that condylar and ramus growth are virtually completed in most patients by this period. Should doubt exist, such guides as bone age, secondary sexual development, and sibling and parent size can be used as a crude index of the remaining growth potential, yet delay could hardly be criticized. We have defined no maximum age limitation, but common sense must prevail in considering patients over 35 years old.

Secondary or associated disease entities must be excluded in an exacting differential diagnosis. The most emphasized and yet the least common is acromegaly. Hemangioma can produce bony overgrowth and occasionally a prognathism; failure to recognize an occult lesion has led to massive hemorrhage at surgery.

CEPHALOMETRIC AND OCCLUSAL ANALYSIS

Once the clinical diagnosis of prognathism is determined, the following ancillary studies are obtained: medical photographs, a cephalogram, dental casts, a Panorex radiograph of the jaws, and a bite registration.

A cephalogram is taken to confirm the anterior displacement of the mandibular basal bone and to assist in estimating the millimeters of retrusion necessary to obtain an esthetic improvement. To achieve this, a soft tissue outline must be incorporated in the cephalometric technique as described. The considerable attention focused on the cephalogram is justified since this parameter, in conjunction with the dental study models, permits simultaneous manipulation of function and esthetics. Thus a balance can be sought between the optimum occlusal alignment which will yield the maximum correction of facial contour.

Cryptic cephalometric formulas, although impressive in growth and development studies, have not proved meaningful in the management of prognathism. The twofold purpose of analysis, the study of basal bone relationships and mensuration, can be obtained with a minimum of geometric tracing. Our cephalometric analysis is determined by construction of standard reference planes and angles. The sella-nasion plane is used to identify the stable cranial base. The lines Na and Nb permit calculation of angles SNA and SNB. The difference between the two, the ANB angle, is a measure of the basal bone alignment and is used to confirm the diagnosis of a prognathism. A negative value of ANB (SNA—SNB) is characteristic of the prognathic deformity. To conclusively eliminate underdevelopment or retrusion of the maxilla as in a relative prognathism, one further observation is required. The value of SNA and SNB must be compared with the norms.

The measurements derived from the cephalometric tracing are then tested on the dental study models. The casts are obtained by taking an alginate impression of the dental arches and pouring in plaster. A bite registration is recorded in soft wax and the models articulated, preferably on a simple articulator or by hand.

The models are used to identify associated malocclusions, particularly an anterior open bite which might only be aggravated by indiscriminate surgery. Gross malalignments or disproportionate occlusal planes should be treated orthodontically prior to surgery. Minor single tooth and cuspal irregularities can be ground into occlusion, but severe disharmony warrants an orthodontic evaluation.

The dental casts are duplicated and the working models are juggled into a posterior occlusion where cuspal interdigitation is maximal. To facilitate this registration, the mandibular model is sectioned across the base, worked into the proposed articulation and fixed with soft wax. If the models are accurately trimmed, the amount of displacement can be directly measured. The millimeters of bony recession permitted for functional occlusion can then be compared with that required to improve the soft tissue profile. Usually a balance between the two is adopted, and satisfactory esthetic and functional results can be anticipated. Nevertheless, an occasional patient with marked prognathism, or prognathism in conjunction with macrogenia, is found, and despite well planned mathematical correction of the malocclusion, a chin prominence persists. This is best appreciated on the working cephalogram using the profile analysis and must be anticipated preoperatively so that the patient may be forewarned that subsequent genioplasty may be required to realize complete correction.

With the discovery of a reasonably functional occlusion on the study models, areas of obvious cuspal interference are identified and ground out preoperatively in the mouth to permit the establishment of a stable occlusion at surgery. Fixation is thereby facilitated and maintained. Postoperative adjustments are routine, but skilled planning before operation will reduce needless sacrifice of tooth structure. When a body osteotomy is planned, the models are sectioned to determine the limits of bony excision required for correction. Teeth in the lines of resection are similarly removed. Templates, fashioned to duplicate the desired excision, are useful intra-orally in mapping the osteotomy lines.

A final adjunct is the Panorex radiograph or complete set of dental films. These are used to exclude nonassociated pathology, to locate the level of the mandibular canal and to appreciate the bony configuration of the mandibular rami. It is axiomatic that dental caries, periodontal disease and related oral pathology be stabilized prior to operation.

FIXATION

The mechanics of intermaxillary fixation frequently hinge on the orientation of the center or the prejudice of the surgeon. Many techniques offer equally satisfactory results; we favor the luxury of orthodontic bands with edgewise arch appliances since most patients will benefit from minor tooth movement, especially leveling, prior to surgery. All such devices are placed prior to surgery, of course. The individual bands, when well fitted, are also kinder to the periodontal tissues than most wires. In those patients requiring extensive preoperative orthodontics, full banding becomes essential.

On the other hand, if orthodontic manipulation is not required, most standard arch bars will suffice. When the number of teeth is limited, cast splints can be fashioned by the dental laboratory from a working model. Regardless of the method selected, preoperative preparation includes application of fixation appliances.

TECHNIQUE OF VERTICAL OSTEOTOMY OF THE RAMUS

This procedure, advocated by many, can be employed in most prognathic patients and is the single most useful procedure for the plastic surgeon. It is contraindicated in open bite. It is distinguished by the opportunity it affords to alter the gonial angle and thereby improve the contour of the lateral profile. It permits unrestricted exposure and avoids wound contamination by oral flora. The ramus mandibularis of the seventh nerve must be carefully protected; otherwise, few anatomical structures are jeopardized.

Under general nasotracheal anesthesia, an incision is begun just below the gonial angle in a prominent skin fold (p. 513). With experience, a wound of 2 to 3 cm. will suffice. The dissection is carried bluntly upward and medially to expose the lower border and angle of the mandible. The lip is observed throughout this phase, as proximity to the mandibular branch of the seventh nerve will be signaled by muscular twitching at the commissure. A nerve stimulator is most useful in identifying possible nerve branches. The periosteum at the angle is scored, and with a curved 2-cm. periosteal elevator the masseter is freed along the lateral ramus from the sigmoid notch posteriorly, anterior dissection being unwarranted. The posterior border is freed and the medial pterygoid similarly elevated to the notch. Dissection here is confined to the posterior medial ramus to avoid injuring the dental nerve and vessels. A hook is next placed in the sigmoid notch and the line of resection, extending from the notch 1 cm. anterior to the angle, is plotted. Using the hook as a guide, the osteotomy line is scored with a tapered burr. The resection is completed using the burr for

the outer two thirds and a saw for the medial plate.

A similar procedure is performed on the opposite side and the mandible displaced posteriorly. It is critical to position the posterior fragment to achieve an overlap with the anterior fragment on the lateral side; the pull of the lateral pterygoid will then insure firm bony contact. The wounds are closed with fine sutures; intermaxillary fixation, usually accomplished with ligatures through edgewise arch appliances, is secured and maintained for eight weeks.

Other more complicated procedures for the treatment of prognathism are described in standard textbooks.

Augmentation Mentoplasty

For many years, while the search for an acceptable prosthetic implant material went on, chin augmentation was accomplished mainly with homologous or autogenous cartilage or bone grafts. Foreign implants were criticized by most plastic surgeons because of their unnatural consistency and tendency to extrude. However, the necessity of obtaining autogenous grafts from the rib cage or the ileum required a second surgical wound which sometimes was more troublesome to the patient than the operation on the chin itself. Furthermore, it was found that autogenous bone grafts to the chin region had a marked tendency to resorb because of the strong molding forces placed on such grafts by the constant mobility and pressure of the soft tissues. Cartilage grafts particularly, whether autogenous or homologous, tended to absorb or warp. Secondary or tertiary operations on the chin were not uncommon following mentoplasty with bone or cartilage, each succeeding operation becoming more difficult through the scar tissue.

The first prosthetic materials that seemed to have some of the desirable properties for chin augmentation were polyethylene and methylmethacrolate. They were used extensively by Rubin et al. (1948), González-Ulloa and Stevens (1968), and others. Unfortunately these substances are difficult to fabricate and shape and they require molding and sizing prior to the operative procedure, although minor adjustments may be made at surgery. They are also extremely hard in consistency, a major objection. While tissue reaction to polyethylene and acrylic is not excessive, it has become evident that other materials developed subsequently (silicone, Teflon and Dacron) are better tolerated and generally less reactive.

With the development of the silicone rubber compounds, augmentation mentoplasty became simplified. During the past decade the use of such implants for genioplasty has become almost universally accepted. Most of the "diehard" bone graft and cartilage graft proponents have abandoned these more complicated techniques for the use of alloplasts in simple chin augmentation.

Silicone rubber (Silastic*) is available in several degrees of firmness or as a fine-celled sponge. Carefully carved and shaped silicone implants seem superior to sponge because immediate shaping and sizing is possible. When sponge is used, the final result cannot be assessed for months because of pressure on the implant by the natural fibrous capsule, with subsequent contraction of the sponge.

Millard (1965) pointed out that there are few operations in the field of cosmetic surgery other than genioplasty in which almost 100 per cent of the patients are pleased with the results. In his series, 15 per cent of patients having rhinoplasty also received chin augmentation. Seventy-five per cent of these patients were not directly conscious of the original chin discrepancy, but all of them were pleased with the final chin implant improvement. The authors' experience, as well as that of many others, certainly confirms these findings.

As a general precept, it is usually unwise for the surgeon to suggest an operation to correct a defect of which the patient is not aware. Chin augmentation is, in our opinion, an exception to this rule. Many patients seeking rhinoplasty are not aware that their chin is small (microgenic) or out of balance with the rest of the face until this fact is pointed out to them. Profile photographs can graphically demonstrate the point, and oriented lateral x-rays (cephalograms) provide further substantiation.

Parents often are aware of a slight "weakness" of the chin in their children but are hesitant to call this fact to the attention of their child or the surgeon. In such instances it behooves the surgeon to point out that augmentation mentoplasty can be almost as important to the result as the nasal plastic operation. In some instances an augmentation mentoplasty may supersede the rhinoplasty in importance. Admittedly this occurs in a very small percentage of cases, but the reservation applies in particular to those patients in whom a rhinoplasty might be fraught with problems and unpredictable results.

Whether it is advisable to do the nasal plastic first followed by mentoplasty, or the reverse, depends upon the type and severity of the deformities of the nose and chin. Both procedures are usually done at the same operative session. However, if the chin is markedly underdeveloped or retruded, it is advisable to operate on this structure first since this change in profile may be helpful in guiding the surgeon in planning nasal reduction. Too often patients are seen who have had simultaneous nasal plastics and chin augmentation in which too much has been removed from the nose and too much added to the chin. This overcorrection of both structures can result in a facial disharmony that is as unbecoming as the original condition.

Horizontal osteotomy and other types of direct bony surgery must be done as a separate operation. Horizontal osteotomy usually requires general anesthesia and a longer operating session. Both factors militate against concomitant rhinoplasty.

The authors employ two techniques for mentoplasty. When augmentation with implants is considered the technique of choice, prefabricated, commercially available silicone rubber implants are used. The implants need not impose a specific size or shape upon the surgeon, as they can be trimmed at the operative table with scissors or scalpel to whatever dimension and shape is desired. The preformed implants reduce operating time and do not impose the nuisance of sculpting an implant from raw blocks.

Close-celled silicone sponge provides excellent results in chin augmentation. If used, the sponge should be slightly oversized to allow for shrinkage from and contraction of the scar capsule and compression of the sponge.

IMPLANT TECHNIQUE

Chin implants can be inserted using the intra-oral approach via the inferior gingivolabial sulcus, or through an incision in the natural horizontal submental chin crease. There are particular indications for each, and they should be noted so that the best results can be achieved with a minimum of complications.

INTRA-ORAL APPROACH

Since Converse (1950) demonstrated the safety and feasibility of introducing autogenous bone grafts through intra-oral incisions, this approach has been widely used. Synthetic implants can also be placed via the intra-oral ap-

---

*Product of Dow-Corning Corporation.

503

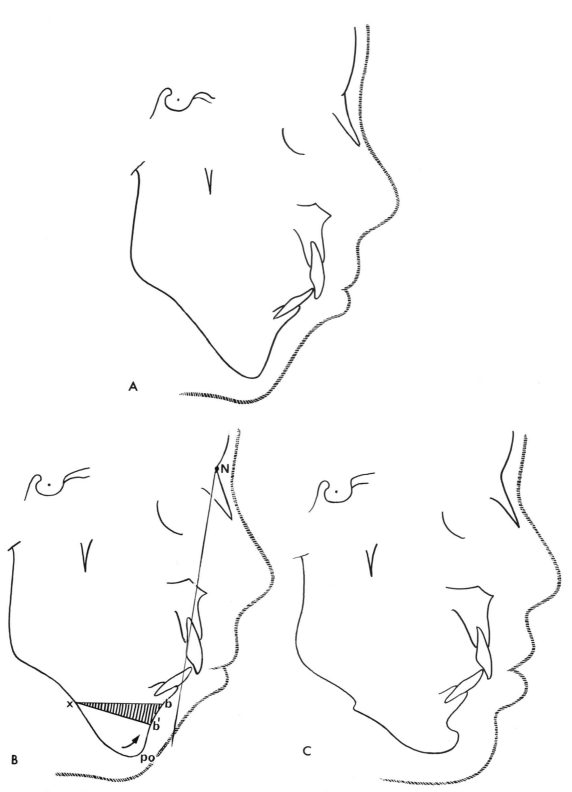

A, Preoperative cephalometric tracing of a young woman with bimaxillary protrusion, facial convexity, excessive facial height, and loss of the labiomental curve. *B*, Cephalometric planning involves determination of the facial plane and the desired new position of "pogonion." Wedge removal to reduce facial height involves elimination of the shaded area and elevation of the mobilized fragment. *C*, Postoperative tracing, showing the improvement in soft tissue contour resulting from wedge removal and advancement of "pogonion." Preoperative and postoperative photographs appear on the opposite page.

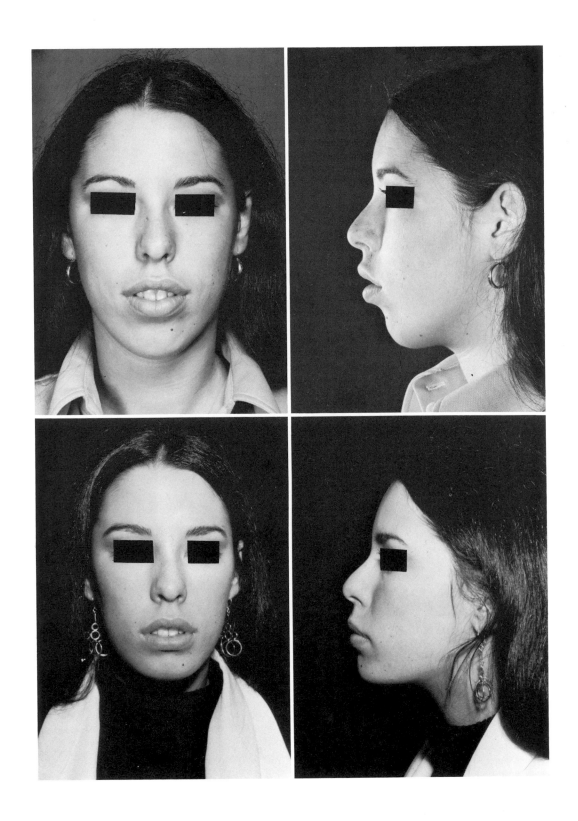

505

proach with a surprisingly low complication rate. It is most helpful to prepare the mouth preoperatively by attending to dental hygiene. The teeth should be scaled and cleaned well. Brushing the teeth with pHisoHex for two or three days before surgery is also of benefit in decreasing wound contamination. Antibiotic coverage is best started in full therapeutic doses 48 hours before surgery and is continued for 10 days postoperatively.

The intra-oral approach described by Converse (1950) is an incision superiorly on the labial side of the lower labiogingival sulcus. It may be made as long as required, leaving a cuff of mucosa on the oral surface of the lip to provide sufficient soft tissue for a tensionless closure. This incision is carried down to bone, and a subperiosteal pocket of suitable size is developed to accept the implant. Pitanguy (1968) favors this basic approach, but emphasizes utilization of the median raphe of the chin musculature to fix the implant in position. He dissects this "ligament" free from its inferior insertion, turns it 180 degrees, and passes it through a notch in the center of the implant for fixation. He believes the notch aids in the formation of a chin dimple. Millard (1971) favors a horizontal incision in the labial mucosa and a vertical separation of the musculature of the lip by blunt dissection extending to the bone, where he fashions lateral extensions of a pocket by blunt dissection. Such a technique has the distinct advantage of providing a mucosal incision of minimal length, well buttressed from beneath by a muscle closure at right angles. The authors favor this approach for implants of smaller size. Larger implants require wide exposure, however, and are best inserted through the submental or external approach.

A useful variation of the intra-oral exposure is the use of two incisions placed at the lateral extensions of the pocket. The implant is placed by "tunneling" between these two incisions.

SUBMENTAL (EXTERNAL) APPROACH

Certain factors militate against optimal results from the intra-oral approach. A short mandibular body (micrognathia) associated with a shallow labial sulcus may cause the implant to be placed in too high a position if placed intra-orally. This results in loss of the natural lip-chin crease (labiomental fold). In addition, the implant is an annoying mass in the labial sulcus which the patient is able to feel with his tongue.

Such a combination of circumstances (a short mandible and shallow sulcus) usually requires the implant to be placed from below (submental incision). This approach permits the surgeon to elevate the periosteum only as high as required for the implant, permitting him to preserve the integrity of the sulcus. In this way the implant can also be placed at a lower level or even along the inferior mandibular margin if desired. As previously stated, large implants are best inserted from an incision in the submental crease so as to prevent excessive tension on the intra-oral suture line which can lead to wound breakdown and extrusion. Accurate positioning of large implants is also facilitated by the external approach.

It is timely to discuss here the oft repeated assumption that implants or grafts can be placed subperiosteally. In our experience they cannot. One need only examine the nonyielding and inelastic nature of periosteum to realize that it cannot be made to stretch and completely cover an implant of appreciable size. The periosteum can certainly be elevated and an implant placed beneath it on the bone, but then only rarely is it possible to close the periosteum over the implant.

Implants may be placed directly on cortical bone, or overlying the periosteum, and this makes little difference in the final result. However, they should *not* be placed in a subcutaneous or intramuscular pocket where they can be readily palpated. Close to the bone will suffice. If the submental approach is used, the surgeon should close the wound in two layers. The deep closure that brings muscles together is most helpful in fixing the implant and protects the skin incision from dehiscence. The danger of extrusion is thus minimized.

DRESSINGS AND POSTOPERATIVE CARE

Elastoplast and adhesive tape splinting are usually applied as a "basketweave" pattern and maintained for two to four days. All dressings are then removed and none are replaced. Wide spectrum antibiotic coverage is maintained for 10 days postoperatively.

When the intra-oral approach is used, only a liquid diet is permitted for three days postoperatively, until the wound is healed.

COMPLICATIONS

Extrusion, malposition, and *bone absorption* are the main complications of augmentation mentoplasty when solid implants are used. Infection can occur, but is rare. When infection does occur, extrusion of the implant is almost certain, although on occasion prompt and vigorous treatment can save implants.

Sponge implants can change in size. This is more of an inconvenience than a complication. Initially sponges fill with serum or fluid, causing swelling of the chin. As the fibrous capsule forms around the implant the sponge contracts slowly, so that the chin size also diminishes. The degree of change is usually not significant and does not contraindicate the use of fine-celled sponge.

Extrusion can occur with any implant, although perhaps not for many months or years after the surgery. Adequate-sized pockets and careful anatomical placement of the implant are the best prophylaxis. Nevertheless, even the most carefully placed implant can shift in position and present as a pressure point either within the mouth or externally at the chin. If the implant becomes extruded it can be replaced. This may not always be necessary, because the residual scar capsule may preserve enough augmentation to please the patient.

Malpositioned implants can be repositioned by adjusting the size and shape of the pocket.

Erosion of bone by onlay implants was reported by Robinson and Shuken (1969). The bone responds to the pressure of the implant by osteolytic activity. Such erosion does not appear to represent a significant contraindication for implants, since apparently it is self-limiting.

HORIZONTAL OSTEOTOMY

The chin can be brought forward surgically by sectioning the mandible in a horizontal plane beneath the alveolar canal (pp. 542 and 543). The severed segment of the mandible with or without muscular attachments is then advanced as far forward as necessary and wired in position to the lower teeth until consolidation has taken place. This technique is an excellent one in solving certain problems such as increased vertical heights or asymmetry.

Horizontal osteotomy of the chin was probably first practiced in Germany during or shortly after World War II, according to references cited by Converse and Wood-Smith (1964) and Hinds and Kent (1969). The operative technique was first reported by Trauner and Obwegeser in the English literature in 1963 in conjunction with a paper on the surgical correction of mandibular deformities of different types. Converse and Wood-Smith discussed variations of the technique and defined five possibilities. These variations and the technique were subsequently strongly endorsed by Hinds and Kent, who recommended it for correction of almost all deformities of the chin to the complete exclusion of the implant technique.

The operation is one of considerably more magnitude than augmentation by implants and carries a significantly higher morbidity, healing time and complication rate. It is also much more inconvenient to the patient. It is, however, the unquestioned operation of choice in those patients who have retrognathia in association with increased vertical height of the mandibular body at the symphysis aptly demonstrated in the patients shown on pages 505 and 509. Such a deformity requires not only horizontal sectioning of the mandible but, in addition, a "piece of pie" (or wedge) is resected from the body and the lower fragment is then brought forward and upward to a position in front of the cut border where it is fixed in position by wiring to a simple orthodontic appliance. The chin prominence is augmented by this procedure while at the same time the height of the mandible is foreshortened. The amount of bone to be resected, as well as the amount of advancement of the lower fragment, can be almost exactly planned from preoperative cephalometric studies.

Horizontal osteotomy is also clearly the technique of choice in asymmetry of the chin (p. 544). Implants in such cases are difficult or impossible to position.

In severe retrusion both horizontal osteotomy and subsequent prosthetic implant may be necessary for optimal results.

TECHNIQUE

The anterior mandible is "degloved" by making an incision on the labial side of the lower sulcus, leaving a sufficient cuff of mucous membrane. The incision is made as far laterally as necessary on either side to gain sufficient exposure of the bone and mental foramen. The mental nerves on either side are carefully dissected clear of investing tissues and guarded from trauma at all times during the procedure.

The subperiosteal dissection continues to the lower border of the mandible where it is often necessary to divide some of the muscular attachments to allow sufficient mobility for forward displacement. The design of the bone cuts is then made by drawing on the bone with blue dye. The osteotomies are done with a Stryker saw and the air-driven drill. If a segment of bone (the "piece of pie") is to be removed, all pieces of bone are saved. These may be used as

507

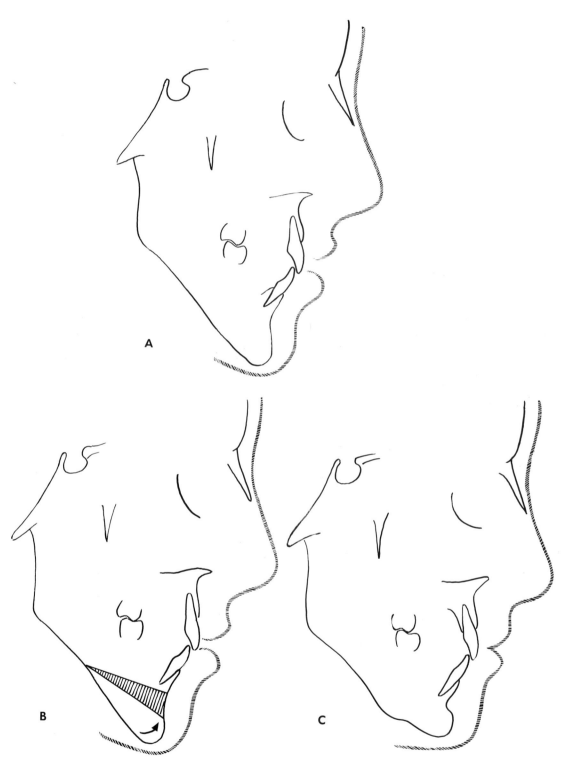

A, Preoperative cephalometric tracing of a patient with excessive facial height and loss of lip competency. Note the loss of the labiomental curve in the preoperative profile photograph on the next page. *B*, Plan for wedge removal and elevation of the mobilized fragment. *C*, Postoperative tracing. Preoperative and postoperative photographs appear on the opposite page.

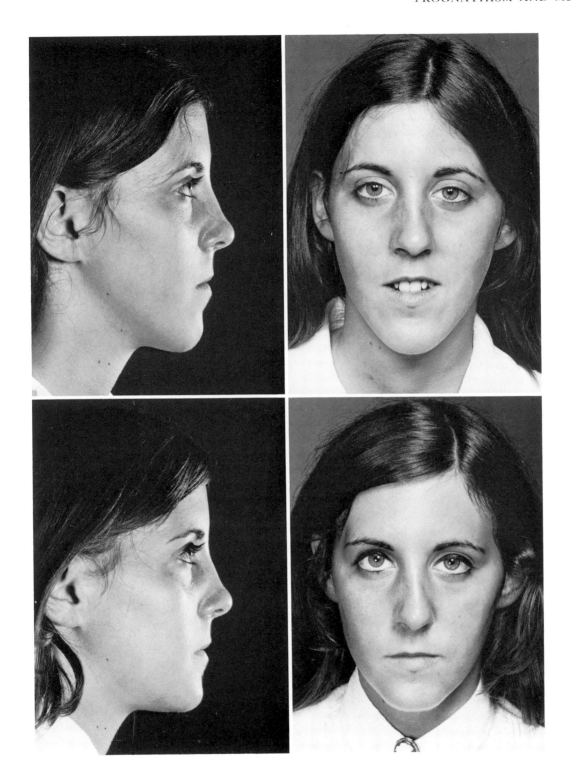

chips to fill gaps between the mobile fragment and the bone of the mandible (p. 544).

It may be necessary, when the fragment is to be advanced forward for a considerable distance, to strip the fragment of most of its anterior soft tissue attachments so that it becomes virtually a free bone graft. Only lingual attachments remain: those of the digastric and genial

muscles. This presents surprisingly few difficulties, and such "grafts" seem to take readily.

Rough bone edges are polished with the drill, and the upper surface of the lower fragment is fitted to the lower edge of the cut mandible in the desired position and relationship. Permanent direct interosseous wiring is rarely necessary, since the mandibular fragment is

509

readily immobilized by wire suspension to pre-fixed orthodontic appliances previously placed in the lower teeth. Drill holes strategically placed in the fragment are required and usually three to four such cable wires are used (p. 543).

The intra-oral mucosal incision is sutured with interrupted sutures of 4–0 chromic catgut, and a simple Barton's bandage is applied. Inter-maxillary fixation is not necessary in such patients.

POSTOPERATIVE CARE

Consolidation occurs within six weeks, during which time the suture line is kept clean by saline, weak peroxide irrigation or mouthwashes. Wide spectrum antibiotics are given for about 10 days postoperatively. The cable wires are removed six to seven weeks postoperatively.

COMPLICATIONS

Temporary hypoesthesia or anesthesia of the chin and lower lip can occur if the mental nerves are excessively stretched or otherwise traumatized. This is usually temporary in nature, but it may persist for several weeks or even months. If the nerve is cut or otherwise irreversibly injured at the time of operation, permanent anesthesia results. Protection of the nerve and its branches during surgery is of prime importance. Should the mental nerve be cut during surgery it should be repaired before closure.

Infection of the wound can be a serious complication, particularly when the mobilized fragment consists of a free piece of bone with only minimal muscular attachments. Sequestration is then a possibility. However, infection is uncommon and has not been a significant problem in our experience. Antibiotic coverage and the establishment of adequate preoperative oral hygiene undoubtedly account for the low incidence of infection.

Irregularities of the mandibular margin are sometimes palpable at the ends of the fragment, but are more of a nuisance than a complication and in time tend to become molded.

SOFT TISSUE CONSIDERATIONS

Lip posture and the location of the soft tissue mass of the chin are extremely important elements in the total facial appearance. They are largely dependent upon jaw form and the relative position of the mandible and the teeth, as noted previously.

The chin mass is of particular importance to the surgeon planning an operative procedure on the mental symphysis. Mandibular osteotomies of various types and implant augmentations have a direct effect on the soft tissues of the anterior muscle mass of the chin and the submental area.

Chin augmentation often has a dramatic effect on the submental soft tissue. A "double chin" (or early "turkey gobbler" effect), which is the result of skin excess only, is sometimes eliminated by simple augmentation as shown in the patient on page 535 (bottom). A salutary effect is achieved when this procedure is done in conjunction with rhytidectomy (pp. 530 and 531). Chin augmentation is being suggested by us more and more frequently to rhytidectomy candidates.

In patients with an excessive submental fat pad, the excess fat, as well as some skin, can be excised at the time a chin implant is introduced through the submental approach.

The anterior soft tissue mass or "chin pad" can be profoundly affected, and the location of this structure and the possible effects of the surgery should be taken into consideration preoperatively. For example, in the "backward divergent" face the mandible may show increased vertical height and a retruded chin point. The chin pad then often rides high and appears most unnatural when the circumoral musculature is brought into action. In such a patient augmentation by implantation alone would increase the forward projection of the chin, but would also exaggerate the unnatural appearance of the chin pad and might possibly elevate it even further.

In such a patient a reduction osteotomy by horizontal section, combined with wedge removal and advancement of the lower segment, usually puts the chin pad in a more normal anatomical relationship. This results in a much more natural facial expression by relaxing the soft tissues of the chin pad. Note the improvement gained in the patient shown on page 505.

Chin Dimple

A central chin "dimple" is considered to be an attractive beauty mark by many. Some prominent personalities in the entertainment industry have been identified by such an indentation. Chin dimples are usually hereditary in nature, but attempts to create them have been made by surgeons. These techniques provide a cicatricial union between the undersurface of the dermis and the underlying bone or periosteum. Alternatively, an implant which has a carved indent in its center to which the overlying soft tissues conform may be inserted (Pitanguy, 1968). These methods can be successful, but the results are inconsistent and thus not predictable.

The method based on producing a scar contracture of dermal adhesion can be disappointing, because even with meticulous attention to anatomic location and detail, such dimples are frequently asymmetrical and unnatural in appearance; they do not move with facial animation.

Natural chin dimples occur almost exactly in the midline and take the shape of a vertical furrow. This symmetry of nature may be most difficult to duplicate by surgery. It is also somewhat risky to attempt to excise musculature and subcutaneous tissue from the dermis in the midline in an attempt to obtain adherence of the dermis to a prosthetic implant. This violates the main safety rule relating to implants, that of adequate soft tissue cover. Local pressure necrosis and the possibility of exposure and extrusion of the implant are complications.

The possibilities of such complications or imperfect results notwithstanding, a chin dimple is frequently demanded by certain patients who are willing to accept the possibility of imperfection. The surgeon is then justified in attempting to form one.

When simultaneous augmentation is not required, the simplest technique is to make a submental incision in the natural skin fold and to undermine the soft tissues of the chin just above the periosteum. A Y-shaped segment of soft tissue, including muscle and subcutaneous tissue, is then excised from the midline of the chin (which, of course, must be carefully marked beforehand) where the desired indentation is planned. This resection extends superficially to the dermis. One or two buried sutures of nylon or chromic catgut are then placed through the undersurface of the dermis and the periosteum of the mandible directly beneath and tied, thus approximating the dermis to the periosteum. Several trial sutures are usually placed until the desired effect is obtained. This manufactured depression can be reinforced by tying a rolled bolus of dry or greased gauze into the external indenture with mattress sutures. Page 546 shows such a patient.

If augmentation mentoplasty is required in addition to a dimple, the technique of Pitanguy (1968) can be used. A suitable prosthesis is carved with a notch in its center. The notch must be placed exactly in the midline over it to fill the contour depression. Some soft tissues can be excised, however, but with great caution and conservatively. When compression bandages are applied over the implant too vigorously the blood supply may be compromised and pressure necrosis of the skin result.

REFERENCES

Ballard, C. F.: The morphological bases of prognosis determination and treatment planning. Dent. Pract. *18*:62, 1967.

Bell, W. H.: Surgical correction of mandibular retrognathism. Amer. J. Orthodont. *52*:518, 1966.

Case, C.: A Practical Treatise on the Technics and Principles of Dental Orthopedia. Chicago, C. S. Case Co., 1921.

Converse, J. M.: Restoration of facial contour by bone grafts introduced through the oral cavity. Plast. Reconstr. Surg. *6*:295, 1950.

Converse, J. M.: Degloving technique. *In* Kanzanjian, V. H., and Converse, J. M. (eds.): The Surgical Treatment of Facial Injuries. Baltimore, The Williams & Wilkins Company, 1959, p. 866.

Converse, J. M., Horowitz, S. L., and Wood-Smith, D.: Deformities of the jaws. *In* Converse, J. M. (ed.): Reconstructive Plastic Surgery. Philadelphia, W. B. Saunders Company, 1964, pp. 869–947.

Converse, J. M., and Wood-Smith, D.: Horizontal osteotomy of the mandible. Plast. Reconstr. Surg. *34*:464, 1964.

González-Ulloa, M., and Stevens, E.: Role of chin correction in profileplasty. Plast. Reconstr. Surg. *41*:477, 1968.

Hinds, E. C., and Kent, J. N.: Genioplasty: The versatility of the horizontal osteotomy. Oral Surg. *27*:690, 1969.

Horowitz, S. L.: The challenge of facial deformity. Dent. Pract. *22*:191, 1972.

Horowitz, S. L., Gerstman, L. J., and Converse, J. M.: Craniofacial relationships in mandibular prognathism. Arch. Oral Biol. *14*:121, 1969.

Horowitz, S. L., and Hixon, E. H.: The Nature of Orthodontic Diagnosis. St. Louis, The C. V. Mosby Co., 1966, Chapters 15 and 17.

Junghans, J. A.: Profile reconstruction with Silastic chin implants. Amer. J. Orthodont. *53*:217, 1967.

Lassus, C.: The horizontal osteotomy of the chin: Its indications. Rev. Stomatol. (Paris) *69*:642, 1968.

Marino, H., and Craviotto, M.: Micrognathia. Treatment with external prosthesis. Plast. Reconstr. Surg. *2*:260, 1947.

Millard, R.: Adjuncts in augmentation mentoplasty and corrective rhinoplasty. Plast. Reconstr. Surg. *36*:48, 1965.

Millard, R.: Augmentation mentoplasty. Surg. Clin. N. Amer. *51*:333, 1971.

Peck, H., and Peck, S.: A concept of facial esthetics. Angle Orthodont. *40*:284, 1970.

Penn, J.: Kiel-bone implants to the chin and nose. Plast. Reconstr. Surg. *42*:303, 1968.

Pitanguy, I.: Augmentation mentoplasty. Plast. Reconstr. Surg. *42*:460, 1968.

Riedel, R. A.: An analysis of dentofacial relationships. Amer. J. Orthodont. *43*:103, 1957.

Rish, B. B.: Profile-plasty. Report on plastic chin implants. Laryngoscope *74*:144, 1964.

Robertson, J. G.: Chin augmentation means of rotation of double chin fat flap. Plast. Reconstr. Surg. *3*:471, 1965.

Robinson, M., and Shuken, R.: Bone resorption under plastic implants. J. Oral Surg. *27*:116, 1969.

Rubin, L. R., Robertson, G. W., and Shapiro, R. N.: Polyethylene in reconstructive surgery. Plast. Reconstr. Surg. *3*:586, 1948.

Trauner, B., and Obwegesser, H.: The surgical correction of mandibular prognathism and retrognathia with consideration of genioplasty. Part I—Surgical procedures to correct mandibular prognathism and reshaping of the chin. Oral Surg. *10*:677, 1957.

Tulley, W. J.: Adverse muscle forces—Their diagnostic significance. Amer. J. Orthodont. *42*:801, 1956.

The technique of vertical osteotomy for correction of prognathism. *A*, A small incision is made in a natural neck crease below the angle of the jaw. *B* and *C*, Dissection is carried down to the inferior margin of the mandible at the angle. A nerve stimulator is employed. The periosteum is incised and elevated. *D*, A fiberoptic retractor is an invaluable aid in any such tunnelling procedure. *E*, The osteotomy is performed with an oscillating saw, aided by an air drill and osteotomes. *F*, The bone is cut posterior to the entrance of the neurovascular bundle (the lingula). *G*, The anterior fragments are retropositioned and placed medial to the posterior fragments in order to prevent medial displacement as a result of the action of the pterygoid muscles. *H*, The final position of the jaws; immobilization is by intermaxillary fixation, and the bone fragments themselves are not wired.

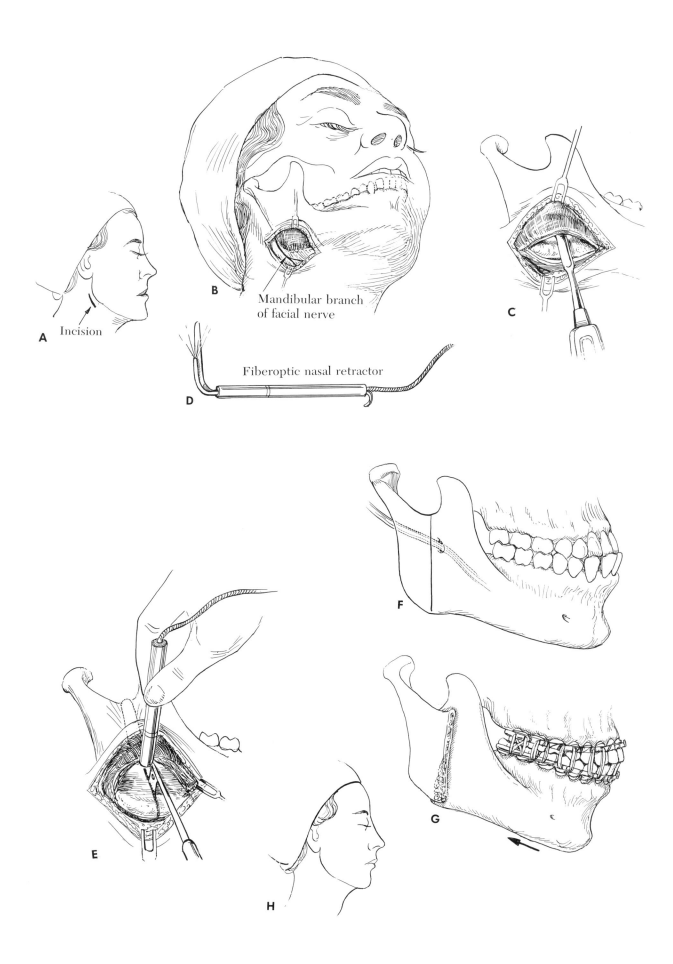

A Incision

B Mandibular branch
of facial nerve

C

D Fiberoptic nasal retractor

E

F

G

H

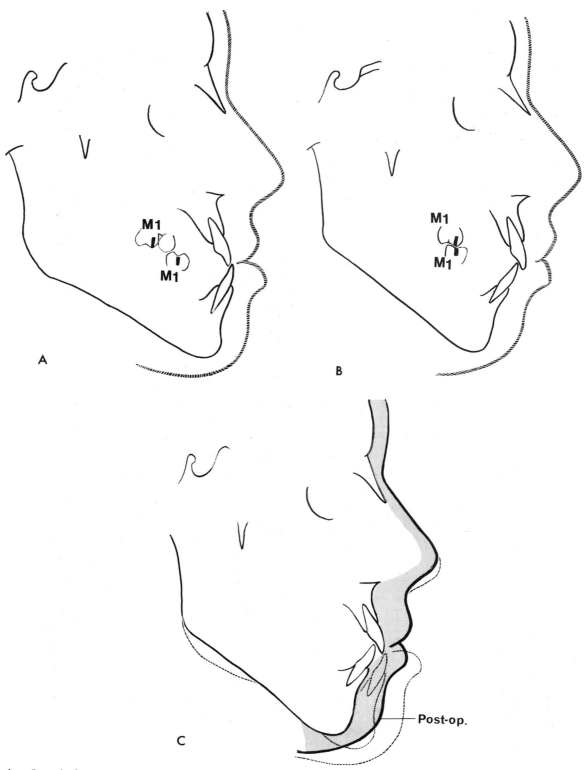

Results of vertical osteotomy: *A*, Preoperative cephalogram tracing, showing typical prognathism with loss of the labiomental curve and Class III (Angle) malocclusion. Note the position of the molars (M₁). *B*, Postoperative cephalogram. *C*, Superimposed cephalograms, showing advancement of the bone and soft tissues. Preoperative and postoperative photographs are on the opposite page.

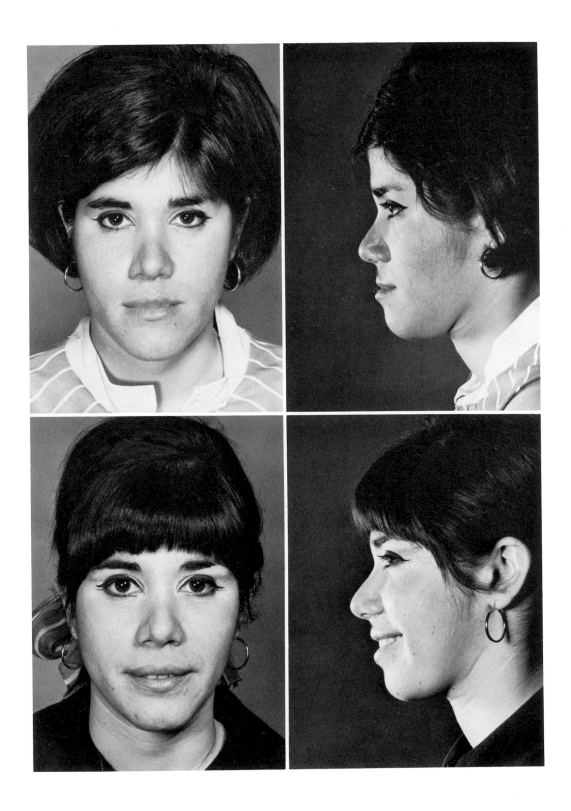

515

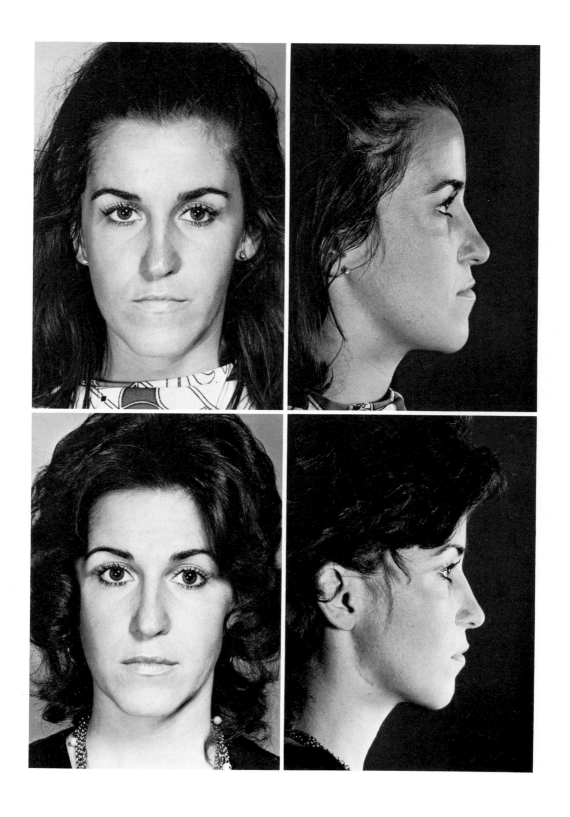

516

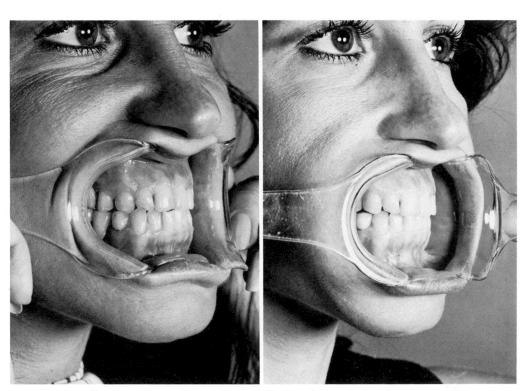

This patient's photographs demonstrate the subtle but effective change in facial appearance that can result from even a slight retropositioning of the mandible after vertical osteotomy. In this patient the mandible was moved back only about 3 mm., according to the tracing and as evidenced by the occlusion photographs, but the facial appearance was markedly softened and improved.

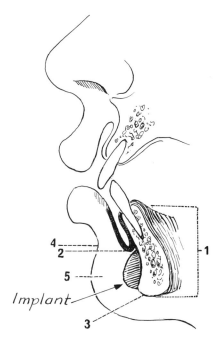

The normal anatomy of the mandible and the adjacent soft tissues plays an important role in determining the success or failure of chin implants. Anatomical factors include (1) vertical height of the mandible at the symphysis; (2) depth of the gingivolabial sulcus; (3) configuration of the lower mandibular rim at the symphysis; (4) development of the labiomental groove; and (5) the amount of soft tissue over the chin.

Implants must be placed into sockets of exact size over the anterior surface of the mandible, so that displacement and resulting malposition and sometimes extrusion cannot occur. It is difficult to increase the length of the chin vertically with prosthetic implants, because they cannot be readily fixed to bone. Attempts to gain length without positive fixation tend to place the implant so that it projects inferiorly beyond the mandibular border, which then acts a fulcrum to the implant's lever, facilitating displacement. When increased vertical length is desired, bone grafts are more suitable, because they can be fixed into position with interosseous wires. Development of a suitable "glue" to fix prosthetic implants to bone would be a great help in alleviating this technical problem.

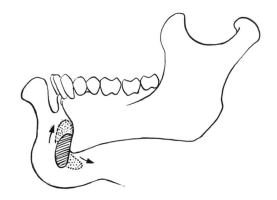

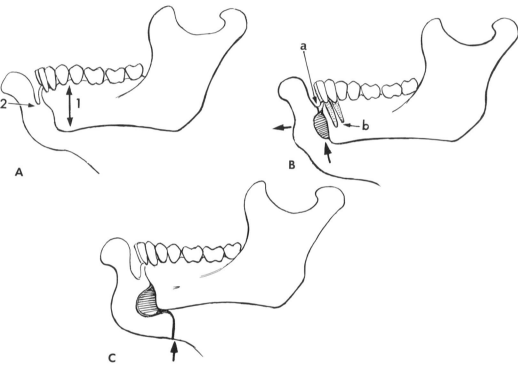

Augmentation mentoplasty is difficult in the presence of certain anatomical variations of the lower jaw, such as decreased vertical height at the symphysis (1 in *A*) and shallowness of the gingivolabial sulcus (2 in *A*). An implant placed too high (as shown in *B*) would elevate the sulcus (*a*), creating an uncomfortable bulge and an unnatural chin shape (arrows). Horizontal osteotomy is also difficult in such patients because the roots of the teeth may extend into the customary plane of section (*b*). The proper placement of an implant in such a circumstance is shown in *C*. The pocket should not be dissected as high as the gingivolabial sulcus. The implant must be placed on the exact tip of the chin and not permitted to slip down. A two-layer soft tissue closure helps to maintain this position.

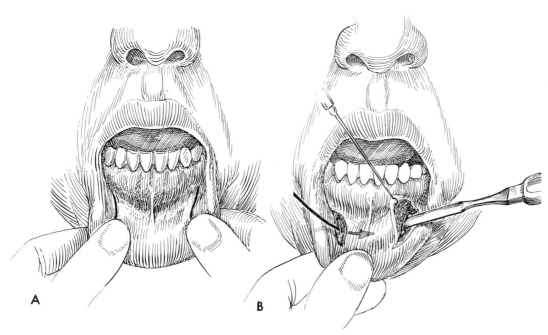

Augmentation mentoplasty by insertion of an alloplastic implant using two incisions placed laterally. The periosteum is raised and a socket is created by a tunnelling procedure. This technique avoids a long horizontal incision directly over the implant, which would increase the likelihood of exposure and extrusion.

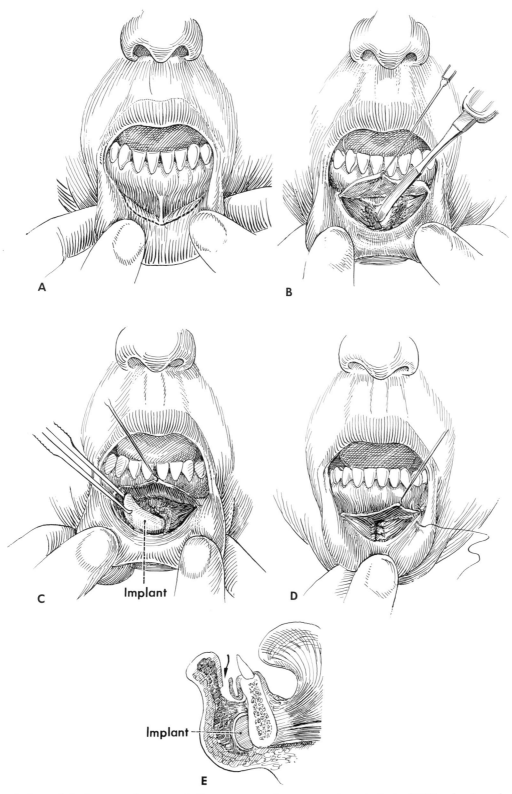

A useful variation of the intra-oral approach for augmentation mentoplasty is that of Millard, who advocates incising the labial mucosa along the sulcus (*A*), but splitting the musculature in a vertical direction (*B*). Closure, therefore, places the deep muscle layer at right angles to the mucosa, which decreases the likelihood of wound breakdown over the implant resulting in extrusion. The implant is shown in its proper position in *E*.

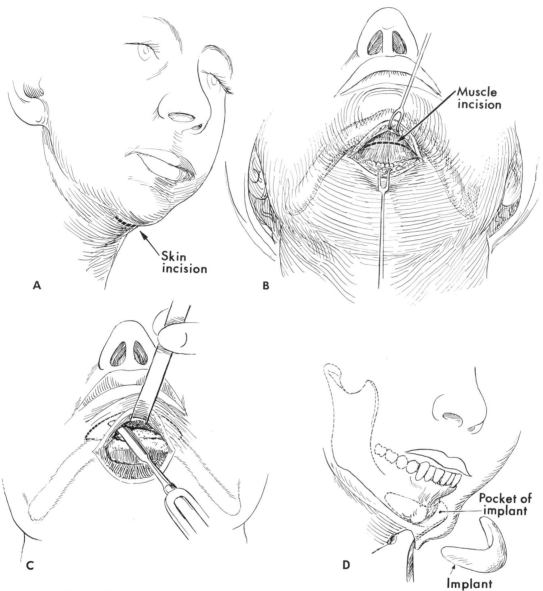

Insertion of a prosthetic chin implant for augmentation by the submental (external) approach. *A*, An incision is placed in the submental crease. *B* and *C*, An exactly sized socket is dissected subperiosteally after the muscle is split. *D*, *E*, *F* and *G*, The socket should be so made that the implant rides along the border of the mandible but does not extend higher than the natural labiomental sulcus (*F*). *H* The periosteum should not be cut free along the lower border of the mandible except over the symphysis, so that the implant cannot slide caudally by a rocking action. *J*, Redundant soft tissue of the submental region is excised. *K* and *L*, The wound is closed in layers.

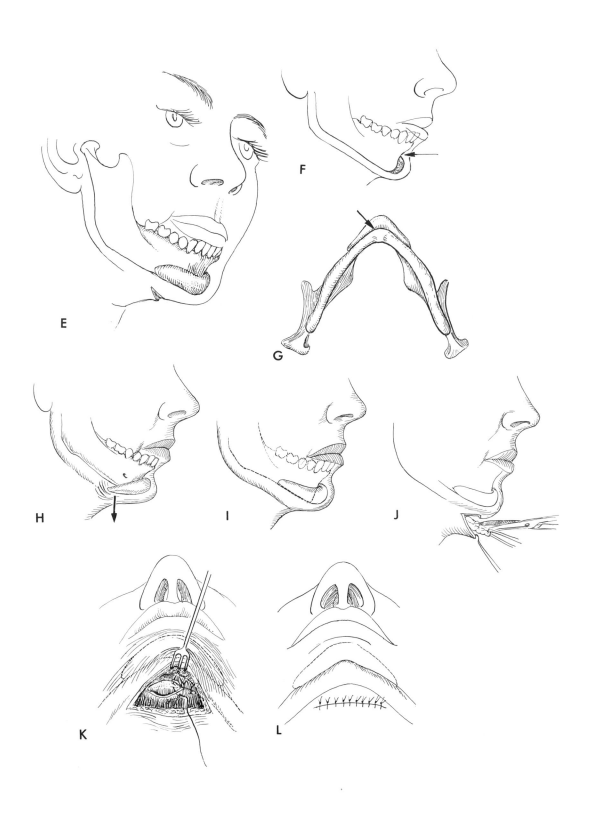

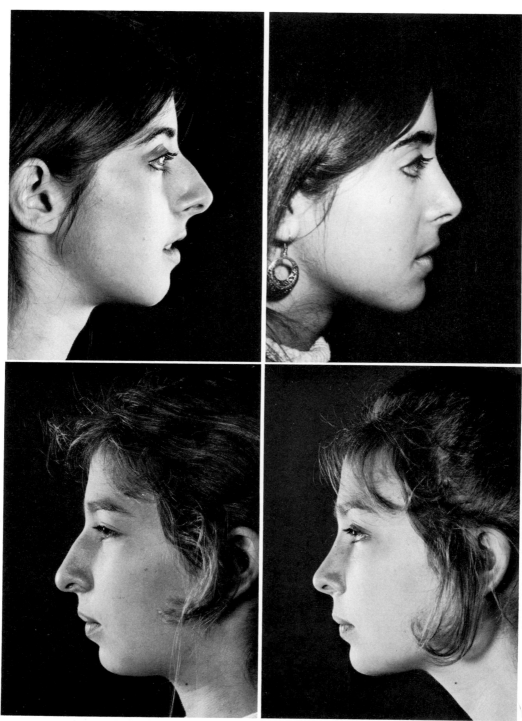

Augmentation mentoplasty with small-sized implants is frequently done at the same time as rhinoplasty. Such implants are easily inserted via the intra-oral approach with little added morbidity. The effect of even such a minor chin build-up is to add measurably to the final result by improving facial balance. Since genioplasty and rhinoplasty are so commonly carried out at the same operation, the surgeon should not hesitate to point out a weak chin to the patient and family during consultation for rhinoplasty. These photographs illustrate typical improvements; note in particular the improvement in lip posture.

524

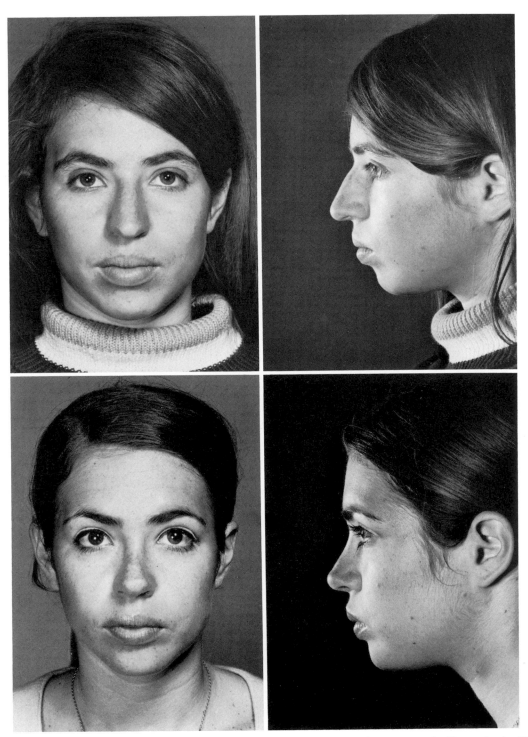

Protrusion of the lips is often caused by bimaxillary protrusion of the teeth or macrocheilia, or both. Chin augmentation cannot alter either of these basic deformities, but it can soften the effect and promote an altogether more pleasant facial appearance. This patient demonstrates the marked improvement that can be effected by augmentation mentoplasty combined with rhinoplasty in the presence of bimaxillary protrusion.

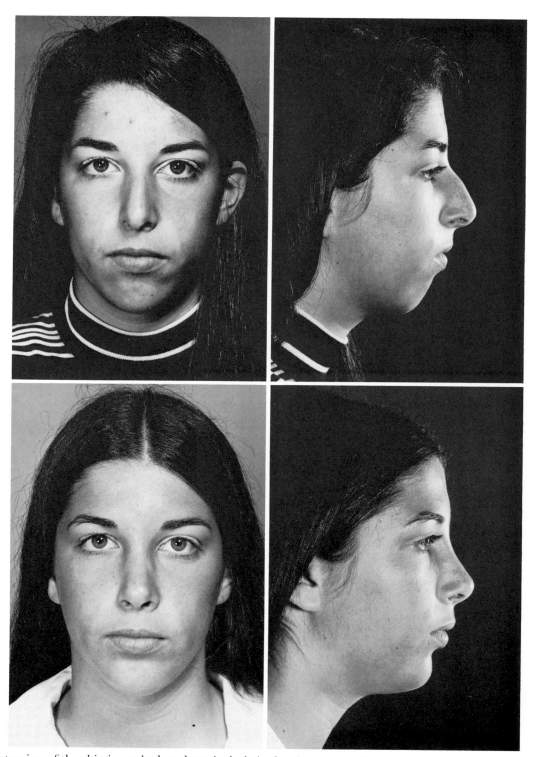

When retrusion of the chin is marked, and particularly in the absence of a Class 2 occlusion, substantial correction can still be achieved at the time of rhinoplasty by the use of larger chin implants. However, these are best inserted through a submental incision, because it is easier to dissect a socket that is properly sized and positioned. It is subsequently easier to place the implant in the proper position.

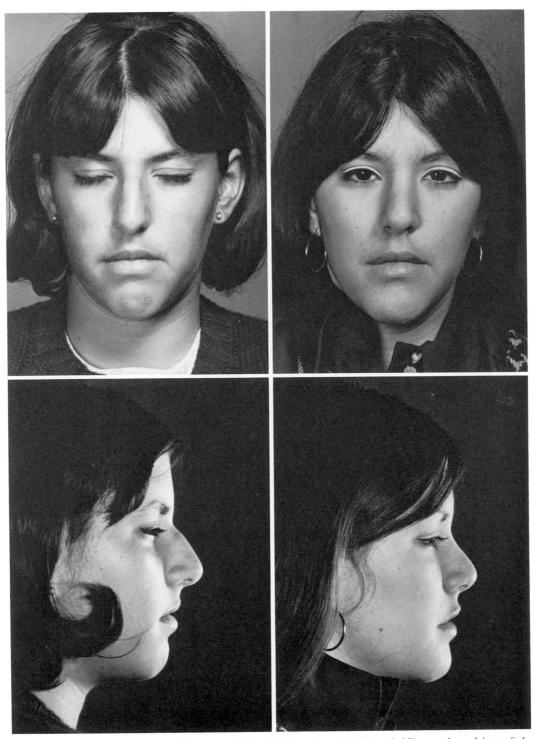

A silicone chin implant in this young lady successfully eliminated unsightly wrinkling or bunching of the muscle mass anterior to the mentum, at the same time achieving a slight but effective augmentation of the chin. The muscle mass at the front of the chin is a complicated interlacing network, and its action can be cosmetically unattractive. Making the pocket for an implant and stripping the soft tissue mass and periosteum from the anterior mandible, as well as positioning the implant itself, seems to eliminate or at least ameliorate this problem in most patients.

527

Microgenia can limit face lift results, and the effect of a cervicofacial rhytidectomy is often enhanced by augmentation mentoplasty. Some patients have never been aware that microgenia is a part of the problem, so that suggesting a chin implant to improve the face lift result is usually welcomed. Other patients are hesitant to inquire about chin correction even though they may have been conscious of a weak chin for many years. In addition, chin implants improve the mentocervical angle. (See also page 198.)

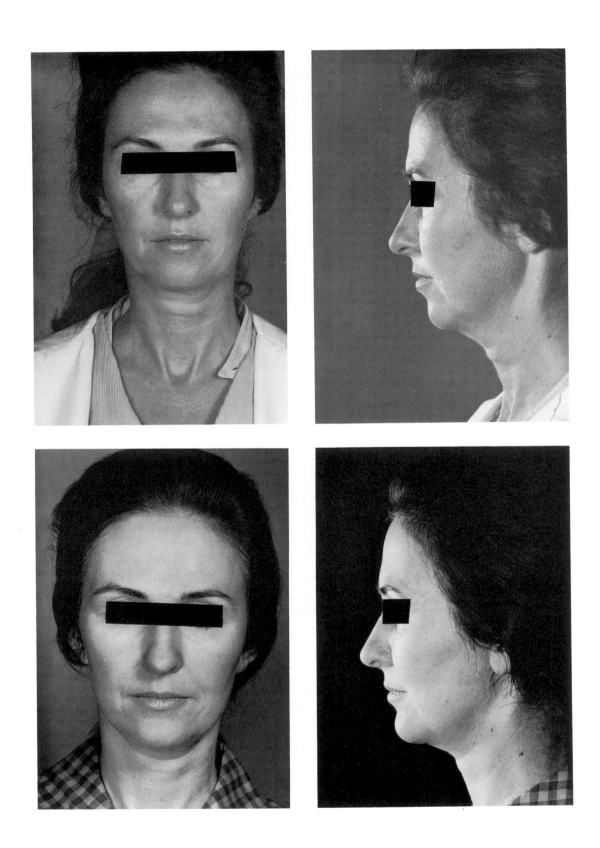

529

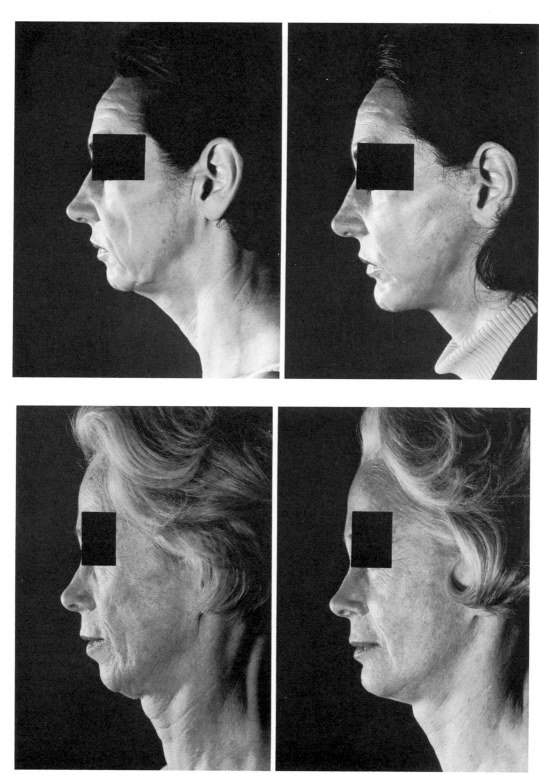

A combination of microgenia (or retrognathia) with marked redundancy and ptosis of the skin along the jaw and upper neck can be adequately corrected only by cervicofacial rhytidectomy and augmentation mentoplasty. Patients in this age group are not good candidates for extensive jaw surgery to restore contour and occlusion. They often had malocclusion for most of their lives and need extensive dental attention. Inasmuch as direct procedures on the mandible are contraindicated, the choice comes down to only implants, which can be placed with ease and which provide excellent contour correction, as seen in these two patients.

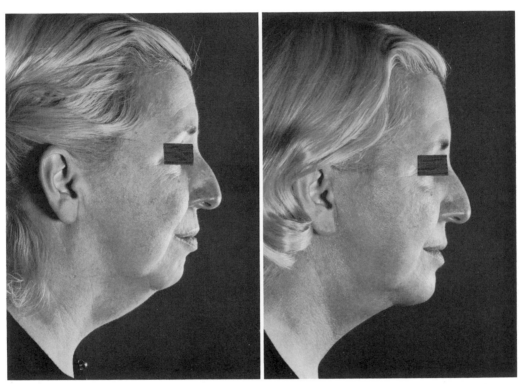

The type of jaw and neck deformity seen in the preoperative photograph of this patient is difficult to correct no matter what the operative technique. A combination of rhytidectomy, chin implant, and direct excision of excessive skin in the submental region and upper neck was required. The same submental incision was used to place the implant and to excise the skin.

This attractive middle-aged woman had been self-conscious about her receding chin for most of her life and had not been aware that augmentation mentoplasty was possible. Osteotomy was not indicated because of the patient's age and the condition of her mouth, but a silicone rubber onlay was placed and produced an excellent correction. Note the improvement in the skin wrinkles on either side of the chin, as well as elimination of muscle bunching of the chin pad itself. The size of the implant required to achieve a correction such as this militates against the intra-oral approach in most instances. A submental incision needs to be only about an inch long.

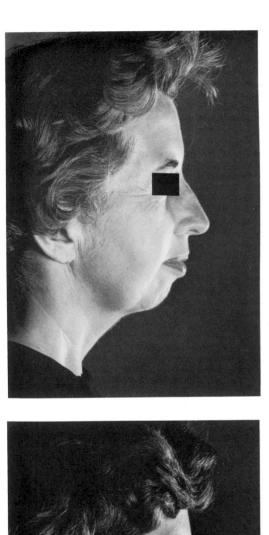
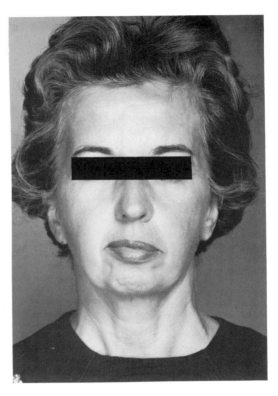
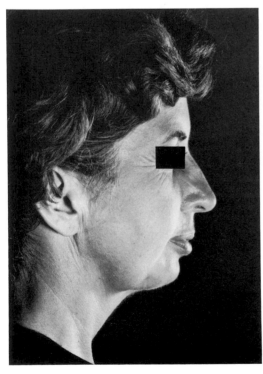
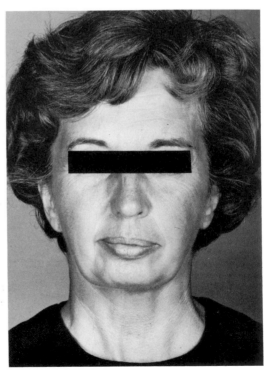

533

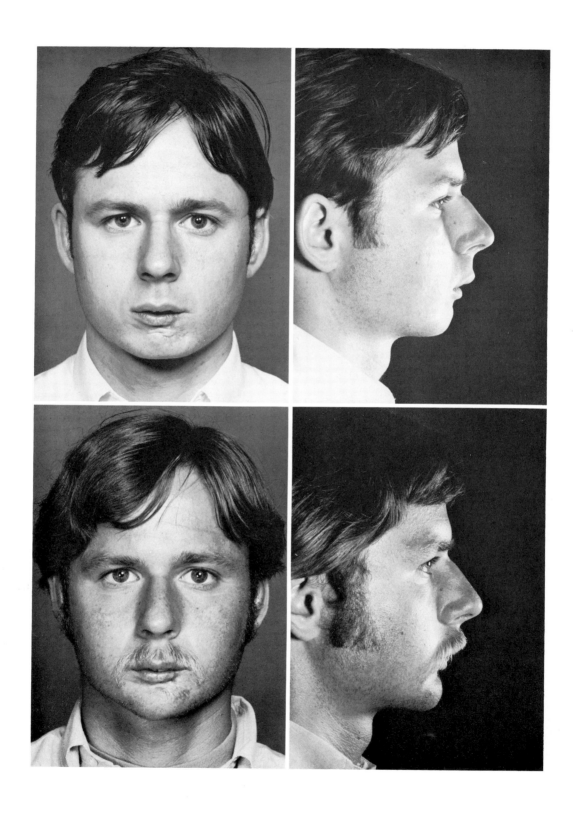

When the soft tissues about the chin have been scarred or otherwise damaged, it is usually advisable to insert implants by the submental route. The submental wound is much better able to withstand the tension created after closure. In this young man there was extensive radiation atrophy with scarring of the soft tissue, mucous membrane, and gingiva, resulting from an unknown dosage of x-rays given to treat a congenital hematoma in early childhood. Significant damage to the entire region was the result, including hypoplasia of the bone with microgenia. A curved silicone rubber implant, inserted from below, was well tolerated. Great care was taken during the operation not to traumatize the mucosa.

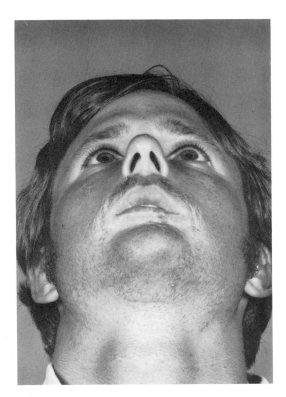

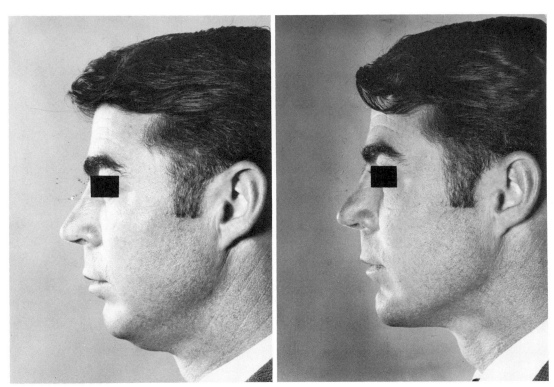

A chin implant is sometimes all that is required to correct a "double chin" caused by an excess of skin without any excess fat. A curved silicone implant inserted by the intra-oral route accomplished such a correction in this 36 year old man, in whom rhytidectomy was not required.

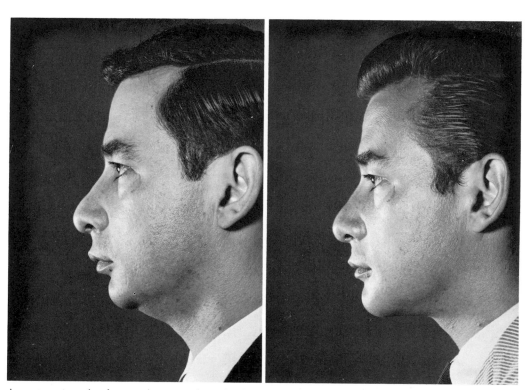

Note the improvement in the cervicomental angle that resulted from chin augmentation in this patient. Minor degrees of double chin are often improved in this way, though this patient posed a difficult problem because the vertical height of his mandible was quite small. The pocket to accommodate the implant must be dissected to exactly the correct size in such a patient, and the implant must be so shaped that it cannot be easily displaced. Bony fixation in such a situation would be highly desirable, but is not as yet possible.

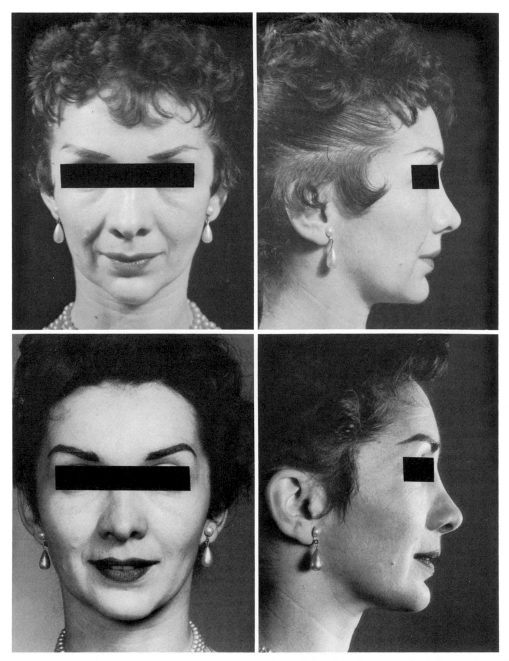

The principal problem in this young woman was not recession of the chin, but a vertical shortening of the mandibular body, as is evident in the preoperative front view. A small chin implant would have been totally inadequate, so augmentation mentoplasty was done instead with autogenous iliac bone grafting. The mandible had to be augmented from angle to angle, and the onlay had to extend below the original inferior margin in order to increase the vertical height. Bone grafts were used because of the difficulty involved in fixing prosthetic implants in place.

Grafts such as those used here may be quite irregular in contour when they are put into position, but over several months, pressure exerted by overlying soft tissue molds the grafts and gives a smooth contour. Prior to the preoperative views seen here, the patient had undergone grafting of cartilage to the chin, which resulted in some forward projection despite a considerable amount of absorption. The front view shows that the only result was a pointed chin. Bone grafts were the only suitable means of improving the situation.

Marked forward projection of the chin in this patient was caused by an overgrowth of the bone at the anterior margin of the symphysis, probably developmental in origin. A large piece of marginal jaw bone was resected through an intra-oral ("degloving") incision, but the procedure was ineffective and little improvement was obtained. This has been our experience in almost all patients with similar deformities. Failure probably occurs because the thick mass of soft tissue that constitutes the chin pad is little affected, if at all, by excision of bone. Vertical osteotomy with retropositioning of the anterior fragments is a superior technique for those whose occlusion permits such a procedure.

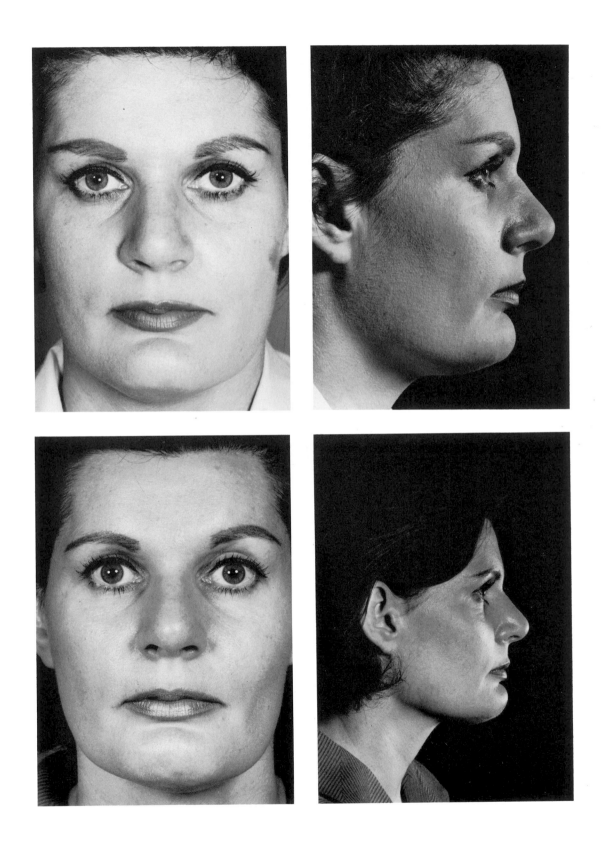

539

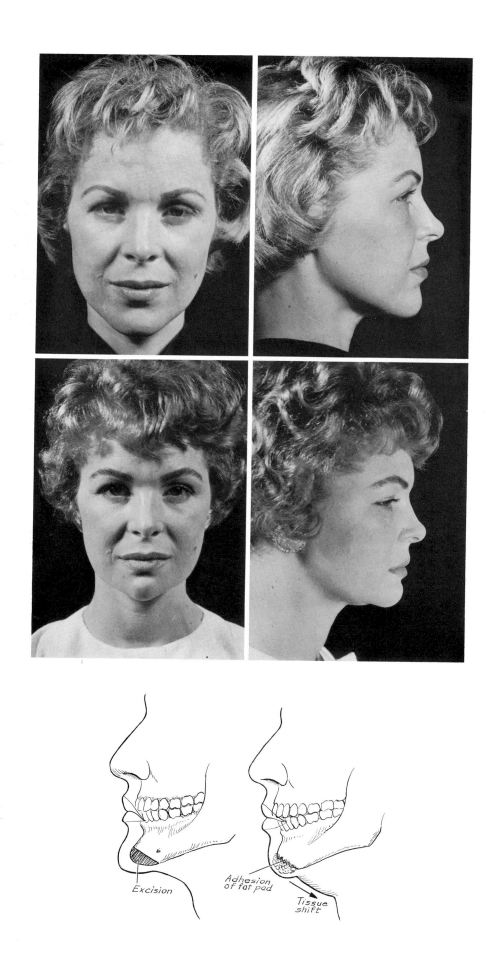

Excision

Adhesion of fat pad

Tissue shift

540

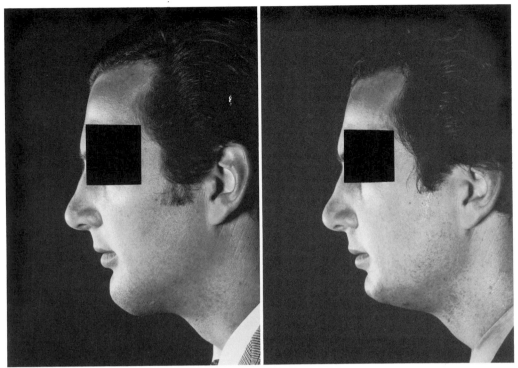

This 28 year old man was operated on by another surgeon for micrognathia. The resulting overcorrection had two factors: The material used for the implant was silicone sponge, but the deformity was not overcorrected to allow for long-term contraction. Sometimes swelling of the sponge persists and contraction never occurs, as in this patient. Moreover, this type of problem is inherently difficult to correct. When the vertical height of the mandible is very short, it is difficult to fix an implant to the anterior surface so that it does not hang below the inferior margin. In this patient the sponge implant was found at a secondary operation to extend well below the mandibular margin, giving the appearance shown in the second photograph. The sponge was removed, yet a reasonable correction was still maintained because of the residual scar. Final postoperative photographs were not obtained.

In patients with increased vertical length of the anterior mandible, it is tempting to excise the lower bony margin of the jaw, a relatively simple procedure that is easily accomplished by the "degloving" technique of Converse. However, the results are usually disappointing. Redundant submental soft tissue creates a postoperative double chin, and adherence of the soft tissue to the raw bony edge beneath can cause contour irregularities and depressions. In this patient the double chin had to be subsequently corrected by excision of excess submental skin.

It has been found desirable to preserve the existing inferior margin of the mandible whenever possible. Horizontal osteotomy with ostectomy of a central segment would undoubtedly have produced a better result in this patient. Maintenance of the lower mandibular margin allows a more natural balance between the mandible and the chin pad and also prevents irregular adherence of soft tissue.

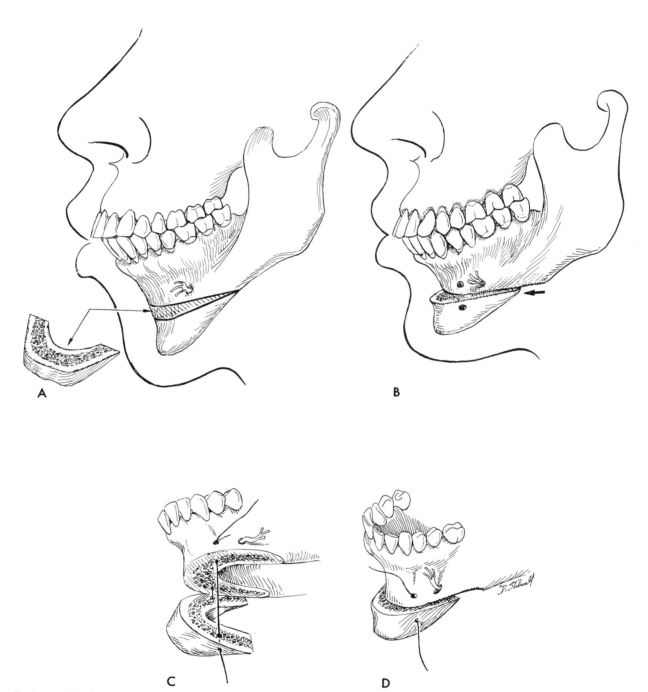

Patients with increased vertical height of the chin benefit most from horizontal osteotomy. *A,* A "piece of pie," of a size predetermined by cephalograms, is resected. *B,* The mandibular segment is set forward into the desired position. *C* and *D,* Interosseous wiring is used for fixation.

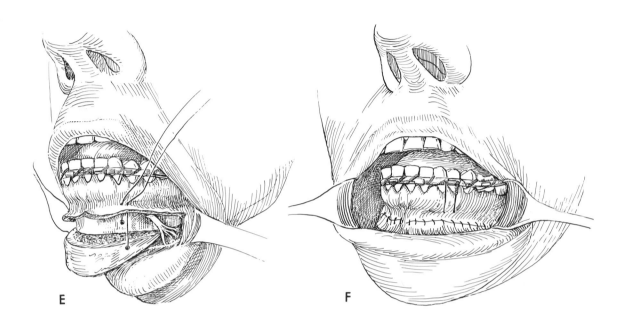

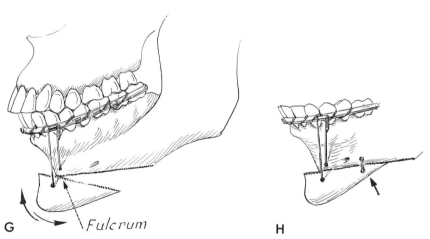

E, It is best to extend the wires through the mucosa as a pull-out. F, The pull-out is tightened around the dental appliance. G and H, Care must be taken to prevent a lever type of action which will displace the fragment. It may be necessary to apply additional wiring (arrow in H) to prevent displacement.

543

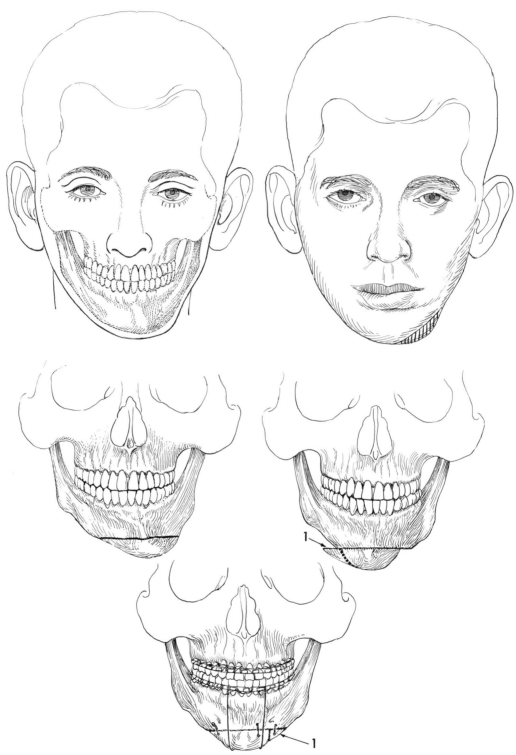

Horizontal osteotomy with lateral repositioning is the technique of choice for correction of severe asymmetry. The extra bone (*1*) can be resected and transferred as a free graft to fill in the opposite side.

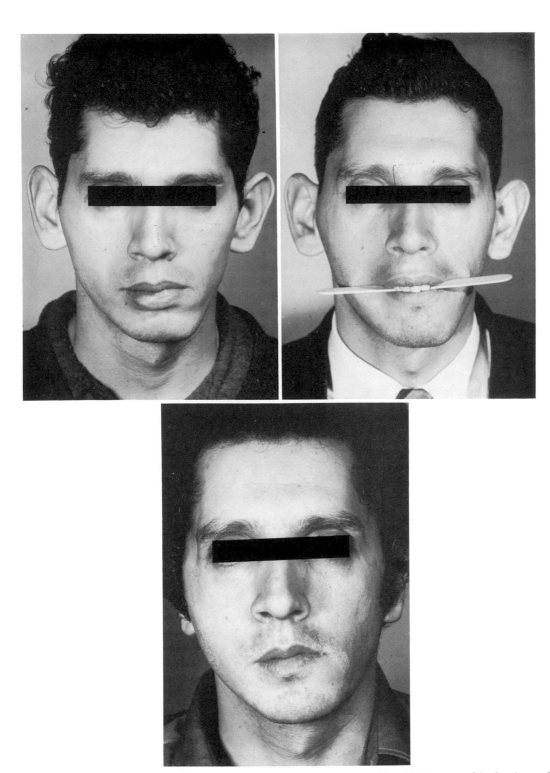

Marked asymmetry of the mandible involving the body and the rami, considerably improved by horizontal osteotomy and a lateral shift.

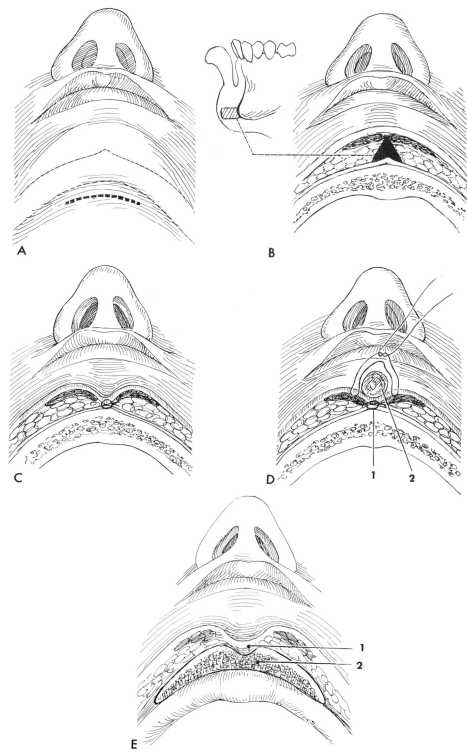

Many people consider dimples to be attractive. Natural dimples are thought to be the result of connection of integumentary fibers with attachments from the dermis to underlying muscle. They are most common in the mobile areas of the cheeks, lower lip, or chin.

Several methods have been tried, but most have been lacking in naturalness of effect because the methods rely on the formation of scar adhesions. The recent technique described by Argamaso seems to be the most promising method so far devised to produce a natural cheek dimple; the method of creating a natural appearing chin dimple still eludes us.

(Legend continued on opposite page.)

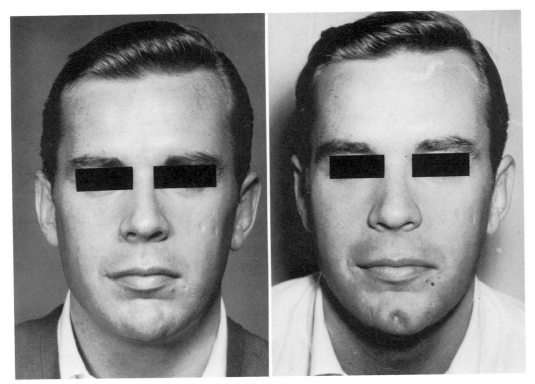

The surgical formation of a chin dimple by the technique illustrated on page 546. The preoperative appearance *(A)* and the postoperative result *(B)* show the disadvantage of this technique, which is the unnatural appearance of the dimple as a result of scar adhesions.

This demonstrates a method of creating a chin dimple by cicatricial adhesions. Through a submental incision *(A)* a wedge of tissue with the base of the periosteum of the anterior surface of the mandible is excised *(B)*. This wedge includes muscle of the midline, and subcutaneous tissue. A buried suture fixes the dermis to the periosteum of the midline *(C)*. A tie-over roll or bolus dressing is used to maintain the depression *(C)*.

Another method of forming a dimple advocated by many is shown in *E*. A notched chin implant is inserted which theoretically imposes a notching or dimple on the overlying soft tissue. This method is usually far less effective in practice than it would seem in principle.

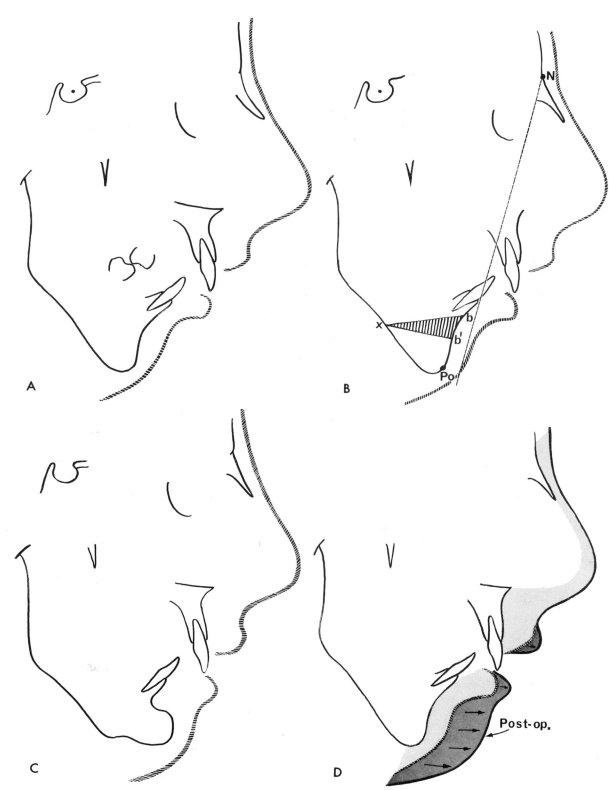

A, Preoperative cephalometric tracing of a young man with micrognathia, a severe maxillomandibular dentoalveolar discrepancy, maxillary hypoplasia, and a nasal deformity. *B,* The operative plan was removal of a wedge (shaded), elevation of the fragment, and consequent advancement of "pogonion" to the facial plane. *C,* Postoperative tracing. *D,* Preoperative and postoperative tracings are superimposed to show the improvement in soft tissue contours. In addition, the patient underwent vertical osteotomy, rhinoplasty, and otoplasty, with the results shown in the postoperative photographs.

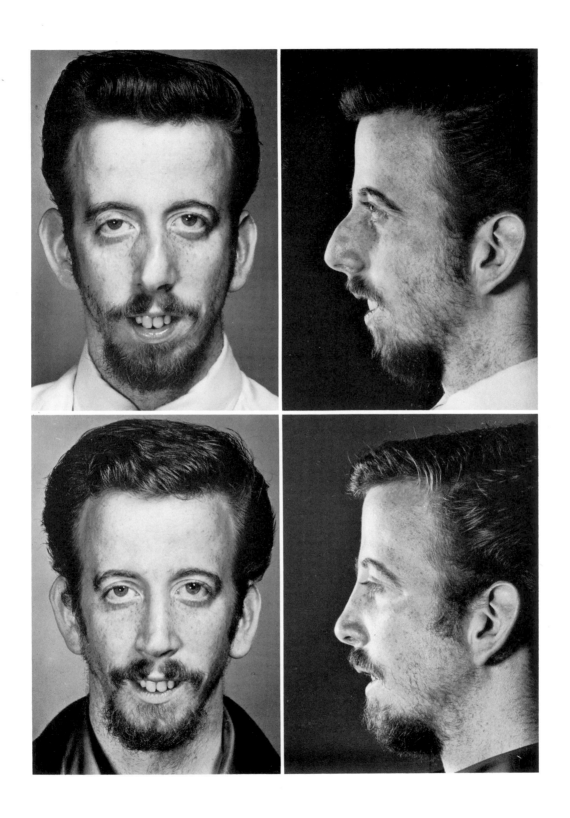

549

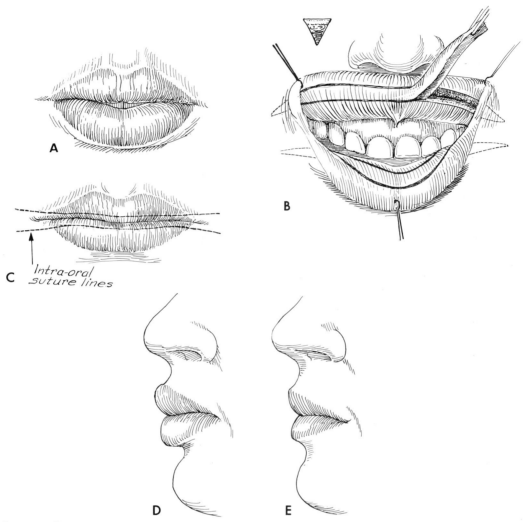

Oversized, protruding, or malpositioned lips can be a distressing facial deformity for many patients. Etiologies include obscure types of low-grade inflammatory reactions, congenital lesions such as hemangiomas or lymphangiomas, and racial characteristics, and many cases are of unknown cause. Protruding lips can also result from protruding teeth, and surgical trimming of the lips will not achieve improvement without correction of the malocclusion.

Many patients have enlarged lips that can be significantly improved by excision of large wedges of soft tissue. If such an excision is done on the mucosal side of the lip, the scar will be invisible. It is often necessary to extend the incision past the commissures on both sides and well into the buccal mucosa, but care must be taken not to interfere with or cross the commissure, because a constricting band may result. Excisions of soft tissue are sometimes carried down to (and may even include) muscle. Undermining is not necessary. Simple interrupted sutures are used for closure.

A and *D* show the extent of a typical problem. The operative plan for lip reduction is quite simple, but certain points are worthy of note. The wedges of tissue (*B*) will vary in width according to the amount of reduction required. *C*, The intra-oral sutures are indicated by the dotted lines and are seen to extend well beyond the commissures.

550

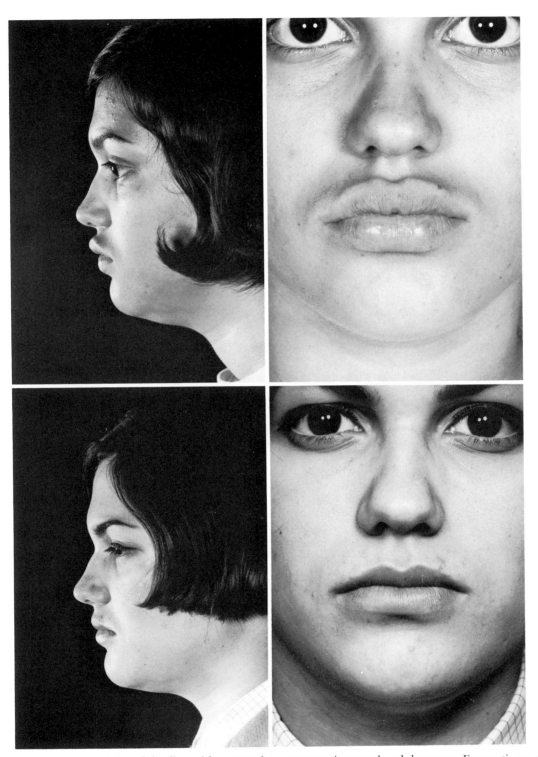

This patient had hypertrophy of the lips with protrusion, present since early adolescence. Excess tissue was excised in the form of a long ellipse from the mucosal surfaces of both lips, down to and including a small strip of muscle. The biopsy was unremarkable except for the equivocal presence of extra mucus glands. The postoperative result has endured for five years without recurrence of the protrusion.

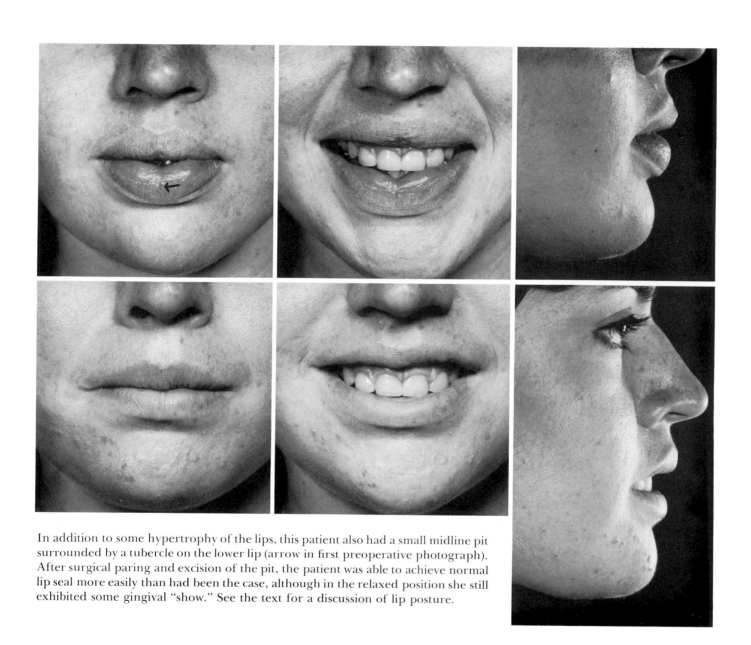

In addition to some hypertrophy of the lips, this patient also had a small midline pit surrounded by a tubercle on the lower lip (arrow in first preoperative photograph). After surgical paring and excision of the pit, the patient was able to achieve normal lip seal more easily than had been the case, although in the relaxed position she still exhibited some gingival "show." See the text for a discussion of lip posture.

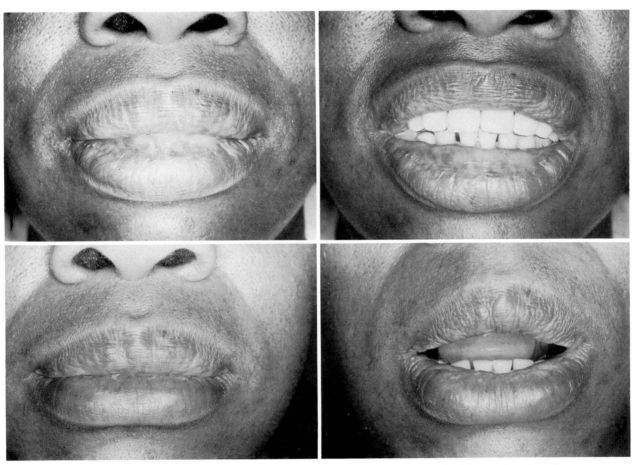

Large lips characteristic of Negro patients can be effectively reduced. With the incisions placed in the mucosa, there is virtually no danger of keloid formation. The excision should not be excessive or the closure too tight, because the lips might not seal.

Chapter 11

OTOPLASTY

DONALD WOOD-SMITH, M.D.

The protruding or lop ear deformity is a common malformation with a frequent concomitant psychological disturbance. These unfortunate children are often the object of misguided ridicule from others, and for this reason we prefer to correct the problem in the four- to six-year age span. At this time the ear growth has neared completion, and we do not find growth deficit to be a problem. In the older patient who has achieved adulthood the lop ear is rarely a problem as he has usually adjusted to his appearance or learned to camouflage the ears by hair styling.

History

Dieffenbach, in 1845, first attempted to correct the protruding ear by simple excision of skin from the postauricular sulcus combined with suture fixation of the ear cartilage to the periosteum of the mastoid region. This method is still employed, with variations, by some surgeons; it forms, in part, the basis of the technique revitalized by Furnas (1968).

Even though many authors credit Morestin (1903) with the first attempts at modification of the cartilage, Ely (1881), Keen (1890), Monks (1891) and Cocheril (1894) had all modified the Dieffenbach technique by both incision and excision of the segments of the conchal cartilage. The foundation of the modern techniques of otoplasty was laid by Luckett, who in 1910 first recognized the importance of the unfurling of the antihelix and the need for correction of this flattening to produce a satisfactory ear contour. This combination of antihelix and conchal correction that is the basis of most present-day techniques was described by MacCollum in 1938 and later refined by Young (1944), who excised segments of the scapha and concha and incised the cartilage along the line of the inferior crus of the antihelix.

Although early results of all these procedures were satisfactory, the sharp margins in the cartilage formed by the simple incisions soon became quite evident as the operative edema regressed; this marred the final result. Many and varied methods were devised in an attempt to correct this technical deficiency. Significant contributions were made by McEvitt (1947), who used multiple parallel incisions along the line of the antihelix; variations of his method were described by Pierce, Klabunde and Bergeron (1947) and Dufourmentel (1958). Holmes (1959) attempted to achieve a similar weakening of the antihelix and correction of contour by the use of multiple incisions in the scalp aspect of the antihelix cartilage to produce a fish-scalelike appearance. The use of surgical abrasion to weaken the antihelix was described by Farrior in 1947 and subsequently championed by Stark and Saunders in 1962. In his improvement of the procedure described by Barsky in 1938, Becker (1952) emphasized the need for removal of the cauda helicus to reduce the cartilaginous protrusion in this region.

These techniques were integrated and refined by Converse, Nigro, Wilson and Johnson

554

in 1956 and were more recently modified by Converse and Wood-Smith in 1963 and 1971.

Mustardé (1963) popularized Owen's method of nonabsorable suture fixation of the cartilage in its corrected position; this technique has gained a wide acceptance because of its simplicity. Furnas (1968) re-emphasized the importance of fixation of the conchal cartilage to the underlying mastoid periosteum in those patients with a relatively well formed antihelix and in whom the primary problem is protrusion of the conchal cartilage. Like the Mustardé, the Furnas technique is popular because of its simplicity; however, indications for its usage are more limited than either the Converse–Wood-Smith or Mustardé techniques.

Modification of the cartilage by surgical weakening of its anterolateral aspect was described by Stenstrom (1963), who utilized multiple incisions combined with excision of a postauricular segment of skin. The anterolateral aspect of the cartilage is approached from the postauricular incision and the procedure completed with the aid of a special scoring instrument. Ju, Li and Crikelair (1963) exposed the cartilage from its lateral aspect, excising and modifying the contour of the cartilage under direct vision; this latter method appears to carry an unwarranted risk of visible scarring.

Anatomy

The auricle usually meets the adjacent scalp at an angle of approximately 30 degrees; the basic structure is a delicate, intricately shaped elastic cartilage with a thin, closely adherent skin covering on its anterolateral aspect. The skin cover is somewhat thicker and less adherent on the scalp aspect of the cartilage and may be readily stripped on this surface. The helix rim arises anteriorly and inferiorly from a crus extending horizontally above the external auditory meatus. The helix continues superiorly and then inferiorly to merge to the cauda helicus and join the lobule of the ear. The antihelix rises superiorly where the anterosuperior and antero-inferior crura join to form the antihelix body; this separates the helix posteriorly from the conchal rim and concha proper. A low shallow fossa of varying prominence, the scapha, lies between the antihelix crura. Enclosed between the two crura is the fossa triangularis.

The conchal cavity composed of cavum below and cymba conchi above meets the anti-helix at the conchal r m and is bounded anteriorly by the tragus and the external auditory meatus, and posteriorly and inferiorly by the antitragus, which is separated from the tragus by the intertragal notch. The lobule exhibits varying degrees of development and attachment to the adjacent scalp and cheek.

The auricle is principally supplied by the superficial temporal and posterior auricular arteries. Sensation is supplied by anterior and posterior branches of the greater auricular nerve, re-enforced by the auriculotemporal and lesser occipital nerves. A portion of the posterior wall of the external auditory meatus is supplied by auricular branches of the vagus nerve.

Pathology

Intelligent planning of the best method of correction of the lop ear deformity requires careful evaluation and analysis of the component parts of the deformity in comparison with the "normal" anatomy. The main characteristics of the lop ear deformity, which may occur singly or in all combinations, are: (1) poorly developed antihelix, (2) overdevelopment of the conchal cartilage, and (3) an increased angle between the lobule and the scalp. The surgeon should carefully analyze these elements of the lop ear deformity in each patient under consideration.

Analysis of the component parts:
A. The antihelix is unfurled in:
   1. The body of the helix
   2. The posterior-superior crus
   3. The body and posterior-superior crus
B. The concha shows excess cartilage:
   1. As uniform excess
   2. In the upper third to upper half
   3. In the lower third to lower half
   4. In both upper and lower thirds
C. The helix rim and conchal rim show size disparity (the cup or shell ear deformity)
D. The lobule shows:
   1. An increased angle of protrusion
   2. An excess size
E. The Machiavellian ear shows:
   1. Poor definition of the helix rim
   2. Usually an excessive ear size
   3. An excess of conchal cartilage
   4. A weak auricular cartilaginous framework
F. The auricle shows a left side to right side size disparity
G. Associated anomalies are:
   1. Darwin's tubercle
   2. Preauricular tubercle
   3. Miscellaneous

The antihelix is commonly unfurled. The superior crus is poorly defined and passes imperceptibly into both the scapha and the triangular fossa, which may appear as a flattened area in contrast to the inferior crus, which is usually well developed. The body of the antihelix is often flattened. Correction requires a partial tubing, with the tube wider superiorly, of the body and the superior crus to form a smooth convexity between the helix and the conchal rim.

Excess of conchal cartilage is found throughout, or the excess may be confined only to the upper third or half or to the lower third or half; cartilage may also be in excess above and below, being of normal contour in the intermediary portion. This variable component must be evaluated before any surgical removal of conchal rim as it governs the conchoscaphal angle and the vertical angle made by the ear with the skull. The importance of adequate removal of conchal rim in the upper and lower thirds cannot be overemphasized to prevent the relatively common postoperative deformity noted on page 563. Frequently there is a relative disparity of conchal rim size to helix rim, giving a "cup" or "shell" appearance. The cause of this disparity may be either an excessive size of conchal rim or a relative shortage of helix. In its fully developed state, this deformity is that of a microtic ear. However, lesser degrees of the deformity are amenable to correction by removal of an adequate amount of conchal cartilage and reshaping of the ear framework.

The lobule may meet the mastoid process at an excessive angle. Correction is achieved by removal of both lobule and mastoid skin and not by an excision of lobule skin alone, which may result in a deformity of the lobule.

The Machiavellian ear represents a total distortion of the auricular anatomy and demonstrates failure of definition of the helix rim, unfurling of crura and the body of the antihelix, excess of conchal cartilage and a general weakness of the whole auricular cartilage (p. 564).

Disparity in size as well as shape may exist between the two ears. If marked, wedge excision of auricular skin and cartilage in the region of the scapha can correct the asymmetry (Tanzer, 1962).

Embryonic vestiges, such as an excessively large Darwin's tubercle or preauricular tags, can be removed at the time of correction of the lop ear deformity, page 565.

The three commonly employed operative techniques are described and illustrated on pages 566 to 577.

Complications and Untoward Results

HEMATOMA

Hematoma is the most immediate problem, and when it occurs, it requires immediate and vigorous treatment. Presence of persistent pain under the dressing heralds this complication and demands immediate removal of the dressing and inspection of the ears. The presence of a hematoma is indicated by a tense and bluish swelling of the retroauricular space; if bleeding has persisted for some time, there will be ecchymosis of the surrounding tissues. The skin sutures should be removed, the blood clot evacuated and all bleeding points coagulated, and the wound closed and a pressure dressing reapplied with great care. Large doses of antibiotics are indicated at this time, as this problem is a common precursor of perichondritis.

PERICHONDRITIS

Perichondritis may occur in the early postoperative phase and usually is a sequel to an undetected and/or inadequately treated hematoma, although this is by no means an essential etiologic factor. Large doses of the appropriate antibiotics are indicated, and the wound should be cultured for a later confirmation of the efficacy of the antibiotic. Adequate drainage is achieved by opening all sutures and carefully irrigating necrotic debris from the wound with hydrogen peroxide solution. Even in the face of such active therapy, a massive destruction of cartilage with severe deformity can result in an ear whose appearance may mimic that of a microtic ear.

INADEQUATE CORRECTION

Inadequate correction is perhaps the most common untoward result of otoplasty; it is, however, often more evident to the surgeon than to the patient and, indeed, it is quite unusual for the patient to be dissatisfied with the result. Contour distortions or asymmetric correction may require secondary operation. The surgeon should approach every procedure with great care, since difficult to control distortions are easy to produce but troublesome to correct. The "telephone" ear deformity is particularly unpleasant since correction will require a "plastering" of the ear to the side of the patient's head, which is a quite unsatisfactory compromise (page 580).

556

HYPERTROPHIC SCARS

Hypertrophic scars in the line of skin incision are frequently seen in the younger patient and are more common in the patient with deeply pigmented skin. Such hypertrophy often resolves with conservative treatment, although intralesional steroid injections may dramatically increase the rate of resolution of the scars in many patients.

We have utilized triamcinolone acetonide, 40 mm. per ml. strength, injecting approximately 0.25 ml. into the hypertrophic scar. The treatment is repeated at weekly intervals when signs of regression appear and we continued for at least four weeks, at which time the time interval may be reduced to two to three weeks, with further injections given as indicated by the resolution of the lesion.

KELOIDS

Keloid of the postauricular incision is one of the most frustrating of all postoperative complications and may require further operative procedures before a solution to the problem is reached. In the early stages of keloid formation the use of intralesional steroid injections of triamcinolone acetonide has proved to be effective in a large percentage of patients. The drug is injected intralesionally on a weekly basis, and if early regression of the keloid has occurred, its use may be extended to every two weeks for some months, tapering off to once a month for a further two to three months before terminating the treatment (page 580).

The use of radiation in this area is fraught with danger, but on occasion has proved to be the only effective means of control of the keloids. When more advanced keloids occur in this region, surgical excision may need to be combined with radiation and delayed skin grafting of the radiated area, with final aid from the use of intralesional triamcinolone acetonide. Problems such as these have proved to be some of the most difficult keloid problems encountered in our practice and ones in which the results of therapy have left much to be desired.

REFERENCES

Barsky, A. J.: Plastic Surgery. Philadelphia, W. B. Saunders Company, 1938, pp. 199–221.

Becker, O. J.: Correction of protruding deformed ear. Brit. J. Plast. Surg. 5:187, 1952.

Cocheril, R.: Essai sur la Restauration du Pavillon de l'Oreille. Paris Thèses. Lille, 1894.

Converse, J. M., Nigro, A., Wilson, F. A., and Johnson, N.: A technique for surgical correction of lop ears. Trans. Amer. Acad. Ophthal. Otolaryng. 59:551, 1956.

Converse, J. M., and Wood-Smith, D.: Technical details in the surgical correction of the lop ear deformity. Plast. Reconstr. Surg. 31:118, 1963.

Dieffenbach, J. E.: Die operative Chirurgie. Leipzig, F. A. Brockhaus, 1845.

Dufourmentel, C.: La greffe cutanée libre tubulée. Ann. Chir. Plast. (Paris) 3:311, 1958.

Ely, E. T.: An operation for prominence of the auricles. Arch. Otolaryng. 10:97, 1881.

Furnas, D. W.: Correction of prominent ears by conchal mastoid sutures. Plast. Reconstr. Surg. 24:189, 1968.

Holmes, E. M.: A new procedure for correcting outstanding ears. Arch. Otolaryng. 69:409, 1959.

Ju, D. M. C., Li, C., and Crikelair, G. F.: The surgical correction of protruding ears. Plast. Reconstr. Surg. 32:283, 1963.

Keen, W. W.: New method of operating for relief of deformity of prominent ears. Ann. Surg. 11:49, 1890.

Luckett, W. H.: A new operation for prominent ears based on the anatomy of the deformity. Surg. Gynec. Obstet. 10:635, 1910.

MacCollum, D. W.: The lop ear. J.A.M.A. 110:1427, 1938.

McEvitt, W. G.: The problem of the protruding ear. Plast. Reconstr. Surg. 2:481, 1947.

Monks, G. H.: Operation for correcting the deformity due to prominent ears. Boston Med. Surg. J. 124:84, 1891.

Morestin, M. H.: De la réposition et du plissement cosmétiques du pavillion de l'oreille. Rev. Orthrop. 4:289, 1903.

Mustardé, J. C.: The correction of prominent ears using simple mattress sutures. Brit. J. Plast. Surg. 16:170, 1963.

Pierce, G. W., Klabunde, E. H., and Bergeron, V. L.: Useful procedures in plastic surgery. Plast. Reconstr. Surg. 2:358, 1947.

Stark, R. B., and Saunders, D. E.: Natural appearance restored to the unduly prominent ear. Brit. J. Plast. Surg. 15:385, 1962.

Stenstrom, S. J.: A "natural" technique for correction of congenitally prominent ears. Plast. Reconstr. Surg. 32:509, 1963.

Tanzer, R. C.: The correction of prominent ears. Plast. Reconstr. Surg. 30:236, 1962.

Wood-Smith, D., and Converse, J. M.: The lop ear deformity. Surg. Clin. N. Amer. 51:417, 1971.

Young, F.: The correction of abnormally prominent ears. Surg. Gynec. Obstet. 78:541, 1944.

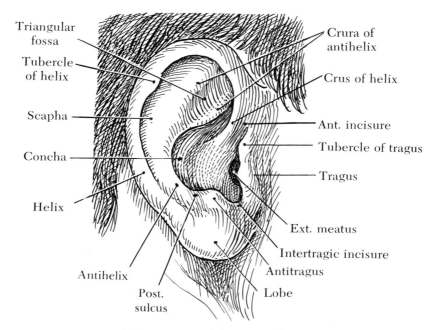

Triangular fossa

Tubercle of helix

Scapha

Concha

Helix

Antihelix

Post. sulcus

Crura of antihelix

Crus of helix

Ant. incisure

Tubercle of tragus

Tragus

Ext. meatus

Intertragic incisure

Antitragus

Lobe

The anatomy of the external ear.

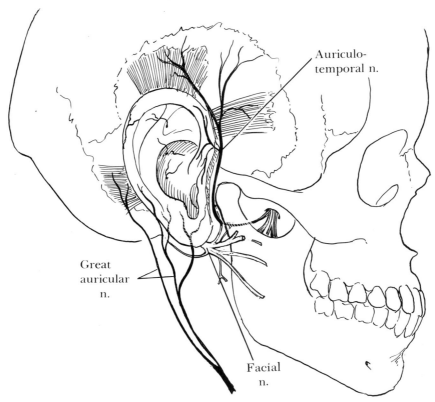

Auriculo-temporal n.

Great auricular n.

Facial n.

The nerve supply of the external ear.

558

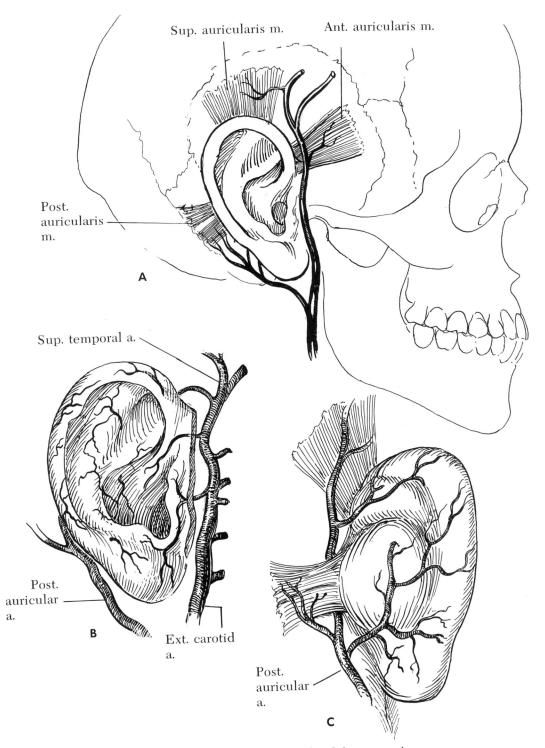

Sup. auricularis m.　　　Ant. auricularis m.

Post.
auricularis
m.

A

Sup. temporal a.

Post.
auricular
a.

B

Ext. carotid
a.

Post.
auricular
a.

C

The musculature and vascular supply of the external ear.

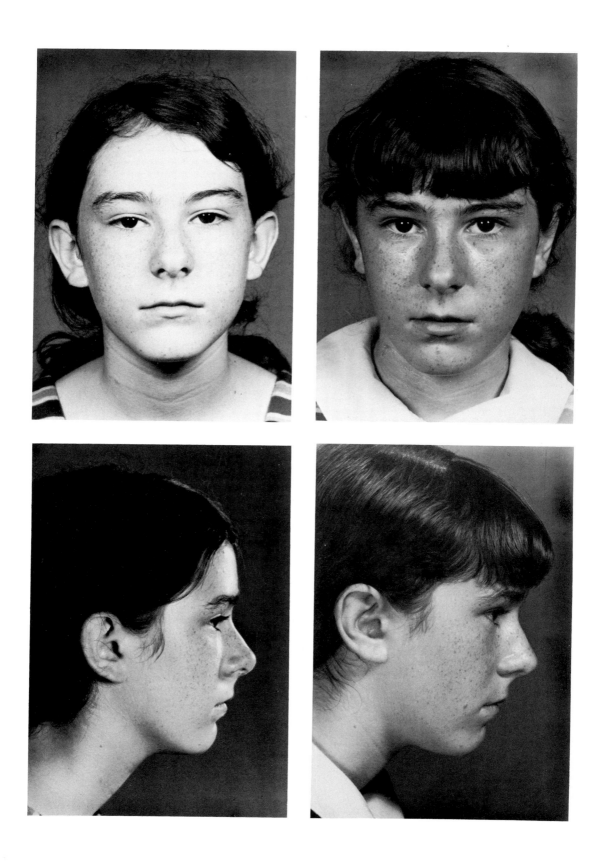

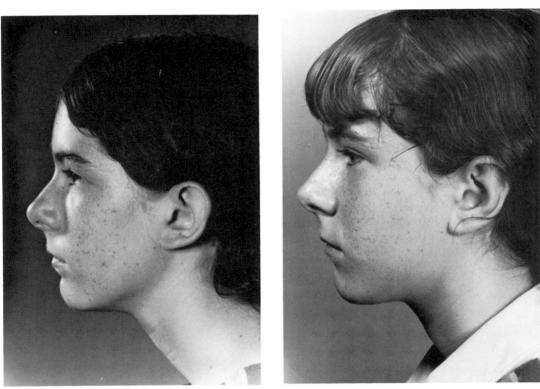

A typical example of lop ear deformity. The postoperative views were taken 12 months after correction by the Converse–Wood-Smith technique.

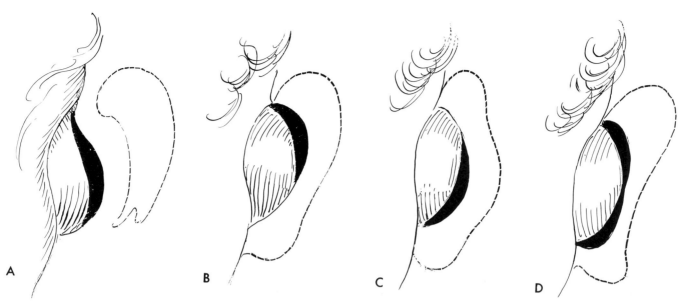

A, Uniform excess of conchal cartilage (black). *B*, Upper third to upper half conchal cartilage excess. *C*, Lower third to lower half excess. *D*, Upper third and lower third excess.

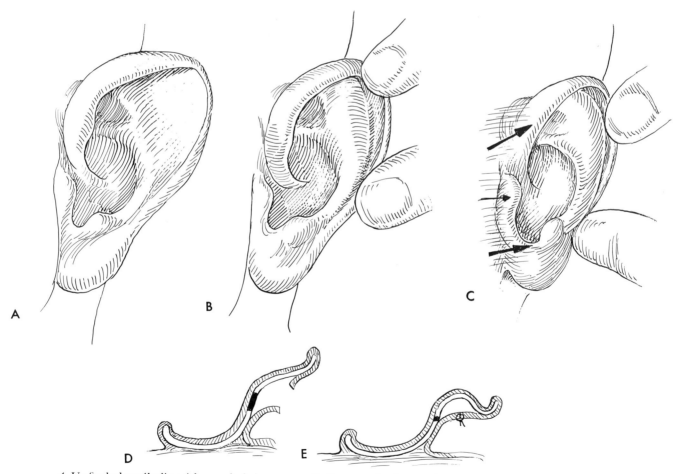

A, Unfurled antihelix with conchal rim excess. *B*, Pressure in the scaphal region forms the antihelix and superior crus. *C*, Further increase of pressure throws the conchal rim into prominence and emphasizes the anterior superior and inferior conchal excess. *D*, The excess conchal rim cartilage and skin. *E*, Representation of the corrected ear.

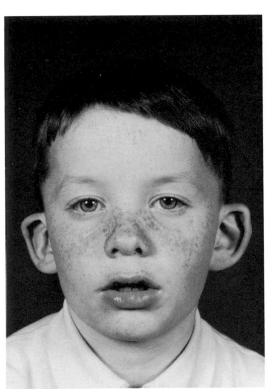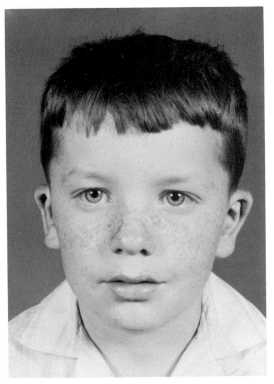

A four year old boy with lop ear deformity corrected by the Converse–Wood-Smith technique, but with inadequate excision of the superior and inferior conchal rim excess.

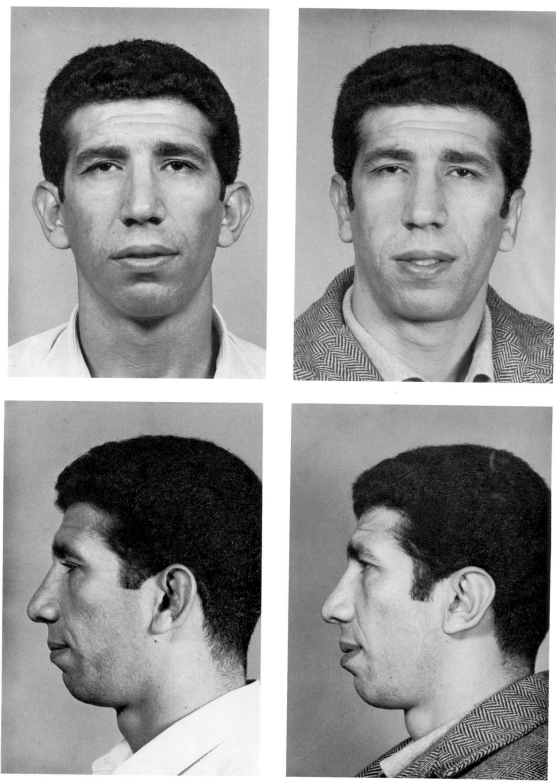

The machiavellian ear, preoperative and postoperative.

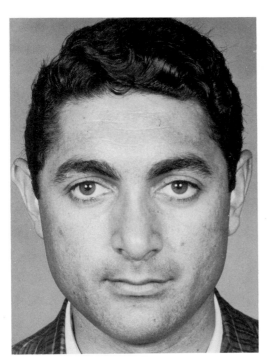 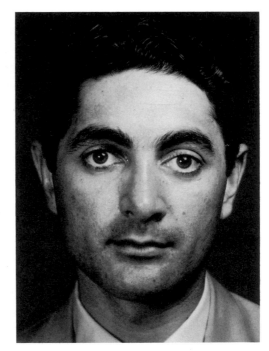

Excessive formation of Darwin's tubercle and mild lop deformity of the right ear, corrected by the Converse–Wood-Smith technique.

(From Converse, J. M., and Wood-Smith, D.: Plast. Reconstr. Surg. *43*:118, 1963. Reproduced with permission.)

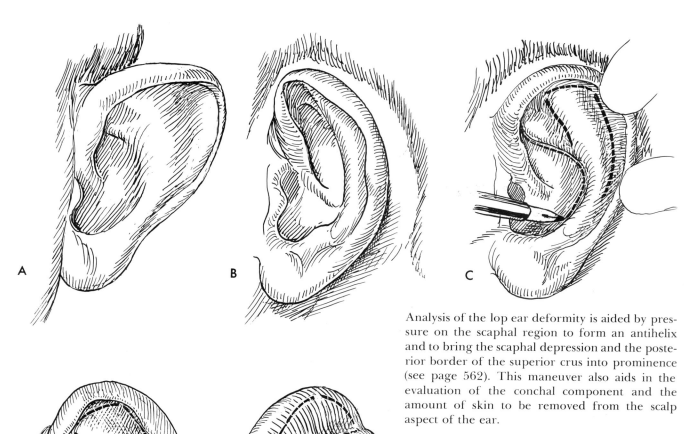

Analysis of the lop ear deformity is aided by pressure on the scaphal region to form an antihelix and to bring the scaphal depression and the posterior border of the superior crus into prominence (see page 562). This maneuver also aids in the evaluation of the conchal component and the amount of skin to be removed from the scalp aspect of the ear.

Local anesthesia is preferred for cooperative patients over the age of six or seven years. However, we do not hesitate to use a general anesthesia in the uncooperative or unduly apprehensive patient. Local anesthesia is achieved by blocking the auricle at its base. Dissection of the postauricular skin and anesthesia of the postauricular area are further aided by the "hydraulic" dissection afforded by local anesthetic infiltration.

The operative field is prepared and draped, and then the procedure outlined above is repeated. The patient's hair is neither clipped nor shaved.

The ear is folded back by gentle pressure in the region of the scapha to produce a tubing of the body of the antihelix and the superior crus of the antihelix. The posterior border of the antihelix and its superior crus are outlined in ink on the anterolateral aspect of the auricle, together with the anterior border of the superior crus, which is thrown into prominence by gentle pressure between the finger and thumb in the region of the junction between the superior and inferior crura (A to C). A third line is marked, parallel and immediately adjacent to the superior helical rim between the two previously marked lines but joining neither. The conchal rim is marked on the anterolateral aspect of the auricle, extending superiorly into the region of the cymba conchae and inferiorly to the external auditory meatus (D and E).

The ear is infiltrated with local anesthetic solution and an ellipse of postauricular skin is removed. The perichondrium is exposed and, after modification of the shape of the cartilage and resection of excess cartilage, suturing of the edges of the skin under some tension will aid as a splint to hold the auricle in its corrected position. The center line of the ellipse to be removed is determined by passing needles from the anterolateral aspect of the auricle through the center line of the body of the antihelix and the superior crus.

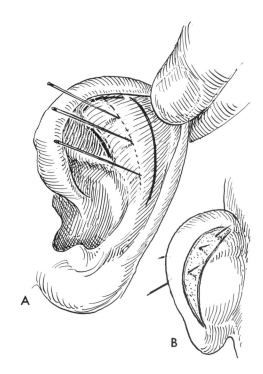

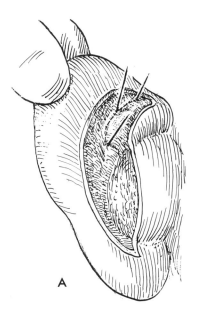

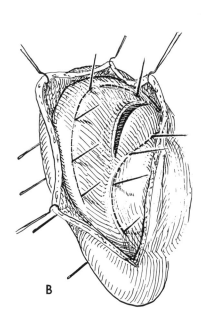

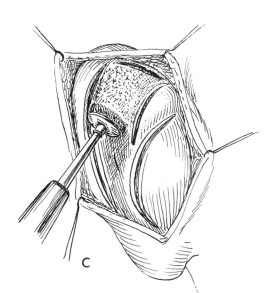

The skin ellipse is removed and hemostasis is secured by electrocoagulation of the bleeding vessels. Skin and subcutaneous tissues are elevated to expose the posterior aspect of the helical rim. Exposure of the perichondrium must extend to the anterosuperior and inferior limits of the conchal rim. The entire posterior aspect of the concha is thus exposed down to its junction with the mastoid process.

By passing straight cutting needles (Keith) from the lateral aspect of the auricle through the postauricular aspect, the posterior border of the antihelix, the superior crus, the superior border of the superior crus, the anterior border of the superior crus, and the conchal rim are outlined. The needles may be left in place and the incisions made to join them, or small ink spots may be placed where the needle points perforate the auricular cartilage.

Incisions are made through the cartilage up to but not including the perichondrium over the anterolateral aspect of the auricular cartilage (A and B). The incisions should not join one another; a gap of a few millimeters is maintained between the ends. The cartilage of the body of the antihelix and the superior crus may require thinning to facilitate folding. An electrically driven rotating wire brush is employed for this purpose (C). The brush removes perichondrium and a layer of cartilage, allowing for its easy folding into a tube. The use of the brush is not always necessary, for the cartilage is often sufficiently weak to permit tubing without such weakening.

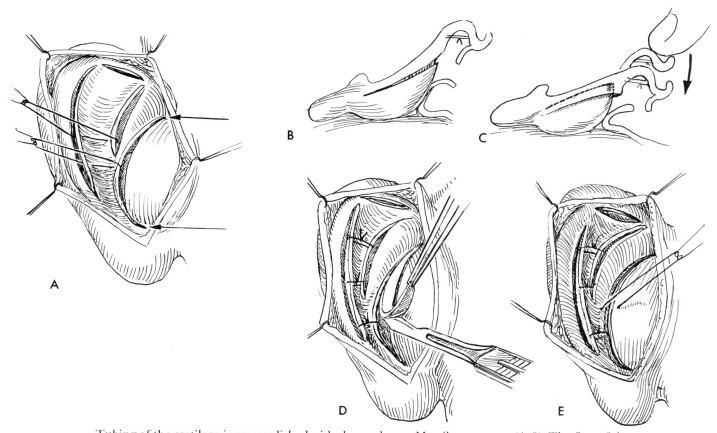

Tubing of the cartilage is accomplished with clear nylon or Mersilene sutures (4–0). The first of these mattress sutures is placed immediately below the junction of the crura of the antihelix where it joins the body of the antihelix. The second is placed in the superior crus of the antihelix immediately above the crural junction. These sutures are tied with sufficient tension to produce the desired contour of the antihelix (A).

The contour of the tube may be maintained by passing straight needles through the tubed cartilage and at the proposed sites of the sutures before the sutures are positioned. By this means the contour of the tube is accurately gauged prior to insertion of the sutures. Once the sutures are in place, the needles are removed.

At this stage, correction of the protruding auricle has been achieved, and with pressure exerted on the scaphal region, the amount of conchal rim resection required to set the auricle back in a satisfactory position can be determined (B and C). An ellipse of conchal cartilage of required size is removed from the medial edge of the rim. Skin lying on the anterolateral aspect of the concha is undermined for a distance of 3 or 4 mm. from the edges of the new conchal rim (D). The edges of the conchal and antihelix cartilages are approximated with a single interrupted 4–0 nylon suture (E).

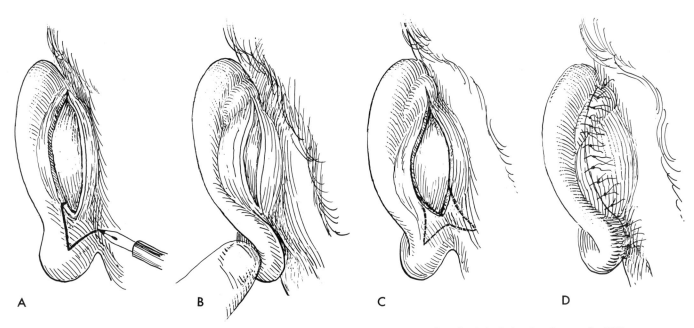

A   B   C   D

When the lobule of the ear protrudes, the skin incision is continued downward to the lobule in the shape of a "V" *(A)*. Pressure of the freshly marked lobe skin against the mastoid skin makes an imprint outlining the mirror image of the skin to be resected *(B to D)*. This W-shaped segment of skin is removed, hemostasis is secured, and the postauricular incision is closed with interrupted 5–0 nylon or 4–0 plain catgut sutures, fitting the small V-shaped incisions together.

A pressure dressing is applied; small pledgets of Acrilan wool (Chemstrand Corp.) or cotton wool soaked in sterile mineral oil are carefully packed within the convolutions of the corrected ear and covered with fluffed-out gauze. More Acrilan wool and a tube gauze head cap are applied, and mild pressure is maintained with a stretchable wrap bandage. The pressure dressing remains undisturbed for a period of five days.

A small fold of excess skin in the conchal fossa usually disappears within two or three months. It can be directly excised if in marked excess, although we have rarely had to do this.

This technique avoids sharp ridges resulting from folding of the cartilage and produces a natural-appearing concha, antihelix, and lobule.

569

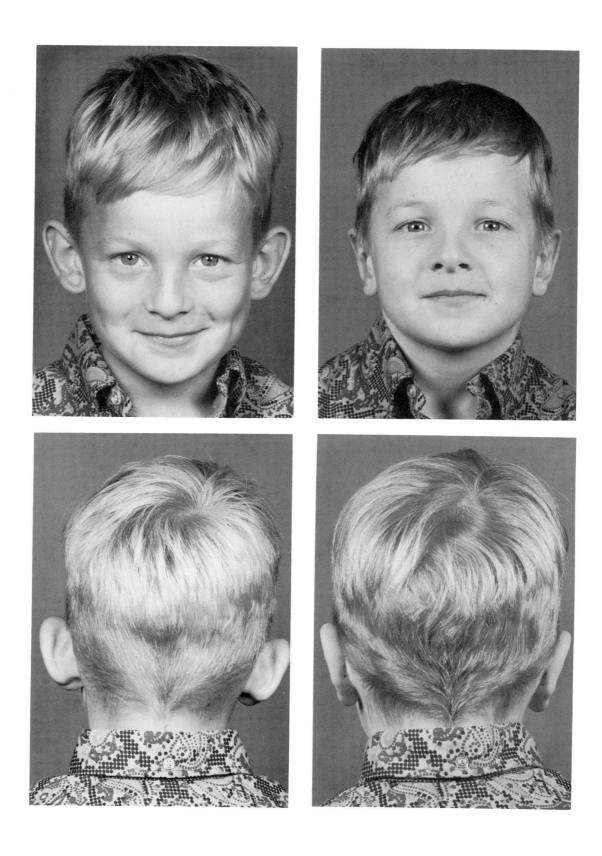

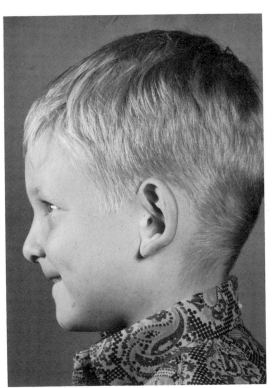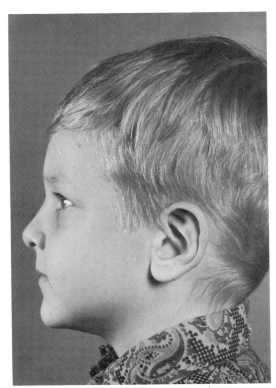

A five year old boy with a typical lop ear deformity. Postoperative views were taken 15 months after correction by the Converse–Wood-Smith technique.

The Mustardé Technique

A method of correcting prominent ears by using buried mattress sutures was described by Mustardé in 1963. It is particularly applicable when the ear cartilage is thin and the ear deformity is not severe. When those conditions are not present, however, we prefer to use the Converse–Wood-Smith technique because more precise correction can be achieved.

It is essential that the perichondrium and adjacent soft tissue be stripped completely from the scalp aspect of the auricle from the point of junction of the concha with the mastoid to the helix rim, so that a smooth correction of the auricle can be made. The line of skin closure should be planned so as not to be in immediate juxtaposition with the buried mattress sutures.

In an ear formed of thin, easily correctable cartilage *(A)*, a new antihelix fold is formed by finger pressure on the auricle, and the center line of the antihelix and the crura of the antihelix are outlined with ink *(B)*. In the small ear, three sutures usually suffice; in the larger ear, four or five buried mattress sutures may be necessary to achieve a smooth contour.

The position of these sutures is marked on the anterior aspect of the ear by ink dots so placed that a portion of cartilage 5 to 10 mm. on either side of the midline is encompassed by the sutures. The points of suture entry are transferred from the auricular skin to the underlying cartilage by passing a 24- or 25-gauge hypodermic needle dipped in marking ink, so that on withdrawal of the needle, the marks of perforation are stained by the dye *(C)*.

An ellipse of skin whose center line lies along the center line of the body of the antihelix and its posterior superior crus is excised down to and including perichondrium. After hemostasis is obtained, the perichondrium is raised from the scalp aspect of the auricle to the helix border and anteriorly to the point of junction of the concha with the underlying mastoid periosteum. This step is important to permit the smooth recontouring of the ear cartilage following insertion of the buried mattress sutures and to prevent the close apposition of the buried sutures to the skin wound.

The mattress sutures are inserted into the marks previously made on the cartilage *(D)*, taking care to encompass the full thickness of the auricular cartilage—including, if possible, the perichondrium on its anterior aspect. We prefer to use 4–0 clear nylon sutures for this purpose, touching the end of the completed knot with the cautery to weld the nylon and insure that it will not unravel; 4–0 white Mersilene is also suitable for this purpose *(E and F)*.

While looking at the anterior aspect of the auricle, the surgeon tightens the knots to produce a satisfactory antihelix contour; we prefer to begin with knots in the region of the body and cauda helicus and proceed superiorly. The sutures should be removed and replaced if a satisfactory contour does not result.

The skin is closed by intradermal 4–0 plain catgut sutures or by a continuous over-and-over 4–0 nylon suture. Protruding lobules can be corrected by the use of the fishtail excision already described (page 569). We do not favor the wedge excision of lobules advocated by Mustardé, for a lobular deformity can result from inadequate correction of the protrusion. Excision of excess conchal cartilage can be easily accomplished in the Mustardé operation, if this is required, and can produce a satisfactory result.

A pressure dressing, using accurately molded pledgets of Acrilan wool or cotton wool soaked in sterile mineral oil, is placed over the ear for seven to 10 days. A slightly elastic sleeping cap, which may be readily made from the upper elasticized end of a woman's stocking, is worn at night to splint the ears for four to six weeks.

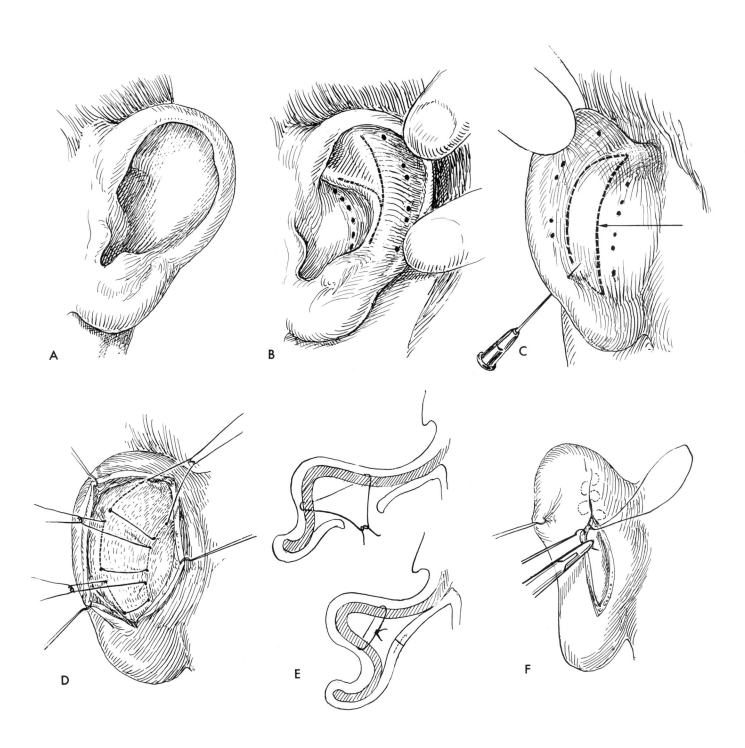

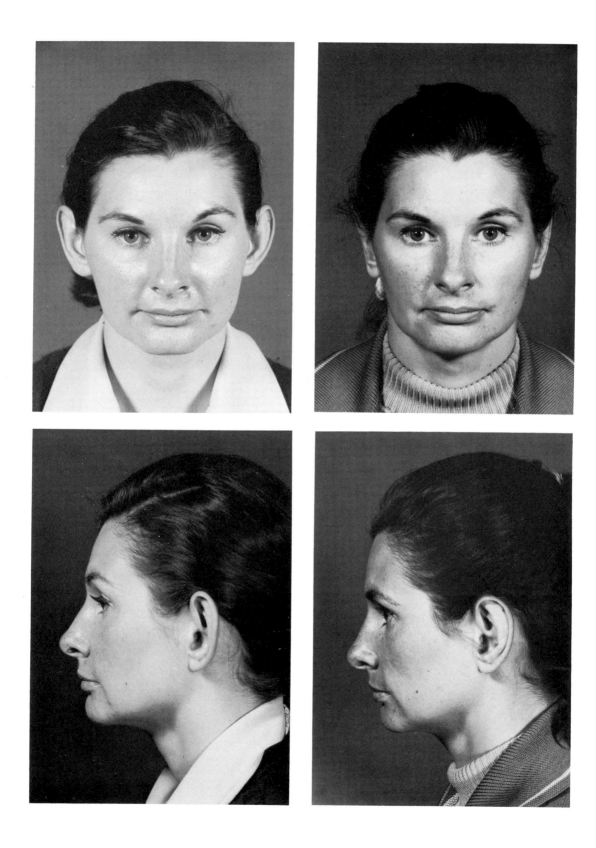

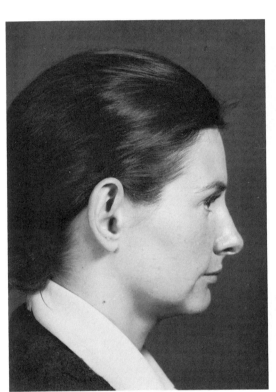 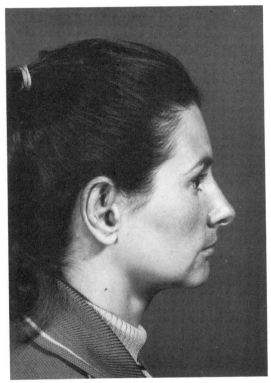

A 25 year old woman with lop ear deformity and thin, easily correctable ear cartilages. The postoperative views were taken two months after correction by the Owens-Mustardé technique.

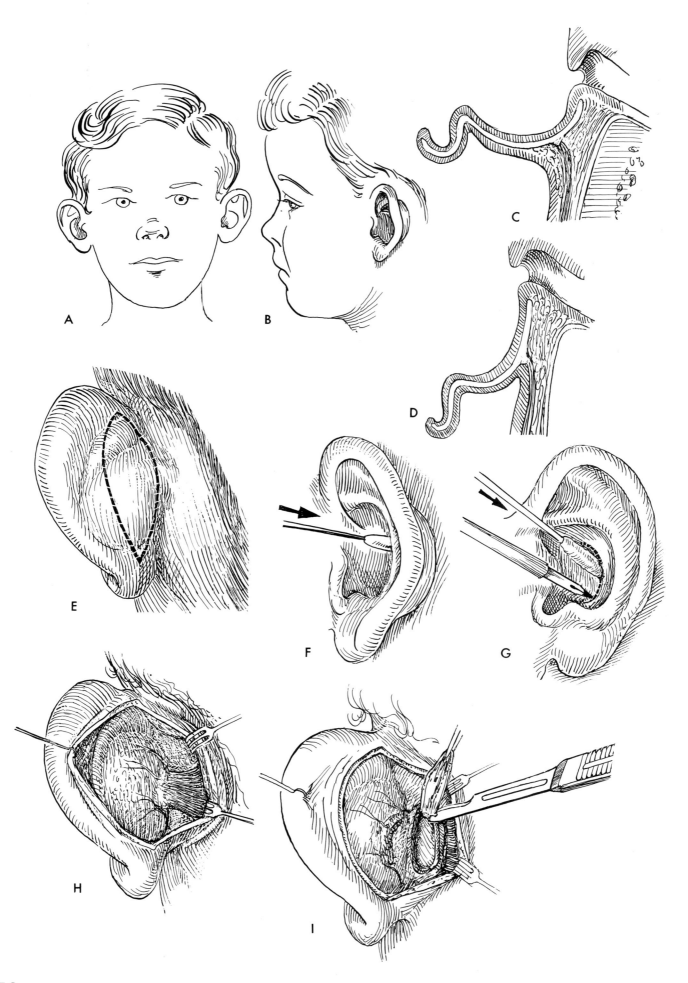

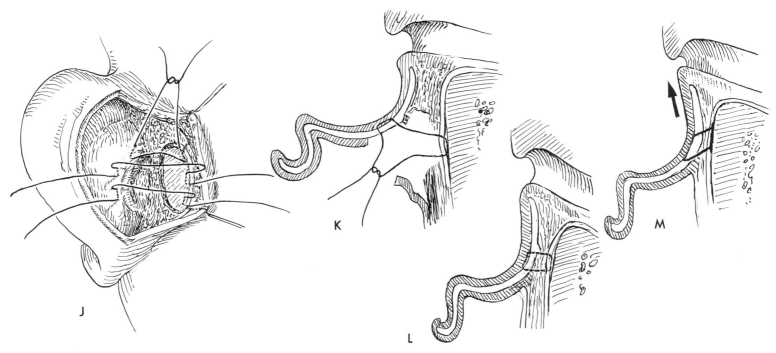

The Furnas Technique

The principal indication for the use of this means of correction of the prominent ear deformity (Furnas, 1968) is the presence of a deeply cupped concha, whose posterior wall is high and detached from the underlying mastoid region, and a relatively well formed antihelix *(A and B)*. In some instances this technique can eliminate the need for excision of a conchal cartilage strip.

A cross-sectional view of the detached concha is shown in *C* and may be compared with normally attached conchal cartilage *(D)*.

The operative technique involves, first, estimation of the degree of detachment of the conchal cartilage and the amount of correction that may be achieved by pressure on the posterior wall of the conchal cavity with a cotton-tipped applicator *(F)*. A line of junction between the posterior concha and the mastoid process, estimated from the point of pressure of the applicator, is marked in the depths of the conchal cavity to serve as an approximate guide to the points of insertion of the concha-mastoid sutures *(G)*.

A posterior auricular segment of skin is excised *(E and H)*. The concha is dissected anteriorly and the fibers of the vestigial posterior auricular muscle and its ligament are divided, with care being taken to preserve the branches of the greater auricular nerve. A segment of the soft tissue overlying the mastoid fascia in this region is removed *(I)*, and the deep fascia over the mastoid process is exposed. The area exposed should be about 1 × 2 cm., and its position is determined by trial and error placement of the conchal cartilage.

Sutures of 4–0 clear nylon are used to approximate and attach the cartilage to the fascia, using the previously placed marks in the depths of the conchal cavity as a rough guide to suture placement. Two or three sutures are generally required, and the thick mastoid periosteum and the full thickness of the conchal cartilage are picked up *(J, K, and L)*. Sutures that are incorrectly placed or that distort the concha are removed and replaced. Care is exerted not to shift the conchal cartilage anteriorly, which will produce a narrowing of the external auditory meatus *(M)*. The sutures are tightened and the final knots are welded by a quick application of the cautery to their ends.

If required, a fold is made in the antihelix, using the Converse–Wood-Smith or Mustardé techniques.

The skin is closed as previously described, and a mild pressure dressing applied for seven to 10 days. The patient should wear a light elastic cap as a splint during sleep for four to six weeks.

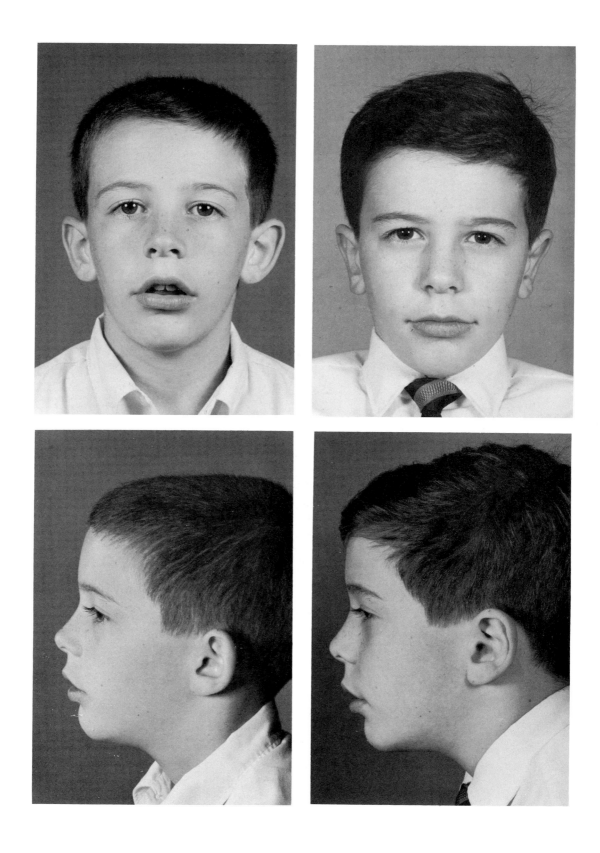

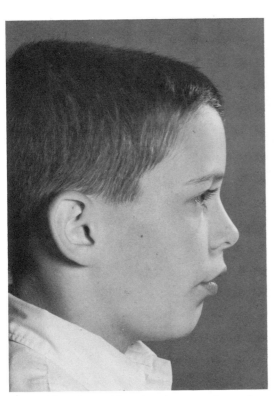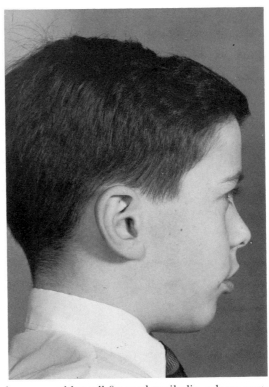

A nine year old patient with a deeply cupped concha and a reasonably well formed antihelix, whose appearance was improved by the Furnas technique. The postoperative photographs were taken six months after the operation.

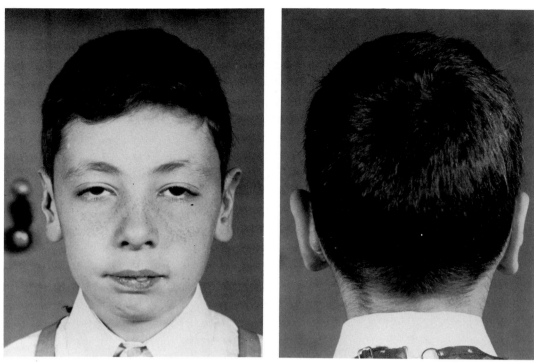

An attempt to correct a "telephone deformity" created this excessive "plastered to head" appearance. Note the postauricular hypertrophic scar on the left.

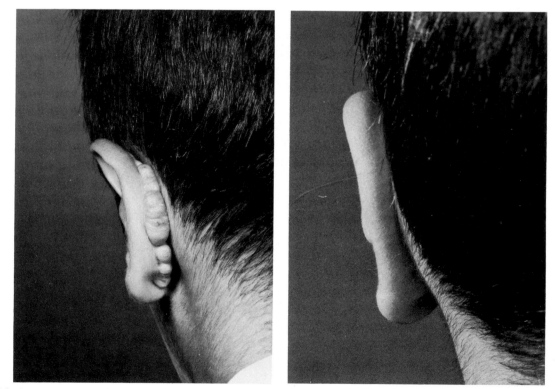

Keloids following correction of bilateral lop ear deformity, corrected by weekly injections of triamcinolone acetonide for three months.

Chapter 12

TREATMENT OF BALDNESS

NORMAN ORENTREICH, M.D.[*]

For many years it was known that autografts of black hair-growing skin transplanted to white haircoat areas of spotted guinea pigs continued to grow black hair. In 1948 the author presented his findings on skin autografts in man to the New York Academy of Sciences. The transposition of autografts was studied in various diseases as well as in common baldness. In the case of the latter, it was found that autografts from the posterior fringe of the scalp (that long maintains hair growth while the rest of the scalp balds) continued to grow as in their original sites when transplanted to the frontal scalp. The basic technique of employing cylindrical punches to make practical use of this fact was published in the Annals of the New York Academy of Sciences, and subsequent refinements have been detailed in recent articles. As a testimonial to effectiveness, the procedure has become widely employed, especially in recent years. Autograft hair growth has been observed for approximately 19 years in early transplanted patients.

However, since not all hair loss is common baldness or some other type suitable for autograft correction, it is worthwhile to review the various alopecias and their treatments before discussing in detail the technique of hair transplantation.

Hair loss can be caused by the deleterious involvement of either the living hair root or the keratinized hair shaft. If only the dead hair shaft is involved, alopecia will be temporary because the underlying follicular apparatus continues to function adequately and will grow new hair. However, an inherently diseased root or toxic factors influencing a functioning follicle can stop hair growth and cause loss of hair followed by: (1) immediate regrowth of new hair; (2) temporary failure to regrow hair; or (3) the persistent inability to regrow hair. If the follicle is completely destroyed, there is permanent loss of hair (Billingham, 1958; Miller, 1971).

Classification of the Alopecias

Congenital alopecia may take the form of complete absence of hair or patches of alopecia existing from birth (Cockayne, 1933). This may be associated with other cutaneous adnexal disorders. Rarely does normal hair develop.

Androgenetic alopecia is produced by androgens, but only in persons genetically predisposed. Male pattern alopecia is the outstanding example of this type. Most hair loss in women (diffuse and patterned) is androgenetic, i.e., the result of a hereditary predisposition to hair loss triggered by endogenous or exogenous androgens (Orentreich, 1966). Each individual hair follicle is genetically predisposed to respond or not to respond to androgenic and other influences that inhibit its growth.

Ninety-five per cent of normal adult men have some hair loss, usually of the patterned type, but frequently a combination of diffuse

*The author wishes to express his thanks to Victor J. Selmanowitz, M.D., and to Miss Helen Conner for their assistance in the preparation of this chapter.

and patterned. Seventy-five per cent of adult women have some hair loss, usually of the so-called diffuse type and only occasionally of the male pattern type. The onset of androgenetic alopecia occurs earlier and the severity is greater in men than in women (Orentreich, 1964).

ALOPECIA ASSOCIATED WITH NEOPLASTIC DISORDERS

Space-occupying masses in the scalp can cause loss of hair by the pressure effects of displacement, dysplasia and atrophy of the hair follicles, or by invasion and replacement of the follicular apparatus. Common cysts of the scalp, which often grow as conglomerates, often pose the pressure problem. Also to be considered are benign neoplasms such as cylindromas (turban tumors) and malignant lesions like leukemic nodular infiltrates (Leider, 1961). When surgical extirpation is indicated, the overlying alopecic skin should simply be observed for the next several months to determine if the hair follicle damage is reversible to the extent of allowing regrowth of hair.

ACQUIRED ALOPECIAS

Acquired alopecias may be of several types: traumatic, hormonal, infectious, neurologic, psychiatric, nutritional, toxic (from poisons or drugs) or strictly dermatologic (Orentreich, 1960).

TRAUMATIC ALOPECIAS. Externally applied pressure (as opposed to internal pressure due to cysts and neoplasms) or pulling on the hairs may be acute or chronic. In acute trauma, with or without laceration, hair loss may occur at the site of injury. This is likely to be permanent if there is scarring. Chronic pressure may also produce localized alopecia. This type of hair loss may be seen after prolonged general anesthesia, especially if the patient is kept in the Trendelenburg position. Edema of the scalp may first be noticed in the area in which temporary hair loss later develops. Pressure and friction on the scalp of infants owing to their lying position will also cause hair loss, which is of a temporary nature. Physical trauma from acute traction by plucking, combing or brushing can cause breakage of the hair shaft or evulsion from the follicle. Breaking of the shaft does not interfere with continuity of growth. Evulsion usually produces a temporary cessation of hair growth. Chronic traction by tight pony-tails, braids, curlers, barrettes, headbands or rubberbands can cause hair loss at the site of tension. If the traction is removed early enough, no follicular damage and resultant permanent alopecia occur. How-

ever, prolonged traction can produce permanent hair loss. Avulsion, which is the tearing away of scalp tissue, can cause not only loss of the hair-bearing follicles and thus permanent alopecia, but also injury to the skull. Burns, from extremes of heat or cold, can be sufficiently severe to have destructive effects on the hair follicle. Hair loss may be permanent if there is necrosis of the follicle-bearing tissue (Stough et al., 1968).

Chemicals may come in contact with the hair and scalp through industry or cosmetics (Harry, 1955). Industrial exposure to sodium and calcium sulfide or dimethylamine can cause hair breakage. The resulting temporary hair loss involves the shaft only and does not interfere with growth. A severe acute chemical dermatitis may also cause temporary hair loss. Only the severest primary irritating action or secondary bacterial infection with cicatrization can explain the permanent hair loss that is seen on rare occasions.

Exposure to x-rays, radium, radioisotopes, atomic bomb fallout or inadvertent short wavelength radiation can produce temporary or permanent alopecia (Van Scott and Reinerston, 1957). In temporary alopecia the epithelial elements are affected. In three to five weeks the hair loss is almost complete, and in 10 weeks hair regrowth may be seen. Ionizing radiation involvement of the more resistant dermal papillae portends permanent hair loss and also invariably produces radiodermatitis.

HORMONAL ALOPECIA. The following clinical entities can produce alopecia: hyperpituitarism, hypopituitarism, hyperthyroidism, hypothyroidism, hypoparathyroidism, hypocorticoidism, diffuse adrenocortical hyperplasia, benign and malignant androgenic adrenocortical tumors, adrenogenital syndrome, benign and malignant androgenic ovarian tumors, puberty, pregnancy, postpartum state, menopause and diabetes mellitus.

INFECTIOUS ALOPECIA. Localized superficial infections seldom cause permanent baldness (Leider, 1961). Deeper infection can cause temporary hair loss owing to breakage of the hair shaft or direct involvement of the follicle. If the follicle is destroyed, scarring is produced and the alopecia is permanent. The following organisms may affect the follicle and cause alopecia: viruses such as those of herpes simplex, herpes zoster, varicella and variola; bacteria such as those causing tuberculosis and leprosy; and pyogenic organisms. The follicles are also destroyed in folliculitis decalvans and acne varioliformis. Fungi usually cause temporary hair loss owing to breakage of the involved hair shaft; certain fungi, such as favus, may destroy the follicles. Kerion may produce permanent hair loss. Alopecia secondary to systemic illnesses, particularly those that cause high fevers, may begin to appear about 10 weeks after the onset of the disease symptoms. The following systemic infections are frequently associated with hair loss: viral, such as influenza; bacterial, such as typhoid fever, scarlet fever, erysipelas and pneumonia; treponemal, such as syphilis; yeast, such as moniliasis; and protozoal, such as malaria.

NEUROGENIC AND PSYCHIATRIC ALOPECIA. There is insufficient evidence to show that neurogenic factors influence the follicle directly. Trichotillomania is the subconscious or conscious pulling out of the hair by the patient (Graham, 1966; Greenberg and Sarner, 1965). Scalp hair, eyebrows and occasionally eyelashes are the hairs most frequently attacked (Orentreich, 1969). This is frequently associated with trichoclasia, the breaking off of the hair. Lichen chronicus circumscriptus (neurodermatitis), which is a chronic itching or rubbing, can cause hair breakage and can produce temporary localized baldness (Orentreich and Selmanowitz, 1970). On the other hand, repeated rubbing or biting of an area can occasionally produce a localized hypertrichosis.

TOXIC (PHARMACOLOGIC OR OCCUPATIONAL) ALOPECIA. Many organic and inorganic chemicals entering the system by inhalation, injection, ingestion or transepidermally may affect hair growth and produce toxic alopecia. Such alopecias may be divided into two groups: (1) toxic nonspecific chemical alopecia, and (2) toxic follicle-specific chemical alopecia. The nonspecific type may be caused by heavy metals, whereas follicle-specific toxic alopecia can be caused by antineoplastic compounds. Baldness produced by these compounds is not likely to be permanent.

NUTRITIONAL ALOPECIA. Nutritional deprivation and metabolic disorder must be severe in order to produce hair loss, which may occur in kwashiorkor, sprue and celiac disease. The common alopecias are not associated with nutritional deficiencies, but anemia, diabetes, hypervitaminosis A and hypovitaminosis A may be factors in producing alopecia.

DERMATOLOGIC ALOPECIA. Alopecia areata and its concentric, guttate, diffuse localized, diffuse generalized, ophiasis, totalis and universalis forms are the many types of bizarre-pattern alopecia of unknown etiology (Kopf and Orentreich, 1957; Orentreich, 1960 and 1966; Van Scott, 1958).

Hair loss usually occurs fairly suddenly and is seldom accompanied by other symptoms, though premonitory paresthesia sometimes occurs and mild erythema of the involved site may be detected early. The pathognomonic "exclamation point" hairs are present during the early active phase of the disorder (Van Scott, 1958). The course of the disease is unpredictable. Single patches usually regrow spontaneously in a few months. Recurrences are common. Extension to alopecia universalis, which occurs rarely, cannot be prognosticated.

Cicatricial alopecias, other than those already mentioned, include a number of cutaneous diseases with atrophy. They are pseudopelade, lupus erythematosus, lichen planus (lichen planopilaris) and scleroderma.

Treatment of the Alopecias

Before considering a surgical ameliorative approach for alopecia, other treatments will be discussed.

HORMONAL THERAPY. With special reference to the scalp generally, estrogens stimulate and androgens inhibit hair growth of the genetically predisposed hair (Orentreich, 1966). The previously mentioned endocrinopathies known to have associated hair loss can be helped either by internal surgical correction, administration of hormones or a combination of both. Hair regrowth may not occur until many months after surgery or institution of appropriate drug therapy. In some cases correction of a hormonal imbalance, as for example in adrenogenital syndrome, will only prevent further hair loss without involving regrowth of hair already lost.

TREATMENT OF INFECTIONS. The best treatment for fungal infections of the scalp is the administration of adequate oral doses of griseofulvin until the microscopic examination of hairs, fungal cultures and the Wood's light fluorescence are negative. Bacterial folliculitis of the scalp is treated with appropriate antibiotics and monitored by culture and sensitivity laboratory tests. Abscesses, furuncles and carbuncles are incised and drained as well.

The systemic infections that influence the hair cycle phases and account for a usually diffuse type of hair loss are likewise treated with the indicated antimicrobials. Since the telogen phase, to which many of the hair follicles may have been reverted, lasts 100 days, it may take three or four months or more before hair regrowth is observed.

TRICHOTILLOMANIA. The "trichotillo test" enables confirmation of the diagnosis of trichotillomania (Greenberg and Sarner, 1965). This test was devised to differentiate between self-inflicted alopecia (which the patient often de-

583

nies) and hair loss at the follicular level. A roughly 5-cm. square area in the alopecic region is coated with collodion in ether, or sprayed with a plastic surgical bandage (Orentreich and Selmanowitz, 1970). The material is allowed to dry, and in the same manner an additional three layers are applied. The patient is advised to leave this area alone and usually manages to comply with this advice, at least partially, because of the adherency of the applied mat. In about three weeks the square area will appear darker through the adherent film. Removal of the film will reveal a 5-cm. square area of short hairs. This area may then again be coated or sprayed to achieve longer length of the hairs, and additional areas may be so coated. Detailed psychiatric evaluations of trichotillomanic patients from our practice may be found in the articles by Graham (1966) and Greenberg and Sarner (1965). Occasionally a neurotic patient will pull off the occlusive patch, and only suturing a patch in place will permit the performance of the trichotillo test (Pearlstein and Orentreich, 1968).

INTRALESIONAL CORTICOSTEROID INJECTIONS. Response to corticosteroid therapy is both diagnostic of and therapeutic for alopecia areata. Intralesional injections of relatively insoluble aqueous suspensions of anti-inflammatory corticosteroids are the treatment of choice for alopecia areata and its variants in terms of extent—alopecia totalis (whole scalp) and alopecia universalis (whole body) (Dillaha and Rothman, 1952 a and b; Dougherty and Schneebeli, 1955; Rony and Cohen, 1955; Orentreich, 1958; Berger and Orentreich, 1960; Orentreich et al., 1960; Orentreich, 1971). Though most corticosteroids are effective, triamcinolone acetonide suspension (concentration 5 mg. per ml.) in a dosage of 0.1 ml. per injection site (1 to 2 cm. apart) is the most practical for acute cases. For chronic, extensive or persistent forms, the longer-acting triamcinolone hexacetonide suspension (concentration 5 mg. per ml.) is beneficial at the same dosage level. Mixtures of both suspensions to make no more than a total of 5 mg. per ml. may be used, depending upon severity and persistence of the condition. Hair regrowth should be evident within four to six weeks, at which time fill-in injections may be given as needed. To avoid local atrophic reactions, previously injected sites should not be reinjected within three months.

The discomfort caused by the injection—the prick of the needle and a burning sensation—is minimized by preparatory freezing with ethyl chloride. Local block anesthesia of the border of the scalp is an effective way of painlessly administering multiple injections of steroid suspension. Jet injection of steroids into the skin produces bruising and discomfort and is not preferable to 30-gauge needle injections.

The regrowing hair usually shows the same texture and pigmentation as the patient's normal hair. Occasionally a patient, usually with alopecia totalis, will claim that the new hair is darker and curlier than it had been.

The application of high potency topical steroids (e.g., 0.2 per cent fluocinolone acetonide cream and 0.5 per cent triamcinolone acetonide cream) under impervious occlusion can be of some minor assistance, but cannot substitute for the subdermal injections (Orentreich, 1958). Likewise, the oral intake of low doses of corticosteroids can be of auxiliary benefit.

Dermatitic cicatricial alopecias such as pseudopelade, discoid lupus erythematosus and lichen planus, if treated at an early inflammatory stage, can also be benefited by intralesional injections of corticosteroids and further assisted by topical application and oral intake of corticosteroids.

Hair Transplantation: Autograft and Homograft Techniques

Recent research has demonstrated that the hair follicles of the frontal scalp regions, where hair recession begins and is most prominent in common baldness, tend to metabolize testosterone differently from those follicles of the occipital fringe corresponding to the region that maintains hair growth the longest (Takashima et al., 1970). With a better understanding of such processes, it is hoped that ultimately the common type of hair loss may be prevented by locally influencing the chemical processes of the susceptible hair follicles. The time when this goal will be reached is not yet predictable, so that presently the surgical transplant method is being employed to the satisfaction of many patients desirous of having their own growing hairs, rather than an artificial prosthesis, to cover their bald areas. Moreover, there will probably always be a place for hair transplantation in the management of traumatic cicatricial alopecias wherein there are no remaining cutaneous appendages in scar tissue sufficiently vascularized to maintain grafts (Orentreich, 1959, 1970; Stough, et al., 1968.)

There are certain forms of alopecia mentioned earlier that should not be treated by utilizing the surgical transplant procedure. For example, in alopecia areata, intralesional injections of steroids (particularly triamcinolone) stimulates regrowth

584

of hair and surgery is not indicated (Dillaha and Rothman, 1952a and b; Rony and Cohen, 1955; Orentreich, 1958; Berger and Orentreich, 1960; Orentreich et al., 1960; Dougherty and Schneebeli, 1955; Orentreich, 1971). If trichotillomania is the cause of baldness, then surgically transplanted hairs are likely to fall prey to the same vagaries as did the previous hairs growing in their natural sites. Most infections of the scalp entail a superficial folliculitis, so that the critical deep portion of the follicular apparatus, including the underlying and crucial dermal papillae, remains viable and capable of growing hair in due time after the infection is eradicated. Following removal of the offending causes, hair may grow in sites of alopecia due to traction or resulting from internal pressure such as from cysts of the scalp. An adequate period of observation for signs of regrowth of hair is mandatory. Adversely affected follicles are often thrown into the telogen phase of the hair growth cycle, which is a resting phase wherein hair growth ceases. This telogen phase lasts about 100 days in the scalp. Then, if hair starts to regrow, it will do so at the rate of 0.1 mm./day, and there will be an additional lag period before short hairs are visible on the surface of the scalp (Myers and Hamilton, 1951; Kligman, 1959; Saitoh et al., 1969; Orentreich, 1969).

The transplant technique has been applied therapeutically for the treatment of hair loss problems such as male pattern alopecia, androgenetic alopecia in women (diffuse and patterned) and the cicatricial alopecias; for that matter, for any indicated state wherein the alopecic receptor sites can sustain autografts from remaining hair-growing donor sites (Orentreich, 1960, 1966; Ayres, 1964; Stough et al., 1968). In the case of avulsion, which was described earlier, if the site is small, immediate replacement of the avulsed skin may be successful.

For common baldness, hair is taken from the donor area (occipital and temporal) and placed in the bald recipient area (frontal and dome). In the hair transplant process "donor dominance" is exhibited by both donor and recipient grafts; that is, they maintain their integrity and characteristics after transplantation; the term "recipient dominance" refers to autografts that develop the characteristics of the recipient sites (Orentreich, 1959).

Selection of patients and planning of the transplant surgery periods should be done considering the following: an examination of the potential of the donor areas and the requirements of the recipient bald sites; the expectations of the patient; the most satisfactory hair style; the number of grafts required; the cost of the procedure; the cosmetic incapacitation dur-

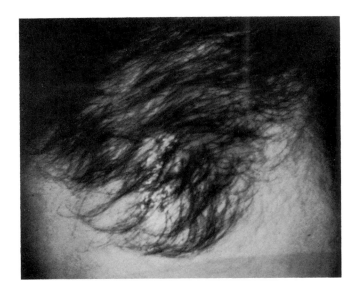

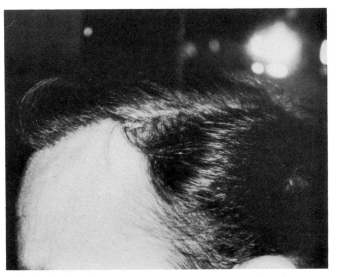

Front of scalp showing multiple grafts several months after transplantation. Two years later frontal scalp grafting shows vigorous full growth of hair.

ing the healing stages; the patient's wound-healing ability; and the patient's general health. Complete blood count and blood sugar levels are determined before transplants are performed. Caution regarding keloid tendencies are particularly warranted in Negro patients. It is a good policy to give the patient a written outline of the principles and the details of the procedure, the sequence of events to expect in wound healing and hair growth, things to avoid, and untoward occurrences that may take place.

STEPS IN TECHNIQUE

First, the donor and recipient sites are cleansed with 70 per cent alcohol. The hair in the donor area is clipped to a length of about 2 mm. above the scalp surface. It is preferable to clip a relatively narrow band running transversely across the scalp to ensure that the donor area can be easily hidden by overlapping hair during the healing period. Shaving the area obliterates visualization of the hair direction (angle inserted into the scalp), which is very important for proper angulation of the punch for removing the skin plugs, and for permitting proper placement in the recipient sites. The donor and recipient areas are sprayed with ethyl chloride and anesthetized by the injection of a 2 per cent lidocaine hydrochloride (Xylocaine) solution. Occasionally 1:100,000 epinephrine in 2 per cent lidocaine hydrochloride is used for excessive bleeders. Metal dental syringes using disposable ampules containing a 2 per cent lidocaine solution are used because their hydraulic characteristics make it easy to inject the scalp tissue. Several ampules are used to produce the area of anesthesia required for the planned procedure.

Punches 2.0, 2.5, 3.0, 3.5 and 4.0 mm. in diameter have been designed for this technique. They differ from the classic skin biopsy punch in

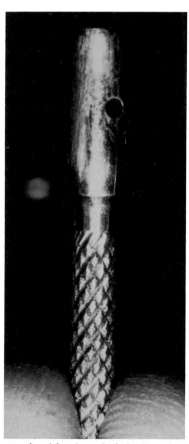

A 4-mm. punch with a knurled shaft and a hole in the cylinder for easy cleaning and to vent air during the incision of the scalp.

(Supplied by Robbins Instrument Company, Chatham, New Jersey.)

these respects: the diameter of the shaft is relatively small, which permits efficient twirling of the punch for rapid cutting; the shaft is knurled to provide a good grip; the cutting head cylinder is relatively straight, in contrast to the truncated arrowhead design of some traditional skin punches; and a small hole is cut at the base of the cylinder to permit cleaning of the cup. The punch most commonly used for hair transplants is 3.5 or 4.0 mm. in diameter. The same size punch is generally used for recipient and donor sites, although a punch 0.5 or 1.0 mm. larger is used occasionally to obtain the donor tissue. Small punches of scalp with hair are used to fill in between the 4-mm. grafts to create a more natural cosmetic effect. Grafts larger than 4 mm. do not heal as well and result in reduced hair density. The bald site is punched using a twirling motion for increased cutting efficiency. The cut is first started at right angles to the scalp, penetrating the skin 1 mm. The punch is then angled in the direction of the hair growth to prepare a site to receive the donor plug with its hairs growing at an angle. When working on the dome of the scalp, the punches are angled radially, pointing to the center of the calyx (the usual pattern for hair on the dome of the scalp). On the frontal scalp the cuts are angled backward since most frontal hair growth is in a forward direction.

DEGREE OF ALOPECIA

The number of plugs cut during each treatment depends on the degree of alopecia, the amount of cosmetic incapacitation the patient is prepared to accept, the frequency at which the treatments are given, the time since the last procedure, and the maximum tolerance of the site for the number of grafts performed.

The advantage of the small full-thickness graft is its tendency to be vascularized in 24 to 48 hours. The first nourishment of the graft is plasma, and the smaller the graft, the more adequate the nourishment. The grafts must not be

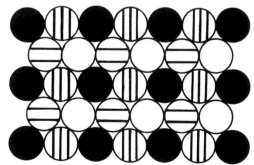

Grafts are separated by the width of the punch diameter. Four procedures are necessary to fill an area completely.

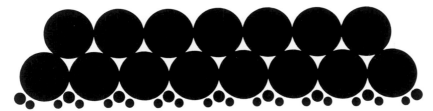

Small punches between 4-mm. grafts to create a more natural hairline.

placed so close together that the vascular insufficiency that occurs in large grafts is produced. Punches are usually separated by the width of the punch diameter to permit an adequate blood supply. After healing, additional plugs can be placed between the previously placed grafts. When doing a single line of grafts (as at the hairline), it is feasible to place the grafts immediately next to each other. Later smaller plugs can be used in the scalloped front line to create a more natural-looking hairline.

Ten to 50 plugs are usually grafted at each visit. A site should be allowed to heal for at least two weeks before additional grafting is performed in the same area. Other sites may be grafted the next day if care is taken not to disturb the previous grafts.

The skin punches removed from the recipient scalp site are discarded. Small tooth forceps are all that is usually needed to remove the grafts after they are cut. If there is a fibrotic anchoring band, small surgical scissors are used to cut the band at its base to release the plug of skin.

Punching the number of plugs needed for the procedure at the donor site is performed at the angle of the hairs in the scalp. They can be cut much closer together than the circular incisions made in the recipient area, leaving enough hair to cover the defect created in the donor area.

The average 4-mm. plug of hair-bearing scalp will contain from 12 to 15 hairs. If the donor scalp hair is very sparse, this number will be less; it is rarely more. The color of the donor hair may be similar to, lighter or darker than the recipient site hair. The degree of graying may also vary.

The hair follicles should be cut parallel to the walls of the cylinder of the punch to prevent their being damaged. An examination of the plugs can easily demonstrate whether the punch is being used at the correct angle.

The donor plugs are removed with a small toothed forceps and are placed immediately in a Petri dish with a 3 by 3 inch square of sterile gauze immersed in sterile physiologic saline or Ringer's solution. The grafts must not be per-

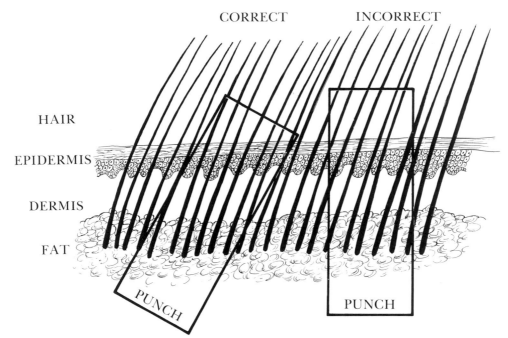

Correct and incorrect angle for cutting donor plugs. Correct method is parallel to hair follicle.

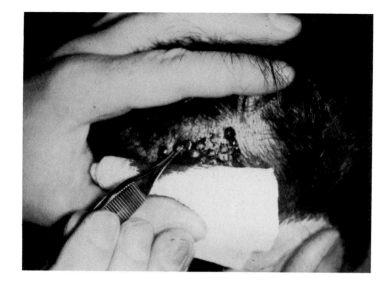

Tooth forceps are used for the removal of donor plugs.

Grafts are placed in a Petri dish of physiologic saline for cleansing.

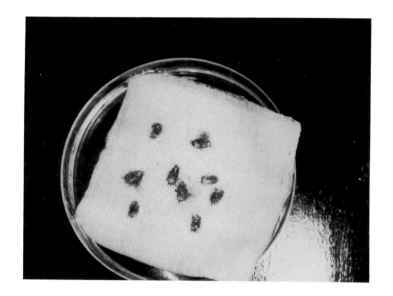

Grafts in recipient sites.

mitted to dry at any time. The skin plugs slip out of the scalp in the donor area with much greater ease than they do in the recipient site. If undue force is required to remove the skin plugs, care must be taken to cut their bases with the points of small surgical scissors well below the hair follicle level.

The donor and recipient areas, after removal of the skin plugs, are covered with wads of gauze, and these are held in place with an elastic cotton bandage. This encourages hemostasis while the donor grafts are prepared. Occasionally, if bleeding is excessive at the donor site, a 3–0 silk suture is placed, sometimes in a figure-of-eight configuration, for hemostasis. Sutures can be removed within the next day or two. Rarely does the recipient site require suture hemostasis. Usually there is no bleeding after 10 or 15 minutes following removal of the plugs. If bleeding starts on insertion of the donor plug, direct pressure is applied with gauze on the donor graft to produce hemostasis. Rarely is it required to suture a graft in its recipient site to stop bleeding. If this is done, the suture is removed the next day. It is possible, in the presence of excessive bleeding, to suture the recipient bleeding site without the graft and to place the graft in this site the next day after removing the suture. The donor graft skin plug is wrapped in sterile gauze, wet with sterile physiologic saline, and placed in the refrigerator (not in the freezing compartment). Grafts will stay viable in this way up to three weeks, provided the gauze is kept moist with sterile physiologic saline.

Before the donor plugs are inserted into the recipient sites, they are cleaned gently while still immersed in saline of all spicules of loose hair. Excess fat and any attached galea aponeurotica are trimmed. Great care must be exercised not to damage the base of the hair follicles. If the dermal papilla of a hair follicle is removed, no hair will grow. The donor grafts are placed in a manner oriented to conform to the angle cut in the scalp, and to produce uniform angulation of the donor hairs in the recipient sites. Additional pressure may be required after placing the grafts for hemostasis. The fibrin clot that forms in minutes holds the plugs in place, and it is unnecessary to use adhesives to hold the grafts in their recipient sites. The treated areas are cleansed with peroxide and water. A thin layer of antibiotic ointment is spread over the implanted autografts. Saran wrap is then applied over the site and is secured with tape. The Saran wrap retains moisture for more rapid healing of the grafts and better epithelialization of their borders, thus minimizing scarring. This

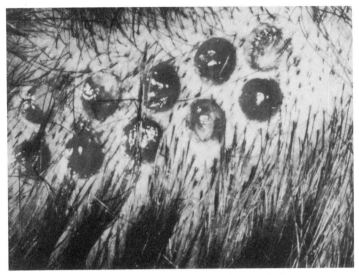

Donor sites prior to combing hair over defect.

type of occlusive dressing also cuts down on crusting on the surface of the grafts, which can be quite thick with gauze dressings. A still further advantage is that the transparent Saran wrap enables final visualization of the placement of the grafts and possible sites of blood oozing before the application of a pressure dressing. This is applied for comfort and security, to prevent movement, and to reduce postoperative bleeding or edema. This type of dressing is usually advisable when the number of grafts transplanted per procedure exceeds 20 skin plugs.

The hair at the donor area is then combed over the donor plug sites. Suturing these holes is unnecessary unless bleeding is excessive. They heal with a minimal cosmetic defect. The hair at the recipient site may be gently combed over the grafts, if there are fewer than 20, to hide their cosmetic effect. If a hair piece prosthesis is worn, it may be carefully fitted into place over no dressing or a light dressing, taking care to make the wig attachments at untreated sites.

POSTOPERATIVE CARE

The patient is advised to drink no alcoholic beverages for the first 24 hours, to perform no strenuous physical activity for the first day and only limited physical activity for five days, and not to disturb the grafts for 10 days. He should also exert great care when combing or brushing near the graft sites; he should avoid shampooing the scalp or showering the head for five days, and should shampoo gently after five days. He should not pick at the grafts, as the crusts

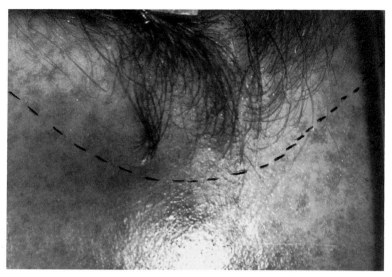

Graft continues to grow while hairline is receding. Graft was initially placed at hairline margin.

will eventually come off with shampooing or bathing. If bleeding occurs he is to apply pressure with gauze or a clean handkerchief directly to the site for 15 minutes. If bleeding persists he should call the physician. The patient should expect mild discomfort, numbness, or altered sensations for weeks after the procedure. He should also be aware that although the hairs in the donor grafts appear to be growing the first month they are really falling out, and he should not expect true hair growth for three months after the procedure is performed. There may be swelling from 24 to 48 hours after the procedure, which may possibly occur on the forehead also.

In the thousands of procedures performed the complications encountered have been: syncope during the procedure (1:100), infection (1:500), hypertrophic or keloidal healing (1:1000) and venous aneurysm or arteriovenous shunt formation (1:5000).

It is now over 19 years since we performed scalp punch autografts on human beings for the first time. The hair in the donor grafts in the recipient sites is still growing, with the characteristics of the donor sites. In thousands of transplant procedures performed by us and by hundreds of other physicians, there has been no instance of donor hair-bearing grafts failing to continue the hair growth initially accomplished if the donor site was in an area of the scalp that was still growing hair. Great care must be taken to select the donor area with an eye toward the future pattern of alopecia formation.

The ability of the grafts to continue to grow hair even when implanted in an area with a receding hairline demonstrates donor dominance.

PRELIMINARY HOMOTRANSPLANTATION TRIALS

The technique of skin punch autotransplantation, used to redistribute hair on the scalp, is very suitable for homograft studies. The growth of hair in the donor graft is irrefutable evidence of a successful take and maintained integrity of the tissues; it dispels any argument that the skin transplanted has been replaced by the host's integument, which is glabrous.

The approximately 21-day period usually encountered in homograft skin rejection is considerably shorter than the 90-day period required for hair growth in a skin graft with intact hair follicles. With an intralesional steroid, administered at the rate of 1 mg. triamcinolone acetonide per 30 days, the rejection phenomenon was suppressed and the hair growing potential was not inhibited. Reducing this dose produced inflammation and rejection. Increasing the dose produced atrophy and suppressed hair growth.

The knowledge gained by dermatologists on the intralesional administration of steroids (Orentreich et al., 1960), combined with the technique of the scalp hair punch grafting, enabled sustained growth of homotransplanted hair for the past year. Further time for observation is required to determine just how long these hairs will continue to grow, if not lifelong.

A method of interrupted exposure to tissue antigens has been employed in an effort to maintain homografts. This method is analogous to that of Macher and Chase (1969a and b), wherein brief exposure of guinea pigs to picryl chloride or dinitrochlorobenzene, followed by excision of the exposed sites, later occasioned a tolerogenic effect to the above chemicals. On re-exposure to the specific chemical in critical dosage, the animals were not sensitized.

Utilizing this principle, homografts from hair scalp have been transplanted to alopecic scalp for 24 hours, removed, and kept in Weymouth's medium at 10° C. for four days. The homografts were then replaced in the same recipient site. Over a year has passed without sloughing of the homografts. Hair shafts remain visible in the donor tissue as evidence of anatomic integrity of the homograft and, hence, a tolerogenic effect. However, the hairs have not grown out, indicating a lack of restoration to full functional capacity. The timing of initial exposure to tissue antigens and subsequent reimplantation of the homograft are now being modified in an attempt to maintain growing properties of homografts.

REFERENCES

Ayres, S., III: Conservative surgical management of male pattern baldness: An evaluation of current techniques. Arch. Derm. 90:493–499, 1964.

Berger, R. A., and Orentreich, N.: Abrupt changes in hair morphology following corticosteroid therapy in alopecia areata. Arch. Derm. 82:408–411, 1960.

Billingham, R. C.: A reconsideration of the phenomenon of hair neogenesis, with particular reference to the healing of cutaneous wounds in adult mammals. In Montagna, W., and Ellis, R. (eds.): The Biology of Hair Growth. New York, Academic Press, 1958, pp. 451–468.

Cockayne, E. A.: Inherited Abnormalities of the Skin and Its Appendages. London, Oxford University Press, 1933.

Dillaha, C. J., and Rothman, S.: Treatment of alopecia areata totalis and universalis with cortisone acetate. J. Invest. Derm. 18:5–6, 1952a.

Dillaha, C. J., and Rothman, S.: Therapeutic experiments in alopecia areata with orally administered cortisone. J.A.M.A. 150:546–550, 1952b.

Dougherty, T. F., and Schneebeli, G. L.: Use of steroids as anti-inflammatory agents. Ann. N.Y. Acad. Sci. 61:328–348, 1955.

Graham, F.: Trichotillomania, a symptom of adolescent identity crisis. Excerpta Med. Int. Congress Series. Psychosomat. Med. 21:239–246, 1966.

Greenberg, H. R., and Sarner, C.: Trichotillomania. Arch. Gen. Psychiat. 12:482–489, 1965.

Harry, R. G.: Modern Cosmeticology. Vol. 1. London, Leonard Hill, Ltd., 1955.

Klfgman, A.: The human hair cycle. J. Invest. Derm. 33:307–316, 1959.

Kopf, A. W., and Orentreich, N.: Alkaline phosphatase in alopecia areata. A.M.A. Arch. Derm. 76:288–295, 1957.

Leider, M.: Practical Pediatric Dermatology. St. Louis, The C. V. Mosby Co., 1961.

Macher, E., and Chase, M. W.: The fate of labeled picryl chloride and dinitro chlorobenzene after sensitizing injections. J. Exper. Med. 129:81–102, 1969a.

Macher, E., and Chase, M. W.: The influence of excision of allergenic depots on onset of delayed hypersensitivity and tolerance. J. Exper. Med. 129:103–121, 1969b.

Miller, S. A.: Hair neogenesis. J. Invest. Derm. 56:1–9, 1971.

Myers, R. J., and Hamilton, J. B.: Regeneration and rate of growth of hairs in man. Ann. N.Y. Acad. Sci. 53:562–568, 1951.

Orentreich, N.: Clinical efficacy of triamcinolone acetonide and hydrocortisone acetate in dermatological patients. Monogr. Ther. 3:161, 1958.

Orentreich, N.: Autografts in alopecias and other selected dermatological conditions. Ann. N.Y. Acad. Sci. 83:463–479, 1959.

Orentreich, N.: Pathogenesis of alopecia. J. Soc. Cosm. Chemists. 11:479–499, 1960.

Orentreich, N.: Alopecia. In Conn, H. F. (ed.): Current Therapy—1964. Philadelphia, W. B. Saunders Company, 1964, pp. 427–430.

Orentreich, N.: Hair problems. J. Amer. Med. Wom. Assoc. 21:481–486, 1966.

Orentreich, N.: Etiology of loss of eyelashes in a child. J.A.M.A. 207:961, 1969a.

Orentreich, N.: Scalp hair replacement in man. In Montagna, W., and Dobson, R. L. (eds.): Hair Growth. New York, Pergamon Press, 1969b, pp. 99–108.

Orentreich, N.: Hair transplants: Long-term results and new advances. Arch. Otolaryng. 92:576–582, 1970.

Orentreich, N.: Disorders of the hair and scalp in childhood. Pediat. Clin. N. Amer., 18(No. 3):953–974, 1971.

Orentreich, N., and Selmanowitz, V. J.: Cosmetic improvement of factitial defects. Med. Trial Tech. Quart., 1970, pp. 172–180.

Orentreich, N., Sturm, H., Weidman, A. L., and Pelzig, A.: Local injections of steroids and hair regrowth in alopecias. Arch. Derm. 82:894–902, 1960.

Pearlstein, H., and Orentreich, N.: Sutured dressing: An adjunct in the treatment of neurotic excoriations. Arch. Derm. 98:508–511, 1968.

Rony, H. R., and Cohen, D. M.: The effect of cortisone in alopecia areata. J. Invest. Derm. 25:285–287, 1955.

Saitoh, M., Uzuka, M., and Sakamoto, M.: Rate of hair growth. In Montagna, W., and Dobson, R. L. (eds.): Hair Growth. New York, Pergamon Press, 1969, pp. 183–201.

Stough, D. B., Berger, R. A., and Orentreich, N.: Surgical improvement of cicatricial alopecias of diverse etiology. Arch. Derm. 97:331–334, 1968.

Takashima, I., Adachi, K., and Montagna, W.: Studies of common baldness in the stumptailed macaque. IV. In vitro. Metabolism of testosterone in the hair follicles. J. Invest. Derm. 55:329–334, 1970.

Van Scott, E. J.: Morphologic changes in pilosebaceous units and anagen hair in alopecia areata. J. Invest. Derm. 31:35, 1958.

Van Scott, E. J., and Reinerston, R. P.: Detection of radiation effects on hair roots of the human scalp. J. Invest. Derm. 29:205–212, 1957.

Chapter 13

HAIR TRANSPLANTATION

CHARLES P. VALLIS, M.D.

Hair transplantation for male pattern baldness has become an increasingly popular operation during the past decade. In carefully selected cases the presently used techniques are quite successful in distributing a significant amount of hair from ageless hair-bearing areas of the scalp to the prematurely bald areas. Hair transplantation has now become the most common cosmetic operative procedure in the male patient.

Several methods have been proposed for the replacement of hair in male pattern baldness. In an attempt to correct the condition, rotation flaps, bipedicle and monopedicle hair-bearing flaps, and partial excision of full segments of hairless skin have all been used (Correa-Inturraspe and Arute, 1957; Lamont, 1957; Limburger, 1959; Adamson et al., 1969). These methods do produce hair growth, but rarely can a flap be taken from an area having hair follicles of high longevity, and the surgical procedures are usually too long and complicated for such a benign condition.

The first really simple and effective method for correcting male pattern baldness was described by Orentreich in 1959. He transplanted small cylinders of autologous full-thickness skin graft from hair-bearing areas to bald areas by means of a skin biopsy punch. This has proved to be an ingenious and extremely appealing procedure to both surgeon and patient because of its utter simplicity.

The author originally described the use of a long strip of full-thickness hair-bearing skin graft from the scalp for the reconstruction of a new frontal hairline (Vallis, 1964, 1967, 1969a and b). When this procedure is used in conjunction with the punch graft method, very gratifying results can be achieved.

In a review of the last 175 male patients with pattern baldness operated on during the past four years, the following significant statistics are found: A total of 601 operative procedures were done. Of these 601 operations, there were 133 strip grafts and 468 punch graft procedures. Of the 175 patients, 68 had a combination of strip grafts and punch grafts. Four had only strip grafts and 103 had only punch grafts.

The ages of the 175 patients ranged between 20 and 58 years. The majority were young adults with premature baldness. Over half the patients in this series had just the punch grafts.

Most patients are not interested in having their original frontal hairline reconstructed. Many simply wish to maintain their existing hairline. Many have marked thinning on top of the scalp and are simply interested in increasing the density of the hair in this area. Many show only a circular patch of baldness in the superior occipital area. In all these cases the punch graft procedure when done alone will add a significant amount of hair.

The strip graft in conjunction with punch grafts has been used primarily in younger individuals with premature loss of hair and obvious recession of the frontal hairline. These patients are anxious to recover as dense a growth as pos-

592

sible in the frontal region. The strip graft operation, when properly executed by a well trained surgeon, provides an acceptable hairline of good density.

Selection of Patients

There are probably more deterrents to than indications for the hair transplant operation, but in carefully selected patients a good growth of hair can be anticipated. Patients with adequate, dense hair of good quality in the donor site may be good candidates. Usually those with dark coarse hair show a better and denser growth than those with fine silky blond hair. Highly motivated patients who understand the limitations and discomfort of the operation are good candidates—especially those who simply want a little more hair than they have and are not looking for miracles.

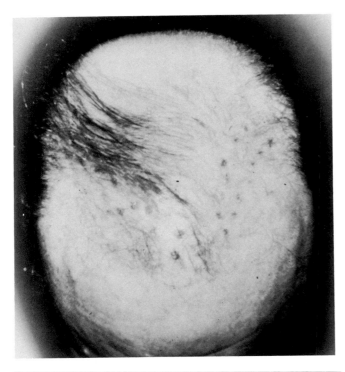

Marked thinning of hair is seen in a 56 year old man. Note the punch grafts in the preoperative view, and the hair growth after five punch-graft procedures in the two later views.

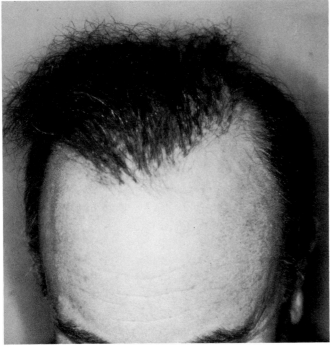

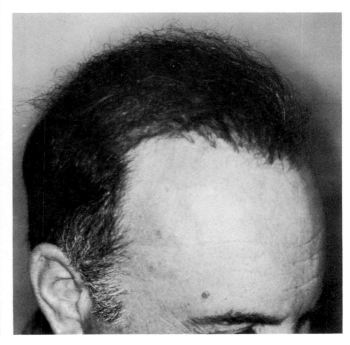

Criteria for Refusing a Patient

Severely bald patients with insufficient hair in the donor site—often just a narrow rim of hair around the parietal and occipital areas—should be refused.

Sparse or thin hair growth in all areas of the scalp is a contraindication.

Many patients with only minimal loss of hair complain that they are losing their hair rapidly, yet they have no real bald patches. They should be told to come back when there is actual recession or baldness.

The prolonged course of the multiple-stage procedures may be a deterrent to many pa-tients. It is essential not to hold anything back from the patient when discussing a proposed hair transplant procedure. It should be explained to him that this is a long series of tedious operative procedures, that considerable patience is required because the new growth is very slow, and that it will be several months before full growth is attained.

Emotionally unstable patients with a history of psychiatric disturbances should be refused.

Patients with any form of severe systemic disease, such as coronary insufficiency or high blood pressure, should not be accepted.

The creation of scars in the donor and recipient areas, although minimal, should be ex-

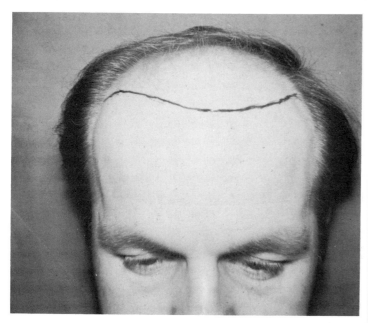

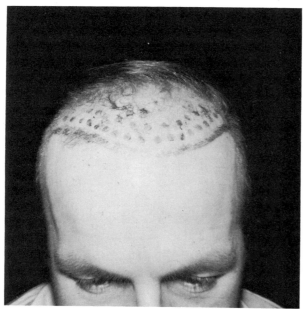

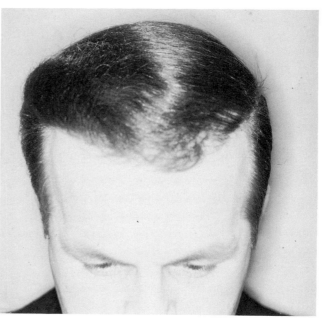

Three successive views showing proposed position of new frontal hairline in a 27 year old man; strip and punch grafts in position; and hair growth after six procedures.

plained to all patients, and is a definite deterrent to some.

Patients with alopecia resulting from a diseased scalp or psychosomatic problems should be referred to a dermatologist. Only hair loss associated with typical pattern baldness or some form of trauma can be helped by the hair transplant techniques.

Description of Techniques

As already stated, the punch graft technique alone is used in the majority of patients. However, in selected patients the strip graft method can add desirable fullness and density to the frontal hairline.

Most of the problems which have been associated with hair transplant surgery are related to the reconstruction of the new frontal hairline. Regardless of which technique is used for the reconstruction of the new frontal hairline, it is important that the position be carefully planned and designed preoperatively. Improperly placed strip or punch grafts create a bizarre and embarrassing effect. It is essential that the proposed new hairline does not run straight across the frontal region. There should be a "widow's peak" with some degree of posterior recession of the hairline on either side to give a more natural appearance. The new hairline should never be placed in front of the temporal hair, regardless of the degree of recession.

Poor results following a strip graft operation can usually be attributed to improper placement of the graft in the frontal area, too narrow a graft, or poor take of the graft, usually due to inept surgical techniques.

Operative Technique for Strip Grafts

The strip grafts should be taken in a horizontal direction from the parietal-occipital area of the scalp. The horizontal direction ensures invisibility of the scar after healing. When taking a strip graft, it is important that the donor incision follow the slant and angulation of the hair follicles. Failure to excise the graft in a direction parallel to the slant of the hairs may destroy several rows of the underlying hair follicles.

The width of the strip graft is very important relative to the ultimate appearance of the hairline. A very narrow strip, although regaining circulation more readily, actually defeats the

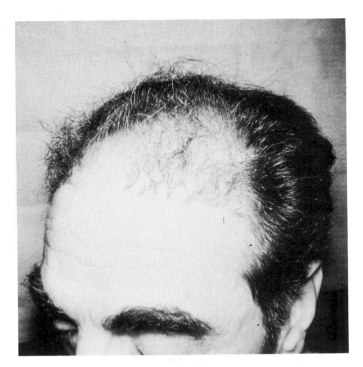

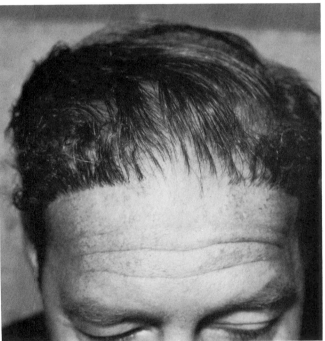

Poorly placed punch grafts in a 52 year old man, and poorly placed strip grafts in a 40 year old man.

purpose of the strip graft operation. The resultant hairline is rather thin and sparse and does not have the density of hair that a wider strip would achieve. The punch graft technique would create a much more presentable hairline than a very narrow strip graft. I have consistently made my strip grafts at least 8 mm., and frequently 9 mm., in width. When these grafts take well, they result in a broad, dense growth of hair which is gratifying to the patient.

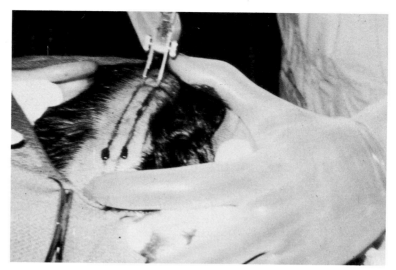

Parallel double blade knife for taking strip graft.

After the strip graft has been removed from the scalp no attempt is made at hemostasis, except for pressure on either side by the assistant. The wound is quickly closed with a continuous 3–0 nylon suture. The graft is carefully pared of excess fascia and fatty tissue, but the paring of the fat should not be too excessive and the hair follicles should not be exposed or damaged. The major circulation for the graft necessarily comes from the sides; consequently an extra amount of fatty tissue under the follicles does not prevent the graft from taking.

The new frontal hairline is usually reconstructed in two stages; one strip is used to span half the frontal scalp on one side, and two weeks later another strip is used for the other side. It is essential that the strips form a complete hairline with no gaps. This is done by overlapping the grafts in the mid forehead. It is possible to span the entire forehead with one long strip, but this lengthens the operating time considerably. These operations are all done under local anesthesia on an outpatient basis. Prolongation under these conditions is an undue strain on the surgeon and the patient.

In preparing the recipient site, a simple incision is made through the skin, subcutaneous tissue and underlying fascia or galea aponeurotica. Complete hemostasis is secured with 4–0 plain catgut ligatures and weak epinephrine packs. Poor hemostasis in the recipient area causes hematomas with ultimate poor take of the graft. Inadequate splitting of the underlying galea aponeurotica in the recipient area will not allow the wound to open widely enough to receive the graft and will ultimately cause constriction of the graft.

The strip grafts should be placed in the wound with the hair follicles pointing inferiorly. If the strip graft is thus placed, when the hair

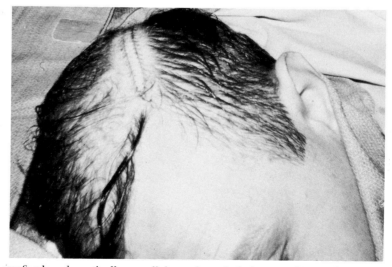

Strip graft placed vertically parallel to where hair is parted in a 27 year old man.

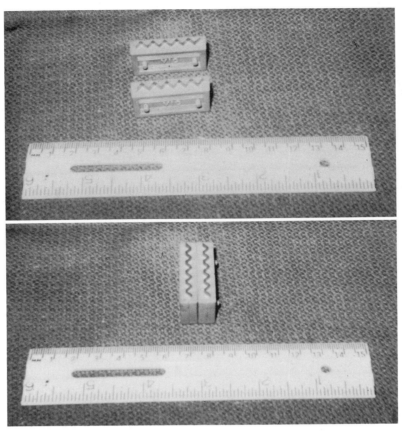

Instrument for making running-W incision, and two instruments joined for taking running-W strip graft.

grows out, there will be a full growth right to the edge of the inferior margin. Also, when the patient combs his hair, the hairs will extend slightly downward before curving superiorly, thus camouflaging the linear edge of the graft. If the graft is not in this position, a pale white linear scar will result along the inferior margin of the graft.

Improper suturing of the graft in the recipient area very frequently results in a poor take of the graft. I have found that a fine continuous 6–0 nylon suture used in the superficial layers of the skin without strangulation, with close coaptation of the skin margins, helps greatly in attaining a good take of the graft.

A circular head bandage is used for pressure over the graft, although a small stent tied over the graft can be used. It is very important that the postoperative dressing not be placed too tightly; a tight dressing will result in embarrassment of the circulation at the site of the graft. An excessively tight dressing will also cause marked periorbital edema and ecchymosis which may last for several weeks after the operation. A rayon dressing is placed initially over the strip graft to prevent adherence to the dressing material. The pressure dressing is kept on for

two days, and then a small dressing is applied over the graft only. Dressings are not required after one week; sutures are removed in 10 days.

A simple instrument was designed to allow the surgeon to take a strip graft of a predetermined and uniform width. It is called the parallel double blade holder for the strip graft. It takes two No. 15 blades and comes in varying widths from 5 to 10 mm. This instrument is used to make the initial incisions in the donor site. The incision is carried through the skin for a few millimeters and then a single blade knife is used to make the deeper incision on either side of the graft. This instrument makes the procedure more exact and effective and shortens the operative time considerably.

The strip graft can also be used in other parts of the scalp besides the frontal hairline. It may be placed vertically on the scalp near and parallel to where the hair is parted. This allows the patient to have more hair to comb over the top of the scalp.

As with any other new operation, constant attempts should be made to improve the operative technique. It is important that a postoperative result closely approaching the normal appearance be obtained. As in all cosmetic

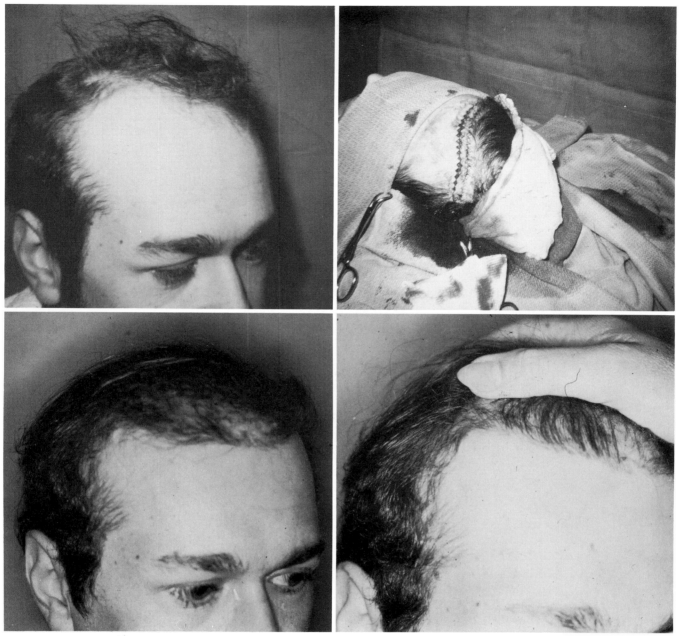

A 24 year old man, seen preoperatively, with a running-W strip graft in position, and after 6 months.

operations, it is imperative that there be no conspicuous signs that an operation has been performed.

The one objection that has been raised against the strip graft procedure is that it forms an unnaturally straight hairline. In my own series of cases this complaint has been voiced only rarely. Actually most patients state that the strip graft, because of the high density of hair that results, really makes the difference by creating the fullness which is so desirable to the patient.

In scar revisions one of the common techniques employed to break up a straight line deformity is to utilize the running-W incision. It occurred to me that if a running-W incision were used to take the strip graft, then any linear appearance of the new frontal hairline would be eliminated.

A new instrument was designed whereby a strip graft with a running-W margin could be taken from the parietal-occipital scalp and then placed in a running-W incision made by the same instrument in the frontal scalp. This technique was employed on four of the patients in this series. These cases were evaluated over a period of six months following surgery.

The instrument is essentially a razor-sharp

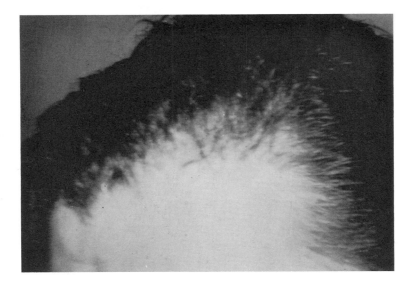

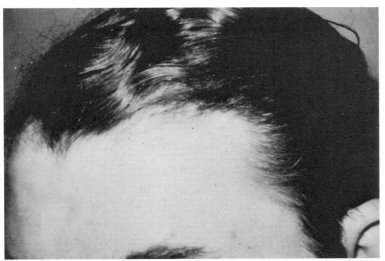

Moderate recession of the hair in a 40 year old man. The postoperative result followed two punch graft procedures.

running-W blade fused to a plastic holder. The blade measures 3 cm. in length. The angle of each triangle is 90 degrees and each limb measures 4 mm. in length. The strip graft in the parietal-occipital area is taken by placing two plastic holders together. This places the running-W blades 8 mm. apart. The parallel blades are then pressed on the scalp on previously marked lines.

The blades are used simply as a "cookie cutter" to make a superficial skin incision. Any desired length of the graft can be made by moving the parallel blades along the scalp. Once the superficial incision is made with this instrument, the remaining portion of the graft is taken with a No. 15 scalpel blade.

The graft is defatted and treated in a fashion similar to the usual strip grafts. The incision in the donor site is repaired with a continuous 3–0 nylon stitch.

A single running-W blade is then used to make the incision in the recipient area. The knife is pressed along the previously designed line on the frontal area of the scalp. A superficial incision is made with the knife. The resulting wound is cut open with a No. 15 scalpel blade, and the incision is carried down through the galea aponeurotica to allow the wound to open wide. The length of the recipient incision is made similar to the length of the strip graft. This is done by counting the number of V's in the incision. The graft fits perfectly in position and is sutured with continuous 6–0 nylon on both sides.

The running-W strip graft method is more tedious and time-consuming than the linear graft technique. However, results in the four patients in which this method was used have shown that the reconstructed frontal hairline has a more natural appearance, although the

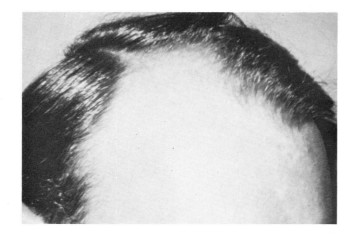

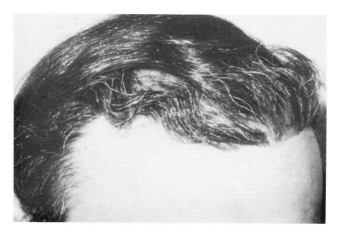

Top, Moderately severe recession in a 37 year old man. *Bottom*, After six procedures.

density of hair growth is not so great as with the linear strip. I feel that this method is worthy of further consideration.

Punch Graft Technique

A complete description of this technique may be found in Chapter 12.

Postoperative Course

The hair follicles in both the strip graft and punch grafts act alike. There is initial growth of hair for about three or four weeks. This hair then falls out as the follicles go into a telogen phase which lasts until two and a half to three months after surgery. The new permanent growth then begins, and the new hair assumes the characteristics of the area from whence it came. Since hair growth proceeds at about 1 cm. per month, a period of six months or more is required before significant hair growth is noted.

In most patients it is necessary to perform the operations so that the interval between procedures does not show an obvious graft which is quite noticeable before hair growth has taken place. It is wise to keep the new grafts close to the existing hairline and to gradually work faceward until a new frontal hairline is established. Unless the patient has long hair or a hairpiece which can camouflage the grafts postoperatively, I usually begin with the punch grafts near the existing hairline and place the strip grafts last.

Complications

If the patients are selected carefully and if the procedures are performed well technically, there should be few complications. In a small percentage of the strip grafts there may not be a complete growth of hair in certain spots. This can be corrected easily by placing small punch grafts in the bald areas of the strip. The same applies for hair growth on the punch grafts. Some punches will grow out a profuse crop of

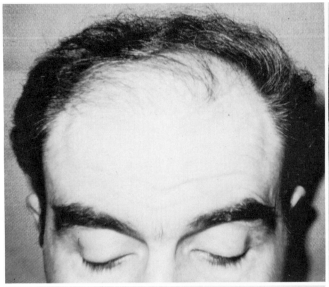

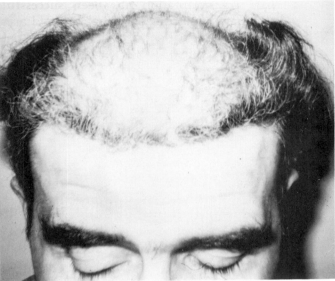

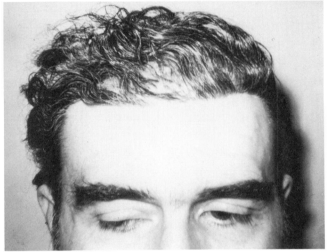

Severe recession in a 40 year old man, treated with strip and punch grafts; results are shown after eight procedures.

hair, while others show sparse growth or remain bare. Usually the initial sets of grafts show the best growth, indicating that after each operation there is some lessening of the blood supply.

The most unpleasant complication is the poorly positioned graft for the frontal hairline. Although it may show a profuse hair growth, it may present an appearance which is esthetically worse than the pre-existing condition. The poorly placed strip graft can usually be repositioned. Poorly placed punch grafts can usually be removed. This is easily done by removing the graft with a punch of similar size and suturing the wound transversely.

Another complication is numbness of the scalp behind the grafts. This numbness is more marked following the strip graft operation. The transverse incision transects the sensory fibers of the supraorbital nerve on both sides, and the numbness will last for several months after surgery. The numbness can be very desirable at first, since subsequent punch grafts can be done with very little additional local anesthesia. Normal sensation eventually returns after a period of eight months to a year.

A raised punch graft presenting a cobblestonelike appearance may sometimes result. This is usually due to a shallow recipient opening or an oversized punch graft which has not been properly defatted. Occasionally small hematomas, especially in the donor site but rarely in the recipient site, have been noted after the punch graft procedure. These can usually be corrected by reopening the wound and suturing it to prevent further bleeding.

Summary

Hair transplantation for male pattern baldness has been done on a large number of patients by dermatologists and plastic surgeons during the past decade. In selected patients

601

hair transplantation has been successful for adequate replacement of hair in bald areas. It must be emphasized, however, that regardless of which technique is used and regardless of the number of operative procedures performed, a full complete growth of hair can never be achieved. This point must be emphasized to every patient in the preoperative discussion.

In most cases the punch graft technique alone is used. However, in selected patients, especially in younger individuals desiring a dense growth in the frontal area, the strip graft in conjunction with the punch grafts can be used. The punch graft technique, when used alone, results in a very satisfactory and significant growth of hair. The strip graft technique is more difficult to perform and should be done only by a skilled surgeon. When the strip graft operation is properly executed, the results are very gratifying.

My most impressive results in this series have been with those who have had the strip graft operation combined with the punch graft method. New ideas relative to the strip graft technique have been discussed. A continued effort should be made by all surgeons to improve the existing techniques so that the most natural-appearing and cosmetically acceptable hair growth can be obtained.

REFERENCES

Adamson, J. E., Horton, C. E., and Mladick, R. A.: The surgical treatment of male pattern baldness. J. Amer. Med. Women's Assoc. 24:897, 1969.

Correa-Inturraspe, M., and Arute, H. N.: Plastic surgery of partial alopecia. Semana med. 19:937, 1957.

Lamont, E. S.: A plastic surgery transformation. West. J. Surg. 65:164, 1957.

Limburger, S.: The surgical treatment of hair loss, Medizinische 35:1559, 1959.

Orentreich, M.: Autographs in alopecias and other selected dermatological conditions. Ann. N.Y. Acad. Sci. 83:463, 1959.

Vallis, C. P.: Surgical treatment of the receding hairline. Plast. Reconst. Surg. 37:247, 1964.

Vallis, C. P.: Surgical treatment of the receding hairline. Plast. Reconst. Surg. 40:138, 1967.

Vallis, C. P.: The strip graft method in hair transplantation. J. Amer. Med. Women's Assoc. 24:890, 1969a.

Vallis, C. P.: Surgical treatment of the receding hairline. Plast. Reconstr. Surg. 44:271, 1969b.

Numbers set in *italics* indicate illustrations.